Nuclear Medicine
The Requisites

The Requisites

Nuclear Medicine

Fourth Edition

Harvey A. Ziessman, MD
Professor of Radiology
Director of Nuclear Medicine Imaging
The Johns Hopkins University
Baltimore, Maryland

Janis P. O'Malley, MD
Associate Professor of Radiology
Director, Division of Nuclear Medicine
University of Alabama at Birmingham
Birmingham, Alabama

James H. Thrall, MD
Radiologist-in-Chief
Massachusetts General Hospital
Juan M. Taveras Professor of Radiology
Harvard Medical School
Boston, Massachusetts

Associate Editor
Frederic H. Fahey, DSc
Director of Nuclear Medicine/PET Physics
Children's Hospital Boston
Associate Professor of Radiology
Harvard Medical School
Division of Nuclear Medicine and Molecular Imaging
Department of Radiology
Children's Hospital Boston
Boston, Massachusetts

ELSEVIER
SAUNDERS

1600 John F. Kennedy Blvd.
Ste 1800
Philadelphia, PA 19103-2899

NUCLEAR MEDICINE: THE REQUISITES   ISBN: 978-0-323-08299-0

Notices

Knowledge and best practice in this field are constantly changing. As new research and experience
broaden our understanding, changes in research methods, professional practices, or medical treatment
may become necessary.

Practitioners and researchers must always rely on their own experience and knowledge in evaluating and using any information, methods, compounds, or experiments described herein. In using such
information or methods, they should be mindful of their own safety and the safety of others, including
parties for whom they have a professional responsibility.

With respect to any drug or pharmaceutical products identified, readers are advised to check the
most current information provided (i) on procedures featured or (ii) by the manufacturer of each
product to be administered, to verify the recommended dose or formula, the method and duration
of administration, and contraindications. It is the responsibility of practitioners, relying on their own
experience and knowledge of their patients, to make diagnoses, to determine dosages and the best
treatment for each individual patient, and to take all appropriate safety precautions.

To the fullest extent of the law, neither the Publisher nor the authors, contributors, or editors as-
sume any liability for any injury and/or damage to persons or property as a matter of products liability,
negligence, or otherwise or from any use or operation of any methods, products, instructions, or ideas
contained in the material herein.

Library of Congress Cataloging-in-Publication Data
Ziessman, Harvey A.
  Nuclear medicine / Harvey A. Ziessman, Janis P. O'Malley, James H. Thrall;
associate editor, Frederic H. Fahey.—4th ed.
    p. ; cm.—(Requisites)
  Includes bibliographical references.
  ISBN 978-0-323-08299-0 (hardcover : alk. paper)
  I. O'Malley, Janis P. II. Thrall, James H. III. Fahey, Frederic H. IV.
Title. V. Series: Requisites series. VI. Series: Requisites in radiology.
  [DNLM: 1. Radionuclide Imaging. 2. Molecular Imaging. 3. Nuclear
Medicine—methods. 4. Radiopharmaceuticals—diagnostic use. 5. Tomography,
Emission-Computed. WN 203]
  616.07′575—dc23

2012051319

Senior Content Strategist: Don Scholz
Content Development Specialist: Margaret Nelson
Publishing Services Manager: Anne Altepeter
Senior Project Manager: Doug Turner
Designer: Steve Stave

Printed in the United States of America

Last digit is the print number: 9 8 7 6 5 4 3

Contributor

Beth A. Harkness, MS, DABR, FACR
Nuclear Medicine Physicist
Henry Ford Health System
Detroit, Michigan
  Chapter 5: Single-Photon Emission Computed Tomography,
  Positron Emission Tomography, and Hybrid Imaging

Foreword

The fourth edition of *Nuclear Medicine: The Requisites* continues to follow the philosophy and format of the first three editions. The basic science chapters are designed to present important principles of physics, instrumentation, and nuclear pharmacy in the context of how they help shape clinical practice. The clinical chapters continue to follow a logical progression from basic principles of tracer distribution and localization to practical clinical applications. The authors believe that understanding tracer mechanisms is fundamental to nuclear medicine practice and that knowledge of how radiopharmaceuticals localize temporally and spatially in normal and diseased tissues is the best deductive tool available for analyzing images and is superior to simply memorizing representative illustrations.

In the time between the publication of the third and fourth editions of this title, the field of nuclear medicine has continued its remarkable development. Single-photon emission computed tomography (SPECT) has morphed increasingly into SPECT/computed tomography (CT), and an increasing number of scanner designs have been developed, primarily for specialized cardiac imaging. Positron emission tomography (PET) has become much more widespread, with larger institutions acquiring their own cyclotrons. It can now be said with confidence that PET/CT has proved to be a substantial advancement, especially in body imaging. PET/magnetic resonance imaging (MRI) is still in its infancy, but enough data are in hand to predict that this integrated method will also become important, although the scale of applications is still unknown. The other revolution in PET is the clinical availability of new radiopharmaceuticals, including agents aimed at Alzheimer disease diagnosis, and literally dozens more tracers are in the pipeline.

Adding new SPECT, PET, PET/CT, and PET/MRI applications to the nuclear medicine armamentarium has injected new, even unprecedented, vitality into the specialty. Readers of *Nuclear Medicine: The Requisites* will feel this vitality almost palpably as they work their way through the book. Among other challenges, the integrated methods of PET/CT and PET/MRI require higher levels of knowledge of anatomic cross-sectional imaging than ever before, as well as more knowledge of the respective technologies. Some of this is beyond the scope of the current book but can be found elsewhere in the Requisites series.

The Requisites in Radiology titles have become old friends to generations of radiologists. The original intent of the series was to provide the resident or fellow with a text that might be reasonably read within several days at the beginning of each subspecialty rotation and perhaps reread several times during subsequent rotations or during board preparation. The series is not intended to be exhaustive but rather to provide the basic conceptual, factual, and interpretive material required for clinical practice. After more than 20 years of experience with the series, it is now clear that the books are also sought out by practicing imaging specialists for the efficiency of their presentation format and the quality of their material. With more people reaching the point of requiring re-certification, the Requisites books should again prove helpful.

Each book in the Requisites series is written by nationally recognized authorities in their respective subspecialty areas. Each author is challenged to present material in the context of today's practice of radiology rather than grafting information about new imaging modalities onto old, out-of-date material. It is our hope in adopting this strategy that readers will find the Requisites titles to be a very efficient way of accessing the most important material.

The first three editions of *Nuclear Medicine: The Requisites* were well received in the radiology and nuclear medicine community. Dr. Ziessman and his colleagues have again done a terrific job in putting together a new and updated edition, and we expect that this edition will be deemed to be as outstanding as its predecessors. We hope that *Nuclear Medicine: The Requisites* will serve residents in radiology as a concise and useful introduction to the subject and will also serve as a very manageable text for review by fellows and practicing nuclear medicine specialists and radiologists.

James H. Thrall, MD
Radiologist-in-Chief
Massachusetts General Hospital
Juan M. Taveras Professor of Radiology
Harvard Medical School
Boston, Massachusetts

Preface

The first edition of *Nuclear Medicine: The Requisites* was published in 1995 and, like the second and third editions, the fourth edition closely follows the philosophy and format of the original—that is, to provide a concise and up-to-date introduction and review of the field of nuclear medicine.

Since the publication of the third edition in 2006, many advances have been made in radiopharmaceuticals and instrumentation, and many are described. Standard use of hybrid positron emission tomography/computed tomography (PET/CT) has become widely accepted, and single-photon emission computed tomography/computed tomography (SPECT/CT) is increasing in clinical use. New radiopharmaceuticals approved by the Food and Drug Administration include I-123 ioflupane (DaTscan), a striatal dopamine transporter used to diagnose parkinsonism, and F-18 florbetapir (Amyvid), an amyloid imaging agent. Many new translational agents are in clinical trials.

Although this edition contains many new images and revised and updated text, the general format of the book has not changed, with Part I discussing basic principles of nuclear medicine and Part II their clinical applications. A major addition to Part I is a new chapter entitled "Molecular Imaging," which introduces the basic concepts of molecular imaging and explains how this rapidly developing field is leading to a future of individualized medicine. A new associate editor, Frederic H. Fahey, DSc, has completely rewritten the Part I chapters "Physics of Nuclear Medicine," "Radiation Detection and Instrumentation," and "Single-Photon Emission Computed Tomography, Positron Emission Tomography, and Hybrid Imaging." The Part II clinical applications chapters "Oncology: Positron Emission Tomography" and the popular "Pearls, Pitfalls, and Frequently Asked Questions" have been extensively revised and updated.

Nuclear Medicine: The Requisites discusses important basic principles and concepts of instrumentation and radiopharmaceuticals. Emphasis is placed on the pharmacokinetics, uptake, distribution, and clearance of radiopharmaceuticals, as well as an understanding of disease pathophysiology, leading naturally to the choice of optimal imaging methods and study interpretation. All the chapters, while rewritten and updated, continue to have the many boxes, tables, and illustrations that aid in learning about this ever-evolving specialty. Intended for the resident in training, as well as for the practicing nuclear radiologist and nuclear medicine physician, the fourth edition of *Nuclear Medicine: The Requisites* provides an organized overview of nuclear medicine pertinent to clinical practice.

Acknowledgments

We thank those who have contributed to the preparation of this book. Selected images were provided by Paco E. Bravo, MD; Christopher J. Palestro, MD; Leonie Gordon, MD; David Mankoff, MD, PhD; Kirk A. Frey, MD, PhD; Alan H. Maurer, MD; Pradeep Bhambhvani, MD; Mark Muzi, MS; and Honggang Liu, MS. Drs. Bravo, Mankoff, and Bhambhvani proofread chapters and made helpful suggestions. We also thank our spouses and family for providing us the time and encouragement for writing this textbook and our residents who continue to teach us.

Harvey A. Ziessman, MD
Janis P. O'Malley, MD
James H. Thrall, MD
Frederic H. Fahey, DSc

Contents

Part I
Basic Principles

CHAPTER 1

Radiopharmaceuticals

Radiopharmaceuticals portray physiology, biochemistry, or pathology in the body without causing any physiological effect. They are referred to as *radiotracers* because they are given in subpharmacological doses that "trace" a particular physiological or pathological process in the body.

This chapter presents general principles regarding radionuclides and radiopharmaceuticals, their production, radiolabeling, quality assurance, dispensing, and radiation safety.

◼ ELEMENTS, RADIONUCLIDES, AND RADIOPHARMACEUTICALS

Most radiopharmaceuticals are a combination of a radioactive molecule, a radionuclide, that permits external detection and a biologically active molecule or drug that acts as a carrier and determines localization and biodistribution. For a few radiotracers (e.g., radioiodine, gallium, and thallium), the radioactive atoms themselves confer the desired localization properties. Both naturally occurring and synthetic molecules can potentially be radiolabeled.

Different types of atoms are called *elements*. Different types of nuclei are termed *nuclides*. An element is characterized by its atomic number (Z)—that is, the number of protons in the nucleus. The atomic number specifies the position of the element in the periodic table (Fig. 1-1). A nuclide is characterized by its atomic number and mass number (A)—that is, protons plus neutrons in the nucleus. Nuclides with the same number of protons are called *isotopes* and belong to the same element (Box 1-1). Unstable nuclides are called *radionuclides*. Radionuclides try to become stable by emitting electromagnetic radiation or charged particles during radioactive decay. Radioactivity is the spontaneous emission of radiation given off by radionuclides.

Radiopharmaceutical mechanisms of localization important to clinical practice are listed in Table 1-1. Understanding the mechanism and rationale for the use of each agent is critical to understanding the normal and pathological findings demonstrated scintigraphically.

Radiopharmaceuticals must be approved by the U.S. Food and Drug Administration (FDA) before they can be commercially produced and used for human clinical or research purposes.

Desired Attributes of Radiopharmaceuticals

Certain characteristics are desirable for clinically useful radiopharmaceuticals. Radionuclide decay should result in gamma emissions of suitable energy (100-200 keV is ideal for gamma cameras and 511 keV for positron emission tomography [PET]) and sufficient abundance (percent likelihood of emissions per decay) for external detection. It should not contain particulate radiation (e.g., beta emissions), which increases patient radiation dose, although beta emissions are suitable for therapeutic radiopharmaceuticals. The effective half-life should be long enough for only the intended application, usually a few hours.

The radionuclide should be *carrier-free*—that is, it is not contaminated by either stable radionuclides or other radionuclides of the same element. Carrier material can negatively influence biodistribution and labeling efficiency. It should have high *specific activity*—that is, radioactivity per unit weight (mCi/mg). A carrier-free radionuclide has the highest specific activity. Technetium-99m most closely matches these desirable features for the gamma camera and fluorine-18 for PET.

The pharmaceutical component should be free of any toxicity or physiological effects. The radiopharmaceutical should not disassociate in vitro or in vivo and should be readily available or easily compounded. The radiopharmaceutical should rapidly and specifically localize according to the intended application. Background clearance should be rapid, leading to good target-to-background ratios.

◼ PRODUCTION OF RADIONUCLIDES

Naturally occurring radionuclides (e.g., uranium, actinium, thorium, radium, and radon) are heavy, toxic elements with very long half-lives (>1000 years). They have no clinical role in diagnostic nuclear medicine. Radionuclides commonly used clinically are artificially produced by nuclear fission or through the bombardment of stable materials by neutrons or charged particles.

Neutron bombardment of enriched uranium-235 results in fission products located in the middle of the atomic chart (Fig. 1-1). Bombardment of medium–atomic-weight nuclides with low-energy neutrons (neutron activation) in a *nuclear reactor* results in neutron-rich radionuclides. Neutron-rich radionuclides (e.g., iodine-131, xenon-133,

Periodic Table of Elements

Period	I A																		VIII A
1	1 H	II A											III A	IV A	V A	VI A	VII A	2 He
2	3 Li	4 Be												5 B	6 C	7 N	8 O	9 F	10 Ne
3	11 Na	12 Mg	III B	IV B	V B	VI B	VII B	—	VIII	—	I B	II B		13 Al	14 Si	15 P	16 S	17 Cl	18 Ar
4	19 K	20 Ca	21 Sc	22 Ti	23 V	24 Cr	25 Mn	26 Fe	27 Co	28 Ni	29 Cu	30 Zn		31 Ga	32 Ge	33 As	34 Se	35 Br	36 Kr
5	37 Rb	38 Sr	39 Y	40 Zr	41 Nb	42 Mo	43 Tc	44 Ru	45 Rh	46 Pd	47 Ag	48 Cd		49 In	50 Sn	51 Sb	52 Te	53 I	54 Xe
6	55 Cs	56 Ba	*	71 Lu	72 Hf	73 Ta	74 W	75 Re	76 Os	77 Ir	78 Pt	79 Au	80 Hg	81 Tl	82 Pb	83 Bi	84 Po	85 At	86 Rn
7	87 Fr	88 Ra	**	103 Lr	104 Rf	105 Db	106 Sg	107 Bh	108 Hs	109 Mt	110 Ds	111 Rg	112 Uub	113 Uut	114 Uuq	115 Uup	116 Uuh	117 Uus	118 Uuo

*Lanthanoids	*	57 La	58 Ce	59 Pr	60 Nd	61 Pm	62 Sm	63 Eu	64 Gd	65 Tb	66 Dy	67 Ho	68 Er	69 Tm	70 Yb
**Actinoids	**	89 Ac	90 Th	91 Pa	92 U	93 Np	94 Pu	95 Am	96 Cm	97 Bk	98 Cf	99 Es	100 Fm	101 Md	102 No

FIGURE 1-1. Periodic table. Highlighted elements have radionuclides commonly used in nuclear medicine.

Box 1-1. Radionuclides and Isotopes

$$\frac{(\text{Protons} + \text{Neutrons})}{(\text{Protons})} \quad {}^{A}_{Z}X \quad {}^{131}_{53}\text{Iodine}$$

$${}^{123}_{53}\text{Iodine} \quad {}^{127}_{53}\text{Iodine}$$

An **element** is characterized by its *atomic number* (Z).
A **nuclide** is characterized by its *mass number* (A) and its *atomic number* (Z).
${}^{131}I$, ${}^{123}I$, and ${}^{127}I$ are **isotopes** of iodine and unstable **radionuclides.**
${}^{127}I$ is stable iodine.

chromium-51, and molybdenum-99) generated through fission or neutron activation undergo beta-minus decay. Charged particle bombardment (with protons, deuterons, alpha particles) to a wide variety of target materials in *cyclotrons* or other special *accelerators* produces proton-rich radionuclides that will undergo positron decay (e.g., carbon-11, nitrogen-13, oxygen-15, fluorine-18) or electron capture (e.g., iodine-123, gallium-67, thallium-201, and indium-111).

The production source and physical characteristics of commonly used radionuclides in clinical nuclear medicine practice are summarized in Tables 1-2 and 1-3.

■ RADIONUCLIDE GENERATORS

One of the practical issues faced in nuclear medicine is the desirability of using relatively short-lived agents (i.e., hours rather than days or weeks) and at the same time the need to have radiopharmaceuticals delivered to hospitals or clinics from commercial sources. One way around

TABLE 1-1 Mechanisms of Radiopharmaceutical Localization

Mechanism	Applications or examples
Compartmental localization	Blood pool imaging, direct cystography
Passive diffusion (concentration dependent)	Blood–brain barrier breakdown, glomerular filtration, cisternography
Capillary blockade (physical entrapment)	Perfusion imaging of lungs
Physical leakage from a luminal compartment	Gastrointestinal bleeding, detection of urinary tract or biliary system leakage
Metabolism	Glucose, fatty acids
Active transport (active cellular uptake)	Hepatobiliary imaging, renal tubular function, thyroid and adrenal imaging
Chemical bonding and adsorption	Skeletal imaging
Cell sequestration	Splenic imaging (heat-damaged red blood cells), white blood cells
Receptor binding and storage	Adrenal medullary imaging, somatostatin receptor imaging
Phagocytosis	Reticuloendothelial system imaging
Antigen-antibody	Tumor imaging
Multiple mechanisms	
Perfusion and active transport	Myocardial imaging
Active transport and metabolism	Thyroid uptake and imaging
Active transport and secretion	Hepatobiliary imaging, salivary gland imaging

TABLE **1-2** Physical Characteristics of Single-Photon Radionuclides Used in Clinical Nuclear Medicine

Radionuclide	Principal mode of decay	Physical half-life	Principal photon energy in keV (abundance) (%)	Production method
Mo-99	Beta minus	2.8 days	740 (12), 780 (4)	Reactor
Tc-99m	Isomeric transition	6 hr	140 (89)	Generator (Mo-99)
I-131	Beta minus	8 days	364 (81)	Reactor
I-123	Electron capture	13.2 hr	159 (83)	Cyclotron
Ga-67	Electron capture	78.3 hr	93 (37), 185 (20), 300 (17), 395 (5)	Cyclotron
Tl-201	Electron capture	73.1 hr	69-83 (Hg x-rays), 135 (2.5), 167 (10)	Cyclotron
In-111	Electron capture	2.8 days	171 (90), 245 (94)	Cyclotron
Xe-127	Electron capture	36 days	172 (26), 203 (7), 375 (17)	Cyclotron
Xe-133	Beta minus	5.2 days	81 (37)	Reactor
Co-57	Electron capture	272 days	122 (86)	Cyclotron

TABLE **1-3** Positron-Emitting Radionuclides: Physical Characteristics

Radionuclide	Physical half-life (min)	Positron energy (MeV)	Range in soft tissue (mm)	Production method
C-11	20	0.96	4.1	Cyclotron
N-13	10	1.19	5.4	Cyclotron
O-15	2	1.73	7.3	Cyclotron
F-18	110	0.635	2.4	Cyclotron
Ga-68	68	1.9	8.1	Generator (Ge-68)
Rb-82	1.3	3.15	15.0	Generator (Sr-82)

TABLE **1-4** Radionuclide Generator Systems and Parent and Daughter Half-Lives

Parent	Parent half-life	Daughter	Daughter half-life
Mo-99	66 hr	Tc-99m	6 hr
Rb-81	4.5 hr	Kr-81m	13 sec
Ge-68	270 days	Ga-68	68 min
Sr-82	25 days	Rb-82	1.3 min

TABLE **1-5** Molybdenum-99/Technetium-99m Generator Systems

Radionuclides	Parent (Mo-99)	Daughter (Tc-99m)
Half-life	66 hr	6 hr
Mode of decay	Beta minus	Isomeric transition
Daughter products	Tc-99m, Tc-99	Tc-99
Principal photon energies*	740 keV, 780 keV	140 keV (89%)
Generator Function		
Composition of ion exchange column	Al_2O_3	
Eluent	Normal saline (0.9%)	
Time from elution to maximum daughter yield	23 hr	

*The decay scheme for Mo-99 is complex, with over 35 gamma rays of different energies given off. The listed energies are those used in clinical practice for radionuclide purity checks.

this dilemma is the use of radionuclide generator systems. These systems consist of a longer-lived parent and a shorter-lived daughter. With this combination of half-lives, the generator can be shipped from a commercial vendor and the daughter product will still have a useful half-life for clinical applications. Although various generator systems have been developed over the years (Table 1-4), to date, the most important is the Mo-99/Tc-99m system.

Molybdenum-99/Technetium-99m Generator Systems

Mo-99 is produced by the fission of U-235. The product is often referred to as *fission moly*. The reaction is U-235 (n, fission) → Mo-99. After Mo-99 is produced in the fission reaction, it is chemically purified and passed on to an ion exchange column composed of alumina (Al_2O_3) (Table 1-5). The column is typically adjusted to an acid pH to promote binding. The positive charge of the alumina binds the molybdate ions firmly. The loaded column is placed in a lead container with tubing attached at each end to permit column elution.

Generator Operation and Yield

The relationship between Mo-99 decay and the ingrowth of Tc-99m is illustrated in Figure 1-2. Maximum buildup of Tc-99m activity occurs at 23 hours after elution. This time point is convenient, especially if sufficient Tc-99m activity is available to accomplish each day's work. Otherwise, the generator can be eluted, or "milked," more than once per day. Partial elution is also illustrated in Figure 1-2. Fifty percent of maximum is reached in approximately 4.5 hours, and 75% of maximum is available at 8.5 hours.

Although greatest attention is paid to the rate of Tc-99m buildup, Tc-99m is constantly decaying, with buildup of stable Tc-99 (or "carrier" Tc-99) in the generator. Generators received after commercial shipment or generators that have not been eluted for several days have significant carrier Tc-99 in the eluate. Because the carrier Tc-99 behaves chemically similarly to Tc-99m, it can compete and adversely affect radiopharmaceutical labeling efficiency. Many labeling procedures require the reduction of Tc-99m from a +7 valence state to a lower valence state. If the eluate contains sufficient carrier Tc-99, complete reduction may not occur, resulting in poor labeling and undesired radiochemical contaminants in the final preparation.

Two types of generator systems are available with respect to elution. "Wet" systems, today most commonly used in regional radiopharmacies, come with a reservoir of normal saline (0.9%) (Fig. 1-3). Elution is accomplished by placing a special sterile vacuum vial on the exit or collection port. The vacuum vial is designed to draw the appropriate amount of saline across the column.

In "dry" systems, common in imaging clinics, a volume-calibrated saline charge is placed on the entry port and a vacuum vial is placed on the collection port (Fig. 1-4). The vacuum draws the saline eluent out of the original vial, across the column, and into the elution vial. Elution volumes are in the range of 5 to 20 mL. Elutions can be performed for add-on or emergency studies that are required in the course of a day (Fig. 1-2). The amount of Tc-99m activity available from a generator decreases each day as a result of decay of the Mo-99 parent (Fig. 1-2). In practice, the 2.8-day half-life of Mo-99 allows generators to be used for 2 weeks.

Quality Control

Rigorous quality control is performed before commercial generator shipment; however, each laboratory must perform quality control steps each time the generator is eluted, to meet various federal and state regulatory guidelines (Table 1-6).

Radionuclide Purity

The only desired radionuclide in the Mo-99/Tc-99m generator eluate is Tc-99m. Any other radionuclide in the sample is considered a radionuclide impurity and is undesirable because it will result in additional radiation exposure to the patient without clinical benefit.

The most common radionuclide contaminant in the generator eluate is the parent radionuclide, Mo-99. Tc-99, the daughter product of the isomeric transition of Tc-99m, is also present but is not considered an impurity or contaminant. Although Tc-99 can be a problem from a chemical standpoint in radiolabeling procedures, it is not a problem from a radiation or health standpoint and is not tested for as a radionuclide impurity. The half-life of Tc-99 is 2.1×10^5 years. It decays to ruthenium-99, which is stable.

The amount of parent Mo-99m in the eluate should be as small as possible, because any contamination by a long-lived radionuclide increases the radiation dose without providing any benefit to the patient. The Nuclear Regulatory Commission (NRC) sets limits on the amount of Mo-99 in the eluate, and this must be tested on each elution. The easiest and most widely used approach is to take advantage of the energetic 740- and 780-keV gamma rays of Mo-99 with dual counting of the specimen. The generator eluate

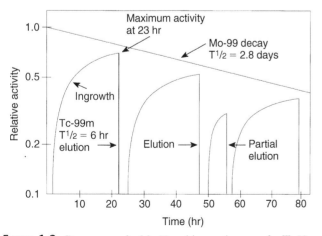

FIGURE 1-2. Decay curve for Mo-99 and ingrowth curves for Tc-99m. Successive elutions, including a partial elution are illustrated. Relative activity is plotted on a logarithmic scale, accounting for the straight line of Mo-99 decay.

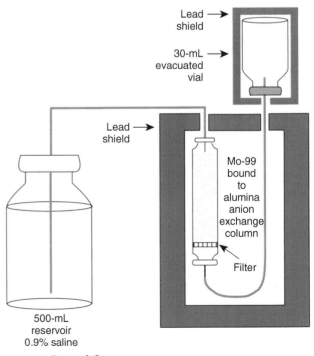

FIGURE 1-3. Wet radionuclide generator system.

is placed in a lead container designed so that all of the 140-keV photons of technetium are absorbed but approximately 50% of the more energetic Mo-99 gamma rays can penetrate. Adjusting the dose calibrator to the Mo-99 setting provides an estimate of the number of microcuries of Mo-99 in the sample. The unshielded sample is then measured on the Tc-99m setting, and a ratio of Mo-99 to Tc-99m activity can be calculated.

The NRC limit is 0.15 μCi of Mo-99 activity per 1 mCi of Tc-99m activity in the administered dose. Because the half-life of Mo-99 is longer than that of Tc-99m, the ratio increases with time. If the initial reading shows near-maximum Mo-99 levels, either the actual dose to be given

to the patient should be restudied before administration or the buildup factor should be computed mathematically. From a practical standpoint, the Mo-99 activity may be taken as unchanged and the Tc-99m decay calculated (Table 1-7). Breakthrough is rare but unpredictable. When it does occur, Mo-99 levels can be far higher than the legal limit.

Chemical Purity

A routine quality assurance step is to measure the generator eluate for the presence of the column packing material, Al_2O_3. Colorimetric qualitative spot testing determines if unacceptable levels are present. Excessive aluminum levels may interfere with the normal distribution of certain radiopharmaceuticals—for example, increased lung activity with Tc-99m sulfur colloid and liver uptake with Tc-99m methylene diphosphonate (Tc-99m MDP).

Radiochemical Purity

When Tc-99m is eluted from the generator, its expected valence state is +7, in the chemical form of pertechnetate (TcO_4^-). The clinical use of sodium pertechnetate as a radiopharmaceutical and the preparation of Tc-99m–labeled pharmaceuticals from commercial kits are based on the +7 oxidation state. The *United States Pharmacopeia* (USP) standard for the generator eluate is that 95% or more of Tc-99m activity be in this +7 state. Reduction states at +4, +5, or +6 result in impurities. These reduction states can be detected by thin-layer chromatography. Problems with radiochemical purity of the generator eluate are infrequently encountered but should be considered if kit labeling is poor. Measures of pharmaceutical purity are summarized in Table 1-8.

■ TECHNETIUM CHEMISTRY AND RADIOPHARMACEUTICAL PREPARATION

Tc-99m is the most commonly used radionuclide because of its ready availability, the favorable energy of its principal

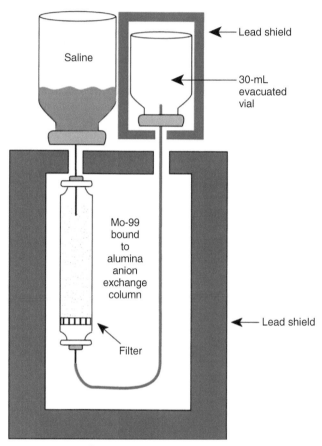

FIGURE 1-4. Dry radionuclide generator system.

TABLE 1-6 Purity Checks: Molybdenum-99/Technetium-99m Generator

Purity checks	Problem	Standard
Radionuclide purity	Excessive Mo-99 in eluent	<0.15 μCi Mo-99/mCi Tc-99m at time of administration
Chemical purity	Al_2O_3 from generator ion exchange column in elution	<10 μg/mL (fission generator) (aurin tricarboxylic acid spot test)
Radiochemical purity	Reduced oxidation states of Tc-99m (i.e., +4, +5, or +6 instead of +7)	95% of Tc-99m activity should be in +7 oxidation state

TABLE 1-7 Physical Decay of Technetium-99m

Time (hr)	Fraction remaining
0	1.000
1	0.891
2	0.794
3	0.708
4	0.631
5	0.532
6	0.501
7	0.447
8	0.398
9	0.355
10	0.316
11	0.282
12	0.251

Tc-99m physical half-life = 6.02 hr.

TABLE **1-8** Measures of Pharmaceutical Purity

Parameter	Definition	Example issues
Chemical purity	Fraction of wanted vs. unwanted chemical in preparation	Amount of alumina breakthrough in Mo-99/Tc-99m generator eluate
Radiochemical purity	Fraction of total radioactivity in desired chemical form	Amount of bound vs. unbound Tc-99m in Tc-99m diphosphonate
Radionuclide purity	Fraction of total radioactivity in the form of desired radionuclide	Ratio of Tc-99m vs. Mo-99 in generator eluate; I-124 in an I-123 preparation
Physical purity	Fraction of total pharmaceutical in desired physical form	Correct particle size distribution in Tc-99m MAA preparation; absence of particulate contaminates in any a solution
Biological purity	Absence of microorganisms and pyrogens	Sterile, pyrogen-free preparations

MAA, Macroaggregated albumin.

TABLE **1-9** Technetium-99m Radiopharmaceuticals

Agent	Application
Tc-99m sodium pertechnetate	Meckel's diverticulum detection, salivary and thyroid gland scintigraphy
Tc-99m sulfur colloid	Lymphoscintigraphy
	Liver/spleen scintigraphy, bone marrow scintigraphy
Tc-99m diphosphonate	Skeletal scintigraphy
Tc-99m macroaggregated albumin (MAA)	Pulmonary perfusion scintigraphy, liver intraarterial perfusion scintigraphy,
Tc-99m red blood cells	Radionuclide ventriculography, gastrointestinal bleeding, hepatic hemangioma
Tc-99m diethylenetriamine-pentaacetic acid (DTPA)	Renal dynamic scintigraphy, lung ventilation (aerosol), glomerular filtration rate
Tc-99m mercaptoacetyltriglycine (MAG₃)	Renal dynamic scintigraphy
Tc-99m dimercaptosuccinic acid (DMSA)	Renal cortical scintigraphy
Tc-99m iminodiacetic acid (HIDA)	Hepatobiliary scintigraphy
Tc-99m sestamibi (Cardiolite)	Myocardial perfusion scintigraphy, breast imaging
Tc-99m tetrofosmin (Myoview)	Myocardial perfusion scintigraphy
Tc-99m exametazime (HMPAO)	Cerebral perfusion scintigraphy, white blood cell labeling
Tc-99m bicisate (ECD)	Cerebral perfusion scintigraphy

ECD, Ethyl cysteinate dimer; *HMPAO*, hexamethylpropyleneamine oxime.

gamma photon (140 keV), its favorable dosimetry with lack of primary particulate radiations, and its nearly ideal half-life (6 hours) for many clinical imaging studies. However, technetium chemistry is challenging. In most labeling procedures, technetium must be reduced from the +7 valence state. The reduction is usually accomplished with stannous ion. One exception is the labeling of Tc-99m sulfur colloid, which requires heating.

The actual final oxidation state of technetium in many radiopharmaceuticals is unclear. Some technetium compounds are chelates, which involve a complex bond at two or more sites on the ligand. Others are used on the basis of their empirical efficacy without complete knowledge of how technetium is being complexed in the final molecule.

The major Tc-99m–labeled radiopharmaceuticals are summarized in Table 1-9. The details of individual technetium radiopharmaceuticals are discussed in the chapters on individual organ systems and include key points in preparation and the recognition of in vivo markers of radiopharmaceutical impurities.

Commercial kits contain a reaction vial with the appropriate amount of stannous ion (tin), the nonradioactive pharmaceutical to be labeled, and other buffering and stabilizing agents. The vials are flushed with nitrogen to prevent atmospheric oxygen interrupting the reaction. The sequence of steps in a sample labeling process is illustrated in Figure 1-5. Sodium pertechnetate is drawn into a syringe and assayed in the dose calibrator. After the Tc-99m activity is confirmed, the sample is added to the reaction vial. The amount of Tc-99m activity added for each product is determined by the number of patient doses desired in the case of a multidose vial, an estimate of the decrease in radioactivity caused by decay between the time of preparation and the estimated time of dosage administration, and the in vitro stability of the product. The completed product is labeled and kept in a special lead-shielded container until it is time to withdraw a sample for administration. Each patient dose is individually assayed before being dispensed.

Excessive oxygen can react directly with the stannous ion, leaving too little reducing power in the kit, which can

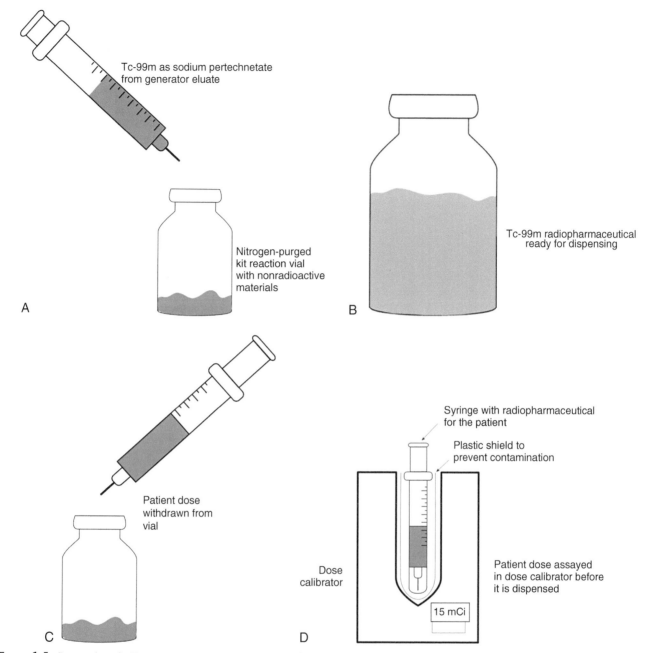

FIGURE 1-5. Preparation of a Tc-99m–labeled radiopharmaceutical. **A,** Tc-99m as sodium pertechnetate is added to the reaction vial. **B,** Tc-99m radiopharmaceutical is ready for dispensing. **C,** The patient dose is withdrawn from the vial. **D,** Each dose is measured in the dose calibrator before it is dispensed.

result in unwanted free Tc-99m pertechnetate in the preparation. A less common problem is radiolysis after kit preparation, also resulting in free pertechnetate. The phenomenon is seen when high amounts of Tc-99m activity are used. The kit preparations are usually designed so that multiple doses can be prepared from one reaction vial.

■ QUALITY ASSURANCE OF TECHNETIUM-99M–LABELED RADIOPHARMACEUTICALS

The difficult nature of technetium chemistry highlights the importance of checking the final product for *radiochemical purity*, defined as the percentage of the total radioactivity in a specimen that is in the specified or desired radiochemical form (Table 1-8). For example, if 5% of the Tc-99m activity remains as free pertechnetate in a radiolabeling procedure, the radiochemical purity would be stated as 95%, assuming no other impurities. Each radiopharmaceutical has a specific radiochemical purity to meet USP standards or FDA requirements, typically 90%. Causes of radiochemical impurities include poor initial labeling, radiolysis, decomposition, pH changes, light exposure, or presence of oxidizing or reducing agents.

The usual approach to assay radiochemical purity in vitro is thin-layer chromatography. Radiochromatography is performed in the same manner as conventional chromatography, by spotting a sample of the test material at one end of a strip. A solvent is then selected for which the desired radiochemical and the potential contaminants have known migration patterns, so the strip can be placed in a dose calibrator for counting. The radiolabel provides an easy means for quantitatively measuring the migration patterns.

In vivo radiochemical impurities contribute to background activity or other unwanted localization and degrade image quality. For many agents, the presence of a radiochemical impurity can be recognized by altered in vivo biodistribution.

For technetium radiopharmaceuticals, the presence of free pertechnetate and insoluble hydrolyzed reduced technetium moieties are tested using instant thin-layer chromatography techniques. For example, using acetone as the solvent, free pertechnetate migrates with the solvent front in a paper and thin-layer chromatography system, whereas Tc-99m diphosphonate and hydrolyzed reduced technetium remain at the origin (Fig. 1-6). For selective testing of hydrolyzed reduced technetium, a silica gel strip is used with saline as the solvent. In this system, both free pertechnetate and Tc-99m diphosphonate move with the solvent front and hydrolyzed reduced technetium again stays at the origin (see Fig. 1-6). This combination of procedures allows measurement of each of the three components. Chromatography systems have been worked out for each major technetium-labeled radiopharmaceutical.

Chromatographic scanners provide detailed strip chart recording of radioactivity distribution. In practice, the easiest way to perform chromatography is simply to cut the chromatography strip into two pieces that can be counted separately.

◼ SINGLE-PHOTON RADIOPHARMACEUTICALS OTHER THAN TC-99M

Radioiodine I-131 and I-123

I-131 as sodium iodide was the first radiopharmaceutical of importance in clinical nuclear medicine. It was used for physiological studies of the thyroid gland for several years in the late 1940s (Table 1-10). Subsequently, it was used to radiolabel radiopharmaceuticals for scintigraphy, including human serum albumin, MAA, hippuran, and meta-iodo-benzyl-guanidine (MIBG). These radiopharmaceuticals are no longer diagnostically used.

The disadvantages of I-131 include relatively high principal photon energy (364 keV), long half-life (8 days), and presence of beta particle emissions. However, it is an important radiopharmaceutical for the treatment of hyperthyroidism and differentiated thyroid cancer.

Whenever possible, I-123 is substituted for I-131 for diagnostic purposes. It has a shorter half-life (13.2 hours) (Table 1-2), and its principal photon energy (159 keV) is better suited to imaging with the gamma camera. It decays by electron capture, and the dosimetry is favorable compared with that of I-131. Even in applications in which imaging over a period of several days allows for improved

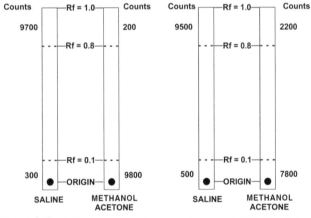

FIGURE 1-6. Radiochromatography for quality control of Tc-99m diphosphonate. The count-activities on the strips are indicated by the numbers beside the strip diagram. The *black dot at the bottom* of each strip represents the origin. *Acceptable (left):* 3% of the activity does not migrate with Tc-99m diphosphonate in saline, and 2% migrates as Tc-99m pertechnetate with the solvent front using methanol: acetone. Thus 5% of the radioactivity is not present at Tc-99m diphosphonate. *Unacceptable (right),* 5% of the activity is present as impurities (saline chromatogram) and 22% as free pertechnetate (methanol: acetone chromatogram). This radiopharmaceutical is of unacceptable quality and should not be used clinically. The *Rf* (rate of flow) of a compound is the distance from the center of its activity on the strip to the origin (site of application) divided by the distance from the solvent front to the origin. An *Rf* of 1 means that the compound moves with the solvent front, whereas an *Rf* of 0 means that the component remains at the origin.

TABLE 1-10 Non–Technetium-99m Radiopharmaceuticals for Single-Photon Imaging

Agent	Application
Diagnostic	
Xe-133 xenon (inert gas)	Pulmonary ventilation scintigraphy
Xe-127 xenon (inert gas)	Pulmonary ventilation scintigraphy
Kr-81m krypton (inert gas)	Pulmonary ventilation scintigraphy
I-123 sodium iodide	Thyroid scintigraphy, thyroid uptake function studies
In-111 oxine leukocytes	Inflammatory disease and infection detection
I-123 meta-iodo-benzyl-guanidine (MIBG)	Adrenal medullary tumor imaging
In-111 pentetreotide (OctreoScan)	Somatostatin receptor tumor imaging
I-123 ioflupane (DaTscan)	Dopamine transporter receptor imaging for Parkinson disease and parkinsonian syndromes
Therapy	
I-131 sodium iodide	Thyroid cancer scintigraphy; thyroid uptake function studies; treatment of Graves disease, toxic nodule, and thyroid cancer
I-131 tositumomab (Bexxar)	B-cell lymphoma imaging and therapy
In-111 ibritumomab (Zevalin)	B-cell lymphoma therapy

target-to-background ratio and thus making I-131 seem advantageous, I-123 is now increasingly replacing I-131— for example, for whole-body thyroid cancer scans and MIBG imaging. I-123 ioflupane (DaTscan) has recently been approved to confirm or exclude the diagnosis of Parkinson disease.

Quality control of radioiodinated pharmaceuticals is necessary to reduce radiation exposure to the thyroid gland. In nonthyroid imaging applications, it is common practice to block the thyroid gland with oral iodine (potassium iodide [SSKI], Lugol solution, or potassium iodide tablets) to prevent thyroid accumulation of any iodine present as a radiochemical impurity or metabolite. Protocols vary, but thyroid blocking medications are started 1 to 12 hours before radiotracer administration in dosages equivalent to at least 100 mg of iodide.

Indium-111

In-111 has proved useful for clinical nuclear medicine (Table 1-10). Its principal photon energies of 172 and 245 keV are favorable, and their abundance is high (>90%). The 2.8-day half-life permits multiple-day sequential imaging. Examples of radiopharmaceuticals include In-111 oxine leukocytes for detection of inflammation and infection and the somatostatin receptor–binding peptide In-111 pentetreotide (OctreoScan) to detect neuroendocrine tumors.

Thallium-201

Tl-201 became available in the mid-1970s for myocardial scintigraphy. It behaves as a potassium analog, with high net clearance (~85%) in its passage through the myocardial capillary bed, which makes it an excellent marker of regional blood flow to viable myocardium.

The major disadvantage of thallium as a radioactive imaging agent is the absence of an ideal photopeak for imaging. The gamma emissions (135 and 167 keV) occur in low abundance (see Table 1-2). The emitted mercury characteristic x-rays in the range of 69 to 83 keV are acquired, as sometimes are the 167-keV gamma emissions. The ability of the gamma scintillation camera to discriminate scattered events from primary photons is suboptimal at this energy. Because of its poor imaging characteristics, Tc-99m–labeled cardiac perfusion radiopharmaceuticals are used.

Radioactive Inert Gases

Radioactive inert gases are used for pulmonary ventilation imaging. Xe-133 is the most commonly used. Its advantage over Tc-99m–labeled aerosols is better distribution into the lung periphery in patients with chronic obstructive lung disease. A disadvantage is the relatively low energy of its principal photon (81 keV), dictating the performance of ventilation scintigraphy before Tc-99m perfusion scintigraphy. Because of its poor imaging characteristics and dosimetry issues, Tc-99m–labeled aerosols are more commonly used. Xe-133 has a 5.2-day half-life, posing radiation safety issues answered to some extent by a xenon trap (charcoal).

Xenon-127 is theoretically superior to Xe-133 because of its higher photon energies (Table 1-2). Thus the ventilation study can be performed after the perfusion scan, limited to the locations of perfusion defects. The high cost of producing Xe-127 and long half-life (36 days) have kept it from wide use.

Krypton-81m has advantages because of its high principal gamma emission (190 keV) and short half-life (13 seconds), allowing for postperfusion imaging and multiple-view acquisition without concern for retained activity or radiation dose. However, the rubidium-81/kr-81m generator system is expensive and must be replaced daily because of its short half-life.

▬ DUAL PHOTON RADIOPHARMACEUTICALS FOR POSITRON EMISSION TOMOGRAPHY

The physical characteristics of commonly used positron-emitting radionuclides are summarized in Table 1-3. Many radiopharmaceuticals have been described for use with PET (Box 1-2). Carbon, nitrogen, and oxygen are found ubiquitously in biological molecules. It is thus theoretically possible to radiolabel almost any molecule of biological interest. F-18 has the advantage of a longer half-life than C-11, N-13, or O-15 and has been used as a label for the glucose analog fluorodeoxyglucose (FDG). F-18 FDG has found widespread clinical application in whole-body tumor imaging and, to a lesser extent, imaging of the brain and heart. The uptake of F-18 FDG is a marker of tumor metabolism and viability.

Box 1-2. **Positron Emission Tomography Selected Radiopharmaceuticals**

PERFUSION AGENTS
O-15 water
N-13 ammonia
Rb-82 chloride

METABOLIC AGENTS
F-18 sodium fluoride
Fe-18 fluorodeoxyglucose
O-15 oxygen
C-11 acetate
C-11 palmitate
N-13 glutamate

TUMOR AGENTS
F-18 fluorodeoxyglucose
C-11 methionine
F-18 fluorothymidine

RECEPTOR-BINDING AGENTS
C-11 carfentanil
C-11 raclopride
F-18 fluoro-L-dopa

BLOOD VOLUME
C-11 carbon monoxide
Ga-68 ethylenediamine tetraacetic acid

AMYLOID-IMAGING AGENT
F-18 florbetapir

Rubidium-82 is available from a generator system with a relatively long-lived parent (strontium-82, $T_{1/2}$ = 25 days) (Table 1-4). Like thallium, it is a potassium analog and used for myocardial perfusion imaging. Its availability from a generator system obviates the need for onsite cyclotron production. One limitation is the high energy (3.15 MeV) of its positron emissions. This results in a relatively long average path in soft tissue before annihilation, degrading the spatial resolution available with the agent. This feature is shared to a lesser extent by O-15.

F-18 florbetapir was recently approved by the FDA for amyloid brain imaging.

The production of most positron-emitting radionuclides and their subsequent incorporation into PET radiopharmaceuticals is expensive and complex, requiring a cyclotron or other special accelerator and relatively elaborate radiochemical-handling equipment. In-house self-contained small cyclotrons with automated chemistry are available but are expensive for most clinical settings. The large, increasing clinical demand and the relatively long 2-hour half-life of F-18 FDG has resulted in its production and distribution by regional radiopharmacies.

■ DISPENSING RADIOPHARMACEUTICALS

Normal Procedures

General radiation safety procedures should be followed in all laboratories (Box 1-3). The dispensing of

---

Box 1-3. Radiation Safety Procedures

Wear laboratory coats in areas where radioactive materials are present.

Wear disposable gloves when handling radioactive materials.

Monitor hands and body for radioactive contamination before leaving the area.

Use syringe and vial shields as necessary.

Do not eat, drink, smoke, apply cosmetics, or store food in areas where radioactive material is stored or used.

Wear personnel monitoring devices in areas with radioactive materials.

Never pipette by mouth.

Dispose of radioactive waste in designated, labeled, and properly shielded receptacles located in a secured area.

Label containers, vials, and syringes containing radioactive materials. When not in use, place in shielded containers or behind lead shielding in a secured area.

Store all sealed sources (floods, dose calibrator sources) in shielded containers in a secured area.

Before administering doses to patients, determine and record activity.

Know what steps to take and the person to contact (radiation safety officer) in the event of a radiation accident, improper operation of radiation safety equipment, or theft or loss of licensed material.

---

radiopharmaceuticals is governed by exacting rules and regulations promulgated by the FDA and NRC, as well as state pharmacy boards and hospital radiation safety committees. Radiopharmaceuticals for clinical use must be approved by the FDA. Radiopharmaceuticals are prescription drugs that cannot be legally administered without being ordered by an authorized individual. The NRC *authorized user* and the radiopharmacy are responsible for confirming the appropriateness of the request, ensuring that the correct radiopharmaceutical designated amount is administered to the patient, and keeping records of both the request and documentation of dosage administration.

Before any material is dispensed, quality assurance measures should be carried out. These are described earlier in this chapter for the Mo-99/Tc-99m generator system and Tc-99m–labeled radiopharmaceuticals. For other agents, the package insert or protocol for formulation and dispensing should be consulted for radiochromatography or other quality control steps that must be performed before dosage administration. Good practice dictates that quality control should always be performed, even when not legally required. Every dose should be physically inspected for any particulate or foreign material (e.g., rubber from the tops of multidose injection vials) before administration. Each dose administered to a patient must be assayed in a dose calibrator. The administered activity should be within ±20% of the prescription request.

Special Considerations

Pregnancy and Lactation

The possibility of pregnancy should be considered for every woman of childbearing age referred to the nuclear medicine service for a diagnostic or therapeutic procedure. Pregnancy alone is not an absolute contraindication to performing a nuclear medicine study. For example, pulmonary embolism is encountered in pregnant women and is associated with potential serious morbidity and mortality. Thus the risk-to-benefit ratio of ventilation-perfusion scintigraphy is high and considered an acceptable procedure in this circumstance. The radiation dosage is kept to a minimum. Tc-99m MAA does not cross the placenta, but xenon does. Radioiodine also crosses the placenta. The fetal thyroid develops the capacity to concentrate radioiodine at 10 to 12 weeks of gestation, and cretinism caused by in utero exposure to therapeutic I-131 may occur.

Women who are lactating and breastfeeding require special attention. The need to suspend breastfeeding is determined by the half-life of the radionuclide and the degree to which it is secreted in breast milk. Radioiodine is secreted by the breast, and breastfeeding should be terminated altogether after the administration of I-131. NRC regulations stipulate that the patient must receive verbal and written instructions to that effect. For I-123, breastfeeding could safely be resumed after 2 days. For Tc-99m agents, 12 to 24 hours is sufficient. Further recommendations regarding breastfeeding for various radiopharmaceuticals are listed in Table 1-11.

Dosage Selection for Pediatric Patients

Various approaches have been used for scaling down the radiopharmaceutical dose administered to children. There is no perfect way to do this because of the differential rate of maturation of body organs and the changing ratio of different body compartments to body weight. Empirically, body surface area correlates better than body weight for dosage selection. Various formulas and nomograms have been developed.

An approximation based on body weight uses the formula:

$$\text{Pediatric dose} = \frac{\text{Patient weight (kg)}}{70 \text{ kg}} \times \text{Adult dose}$$

Another alternative is the use of *Webster's rule*:

$$\text{Pediatric dose} = \frac{\text{Age in years} + 1}{\text{Age in years} + 7} \times \text{Adult dose}$$

This formula is not useful for infants. Moreover, in some cases a calculated dose may not be adequate to obtain a diagnostically useful study and physician judgment must be used. For example, a newborn infant with suspected biliary atresia may require 24-hour delayed Tc-99m HIDA imaging, which is not feasible if the dose is too low. Therefore a minimum dose for each radiopharmaceutical should be established.

The concept *As Low As Reasonably Achievable (ALARA)* has always been a basic tenet in nuclear medicine regarding the administered dose. This concept has been recently reemphasized for pediatric diagnostic imaging. It has been restated as *the lowest absorbed radiation dose that is consistent with quality imaging*. Expert consensus recommendations for pediatric administered doses are listed in Table 1-12.

Nuclear Regulatory Commission and Agreement States

The NRC regulates all reactor by-product materials with regard to use and disposal, radiation safety of personnel using them, and the public. Certain states, termed *Agreement States*, have entered into regulatory agreements with the NRC that give them the authority to license and inspect by-products, sources, or special nuclear material used or possessed within their borders. Currently more than 40 states are Agreement States, and the number is growing. These states agree to set regulations at least as strict as those of the NRC, but they may have stricter rules.

Authorized User

An Authorized User is a person with documented training and experience in the safe handling and use of radioactive materials for medical use who is authorized to order, receive, store, and administer radiopharmaceuticals. Two general paths exist for becoming an authorized user: certification by specialty board or training and work experience. The NRC has defined requirements for becoming an authorized user based on the type of use for the radiopharmaceutical—uptake and dilution, imaging and localization, and therapy (Box 1-4). Once Authorized User eligible status is achieved, the candidate can apply to bodies such as the hospital Radiation Safety Committee and the Radiation Safety Officer to become an authorized user with a radioactive materials license.

Medical Event

The NRC defines a *medical event* as a radiopharmaceutical dose administration involving the wrong patient, wrong radiopharmaceutical, wrong route of administration, or administered dose differing from the prescribed dose when the effective dose equivalent to the patient exceeds 5 rem to the whole body or 50 rem to any individual organ (Box 1-5). The definition and procedures for handling misadministrations of radiopharmaceuticals are set out in the

TABLE 1-11 Recommendations for Radiopharmaceuticals Excreted in Breast Milk

Radiopharmaceutical	Administered activity mCi (MBq)	Counseling adivsed	Withhold breast-feeding
Ga-67 citrate	5.0 (185)	Yes	Cessation
I-131 sodium iodide	0.02 (0.7)	Yes	Cessation
I-123 sodium iodide	0.4 (14.8)	Yes	48 hr
I-123 MIBG	10 (370.0)	Yes	48 hr
Tl-201	3 (111)	Yes	96 hr
In-111 leukocytes	5 (185)	Yes	48 hr
Tc-99m MAA	4 (148)	Yes	12 hr
Tc-99m red blood cells	20 (740)	Yes	12 hr
Tc-99m pertechnetate	5 (185)	Yes	4 hr

Modified with permission from Stabin MG, Breitz HB. Breast milk excretion of radiopharmaceuticals: mechanisms, findings, and radiation dosimetry. *J Nucl Med.* 2000;41:863-873.
MAA, Macroaggregated albumin; *MIBG*, meta-iodo-benzyl-guanidine.

TABLE 1-12 Consensus Recommendations for Administered Activities in Children

Radiopharmaceutical	Recommended administered activity mCi/kg (MBq/kg)	Minimum activity mCi (MBq)	Maximum activity mCi (MBq)
I-123 MIBG	0.14 (5.2)	1.0 (37)	10 (370)
Tc-99m MDP	0.25 (9.3)	1.0 (37)	
F-18 FDG	0.10-0.14 (3.7-5.2)	1.0 (37)	
Body			
Brain	0.10 (3.7)		
Tc-99m DMSA	0.05 (1.85)	0.5 (18.5)	
Tc-99m MAG3	0.10 (3.7)	4.0 (148)	4 (148)
Tc-99m HIDA	0.05 (1.85)	0.5 (18.5)	
Tc-99m MAA	0.07 (2.59)	0.4 (14.8)	
Tc-99m pertechnetate	0.05 (1.85)	0.25 (9.25)	
F-18 sodium fluoride	0.06 (2.22)	0.5 (18.5)	1.0 (≤37)
Tc-99m (cystography)		0.25 (9.25)	1.0 (37)
Tc-99m SC (liquid GE)		0.25 (9.25)	0.5 (18.5)
Tc-99m SC (solid GE) (GE, gastric emptying)			

Modified from Gelfand MJ, Parisi MT, Treves ST; Pediatric Nuclear Medicine Dose Reduction Workgroup. Pediatric radiopharmaceutical administered doses: 2010 North American consensus guidelines. *J Nucl Med.* 2011;52(2):318-322.
DMSA, Dimercaptosuccinic acid; *FDG*, fluorodeoxyglucose; *GE*, ; *HIDA*, hepatobiliary iminodiacetic acid; *MAA*, macroaggregated albumin; *MDP*, methylene diphosphonate; *MIBG*, meta-iodo-benzyl-guanidine; *SC*, .

Box 1-4. Nuclear Regulatory Commission 10 CFR Part 35: Medical Use of By-Product Material

35.190 Training for uptake, dilution, and excretion studies

35.290 Training for imaging and localization studies

35.390 Training for any therapy requiring a written directive

35.392 I-131 ≤33 mCi

35.394 I-131 >33 mCi

35.396 Parental administration of a beta emitter

Box 1-5. Annual Dose Limits for Radiation Exposure (Nuclear Regulatory Commission Regulations)

ADULT OCCUPATIONAL

5 rem (0.05 Sv) total effective dose equivalent

50 rem (0.5 Sv) to any organ or tissue or extremity

15 rems (0.15 Sv) to the lens of the eye

MINORS (<18 YEARS OF AGE) OCCUPATIONAL

10% of those for adult workers

EMBRYO/FETUS OCCUPATIONAL

0.5 rem (5 mSv) during pregnancy

MEMBERS OF THE PUBLIC

0.1 rem (1 mSv)

2 mrem (0.02 mSv) in any hour (average)

Box 1-6. Procedure for Radioactive Spill

1. Notify all persons in the area that a spill has occurred.
2. Prevent the spread of contamination by isolating the area and covering the spill (absorbent paper).
3. If clothing is contaminated, remove and place in plastic bag.
4. If an individual is contaminated, rinse contaminated region with lukewarm water and wash with soap.
5. Notify the radiation safety officer.
6. Wear gloves, disposable laboratory coat, and booties to clean up spill with absorbent paper.
7. Put all contaminated absorbent paper in labeled radioactive waste container.
8. Check the area or contaminated individual with appropriate radiation survey meter.

Code of Federal Regulations (10 CFR-35); however, the terminology was changed in 2002. What was previously called a *misadministration* is now called a *medical event*. Many of the prior misadministrations no longer have to be reported to the NRC or state.

Medical events are extremely unlikely to occur as a result of any diagnostic nuclear medicine procedure. Most will be related to radioiodine I-131. However, when a medical event is recognized, regulations for reporting the event and management of the patient must be followed. The details are determined in part by the kind of material involved and amount of the adverse exposure of the patient. All medical events must be reported to the radiation safety officer, regulatory agency, referring physician, and affected patient. Complete records on each event must be retained and available for NRC review for 10 years.

Adverse Reactions to Diagnostic Radiopharmaceuticals

Adverse reactions to radiopharmaceuticals are extremely rare because the pharmaceutical is formulated in a subpharmacological dose that should not cause a physiological effect. When they occur, they are usually mild and rarely fatal. Of concern is the possibility of reactions caused by the development of human antimouse antibodies (HAMA) after repeated exposure to radiolabeled antibody imaging agents. This has been a factor in the FDA's slow approval for radiolabeled antibodies. Tc-99m fanolesomab (NeutroSPEC) had approval withdrawn as a

result of possible serious adverse effects. In-111 capromab pendetide (ProstaScint) and In-111 and Y-90 ibritumomab (Zevalin) and I-131 tositumomab (Bexxar) have proved safe.

▬ RADIATION ACCIDENTS (SPILLS)

In a busy nuclear medicine practice, accidental spills of radioactive material invariably occur. The spills are divided into minor and major categories, depending on the radionuclide and the amount spilled. For I-131, incidents involving less than 1 mCi are considered minor; spills more than that are considered major. For Tc-99m, Tl-201, and Ga-67, a major spill is considered to be more than 100 mCi.

The basic principles of responding to both kinds of spills are the same (Box 1-6). For minor spills, people in the area are warned that the spill has occurred. Attempts are made to prevent the spread of the spilled material. Absorbent paper is used to cover the spilled material. Minor spills can be cleaned up using soap and water, disposable gloves, and remote handling devices. All contaminated material, including gloves and other objects, should be disposed of in designated bags. The area should be continually surveyed until the reading from a Geiger-Müller (GM) survey meter is at background levels. All personnel involved should also be monitored, including hands, shoes, and clothing. The spill must be reported to the institution's radiation safety officer.

For major spills, the area is cleared immediately. Attempts are made to prevent further spread with absorbent pads, and, if possible, the radioactivity is shielded. The room is sealed off, and the radiation safety officer is notified immediately. The radiation safety officer typically directs further response—for example, when and how to proceed with cleanup and decontamination.

In dealing with both minor and major spills, an attempt is made to keep radiation exposure of patients, hospital staff, and the environment to a minimum. The radiation safety officer must restrict access to the area until it is safe for patients and personnel. However, no absolute guidelines exist to provide a definitive approach to every spill.

Each laboratory is responsible for developing its own set of written procedures. The radiation safety officer must restrict access to the area until it is safe for patients and personnel.

■ QUALITY CONTROL IN THE NUCLEAR PHARMACY

Selected quality control procedures for Tc-99m–labeled radiopharmaceuticals and for Mo-99/Tc-99m generator systems are described earlier in this chapter. Considerations of radiochemical and radionuclide purity also apply to other single-photon agents and positron radiopharmaceuticals (see Table 1-8). Radiochemical purity is important for radioiodinated agents because of the potential for uptake of free radioiodine by the thyroid gland if the radiolabel disassociates from the carrier molecule. Other quality control procedures are aimed at ensuring the sterility and apyrogenicity of administered radiopharmaceuticals. Quality control monitoring of the dose calibrator performance is important to ensure that administered doses are within prescribed amounts.

Sterility and Pyrogen Testing

Sterility implies the absence of living organisms (see Table 1-8). *Apyrogenicity* implies the absence of metabolic products such as endotoxins. Because many radiopharmaceuticals are prepared just before use, definitive testing before they are administered to the patient is impractical, which doubles the need for careful aseptic technique in the nuclear pharmacy.

Autoclaving is a well-known means of sterilization of preparation vials and other utensils and materials, but it is not useful for radiopharmaceuticals. When terminal sterilization is required, various membrane filtration methods are used. Special filters with pore diameters smaller than microorganisms have been developed for this purpose. A filter pore size of 0.22 μm is necessary to sterilize a solution. It traps bacteria, including small organisms such as *Pseudomonas.*

Sterility testing standards have been defined by the USP. Standard media, including thioglycollate and soybean-casein digest media, are used for different categories of microorganisms, including aerobic and anaerobic bacteria and fungi.

Pyrogens are protein or polysaccharide metabolites of microorganisms or other contaminating substances that cause febrile reactions (see Table 1-8). They can be present even in sterile preparations. The typical clinical syndrome is fever, chills, joint pain, and headache developing minutes to a few hours after injection. The USP test for pyrogen testing uses limulus amebocyte lysate. It is based on the observation that amebocyte lysate preparations from the blood of horseshoe crabs become opaque in the presence of pyrogens.

Radiopharmaceutical Dose Calibrators

The dose calibrator is an important instrument in the radiopharmacy and is subject to quality control requirements. Four basic measurements are included: accuracy, linearity, precision or constancy, and geometry. All of these tests must be performed at installation and after repair.

Accuracy

Accuracy is measured by using reference standard sources obtained from the National Institute of Standards and Technology. The test is performed annually, and two different radioactive sources are used. If the measured activity in the dose calibrator varies from the standard or theoretical activity by more than 10%, the device must be recalibrated.

Linearity

The linearity test is designed to determine the response of the calibrator over a range of measured activities. A common approach is to take a sample of Tc-99m pertechnetate and sequentially measure it during radioactive decay. Because the change in activity with time is a definable physical parameter, any deviation in the observed assay value indicates equipment malfunction and nonlinearity. An alternative approach is to use precalibrated lead attenuators with sequential measurements of the same specimen. This test is performed quarterly.

Precision or Constancy

The precision, or constancy, test measures the dose calibrator's ability to measure the same specimen over time. A long-lived standard such as barium-133 (356 keV, $T_{1/2}$ 10.7 years), cesium-137 (662 keV, $T_{1/2}$ 30 years), or cobalt-57 (122 kev, $T_{1/2}$ 271 days) is used. The test is performed daily, and results should be within 10% of the reference standard value.

Geometry

The geometric test is performed during acceptance testing of the dose calibrator. The issue is that the same amount of radioactivity contained in different volumes of sample can result in different measured or observed radioactivities. For a given dose calibrator, if readings vary by more than 10% from one volume to another, correction factors are calculated. For convenience, the correction factors are based on the most commonly measured volume of material, which is typically determined from day-to-day clinical use of the dose calibrator.

■ RECEIVING RADIOACTIVE PACKAGES

Packages containing radioactive materials must be labeled according to the amount of measured activity at the surface and at 1 m (Table 1-13). Packaging is required to pass rigorous durability testing: drop test, corner drop test, compression, and water spray for 30 minutes. The U.S. Department of Transportation sets guidelines for regulations concerning not only package labeling but also transport rules concerning air and truck shipments. Placards are required on all sides of any truck carrying packages in the Level III Yellow label category.

TABLE 1-13 Survey Limits for Radioactive Material Package Receipt

Test	Exposure Limits
Surface survey	<200 mR/hr
Activity at 1 m	<10 mR/hr
Wipe test	6600 dpm/300 cm^2

Once a radioactive package has been received, it must be monitored for contamination within 3 hours from delivery during normal working hours or within 3 hours of the beginning of the next working day. An inspection is first done, looking for signs of damage or leakage. Then an external survey is performed with a GM counter at the surface and at 1 m. Finally, a wipe test is performed, swabbing 300 cm^2 of the surface with absorbent paper and counting in a scintillation counter. The sender must be notified of any package exceeding limits (Table 1-14), and records of the survey must be kept, including date, name of the person performing the survey, survey readings, manufacturer, lot number, type of product and amount, and time of calibration.

▬ RADIATION DOSIMETRY

The amount of radioactivity that can be administered for scintigraphic procedures performed in clinical nuclear medicine is limited by the amount of radiation exposure received by the patient. The patient radiation exposure is determined by the percent localization of the administered dose in each organ of the body, the time course of retention in each organ, and the size and relative distribution of the organs in the body. This information is obtained from biodistribution and pharmacokinetic studies during the development and regulatory approval process for a new radiopharmaceutical. For each radiopharmaceutical, estimates of radiation absorbed doses are made as part of the approval process and contained in the package insert (Table 1-15).

The radiation absorbed dose *(rads)* to any organ in the body depends on biological factors (percent uptake, biological half-life) and physical factors (amount and nature of emitted radiations from the radionuclide). One rad is equal to the absorption of 100 ergs per gram of tissue. The formula for calculating the radiation absorbed dose is:

$$D (r_k \leftarrow r_h) = \tilde{A}_b \, S \, (r_k \leftarrow r_h)$$

The formula states that the absorbed dose in a region k resulting from activity from a source region b is equal to the cumulative radioactivity given in microcurie-hours in the source region ($\tilde{A}$) times the mean absorbed dose per unit of cumulative activity in rads per microcurie-hour (S). The cumulative activity is determined from experimental measurements of uptake and retention in the different source regions. The mean absorbed dose per unit of cumulative activity is based on physical measurements and is determined by radiations emanating from the radionuclide.

The total absorbed dose to a region or organ is the sum from all source regions around it and from activity within the target organ. For example, a calculation of the absorbed dose to the myocardium in a Tc-99m tetrofosmin scan must

TABLE 1-14 Radioactive Package Labeling Categories

| Label category | Exposure | |
	Surface (mR/hr)	At 1 m (mR/hr)
I White	<0.5	—
II Yellow	>0.5 to ≤50	<1
III Yellow	>50 to ≤200	>1 to ≤10
Not Allowed	>200	>10

TABLE 1-15 Radiation Doses From Common Diagnostic Nuclear Medicine Procedures

Radionuclide (rem)	Agent	Activity (mCi)	Highest dose (rads) (organ)	Effective dose equivalent (rem)
F-18	FDG	10	5.9 (bladder)	0.7
Ga-67	Citrate	5	11.8 (bone surface)	1.9
Tc-99m	HIDA	5	2.0 (gallbladder)	0.3
	HMPAO	20	2.5 (kidneys)	0.7
	MAA	4	1.0 (lungs)	0.2
	MDP	20	4.7 (bone surface)	0.4
	MAG3	20	8.1 (bladder wall)	0.5
	Sestamibi	20	2.7 (gallbladder)	0.7
	Tetrofosmin	20	2.7 (gallbladder)	0.6
	Sulfur colloid	8	2.2 (spleen)	0.3
In-111	Leukocytes	0.5	10.9 (spleen)	1.2
I-123	Sodium iodide (25% uptake)	0.2	2.6 (thyroid)	0.2
I-123	MIBG	10.0	0.1 (liver)	0.07
Xe-133	Inert gas	15	0.06 (lungs)	0.04
Tl-201	Chloride	3	4.6 (thyroid)	1.2

Data from Siegel JA: *Guide for Diagnostic Nuclear Medicine and Radiopharmaceutical Therapy.* Reston, VA, Society of Nuclear Medicine, 2004.
SI conversion: 1 rem = 0.01 Sv; 1 mCi = 37 MBq.
FDG, Fluorodeoxyglucose; *HIDA,* hepatobiliary iminodiacetic acid; *HMPAO,* hexamethylpropyleneamine oxime; *MAA,* macroaggregated albumin; *MDP,* methylene diphosphonate; *MIBG,* meta-iodo-benzyl-guanidine.

take into account contributions from radioactivity localizing in the myocardium and from radioactivity in the lung, blood, liver, intestines, kidneys, and general background soft tissues. The percentage uptake and the biological behavior are different in each of those tissues. The amount of radiation reaching the myocardium is also different, depending on the geometry of the source organ and its distance from the heart. The formula is applied for each source region, and the individual contributions are summed.

Factors that affect dosimetry include the amount of activity administered originally, the biodistribution in one patient versus another, the route of administration, the rate of elimination, the size of the patient, and the presence of pathological processes. For example, for radiopharmaceuticals cleared by the kidney, radiation exposure is greater in patients with renal failure. Another example is the differing percentage uptakes of radioiodine in the thyroid depending on whether a patient is hyperthyroid, euthyroid, or hypothyroid.

The radiation absorbed dose (rads or Gray) does not describe the biological effects of different types of radiation. The equivalent dose (rem or Sievert) relates the absorbed dose in human tissue to the effective biological damage of the radiation. Not all radiation has the same biological effect, even for the same amount of absorbed dose. To determine the equivalent dose, the absorbed dose (rads or Gray) must be multiplied by a quality factor unique to the type of incident radiation.

Effective dose is calculated by multiplying actual organ doses by "risk weighting factors" that give each organ's relative radiosensitivity to developing cancer and adding up the total of all the numbers, which is the effective whole-body dose or just effective dose. These weighting factors are designed so that this effective dose represents the dose that the total body could receive (uniformly) that would give the same cancer risk as various organs getting different doses. The effective dose can be used to compare radiation doses of various imaging modalities.

Estimates of radiation-absorbed dose for each major radiopharmaceutical are provided in tabular form in the specific organ system chapters.

▬ SUGGESTED READING

Cherry SR, Sorenson JA, Phelps ME. *Physics in Nuclear Medicine*. 3rd ed. Philadelphia: W.B. Saunders; 2003.

Christian PE, Waterstram-Rich KM, eds. *Nuclear Medicine and PET/CT: Technology and Techniques*. 7th ed. St. Louis: Mosby; 2012.

Fahey FH, Treves ST, Adelstein SJ. Minimizing and communicating radiation risk in pediatric nuclear medicine. *J Nucl Med*. 2011;52(8):1240-1251.

Gelfand MJ, Parisi MT, Treves ST. Pediatric Nuclear Medicine Dose Reduction Workgroup. Pediatric radiopharmaceutical administered doses: 2010 North American consensus guidelines. *J Nucl Med*. 2011;52(2):318-322.

Mettler FA, Huda W, Yoshizumi TT, Mahesh M. Effective doses in radiology and diagnostic nuclear medicine: a catalog. *Radiology*. 2008;248(1):254-263.

Saha GB. *Fundamentals of Nuclear Pharmacy*. 6th ed. New York: Springer; 2010.

Siegel JA. *Guide for Diagnostic Nuclear Medicine and Radiopharmaceutical Therapy*. Reston, VA: Society of Nuclear Medicine; 2004.

Stabin MG, Breitz HB. Breast milk excretion of radiopharmaceuticals: mechanisms, findings, and radiation dosimetry. *J Nucl Med*. 2000;41(5):863-873.

CHAPTER 2

Molecular Imaging

Nuclear medicine has always involved molecular imaging (MI). By combining a detectable label, such as a radiotracer, with a molecule of physiological importance, many different cellular function parameters can be assessed. In fact, MI has been defined as the visualization, characterization, and measurement of biological processes. It can diagnose disease and assess therapeutic response, long before changes can be seen with computed tomography (CT) at the anatomical level. The fact that MI allows noninvasive assessment and quantification is especially desirable when following patients over time. Small differences among patients can be identified so treatments can be specifically modified for the needs of the individual. This move toward "personalized medicine" may also involve more accurate identification of research subjects, leading to more successful and cost-effective clinical trials in the future.

In the past, a fairly sharp divide existed between MI uses in preclinical research and those for clinical imaging and therapy. More recently, the process of advancing translational research has become an important focus of the MI community, and the line between the laboratory and clinic has blurred. Some of the definitions involved in MI are listed in Box 2-1.

Many nuclear medicine techniques have played a role bridging the gap between the worlds of research and clinical practice. The widespread acceptance and use of fluorine-18 fluorodeoxyglucose (F-18 FDG) positron emission tomography with computed tomography (PET/CT) has highlighted the importance of MI and has spearheaded a revolution in imaging and therapy. The addition of multimodality equipment, such as single-photon emission computed tomography with computed tomography (SPECT/CT), PET/CT, and now PET/magnetic resonance (PET/MR), continues to drive the field forward.

Multiple new agents currently undergoing clinical trials will move through the approval process and help transform the way we think about imaging. MI and therapy will be revolutionized with new quantitative assays directed at wide-ranging targets, including gene expression, membrane receptors, and protein upregulation, as well as tumor metabolism, perfusion, and hypoxia.

IMAGING TECHNIQUES

Many different parameters of cellular function can be imaged using MI techniques. A list of these techniques is provided in Table 2-1. The many potential benefits and limitations demonstrated by each of these techniques determine their usage. Increasingly, imaging forms may be combined as hybrid instruments with anatomical modalities such as CT that allow superior localization of the biomarker being detected.

Box 2-1. Molecular Imaging Definitions

Apoptosis: Programmed cell death, which is the way the body disposes of damaged, old, or unwanted cells.

Pharmacodynamics: Study of the effects of a drug on a living organism, including relationship between the drug dose and its effect.

Pharmacogenetics: Study of how a body reacts to a drug based on an individual's genetic makeup.

Pharmacokinetics: Study of how living tissues process drugs, including alterations in chemical makeup and drug absorption, distribution, metabolism, and excretion. This may involve tagging a drug with a probe or radiotracer.

Reporter gene system: Engineered genes that encode a product that can be easily assayed to assess a process being monitored after the genes are transfected into cells.

Signal amplification: Use of enzymes to activate contrast agent (e.g., protease activation optical agents).

Target identification—DNA microarray: Efficient method for identifying potential targets by detecting mRNA expression. Further target validation needed because posttranscriptional and posttranslational processing means proteins are not always expressed.

Target identification—genomics: The study of DNA sequences, genes, and their control and expression.

Target identification—proteonomics: High-throughput methods to quantitatively determine tissue protein expression (alternative to DNA microarray). Mass spectrometry–based proteonomics using cell lines or tissue samples or immunohistochemistry of diseased or unaffected tissues can be used in tissue arrays.

Target validation: Once the target is identified, expression and subcellular localization are evaluated in a variety of tissues.

Translational medicine: The process of moving basic laboratory research into clinical practice, including necessary patient testing and clinical trials to ensure safety.

Tumor marker: Substances that may be used to identify and monitor cancer. They may be materials released into blood or urine in response to cancer or may be labeled for identification with molecular imaging techniques.

TABLE 2-1 Functional and Molecular Imaging Modalities

Modality	Advantages	Disadvantages
PET	High sensitivity Highly quantitative Temporal monitoring possible Many translational agents under development	Radiation Cyclotron on site for short-lived agents Spatial resolution relatively low
SPECT	Widely available Many probes	Lower spatial resolution and less quantitative than PET Some radiation
Optical imaging	High spatial resolution possible Good sensitivity Quick and inexpensive	Limited detection depth Limited clinical use
MRS	Sensitive Native molecules, no contrast needed	Limited region examined
MRI	High resolution	Lower temporal resolution Sensitivity lower
Ultrasound with contrast	Portable No radiation Low cost High frequency with microbubbles provides good spatial resolution Real-time temporal monitoring	Microbubbles research only Sensitivity lower Quantitative ability low

MRI, Magnetic resonance imaging; *MRS*, magnetic resonance spectroscopy; *PET*, positron emission tomography; *SPECT*, single-photon emission computed tomography.

Radionuclide Imaging

SPECT and PET offer obvious advantages because of their sensitivity for radiolabeled probe detection. Although PET offers some potential advantages over SPECT, such as improved resolution and quantitative capabilities, SPECT is often more practical because it is less expensive and widely available. The combination of either technology with CT allows improved accuracy. Micro-PET and micro-SPECT systems are available for smaller animals. New dedicated clinical breast positron emission mammography (PEM) cameras recently have shown improved accuracy over whole-body PET-CT scanners in assessing primary breast tumors with F-18 FDG, and single-photon breast-specific gamma imaging (BSGI) or molecular breast imaging (MBI) cameras for technetium-99m sestamibi imaging have begun to find increased clinical demand.

Magnetic Resonance Imaging

Magnetic Resonance Spectroscopy

Magnetic resonance spectroscopy (MRS) has been able to assess the molecular composition of tissues. Radiofrequency pulses are applied that excite atoms such as hydrogen-1. It is possible to monitor concentrations of molecules, including choline, *N*-acetylaspartate, and creatinine, by the signals detected. Although other nuclei exhibit low signal-to-noise ratios with MRS, a process termed *hyperpolarization* allows the use of helium-3 and xenon-129 in lung perfusion

examinations and carbon-13–labeled molecules, such as C-13 pyruvate, to map tumor metabolism. Applications of MRS are wide ranging, but its utility is limited in comparison to the sensitivity of PET. Although PET can detect nanomolar concentrations of radiotracers, MR sensitivity is in the millimolar range.

Diffusion Magnetic Resonance Imaging

Not only are the high soft tissue contrast, anatomical resolution, and contrast enhancement capabilities of MRI useful but new imaging sequences are also able to assess some functional tissue characteristics. One of these, diffusion weighted MR (DW-MR), is being investigated as a means of characterizing, staging, and assessing therapy in some tumors. DW-MR makes use of the fact that water molecules are more mobile when tissues are less cellular. Based on the DW-MR, an apparent diffusion coefficient (ADC) value is calculated. Lower ADC values have been shown in tumors, such as glioblastomas, with poorer prognosis.

Optical Imaging

Because the low energy of light is attenuated and scattered by soft tissues, optical imaging of biological processes is limited to preclinical work with small animals (usually mice) or very superficial targets (such as in endoscopy). However, it offers several advantages by being inexpensive, flexible, and sensitive. Technical advancements in detectors have resulted in improved sensitivity and resolution, as have multimodality cameras combining SPECT, PET, and CT. The two major categories of optical imaging are bioluminescence and fluorescent imaging.

An example of bioluminescence involves the enzyme luciferase, which is responsible for the glow in insects such as the firefly, jellyfish, and some bacteria. This enzyme is placed into the DNA of cells, animals, or models of disease as a reporter gene. The substrate, D-luciferin, is administered, and a chemical reaction results in low levels of a spectrum of emissions. However, background noise is almost nonexistent because little light is emitted from the imaged tissues. Despite its disadvantages, this has become an integral technique for preclinical imaging.

Fluorescence imaging uses a fluorescent protein—a fluorophore—that is excited by an external light source. The fluorescent protein can be genetically engineered into an animal, or a molecule of interest can be labeled with fluorophore fluorescent particles. Unlike bioluminescence, in which the signal detected is proportional to the number of luminescent cells, fluorescence signal maybe more difficult to quantify because it is affected by the number of fluorescent cells and the intensity of the external light used for excitation. The quantum yield of the signal in fluorescence is orders of magnitude higher than for bioluminescence and does not require administration of a substrate. Photoproteins such as green fluorescent protein (GFP) have been available for years. New proteins with emission spectra peaks in the near-infrared (NIR) wavelengths, or NIR fluorochromes, have expanded the range of this technique, showing less absorption. It is possible to image multiple targets of interest at one time. Use of this technique has been extended beyond small animal preclinical research. For example, diffuse optical imaging and diffuse optical spectroscopy using NIR light has been used to detect tumors and monitor effects of neoadjuvant chemotherapy in breast cancer.

Ultrasound

Recent advances in ultrasound contrast enhancement include the use of microbubble technology and high-frequency ultrasound. Small gas bubbles can be stabilized with a lipid, albumin, or polymer shell. For imaging, microbubbles have been conjugated onto many molecules, such as peptides and antibodies. Also, the microbubbles can be used to deliver a therapeutic payload. This could include gene therapy and cancer treatments. Perfluorocarbon-filled microbubbles allow optimal conditions for targeting and drug delivery.

▬ BIOMARKERS

Background

To assess cellular function noninvasively, it is important to identify biomarkers, specific characteristics of a disease or cellular process that can be measured. Biomarkers can help predict which patients are likely to respond to a specific therapy, such as patients who possess a necessary receptor. Response biomarkers can be used to follow changes in a disease over time. The development of standardized imaging biomarkers is growing. Many multicenter and corporate trials now incorporate measurements of various biomarkers by CT, ultrasound, or MR. Criteria such as the revised Response Evaluation Criteria in Solid Tumors (RECIST) have been put into general use to standardize the way size and tumor volume measurements are obtained and reported. The inclusion of F-18 FDG PET-CT criteria into clinical trials is rapidly growing, and recommendations about standardized PET reporting as a biomarker (i.e., PET RECIST [PRECIST]) have been made.

In addition to F-18 FDG, many other cellular function parameters are being investigated as potential biomarker targets. These include cell proliferation, peptide and membrane biosynthesis, receptor expression, hypoxia, angiogenesis, apoptosis, and gene transfection (Table 2-2). When developing a nuclear probe, target selection is critical. For imaging, the target must be specific for the disease, reflect disease extent, and be accessible to the probe. Probe accumulation, on the other hand, must reflect the extent of disease. Both intracellular and extracellular targets have been successfully used, and many probes employ existing receptor ligands, antibodies, or enzymes as their foundation. Unlike targets such as receptors, in which one imaging molecule per target will be localized, the use of an enzyme approach results in signal amplification with many imaging molecules per target molecule.

Cell Metabolism: Florine-18 Fluorodeoxyglucose

The glucose analog F-18 FDG is a sensitive marker for many tumors, reflecting increased tumor glycolysis. F-18 FDG has been proven useful for tumor diagnosis, staging, and therapy monitoring. However, in some situations, F-18

FDG is not the optimal imaging agent. Many cancers, such as well-differentiated and slowly growing tumors, do not accumulate F-18 FDG to a significant extent. F-18 FDG also lacks specificity, showing accumulation in inflammatory and infectious processes.

Cell Proliferation: Florine-18 Fluorothymidine

A biomarker mirroring DNA synthesis could show increased specificity for tumors compared to F-18 FDG. The pyrimidine nucleoside thymidine is the logical choice because it is taken up proportionally to DNA synthesis but is not a precursor of mRNA. Thymidine kinase 1 (TK1) phosphorylates thymidine taken up into the cell, and the activity of TK1 roughly serves as a marker of DNA synthesis. However, the picture is complicated by the fact that

TABLE 2-2 Functional Imaging Assays with Positron Emission Tomography and Single-Photon Emission Computed Tomography

Cellular Parameter	Agent	Clinical (C) Translational (T) Preclinical (P)
Metabolism	F-18 fluorodeoxyglucose	C
Proliferation	F-18 fluorothymidine (FLT)	T
Biosynthesis	C-11 choline	T
	C-11 acetate	T
Amino acid transport, metabolism, and peptide synthesis	C-11 methionine	T
	F-18 fluoroethyltyrosine (FET)	T
	F-18 DOPA	T
Receptor expression	In-111 pentetreotide	C
	Ga-68 DOTA-TOC	T
	Ga-68-DOTA-F(ab')₂-herceptin	T
	In-111-DTPA-trastuzumab	T
	F-18 16α-17β-fluoroestradiol (FES)	T
	F-18 fluorodihydrotestosterone	T
Antigen expression	In-111 ibritumomab tiuxetan (CD 20+)	C
	In-111 capromab pendetide (prostate-specific membrane antigen)	C
Blood flow	O-15 water	P, T
Angiogenesis	F-18 galacto-RGD	T
Epidermal growth factor receptor (EGFR)	In-111-DTPA-EGF	T
	Ga-68-DOTA-EGF	T
Apoptosis	Tc-99m annexin-V	T
Hypoxia	F-18 fluoromisonidazole (FMISO)	T
	Cu-64 ATSM	T
Transgene expression	F-18 FHBG monitor gene Rx	P

FHBG, Fluoropencicyclovir; *RGD,* arginine-glycine-aspartic acid.
*Some sites outside of the United States clinically applied.

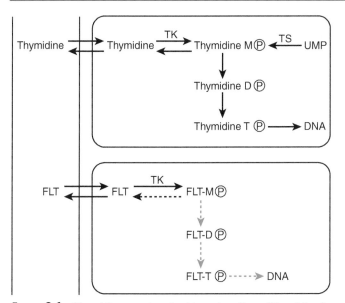

FIGURE 2-1. Thymidine as an imaging biomarker. *Upper,* Thymidine is taken up into the cell and phosphorylated by thymidine kinase 1 (TK) in the external salvage pathway. Cells also perform endogenous de novo synthesis with deoxyuridine *(UMP)* and the enzyme thymidylate synthase *(TS)*. *Lower,* F-18–labeled thymidine *(FLT)* is taken up into the cell, phosphorylated, and trapped similar to thymidine. However, as the *dashed arrows* suggest, FLT is not further metabolized and is not incorporated into DNA. *FLT-D,* difluorothymidine; *FLT-M,* monofluorothymidine; *FLT-T,* trifluorothymidine; *P (circled),* phosphate.

thymidine is also incorporated into DNA via a second pathway involving de novo synthesis from the nucleotide deoxyuridine (Fig. 2-1). Cells and tumors can vary in the use of the targeted extrinsic salvage pathway versus de novo synthesis. In addition, mitochondrial uptake, which occurs independently of cellular division but at a relatively low background level, adds to the complexity. Despite difficulties caused by complicated thymidine metabolism, TK1 activity significantly increases in cancer, which is critical for the success of an imaging probe.

Several different thymidine analog compounds have been developed. The first radiotracer evaluated in vivo for the imaging of cellular proliferation was carbon-11 thymidine. The short half-life of the C-11 label and rapid catabolism, resulting in labeled metabolites, limited utility. Different F-18–labeled thymidine analogs have been investigated. Currently, the most widely used and promising proliferation agent is F-18 fluorothymidine (FLT). Once phosphorylated by TK1, F-18 FLT is essentially trapped within the cell. Unlike thymidine, hydrogen-3 thymidine, or C-11 thymidine, F-18 FLT is not further metabolized and is not incorporated into DNA.

The normal distribution of FLT differs from that of F-18 FDG. Activity is lower in the mediastinum and bowel and very low in the brain. Marked marrow uptake and significant background liver activity are seen (Fig. 2-2, *A*). Obviously, the areas with high background activity create challenges for the visualization of metastases, particularly in the bones (Fig. 2-2, *B*). In addition, F-18 FLT does not accumulate to any significant extent when the blood–brain barrier is intact, so sensitivity is poor for low-grade tumors

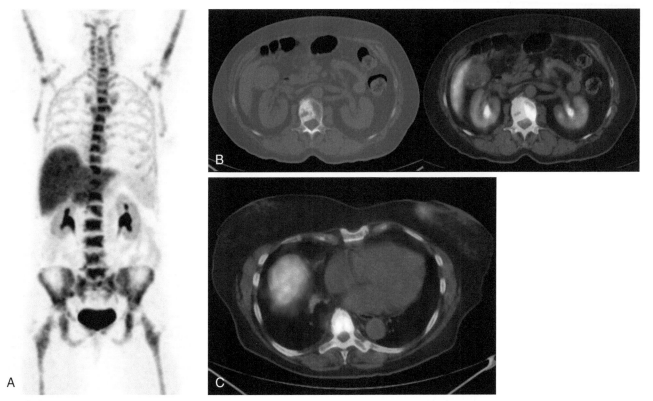

FIGURE 2-2. F-18 fluorothymidine (F-18 FLT) in newly diagnosed breast carcinoma. **A,** Maximum intensity projection image shows expected intense uptake in the bones, moderate activity in the liver, and very low uptake in the brain. **B,** Axial PET and CT images in the same patient show a lack of radiotracer activity in a sclerotic osseous metastasis. **C,** Radiotracer activity was present in the primary tumor in the left medial breast.

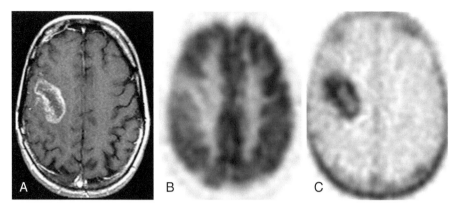

Figure 2-3. F-18 fluorothymidine in glioma. **A,** T1-weighted, gadolinium-enhanced MRI of the brain shows a large, enhancing tumor in the right frontoparietal cortex. **B,** F-18 FDG PET image at the same level is deceptive, showing little activity. **C,** However, significant accumulation of F-18 FLT more accurately represents tumor activity. (Courtesy Mark Muzi.)

and those that do not show significant contrast enhancement on MRI or CT. It has been determined by examining parameters such as Ki-67 in many tumors, including breast cancer, non–small cell lung cancer, and high-grade brain tumors (Fig. 2-3), that F-18 FLT uptake does in fact correlate with DNA synthesis (Fig 2-2, *C*). Promising early studies suggest FLT will be useful in monitoring chemotherapy response in breast cancer and possibly other tumors.

Considered an investigational drug by the U.S. Food and Drug Administration (FDA), examinations are not reimbursable under private or government insurance plans and use of FLT requires an investigational new drug (IND) application be in place. To promote development of FLT as a potential clinical tool, the National Cancer Institute (NCI) of the National Institutes of Health (NIH) developed an IND application for F-18 FLT. Multicenter trials using FLT are under way through the American College of Radiology Imaging Network (ACRIN). FLT can now be purchased through commercial vendors.

Biosynthesis

Amino Acid Transport and Metabolism and Peptide Synthesis

In addition to cellular proliferation, other parameters may better reflect tumor growth in some cases than F-18 FDG. Using amino acids as radiolabeled probes allows assessment of amino acid transport and metabolism and peptide biosynthesis. Many studies have been published examining the utility of radiolabeled amino acids in evaluation of brain tumors, an area of limitation for F-18 FDG. Some agents, such as C-11 methionine and F-18 fluoroethyltyrosine (F-18 FET), have shown increased sensitivity for gliomas over FLT. This is particularly true in the case of low-grade gliomas and tumors failing to exhibit MR enhancement. However, C-11 methionine has been seen to accumulate in cases of infection, particularly when severe, limiting specificity. C-11 methionine has also been used to examine prostate cancer with some success. F-18 DOPA not only has significantly higher sensitivities and specificities for various brain tumors than F-18 FDG but is also superior for detection of neuroendocrine cancers.

Lipid Metabolism and Phospholipid Synthesis

In addition to increased glycolytic activity, tumors can show increased fatty acid metabolism and lipid biosynthesis

during the production of membranes. These dividing cells show an increased expression of fatty acid synthase (FAS) and choline kinase in two related paths for phospholipid production. Several trials have been done with radiolabeled C-11 acetate, C-11 choline, and more recently F-18 choline in prostate cancer. This is an area of particular interest given the limitations of F-18 FDG in this disease. These agents show uptake in primary prostate cancer with good discrimination from the bladder because there is no urinary excretion, and they have been used with some success to assess metastasis. Choline uptake does not appear to correlate with tumor grade, and false positive findings could result from accumulation in benign conditions of the prostate. Uses for these agents in other cancers continue to be investigated.

Hypoxia

Tumor hypoxia is an important prognostic factor in a wide range of tumors; its presence predicts recurrence, metastasis, and decreased survival. Tumor hypoxia is an established resistance factor for radiotherapy and is increasingly recognized as promoting resistance to systemic cancer therapies. Hypoxia promotes a more aggressive and resistant cancer phenotype, mediated by the transcription factor hypoxia-inducible factor 1 (HIF-1), which leads to cell cycle arrest, angiogenesis, and accelerated glycolysis. Noninvasive imaging studies have been examining tumor hypoxia for years; currently, two promising PET agents are undergoing multicenter clinical trials in the United States—F-18 fluoromisonidazole (FMISO) and copper-64 diacetyl-bis(N4-methylthiosemicarbazone) or Cu-64 ATSM.

Florine-18 Fluoromisonidazole

The nitroimidazoles are a class of hypoxia compounds that have been studied for years. In the viable cell, they are reduced to the RNO_2 radical without regard to oxygen concentrations. However, when oxygen is present, the radical is reoxidized and uncharged misonidazole diffuses out of the cell. In situations in which oxygen levels are low, the radical is further reduced and is trapped after binding to intracellular molecules.

F-18 fluoromisonidazole (FMISO) is the most extensively studied nitroimidazole for in vivo imaging. It readily diffuses into cells because of its lipophilic nature. Tissue nitroreductases lead to the generation of radical anions, which are quickly eliminated in the presence of

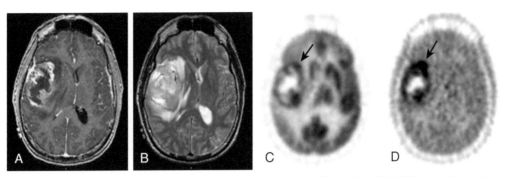

FIGURE 2-4. F-18 fluoromisonidazole (FMISO) tumor hypoxia. T1-weighted, gadolinium (**A**) and flare (**B**) MRI images of the brain reveal an aggressive-appearing enhancing tumor with mass effect and edema in the right cortex. **C,** F-18 FDG PET does show a peripheral ring of increased metabolic activity peripherally *(arrow).* **D,** F-18 FMISO images of the same area show significant hypoxic areas in the tumor *(arrow),* some more prominent than on F-18 FDG. Hypoxic areas are likely to be more resistant to chemotherapy and radiation.

oxygen; however, in the absence of oxygen, these radicals bind to tissue macromolecules and are retained. Thus, after equilibration, typically around 2 hours after injection, the accumulation of F-18 FMISO indicates tissue sites lacking oxygen. F-18 FMISO has been evaluated in several tumors, including head and neck cancer and glioblastoma (Fig. 2-4), and, like F-18 FLT, is the subject of an NCI IND to promote research investigations.

Copper-64 ATSM
The other major class of hypoxia imaging agent is based on metal chelates of dithiocarbazones. Copper(II)-diacetyl-bis(N4-methylthiosemicarbazone) (Cu-ATSM) can be radiolabeled with copper-60 ($T_{1/2}$ = 23.7 minutes), copper-62 ($T_{1/2}$ = 9.74 minutes), or Cu-64 ($T_{1/2}$ = 12.7 hours). The half-life of Cu-64 ATSM is better for clinical use and commercial distribution. Like F-18 FMISO, Cu-64 ATSM is reduced after entering the cell. The resulting unstable compound is reoxidized in the presence of oxygen and freely diffuses from the cell. In hypoxic tissues, the copper dissociates from the chelate and becomes irreversibly trapped.

Hypoxia Imaging Applications
Studies using the hypoxia agents include Cu-64 ATSM in cervical cancer and F-18 FMISO in head and neck cancer, non–small cell lung cancer, and gliomas. In glioblastoma, hypoxia is of particular interest given the necrotic nature of the tumor and a typical hypercellular rim that has been shown to be hypoxic. Aggressiveness of gliomas has been related to the presence of hypoxia. Although it is unclear whether F-18 FMISO will be able to predict outcomes, limited studies suggest it may guide therapy in different ways. For example, the antineoplastic therapeutic agent tirapazamine is activated by reductases to form free radicals in hypoxic cells, inducing DNA damage and sensitizing tumors to other therapy. Given the side effects of this agent, identifying appropriate candidates is essential. Hypoxia imaging has also been used in some trials examining ways to improve external beam radiation planning.

Angiogenesis
Vascular endothelial growth factor (VEGF) is overexpressed in many cancer cells, reflecting the ability of tumors to induce neovascularity. Treatment with bevacizumab

(rhuMAb VEGF, Avastin), the first FDA-approved antiangiogenesis drug, has shown success at treating non–small cell lung cancer, metastatic colorectal cancer, and breast cancer when combined with conventional chemotherapy drugs.

Noninvasive monitoring of angiogenesis is still in the early stages of development. Several radiolabeled forms of the VEGF molecule, including the SPECT agent iodine-123 VEGF and PET agents with such as zirconium-89 VEGF or the Cu-64 labeled epidermal growth factor agent, Cu-64 DOTA-EGF, have been used to monitor therapy in preclinical and limited clinical trials.

Imaging new vessel formation extends beyond VEGF. Although hypoxia induces expression of VEGF, regulation is a multistep process and occurs through a variety of factors. One of these is $\alpha_v\beta_3$ integrin, which mediates activated endothelial cell migration of during vessel formation and is a specific marker for neovessels. Therefore monitoring $\alpha_v\beta_{33}$ expression through the use of nuclear techniques has gained interest.

Several proteins, such a fibrinogen, interact with $\alpha_v\beta_3$ integrin through the amino sequence arginine-glycine-aspartic acid (RGD). Strategies to radiolabel RDG and to develop improved imaging agents have been under way for several years. Glycosylation of the RGD has been one approach to show benefit. A product of this work, F-18 galacto-RGD shows improved retention in tumors and overall kinetics. Other PET, SPECT, and therapy agents also have been formed using the RGD molecule.

Receptor Expression

Somatostatin Receptors
Somatostatin receptors (SSTRs) are found in a variety of tissues, including the gastrointestinal tract and brain. SSTRs are also expressed in numerous tumors, such as neuroendocrine tumors (carcinoid, insulinoma, pheochromocytoma, etc.), lung cancer, meningioma, and lymphoma. Most of the work to date involves targeting one of the most commonly expressed of the six known receptor subtypes—type 2. In addition to clinical imaging with indium-111 pentetreotide (Octreoscan), an 8-amino-acid somatostatin analog, improved accuracy has been shown with several PET-labeled peptides including: Ga-68 DOTA-Tyr³ octreotide (Ga-68 DOTA-TOC), Ga-68 DOTA-Tyr³

octreotate, and Ga-68 DOTA-1-NaI^3 octeotide (Ga-68 DOTA-NOC). These agents all bind to SSTR receptor 2, but Ga-68 DOTA-NOC also has affinity for subtypes 3 and 5 and Ga-68 DOTA-TOC also binds to subtype 5.

Great interest has been shown in therapeutic aspects of somatostatin receptor binding. In addition to trials using In-111 pentetreotide, good response has been shown with beta-emitters, including yttrium-90 and lutetieum-177. Trials with these agents are more prevalent in Europe, where the regulatory environment can be more conducive to early clinical trials.

Hormone Receptors

Given the fact that hormonal therapy plays an important role in treatment of breast and prostate cancer, it is no surprise that targeting these receptors with radiolabeled probes has become of interest. Although receptor status is easily determined by tissue biopsy, it is more difficult to assess the status of metastases. This is of particular importance because receptor-positive primary tumors may show variable expression after metastasizing or recurring.

F-18 16β-fluoro-5α-dihydrotestosterone (F-18 FDHT) has been used to detect androgen receptors in primary prostate cancer tumors and metastatic disease in early clinical trials. More work has been done in breast cancer receptor targeting. F-18 16α-17β-fluoroestradiol (F-18 FES) has shown the greatest promise for estrogen receptor labeling. F-18 FES uptake has been correlated with patient prognosis and response to aromatase inhibitors. For HER2 (ErB2) receptor assessment, antibody-based probes using both SPECT and PET radiolabels have shown the greatest utility thus far. Several different agents, including In-111 trastuzumab, Zr-89 trastuzumab, and a Ga-68 labeled F(ab')$_2$ fragment, are under investigation.

Apoptosis

Apoptosis, or programmed cell death, is the primary method by which old or unneeded cells are removed from the body and is believed to be a major mechanism by which anticancer treatments work. It is a very different process from necrotic cell death associated with tumors, trauma, or infection. Apoptosis depends on signals, such as extrinsic tumor necrosis factor, to initiate a cascade response related to a series of caspases. Apoptotic cells will express surface phosphatidylserine, which can serve as a target for imaging probes. The first imaging probe for apoptosis involved Tc-99m labeling of the peptide annexin V. Additional probes have been investigated, and nonnuclear techniques such as MRS examining factors such as changes in choline have been explored. Because chemotherapy agents often induce tumor cell death through apoptosis, imaging could identify areas at risk for therapy resistance. Additionally, apoptosis plays an important role in cardiovascular disease. However, imaging remains a preclinical investigational tool at this time.

Future Applications: Nanotechnology

Nanoparticles are a rapidly developing and exciting area of investigation. These tiny organic and inorganic particles, ranging in size from 1 to 100 nm, are another area blurring the boundaries between imaging and therapy. Numerous different nanoparticles have been used in imaging and therapeutic applications. They can be used as imaging contrast agents and also can deliver therapy, with many being responsive to conditions associated with tumor expression or even factors such as pH. Rare earth–labeled nanoparticles can be used for optical imaging and MRI, and PET imaging is possible using radiolabels such as F-18 and Cu-64.

▄ REPORTER GENE IMAGING AND GENE THERAPY

Recombinant DNA technology has resulted in the ability to insert genes into DNA to study basic biology and as an approach for gene-based therapy. Often, it is not possible to directly image a target of interest such as levels of expression of a therapeutic gene. The idea of using reporter genes—that is, diagnostic genes linked to another gene of interest designed to indicate when a particular transgene is expressed—was developed for basic cellular and molecular research using approaches such as GFP. The idea has been translated to imaging using optical reporters and reporters designed for use with radionuclide labels, such as the viral thymidine kinase gene from the herpes simplex virus type 1 *(HSVtk1)*. This technique can be used to monitor gene therapy in humans with a reporter gene linked to genes intended for gene therapy that could noninvasively report on the success of transfection of the therapeutic gene in target tissues.

Strategy

Many different viral vectors have been used to transfer genetic material into a host cell, although the most common is the herpes simplex virus type I (HSV1). Several HSV1 characteristics make it a useful vector. It is highly infectious, with a broad range of targets on the host cell. It also possesses many nonessential genes, which can be deleted without compromising its ability to infect and replicate, making room for genes of interest. Researchers can construct a plasmid and use viral vector transport to insert a reporter gene into the system being observed. Imaging can be done with a targeted reporter probe that is trapped within a cell carrying one of these reporter genes. For example, in preclinical work, the gene for luciferase can be inserted into cells and then optical imaging can monitor expression in transfected cells. Two main categories of reporter gene strategies exist—those using receptors and those using enzymes.

It is possible to insert reporter genes to produce receptors, and the degree of receptor expression can be imaged, reflecting the cellular activity. Although challenges exist, such as developing probes with sufficient binding affinity, these receptors make excellent imaging targets, easily accessible on the cell surface. Several well-characterized reporter systems are being used in clinical trials including D$_2$ dopaminergic and somatostatin receptors.

Enzyme-based reporter systems are more commonly used than receptor systems, providing the advantage of signal amplification. Rather than the one-to-one relationship seen in receptor imaging, one enzyme molecule can act on numerous substrate molecules. The enzyme most widely used in reporter gene imaging is based on HSV1-tk. Once a cell is transfected, expression of HSV1-tk results in an enzyme with several potential substrates, including ganciclovir, 5-iododeoxyuridine, and 1-(2'-deoxy-2'fluoro-1-β-D-arabinofuranosyl-5-iodouracil (FIAU). These can be radiolabeled with agents ranging from iodine (iodine-124 FIAU, I-123 FIAU) to F-18 (F-18 fluoroganciclovir).

Monitoring Gene Therapy

One exciting area of research concerns the possibility to use recombinant gene technology as a mechanism for therapy. These therapies could provide novel solutions for treating disease such as cancer. However, to be able to develop such protocols, accurate monitoring methods are needed. By linking a therapeutic gene with an imaging reporter gene, this would be possible in vivo using noninvasive means with PET or SPECT.

In treatment, for example, a cell transfected with HSV1-tk could be killed by administering a prodrug substrate, such as ganciclovir, which would form a toxic compound inside the cell when acted on by HSV1-tk. Alternatively, cells could be transfected with the gene for a receptor, such as the somatostatin receptor, along with a therapeutic gene. The distribution of the gene could be assessed with In-111 octreotide or Ga-68 DOTA-TOC and activity followed over time to assess therapy effect.

▬ IMAGING BIOMARKERS AND NEW DRUG DEVELOPMENT

Until recently, methods used to identify a target for a cancer therapy agent or to monitor its effects have relied on assays using tissue or blood samples. A noninvasive, imaging-based assay offers several potential benefits. This includes the quantitation possible with PET without perturbing the system being analyzed as with biopsy so that accurate serial measurements are possible. In addition, imaging biomarkers are an important component in the move toward "personalized" cancer therapy.

To determine if a therapy will be successful, MI targets can be identified that will predict whether a patient will respond. One example of this would be identifying HER2 overexpression in a patient with breast cancer to decide if therapies such as trastuzumab directed against HER2 will be effective. In addition to the uses of MI in determining potential therapy targets, it also can help assess drug pharmacodynamics and the response, if any, to a certain drug. This knowledge can help prevent unnecessary treatments and undesirable delays in starting appropriate therapies.

As potential new drugs move through the development process into clinical trials, many factors need to be considered (Fig. 2-5). In phase I and II (early phase) trials, small numbers of patients are evaluated at a limited number of sites to confirm the effects of the drug and that appropriate patients are selected for the therapy. These trials often involve evaluating complex kinetics of the drug. MI techniques using short-lived labels such as C-11 are useful for rapid, serial studies needed to assess kinetics and drug transport. These early-phase trials also look at the effects of a drug on the tumor and on normal tissue to assess safety. Finally, it is critical to determine if the drug will affect the biodistribution or clearance of the imaging probe being used, because this could alter measurements.

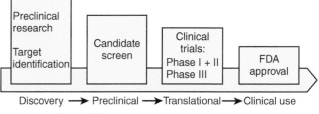

FIGURE 2-5. Stages of new drug development.

In phase II and III (late phase) trials, imaging biomarkers can be helpful indicators of early response or might even act as surrogate end points. In many cases, tumors will show a response rapidly with an MI agent, even when the tumor mass appears unchanged on conventional imaging, such as CT. These larger trials require tightly controlled protocols at multiple centers, so the imaging markers used must be more widely available. PET agents labeled with F-18, Cu-64, or I-124 have sufficiently long half-lives to can be easily shipped from regional cyclotron and production centers.

The increasing expense of taking a new agent through the FDA approval process into clinical use demands careful selection and monitoring protocols. From preliminary target identification, discovering sensitive populations, and monitoring therapeutic effects in clinical trials, noninvasive imaging techniques are playing an increasingly important role in this process.

▬ SUGGESTED READING

Blankenberg FG, Norfray JF. Multimodality molecular imaging of apoptosis in oncology. *AJR Am J Roentgenol.* 2011;197(2):308-317.

Contag CH. In vivo pathology: seeing with molecular specificity and cellular resolution in the living body. *Ann Rev Pathol Mech Dis.* 2007;2:277-305.

Dunphy MP, Lewis JS. Radiopharmaceuticals in preclinical and clinical development for monitoring therapy with PET. *J Nucl Med.* 2009;50(suppl 1): 106S-121S.

Ferrara K, Pollard R, Borden M. Ultrasound microbubble contrast agents: fundamentals and application to gene and drug delivery. *Annu Rev Biomed Eng.* 2007;9:415-447.

Hylton N. Dynamic contrast-enhanced magnetic resonance imaging as an imaging biomarker. *J Clin Oncol.* 2006;24(10):3293-3298.

Kang JH, Chung JK. Molecular-genetic imaging based on reporter gene expression. *J Nucl Med.* 2008;49(suppl 2):164S-179S.

Ledezma CJ, Chen W, Sai V, et al. ¹⁸F-FDOPA PET/MRI fusion in patients with primary/recurrent brain gliomas: initial experience. *Eur J Radiol.* 2009;71(2):242-248.

Mankoff DA, Link JM, Linden HM, Sundararajn L, Krohn KA. Tumor receptor imaging. *J Nucl Med.* 2008;49(suppl 2):149S-163S.

Nishino M, Jagannathan JP, Ramaiya NH, Van den Abbeele AD. Revised RECIST guideline version 1.1: what oncologists want to know and what radiologists need to know. *AJR Am J Roentgenol.* 2010;195(2):281-289.

Plathow C, Weber WA. Tumor cell metabolism imaging. *J Nucl Med.* 2008;49(suppl 2):43S-63S.

Rohren EM, Macapinlac HA. PET imaging of prostate cancer: other tracers. *PET Clin.* 2009;4:185-192.

Salsov A, Tammisetti VS, Grierson J, Vesselle H, FLT. Measuring tumor cell proliferation in vivo with positron emission tomography and 3'-deoxy-3'[¹⁸F] fluorothymidine. *Semin Nucl Med.* 2007;37(6):429-439.

Tromberg BJ, Cerussi A, Shah N, et al. Imaging in breast cancer: diffuse optics in breast cancer: detecting tumors in premenopausal women and monitoring neoadjuvant chemotherapy. *Breast Cancer Res.* 2005;7(6):279-285.

Vallabhajosula S, Solnes L, Vallabhajosula B. A broad overview of positron emission tomography radiopharmaceutical and clinical applications: what is new? *Semin Nucl Med.* 2011;41(4):246-264.

Virgolini I, Ambrosini V, Bomanji JB, et al. Procedure guidelines for PET/CT imaging with 68Ga-DOTA-conjugated peptides: 68Ga-DOTA-TOC, 68Ga-DOTA-NOC, 68Ga-DOTA-TATE. *Eur J Nucl Med Mol Imaging.* 2010;37(10):2004-2010.

Wahl RL, Jacene H, Kasamon Y, Lodge MA. From RECIST to PERCIST: evolving considerations for PET response criteria in solid tumors. *J Nucl Med.* 2009;50(suppl 1):122S-150S.

CHAPTER 3

Physics of Nuclear Medicine

Nuclear medicine involves the administration of radiopharmaceuticals to patients for diagnostic and therapeutic purposes. For diagnostic imaging, radiation emitted from these radiopharmaceuticals must be detected by external detectors to determine its in vivo distribution. For therapeutic nuclear medicine, some of the emitted radiation must be absorbed by targeted tissues to achieve the desired effect. In both cases, an understanding of the nature of the radioactivity, the amount administered, the radiation emissions, and how it interacts with matter is essential. The essential aspects of the basic physics of nuclear medicine will be discussed in this chapter.

■ ATOMIC STRUCTURE OF MATTER

Structure of the Atomic Nucleus

All matter consists of atoms that contain a nucleus and orbiting electrons (Fig. 3-1). The nucleus consists of two kinds of atomic particles called *protons* and *neutrons*, collectively known as *nucleons*. The protons have a mass of 1.67×10^{-27} kg and a positive electronic charge of 1.6×10^{-19} coulombs (C). The neutrons have a mass similar to that of the protons and are electrically neutral. Electrons are substantially less massive than either the proton or the neutron (Table 3-1), with an electric charge similar to the proton; however, the charge is negative rather than positive. All of the electric charge within the nucleus is positive, which provides a repulsive force pushing the nucleus apart. Each nucleon provides a nuclear attractive force that acts to pull the nucleus together.

Atoms of a particular element are characterized by a certain number of protons in the nucleus. Thus all carbon atoms have 6 protons, all oxygen atoms have 8 protons, and all iodine atoms have 53 protons. The number of nuclear protons is referred to as the *atomic number, Z*. Atoms of a particular element may have a varying number of neutrons. For example, some atoms of oxygen may have 8 neutrons and others may have 7 or 10 neutrons in addition to their 8 protons. The number of neutrons in the nucleus is referred to as the *neutron number, N*, and the total number of nucleons is referred to as the *atomic mass, A*. Thus A is the sum of Z and N. In the oxygen example, A would be 15, 16, and 18 for atoms that have 7, 8, or 10 neutrons, respectively, in addition to their 8 protons. One of Albert Einstein's essential observations was the equivalence of mass and energy as described by his famous $E = mc^2$ equation. If the mass of the nucleus is considered in kilograms, it is less than the sum of the nucleons it comprises. This difference in mass is manifest in the nuclear binding energy that holds the nucleus together.

A nuclear entity defined by a particular number of protons and neutrons (Z and N number) is referred to as a *nuclide*. Alternatively, the Z and the A numbers also define the nuclide because the N number can be inferred by taking the difference of A and Z (N = A – Z). A nuclide can be represented by the elemental name or symbol (e.g., iodine or I) and the A number augmented by the Z and N numbers. For example, consider a particular nuclide of iodine with 53 protons (Z = 53) and 78 neutrons (N = 78), for a total of 131 nucleons (A = Z + N = 131). This nuclide, iodine-131, is given the symbols ^{131}I or $^{131}_{53}$I$_{78}$.

The element iodine has a Z number of 53, and the N number can be inferred from the difference of A and Z; thus it is sufficient to use the I-131 or ^{131}I designations. Nuclides of the same element (or similar Z numbers) are isotopes—for example, I-131, I-123, and I-125. This can be remembered because *isotope* has the letter *p* in it; isotopes have similar numbers of protons (or Z). Nuclides with a similar N number are isotones, which can be remembered because *isotone* has the letter *n* in it. Examples of isotones are ^{131}I^{78} and ^{130}Xe^{78}. Nuclides with a similar A number are isobars. This can be recalled because *isobar* has the letter *a* in it. Examples of isobars are I-131 and Xenon-131. Finally, the nuclei of atoms can configure themselves into different energy levels in a manner analogous to that of the electronic energy levels. Nuclides with similar Z and N numbers, and thus similar A numbers, but different energy levels, are isomers, which can be remembered because the word *isomer* has the letter *e* in it. For example, technetium-99 and its metastable state, Tc-99m, are isomers.

Electronic Structure of the Nucleus

In addition to the nucleus, the atom also contains orbiting electrons (Fig. 3-2). In the case of an electrically neutral atom, the number of orbiting electrons is equal to the number of nuclear protons. If this is not the case, the atom will be ionized and will exhibit a net electric charge. The orbital electrons (Table 3-2) arrange themselves into particular discrete orbital shells. The innermost shell is referred to as the *K shell*, and subsequent shells are referred to as *L, M, N*, and so on. The K shell contains 2 electrons and the L shell 8, and varying numbers occur thereafter. The binding energy is higher for the inner shells; and the binding energy of a particular shell also depends on the Z number of atom and thus is characteristic of a particular element.

■ ELECTROMAGNETIC RADIATION

The electromagnetic spectrum represents a wide range of radiative energy. The way these radiations act depends on the particular situation—in some cases like waves and in other cases like particles referred to as *photons*. This duality of the nature of electromagnetic radiation was one of the fundamental observations of modern physics at the

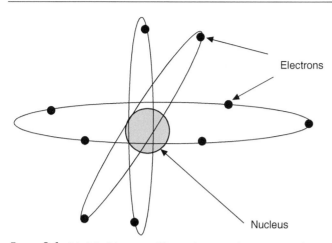

FIGURE 3-1. Model of the atom. The nucleus contains protons and neutrons and has a radius of 10^{-14} m. The protons in the nucleus carry a positive charge. The orbital electrons carry a negative charge.

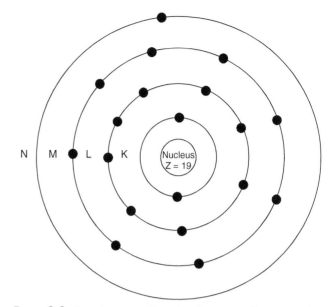

FIGURE 3-2. Potassium atom. Potassium has an atomic number of 19, with 19 protons in the nucleus and 19 orbital electrons.

TABLE 3-1 Summary of Physical Constants

Speed of light in a vacuum (c)	3.0×10^8 m/sec
Elementary charge (e) 1.602×10^{-19} coulomb	4.803×10^{-10} esu
Rest mass of electron	9.11×10^{-28} g
Rest mass of proton	1.67×10^{-24} g
Planck's constant (h)	6.63×10^{-27} erg sec
Avogadro's number	$6.02 \times 10^{23} \dfrac{\text{Molecules}}{\text{Gram mole}}$
1 electron volt (eV)	1.602×10^{-12} erg
1 calorie (cal)	4.18×10^7 erg
1 angstrom (Å)	10^{-10} m
Euler number (e) (base of natural logarithms)	2.718
Atomic mass unit (U)	1.66×10^{-24} g (½ the mass of a carbon-12 atom)

TABLE 3-2 Terms Used to Describe Electrons

Term	Comment
Electron	Basic elementary particle
Orbital electron	Electron in one of the shells or orbits in an atom
Valence electron	Electron in the outermost shell of an atom; responsible for chemical characteristics and reactivity
Auger electron	Electron ejected from an atomic orbit by energy released during an electron transition
Photoelectron	Electron ejected from an atomic orbit as a consequence of an interaction with a photon (photoelectric interaction) and complete absorption of the photon's energy
Conversion electron	Electron ejected from an atomic orbit because of internal conversion phenomenon as energy is given off by an unstable nucleus

turn of the twentieth century. The relationship of the photon energy to the frequency of the electromagnetic wave is given by $E = h\nu$, where E is energy, ν is frequency and h is the Plank constant.

The electromagnetic spectrum includes a variety of entities, including radio waves, microwaves, visible light, infrared and ultraviolet radiation, x-rays, and gamma rays (Fig. 3-3). The differences in these types of radiation are their photon energy and frequencies. For example, x-ray and gamma ray photons have substantially higher energy and frequency than radio, microwave, and visible radiation. The difference among colors of visible light is photon energy, with blue light having higher energy than red light. The unit of energy typically used in atomic and nuclear physics is the electron volt (eV), which is the amount of energy an electron garners when crossing an electronic potential difference of 1 volt. One eV is equivalent to 1.6×10^{-19} joules. Visible light has energy slightly less than 1 eV. X-rays and gamma rays are in the energy range from

several thousand eV (or keV) to tens of millions eV (or megaelectron volts [MeV]). It is interesting to note that the resulting frequencies for x-rays and gamma rays (between 10^{-15} to 10^{-10} m) is on the same order as the nucleus and the atom, respectively, and thus it would reasonable that these entities would interact on the nuclear and atomic levels.

The energy range of x-rays and gamma rays overlap substantially. What is the difference between these entities, if not energy? In truth, it is not energy that separates these, but how they are produced. High-energy photons generated by transitions in the orbits of atomic electrons or by the deacceleration of charged particles are referred to as *x-rays*, and photons generated by nuclear transitions are referred to as *gamma rays*. Once produced, nothing distinguishes between an x-ray and a gamma ray. A 100-keV x-ray is absolutely identical and

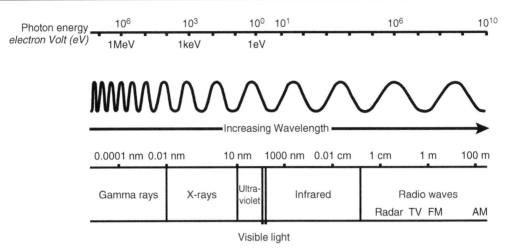

Figure 3-3. Electromagnetic energy spectrum. Photon energies (eV) and wavelengths of x-rays and gamma ultraviolet, visible light, infrared, and radio waves.

indistinguishable from a 100-keV gamma ray. Thus it is important to consider the differences when evaluating the production of these photons and their characterization and magnitude of intensity. However, they may be simply considered high-energy photons of certain energies when considering how x-rays and gamma rays interact in matter, how they are detected, and what effects they may have on biological tissues.

Production of X-Rays

X-rays are produced in two ways: (1) as a result of the transition of atomic electrons from one orbit to another and (2) as a result of the deacceleration of charged particles, typically electrons, and usually as a result of columbic interactions with collections of other charged particles. In the first instance, electrons may move from one atomic orbit to another—for example, from the L or M shell to the K shell. The binding energy of the inner shell—in this case the K shell—is higher than that of the outer shells, and thus when an electron moves from an outer shell to an inner shell, the difference in energy is manifest with the emission of energy, in the context of fluorescent x-rays or the ejection of other outer electrons, referred to as *Auger* electrons. In the case of fluorescent x-rays, the x-ray energy will be given by the difference in binding energies of the 2 shells involved. Consider the case of fluorescent x-rays from electronic transitions within an iodine atom. The binding energies of the K, L, and M shells are 35, 5, and 1 keV, respectively. Thus the energy of the fluorescent x-rays resulting from the transition of electrons from the L to K shell (referred to as K_α *fluorescent x-rays*) is 30 keV (= 35 – 5 keV) and that from the transition from M to K shell (referred to as K_β *x-rays*) is 34 keV (= 35 – 1 keV). In addition to K x-rays, L, M, and other x-rays can be produced, but these will be of lower energies given the reduced binding energies of these outer shells.

An alternative to the emission of fluorescent x-rays is the emission of Auger electrons from the outer shells. The kinetic energy of the resultant Auger electrons is the difference in the binding energies of the electron shells of the transition of the initial electron reduced by the binding energy of the emitted Auger electron.

$$KE_{Auger} = BE_{Inner} - BE_{Outer} - BE_{Auger}$$

where *KE* is the Auger electron kinetic energy and *BE* is the binding energy of the orbiting electrons. The probability that a fluorescent x-ray rather than an Auger electron will be emitted is higher in cases in which the electrons are more tightly bound—that is, have higher binding energies. Thus transitions involving inner shells and in atoms with higher Z numbers are more likely to emit fluorescent x-rays than Auger electrons. Conversely, transitions involving outer shells are more likely to result in the emission of Auger electrons. Therefore a vacancy in an inner shell that may result initially in the emission of a fluorescent x-ray, leading to a vacancy in an outer shell, will also result in further emissions, which are likely to be Auger electrons as the transitions move toward the outer shells. In this case, for each vacancy in the K shell, 1 or 2 x-rays and several (perhaps as many as 8-10) Auger electrons will be emitted.

The second manner in which x-rays can be produced is with the deacceleration of charged particles. In nuclear medicine, the charged particles of most interest are electrons and beta particles. This is referred to as *bremsstrahlung* (braking) radiation—that is, the radiation emitted as the electron is slowing. This deacceleration is typically realized as the electron undergoes electronic or coulombic interactions with the positively charged nucleus as it passes through matter. The magnitude of the bremsstrahlung production increases linearly with the kinetic energy of the incident electron and the Z number of the target material on which the electron is impinging. Thus bremsstrahlung x-ray production is more likely to occur at higher energies and with high Z targets. As a result, radiographic systems generate x-rays by directing an energetic electron beam into a tungsten (Z = 74) target.

■ RADIOACTIVITY AND RADIOACTIVE DECAY

The nucleons in the atomic nucleus can arrange themselves in multiple configurations that have different energy

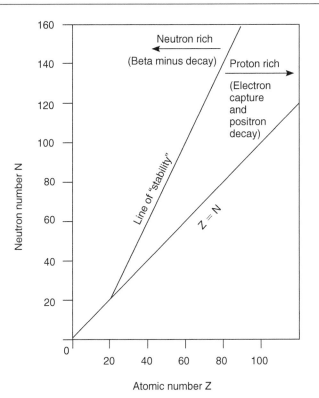

FIGURE 3-4. Graph of neutrons (N) versus protons (P) for various nuclides. For low atomic number elements, the two are roughly equal (Z = N). With increasing atomic number, the relative number of neutrons increases. Stable nuclear species tend to occur along the "line of stability."

levels. Many of these configurations are unstable, and the nucleus will tend to rearrange itself to establish a more stable configuration. This situation is referred to as *radioactivity,* and the process by which an unstable nucleus transforms itself into a nucleus at a lower energy is referred to as *radioactive decay.* Nuclides that are unstable and may tend to undergo radioactive decay are called *radioactive nuclides* or *radionuclides.* Those that are stable and will not undergo further decay are referred to as *stable nuclides.* The initial nuclide is referred to as the *parent* nuclide and the resultant nuclide as the *daughter* nuclide. Although the daughter nucleus that results from a radioactive decay has a lower energy than the parent nucleus, it may not be stable and thus subsequent radioactive decays may result.

Figure 3-4 shows a plot of the stable nuclides as a function of the Z number on the x-axis and the N number on the y axis. At low values of Z and N, these tend to be equal for stable nuclides such as carbon-12, nitrogen-14, and oxygen-16. However, as the nucleus becomes larger, the repulsive force of the nuclear protons continues to grow and more neutrons are necessary in the stable nucleus to provide additional attractive nuclear force. Other factors, beyond the scope of this book, also contribute to the stability and instability of the nucleus. For example, nuclides with even numbers of protons and neutrons tend to be more stable than those with odd Z and N configurations. These factors lead to variations with respect to stable nuclides for a particular Z and N value. The unstable nuclides fall to either the right or the left of the line of stability in Figure 3-4. The unstable nuclides to the right are considered proton rich, and those to the left are

neutron rich. In either case, these unstable radionuclides will tend to decay to entities that are closer to the curve of stability. Proton-rich radionuclides tend to decay in a manner that will reduce the Z number and increase the N number. Conversely, neutron-rich radionuclides will tend to decay in a way that increases the Z number and reduces the N number.

Modes of Radioactive Decay

The radioactive atom can decay in multiple ways, with the emission of energy in the form of electromagnetic radiation or the kinetic energy of an emitted charged particle. A variety of factors are involved, including whether the nucleus is proton rich or neutron rich. These modes of radioactivity will be reviewed, with particular emphasis on those most pertinent for nuclear medicine.

A common approach in representing radioactive decay is a figure referred to as the *decay scheme* (Figs. 3-5 through 3-9 and 3-11). Higher energy levels are toward the top of the figure, and higher Z numbers are to the right of the figure. The decay scheme illustrates the transition from the parent to the daughter nuclide. Transitions that lead to a reduction in energy are represented by an arrow pointing down. If it also results in a nuclide with either a decrease or increase in the Z number of the daughter compared to the parent, the arrow will point to the lower left or lower right of the figure, respectively.

In *alpha decay,* an unstable heavy atom may decay to a nuclide closer to the curve of stability by emitting an alpha particle consisting of 2 protons and 2 neutrons—that is, the alpha particle is essentially the same as an ionized helium atom. The daughter nucleus also may not be stable, and thus the emission of an alpha particle often will lead to the emission of a series of radiations until the resultant nucleus is stable. The decay scheme for the decay of radium-226 to radon-222 is shown in Figure 3-5. Alpha particles are densely ionizing and thus tend to deposit their energy over a very short distance, a small fraction of a millimeter. For this reason, alpha particles emitted from outside are unlikely to be able to enter the body and thus typically pose a limited health risk, whereas those that are internally deposited are not likely to exit the body and thus are not useful for imaging. However, if agents involving alpha emitters can be distributed to selected tumors, they have the potential to be very effective for therapeutic applications because the alpha particle can lead to substantial cell death.

Neutron-rich radionuclides decay in such a manner as to approach the line of stability (Fig. 3-4). In general, this leads to a transition that results in an increase in the Z number and a decrease in the N number. The emission of a negative *beta particle* leads to an isobaric transition—that is, no change in A, the atomic mass, which results in the reduction of N and an increase in Z by 1. This is referred to as *beta* or *beta-minus decay.* The negative beta particle is indistinguishable from an electron with the same mass and electric charge. The only difference between the two entities is that if it is emitted from the nucleus, it is a beta particle, and if it orbits around the nucleus, it is an electron. For example, I-131 decays through beta-minus decay (Fig. 3-6). In beta-minus decay, a second particle, called the *antineutrino,* is also emitted that shares the transition energy. The antineutrino is very difficult to measure because it has virtually no mass or charge associated with it, only energy. However, the result is that the beta particle is emitted with a continuous kinetic energy distribution. Sometimes the beta particle will be emitted with most of the transition energy, and in other cases most of the energy is emitted with the antineutrino. All possible sharing of energy between the two entities is also possible. The maximum kinetic energy of the beta particle (E_{max}) is defined by the difference in the energy levels of the parent and daughter nuclides (Fig. 3-6). The average beta particle kinetic energy is estimated as one third of E_{max} ($E\beta \approx E_{max}/3$). Radionuclides of interest in nuclear medicine that decay by beta-minus decay include phosphous-32, molybdenum-99, and I-131. These radionuclides are either derived from fission products of a nuclear reactor *(fission produced)* or generated using neutron activation from a nuclear reactor *(reactor produced)*.

Proton-rich radionuclides will transform such that the daughter nuclide will have a lower Z and a higher N number. Two decay modes can accomplish this—*beta plus decay* and *electron capture*. In beta plus decay, a positively charged beta particle, also referred to as a *positron*, is emitted from the parent nucleus. This is also referred to as *positron decay*. The resulting daughter nucleus has one fewer proton and one more neutron than the parent nucleus. The atomic mass, A, does not change; therefore this is an isobaric transition. The positron has the same mass as the beta-minus particle or the electron. Its charge is of the same magnitude as that of the electron, but it is positively rather than negatively charged. In fact, the positron is the *antiparticle* of the electron; if they are brought into close contact with each other, they will *annihilate*, transforming the mass of the 2 particles to energy in the form of two 511-keV photons. The 511-keV value derives from the energy equivalence of the electron mass using Einstein's equation ($E = mc^2$). This annihilation process is the basis of positron emission tomography, as will be discussed in a subsequent chapter.

In positron decay, a neutrino is emitted in addition to the positron and the kinetic energy is shared between the two particles in a manner similar to beta-minus decay. The neutrino also is very difficult to measure because it has minimal mass and no electric charge. Like the negative beta particle, the average kinetic positron energy is one

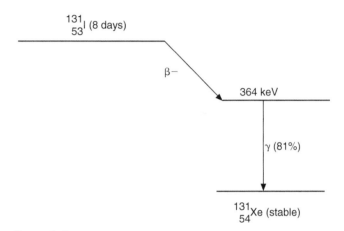

FIGURE 3-6. Decay scheme for iodine-131. Decay is by negatron emission. In negatron or beta-minus decay the atomic mass does not change (isobaric transition). The atomic number increases by 1. The daughter, Xe-131, has one more proton in the nucleus.

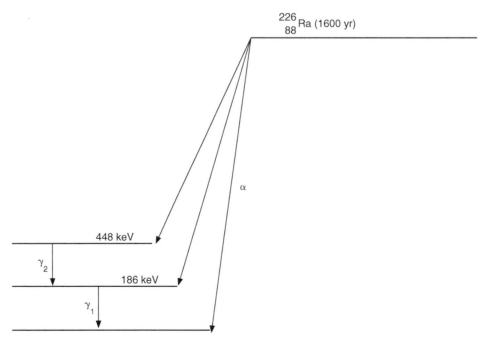

FIGURE 3-5. Decay scheme for radium-226. Decay is by alpha particle emission to the daughter product Rn-222. The emission of an alpha particle results in a decrease in atomic number of 2 and a decrease in atomic mass of 4.

third of E_{max}. For positron decay to occur, the transition energy must be in excess of 1022 keV (twice 511 keV). This energy threshold is to overcome the production of the positron as well as the additional orbital electron to maintain electric neutrality. Radionuclides of interest in nuclear medicine that undergo positron decay include fluorine-18 (Fig. 3-7), nitrogen-13, carbon-11, gallium-68, and rubidium-82. These radionuclides are typically produced using a cyclotron.

An alternative to beta plus decay for proton-rich radionuclides is electron capture. In this process, an inner-shell, orbital electron is absorbed into the nucleus, leading to the reduction of Z and increase of N by 1, similar to positron decay. However, no energy threshold exists for electron capture to occur; thus, in cases in which the transition energy is less than the 1022 keV threshold, electron capture is the only possible process, but when it is greater than 1022 keV, either positron decay or electron capture is possible. For F-18, positron decay occurs 97% of the time and electron capture occurs 3% of the time. The capture of an orbital electron leads to an inner-shell vacancy, which in turn leads to the emission of fluorescent x-rays and Auger electrons. Radionuclides of interest in nuclear medicine that decay through electron capture exclusively include thallium-201 (Fig. 3-8), gallium-67, and indium-111, which are produced in a cyclotron.

The radioactive daughter may still be in an excited state, and thus further radioactive decays may occur. These radioactive daughters may decay to yet another radionuclide, but in some cases, they decay from one energy level to another while remaining the same nuclide (same Z and N numbers). This is referred to as an *isomeric transition* because the nuclide decays from one isomer (energy level) to another. This transition may result in the emission of a gamma ray, the energy of which is determined by the difference in the initial and eventual energy levels. In some cases, this transition may alternatively result in the emission of an orbital electron in a process called *internal conversion*. The kinetic energy of these emitted *conversion electrons* is the difference in the two energy levels minus the electron's binding energy.

After the decay of I-131, its daughter, Xe-131, is in an excited state and almost immediately decays by isomeric transition with the emission of a 364-keV gamma ray (Fig. 3-6). In another example, Mo-99 decays to an excited state of Tc-99. If the daughter nucleus remains in this state for a considerable amount of time (>1 second), the state is said to be *metastable* (i.e., almost stable). The metastable state of Tc-99 has a 6-hour half-life and is referred to as *Tc-99m*. Tc-99m is the most commonly used radionuclide in nuclear medicine, in part because of its reasonable half-life, gamma ray energy (140 keV), and decay scheme (Fig. 3-9) and because it emits mostly gamma rays with a few conversion electrons but no beta or alpha particles.

Radioactive Decay

Consider a sample that contains a certain number (N) of radioactive atoms of a particular radionuclide. In time, these parent radioactive atoms will decay to atoms of the daughter nuclide. The atoms in the sample will not all decay at the same time. The period from some point in time until radioactive decay of a particular radionuclide is a random variable with a *mean time*, T_m, that is characteristic of that radionuclide. The reciprocal of T_m is referred to as the *decay constant*, λ, also characteristic of the particular radionuclide.

$$\lambda = 1 / T_m$$

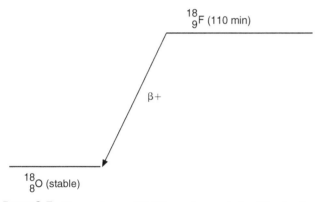

FIGURE 3-7. Decay scheme of F-18 by positron emission. The daughter product, O-18, has one fewer proton in the nucleus. Positron decay is another example of an isobaric transition without change in atomic mass between parent and daughter.

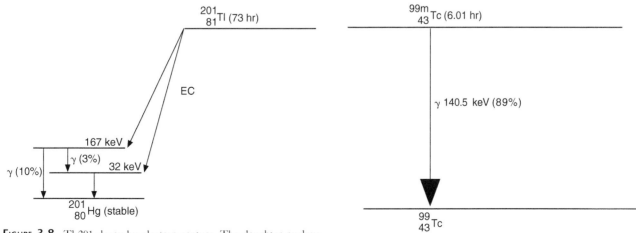

FIGURE 3-8. Tl-201 decay by electron capture. The daughter nucleus (Hg-201) has one fewer proton than the parent.

FIGURE 3-9. Isomeric transition of Tc-99m to Tc-99.

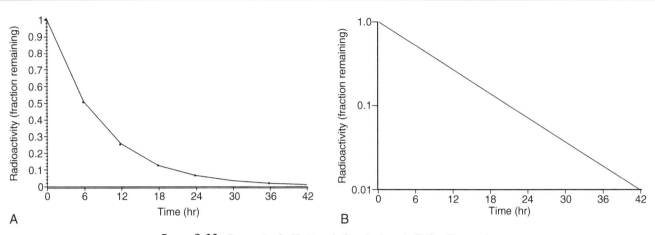

Figure 3-10. Decay plot for Tc-99m. **A**, Standard graph. **B**, Semilog graph.

The decay constant also can be described as the fraction of the radioactive atoms that decay per unit time over a very short duration (much less than T_m). Thus the number of atoms, dN, that decay in a small time interval, dt, is given by:

$$dN = -\lambda\, N\, dt$$

Integrating this equation over time leads to:

$$N = N_o\, e^{-\lambda t}$$

where N_o is the initial number of radioactive atoms and N is the number remaining after some time, t.

This equation describes exponential decay in which a certain fraction of the material is lost in a set period. This fraction is referred to as the *decay fraction*, DF.

$$DF = e^{-\lambda t}$$

Thus the number of radioactive atoms remaining, N, is also given by:

$$N = N_o \times DF$$

Also, the number of atoms that have decayed in time, t, is given by N_d.

$$N_d = N_o \times (1 - DF)$$

The time necessary for half of the material to decay can be defined as the *half-life*. The half-life is related to the mean life and the decay constant by the following equations:

$$T_{1/2} = \ln(2)\, T_m = 0.693\, T_m = 0.693/\lambda$$

Alternatively one can determine the decay constant from the half-life by:

$$\lambda = 0.693/T_{1/2}$$

One can also express the radioactive decay equation using the half-life:

$$N = N_o\, e^{-0.693\, t/T_{1/2}}$$

If a sample contains 10,000 radioactive atoms at a particular point in time, one half-life later, there will be 5000 atoms, another half-life later there will be 2500 atoms, and so on. This process of a certain fraction of the material decaying in a certain time is representative of exponential decay (Fig. 3-10). When graphed using a log scale on the y axis (semilog plot), the result is a straight line with the negative slope equal in magnitude to the decay constant (Fig. 3-10, *B*).

The quantity that specifies the amount of radioactivity, defined as the *activity*, is the number of nuclear transformations—decays or disintegrations—per unit time. The activity is characterized by the number of radioactive atoms in the sample, N, divided by the mean time to radioactive decay, T_m.

$$A = N/T_m$$

Activity is thus the product of the decay constant and the number of radioactive atoms.

$$A = \lambda\, N$$

Conversely, if the amount of activity of a particular radionuclide is known, the number of radioactive atoms can be calculated.

$$N = A/\lambda$$

Because the activity is directly related to the number of radioactive atoms, all of the equations for radioactive decay apply to activity, as well as the number.

$$A = A_o\, e^{-\lambda t}$$

and

$$A = A_o\, e^{-0.693 t/T_{1/2}}$$

The units associated with activity are the *becquerel* (1 Bq = 1 disintegration per second) and the *curie* (1 Ci = 3.7×10^{10} disintegrations per second) (Box 3-1).

$$1\ mCi = 37\ MBq \quad \text{and} \quad 1 MBq = 27\ \mu Ci$$

Box 3-1. Conversion of International System and Conventional Units of Radioactivity

CONVENTIONAL UNIT

1 curie (Ci) = 3.7×10^{10} disintegrations per second (dps)

SI UNIT

1 becquerel (Bq) = 1 dps

CURIES → BECQUERELS

1 Ci = 3.7×10^{10} dps = 37 GBq
1 mCi = 3.7×10^{7} dps = 37 MBq
1 μCi = 3.7×10^{4} dps = 37 KBq

BECQUERELS → CURIES

1 Bq = 1 dps = 2.7×10^{-11} Ci = 27 pCi
1 MBq = 10^{6} dps = 2.7×10^{-5} Ci = 0.027 mCi
1 GBq = 10^{9} dps = 27 mCi

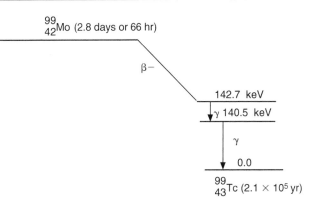

FIGURE 3-11. Decay scheme of Mo-99. Beta-minus emission to Tc-99m, followed by isomeric transition to Tc-99.

Example 1. The radiopharmacy is preparing a dose of a I-123–labeled agent (12-hour half-life) for the clinic. If 10 mCi is to be administered at 1 PM, how much activity should be placed in the syringe at 7 AM?

$$A = A_o\, e^{-0.693\, t/T_{1/2}}, \text{ thus } 10 = A_o\, e^{-0.693\, 6\,hr/12\,hr}$$
$$A_o = 10 / e^{-0.693\, 6\,hr/12\,hr} = 10 / 0.707 = 14.1 \text{ mCi}$$

Example 2. The staff at the nuclear medicine clinic is testing their equipment with a cobalt-57 source (270-day half-life) that was calibrated to contain 200 MBq on January 1 of this year. How much activity remains on September 1 (243 days)?

$$A = A_o\, e^{-0.693\, t/T_{1/2}}, \text{ thus } A = 200\, e^{-0.693\, 243\,days/270\,days}$$
$$= 200 \times 0.536 = 107 \text{ MBq}$$

In many instances, the radioactive daughter is in turn radioactive; however, it has a half-life different from that of the parent. In certain cases, when the half-life of the daughter is smaller than that of the parent, the amount of radioactivity of the two entities reaches *equilibrium*—that is, the ratio of the two activities becomes constant and this ratio depends on the relative values of the two half-lives. If the half-life of the daughter is very much shorter than that of the parent (e.g., by more than a factor of 100), the two entities can reach secular equilibrium—at which the activities of the two are equal. Essentially, as soon as the parent atom decays, the resultant daughter atom subsequently decays and thus two numbers of disintegrations are the same. Strontium-82 (25 days) that decays to Rb-82 (73 seconds) can reach secular equilibrium.

In another special case, if the half-life of the parent is somewhat longer than that of the daughter (e.g., by a factor of 10), then, after reaching equilibrium, the activity of the daughter is slightly greater than that of the parent, with the ratio determined by the ratio $T_p/(T_p - T_d)$, where T_p and T_d are the half-lives of the parent and daughter, respectively. This situation is referred to as *transient equilibrium*. The decay of Mo-99 (66-hour half-life) to Tc-99m (6-hour half-life) and eventually to Tc-99 can reach

transient equilibrium (Fig. 3-11). The time to reach equilibrium, if initially no activity of the daughter present, is about 4 half-lives. For Mo-99–Tc-99m–Tc-99, about 24 hours is required to reach equilibrium.

■ INTERACTIONS BETWEEN RADIATION AND MATTER

To understand detection, attenuation, and biological effects of radiation, it is important to understand how electromagnetic radiation and charged particles interact with matter. Radiation deposits energy in matter through a series of ionizations and excitations. Knowing how this occurs and under what conditions yields better comprehension of the best approaches for detecting and imaging radiation, how to compensate for attenuation and scatter, and how to estimate the radiation dose to the patient.

Gamma rays and x-rays are the radiations of specific interest in nuclear medicine. However, these entities are considered indirectly ionizing radiation in that they transfer their energy to charged particles, specifically electrons, which lead to most of the ionization and excitation within the matter of interest. Thus it is important also to understand the interaction of charged particles and matter.

Charged Particle Interactions with Matter

The interaction of charged particles, including electrons, primarily involves electric forces between the particles and the atoms constituting the material on which these particles impinge. These interactions may be with the nucleus, leading to the emission of electromagnetic radiation, or to the excitation and ionization of orbital electrons. These interactions lead to the deposition of energy within the material. This is essential in the context of radiation detection, but also may lead to detrimental health effects if the energy deposition is in sensitive areas such as cellular DNA. For these reasons, the ability to estimate the amount of deposited energy relies on our understanding the nature of the interactions of charged particles interactions with matter.

As described in the section on the production of x-rays, electrons passing close to the nucleus undergo deacceleration, leading to the emission of bremsstrahlung radiation and thus a loss of electron energy as they pass through the matter. These electronic energy losses are referred to as *radiative losses*. The magnitude of these losses is directly proportional to the energy of the impinging electrons and the atomic number (Z number) of the target material.

In the case of clinical administration of pure beta emitters, bremsstrahlung radiation can be used to image the in vivo distribution of the radiopharmaceutical. This can be of particular use when evaluating administration of beta-emitting radiopharmaceuticals for therapeutic applications. As the emitted beta particles pass through the patient, they lead to the emission of bremsstrahlung radiation that can be imaged. In general, the result is a very-low-quality image compared to that of direct emission of x-rays or gamma rays, but it can be helpful in attaining a general impression of the beta-emitting radiopharmaceutical distribution.

In addition, as electrons pass through matter, their charge interacts with the negative charges of the atomic orbital electrons. For impinging electrons and negative beta particles this is a repulsive force, and for positrons (i.e., positive beta particles) this is an attractive force. These interactions lead to excitations and ionizations of the orbital electrons. The electronic excitations may lead to the emission of electromagnetic radiation with a wide range of energies, including visible or ultraviolet radiation, and may depend on the structural considerations, such as whether the atoms are incorporated into a crystal. These emissions are essential in the case of scintillation detectors.

The incident electron can lead to a large number of ionizations as it passes through matter, producing a large number of ionized electrons and atoms. The large majority of the resultant ionized electrons are of low energy. However, some of these interactions result in high-energy electrons sometimes referred to as *delta rays* that in turn cause ionizations. In the energies of practical interest in nuclear medicine, nearly all of the electronic energy is expended in excitation and ionization or collisional losses compared to radiative losses. The rate at which the charged particle loses energy per unit path length is referred to as the *stopping power*. A related quantity is the linear energy transfer (LET), which is the amount of energy deposited locally (i.e., not including the energy lost to energetic electrons or delta rays, per unit path length). Radiation with a higher LET has been shown to be more effective in causing biological damage. The stopping power and LET depend on the type of radiation, its energy, and the density of the material through which it travels. For example, alpha particles have a higher LET than electrons, low-energy electrons have higher stopping power than those with higher energy, and energy deposition is higher in more dense material than it is in less dense material.

The range of the charged particle is the distance from the point at which it was emitted to the point at which it has lost all of its energy. The range is the straight line distance between the two points compared to the path length that follows the actual path of the particle. For electrons, the path length may be about twice the range. The range depends on the type of charged particle, its initial energy, and the material through which it is passing. In soft tissue, alpha particles have a range of a fraction of a millimeter and electrons and beta particles have ranges of several millimeters to several centimeters, depending on the initial energy.

Photon Interactions in Matter

Small bundles of electromagnetic energy are referred to as *photons*. As photons in the x-ray or gamma ray energy range pass through matter, they can interact with the nucleus, the orbital electrons, or the complete atom as a whole. At energy levels of just a few kiloelectron volts, the photons can be scattered in a manner that does not result in energy deposition referred to as *Rayleigh scattering*. At energy levels of several megaelectron volts, the photon can interact with the nuclear field in a manner that leads to the production of an electron and a positron. This interaction is known as *pair production*. However, in the energy range of most interest in nuclear medicine, from several tens of kiloelectron volts to approximately 1 MeV, the two most prominent modes of photon interaction are the photoelectric effect and Compton scattering. Thus the rest of this section will specifically discuss these two interactions.

In the photoelectric effect (Fig. 3-12), the photon interacts with an atomic orbital electron, leading to the liberation of the electron and a subsequent electron shell vacancy. The liberated electron, referred to as the *photoelectron*, is ejected with a kinetic energy equal to the energy of the incident photon minus the binding energy associated with the electron's initial orbital shell. Thus the incident electron must have sufficient energy to overcome the electron binding energy for a particular shell. The probability of the photoelectric effect decreases dramatically with increasing incident photon energy. It is perhaps counterintuitive that more tightly bound electrons are more likely to be involved in a photoelectric interaction. As a result, atomic electrons from materials with high Z numbers are much more likely to undergo a photoelectric interaction than those from lower Z materials. Thus to first order, the probability of a photoelectric interaction is given by:

$$P_{PE} \, \alpha \, Z^4 / E^3$$

where P_{PE} is the probability of a photoelectric interaction, Z is the Z number of the material in question and E is the energy of the incident photon. In addition, the probability of photoelectric interaction is highest for the electrons in the innermost shell with a binding energy less than the incident photon energy. Thus electrons in the orbital shell with binding energy just less than the incident photon energy are the most likely to interact. A photoelectric interaction causes an inner shell vacancy as the electron is ejected, which leads to emission of fluorescent x-rays and Auger electrons.

In Compton scattering, the incident photon interacts with an electron, resulting in some of the photon's energy transferring to the electron such that the photon loses some energy and changes direction (Fig. 3-13). The lost energy is manifest as the kinetic energy of the Compton scattered photon. The amount of energy transferred from the photon to the electron depends on the angle of scatter, with a small amount of energy transferred for small-angle scattering and more with large-angle scattering. The angular distribution

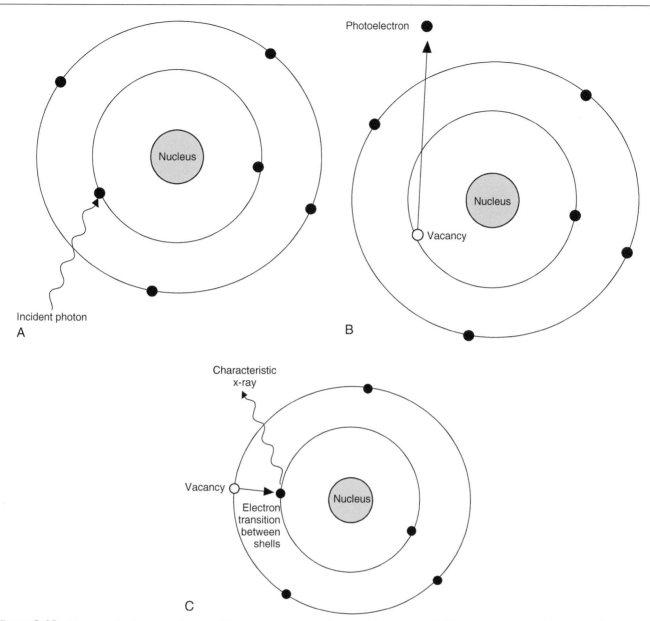

FIGURE 3-12. Photoelectric absorption. **A,** An incident photon interacts with an orbital electron. **B,** The electron is ejected from its shell, creating a vacancy. The electron is either ejected from the atom or moved to a shell farther from the nucleus. **C,** The orbital vacancy is filled by the transition of an electron from a more distant shell. A characteristic x-ray is given off as a consequence of this transition.

of scatter depends on the incident photon energy. With lower energies, the scattering tends to be more isotropic, whereas it is more forward scattered with higher-photon energies. Unlike the photoelectric effect, no preference is seen for tightly bound electrons; thus most Compton interactions involve outer-shell, loosely bound electrons. In most cases, the electron can be considered free. Thus the probability of Compton interaction mostly depends on the electron density (electrons per milliliter) and is not strongly dependent on energy or Z number.

Whether a photoelectric or Compton event is more likely depends on the incident photon energy and the material in question. Photoelectric effect will tend to be the predominant mode of interaction at lower energies and with materials with higher Z numbers, whereas Compton scatter will be predominant at moderate photon energies and lower Z numbers. At higher energies, pair production becomes the

most likely interaction. Figure 3-14 demonstrates the most prominent modes of interaction as a function of photon energy and Z number of the material of interest. As can be seen, for soft tissue (effective $Z \approx 7$), sodium iodide (effective $Z \approx 53$), and lead ($Z = 72$), the photoelectric effect is the predominant mode of interaction up to photon energies of approximately 30, 300, and 500 keV, respectively. At energies greater than this and less than 1 MeV, Compton scatter is the most likely mode of interaction.

Consider a thickness (Δx) of a particular material thin enough that the probability of interaction of a photon of a certain energy with the material is small, less than 1%. The linear attenuation coefficient, μ, can then be defined as the probability of interaction by either the photoelectric effect or Compton scatter divided by the material thickness.

$$\mu(cm^{-1}) = (P_{PE} + P_{CS}) / \Delta x$$

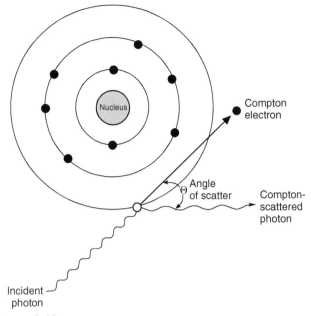

FIGURE 3-13. Compton scatter. An incident photon interacts with an outer or loosely bound electron. The photon gives up a portion of its energy to the electron and undergoes a change in direction at a lower energy.

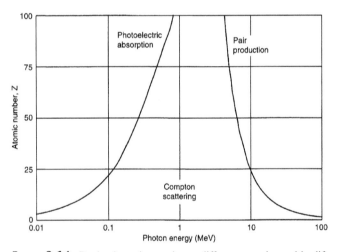

FIGURE 3-14. Predominant interaction at different energies and in different materials. This graph shows where the photoelectric effect, Compton scattering, or pair production as a function of the atomic number, Z (i.e., the number of nuclear protons) and the photon energy (in MeV). (Cherry SR, Sorenson JA, Phelps ME. *Physics in Nuclear Medicine*. 3rd ed. Philadelphia: WB Saunders; 2003:84.)

where P_{PE} and P_{CS}, respectively, are the probabilities of the photoelectric effect or Compton scattering occurring in the material. For N_o photons impinging on a slab of material with thickness, x, the number of photons traversing the material without interaction is:

$$N = N_o\, e^{-\mu x}$$

Thus $e^{-\mu x}$ is the fraction of incident photons that do not interact. This equation is similar to that for radioactive decay but with the exponent being μx rather than λt. If N

is the number traversing without interaction, then the number interacting in the material, N_i, is:

$$N_i = N_o(1 - e^{-\mu x})$$

Thus $e^{-\mu x}$ is the fraction of incident photons that does not interact in the material, and $(1 - e^{-\mu x})$ is the fraction that does interact. The equation can also be used to estimate the fraction of the photon beam intensity (number of photons incident per unit area per second), exposure rate (milliroentgen [mR] per hour), or air kinetic energy released per unit material (kerma) rate (milligray [mGy] per hour) that traverses a barrier.

$$I = Io\, e^{-\mu x}$$

Note that this will be less than the beam intensity on the other side of the barrier, which will include not only the beam without interaction but also the portion of the beam that has been forward scattered. The total beam intensity, I_{TOT}, is given by:

$$I_{TOT} = Io\, B\, e^{-\mu x}$$

where *B* is referred to as the *build-up factor*, which is the ratio of the total beam intensity divided by the unattenuated beam. The build-up factor depends on the thickness and material of absorbing material and the energy of the incident photon beam.

Radiation Dosimetry

Quantities that have been defined by the International Council on Radiological Units (ICRU); for each quantity, a particular unit of measurement has been defined. In an example in another context, temperature would be considered a quantity and the unit used to measure it would be degrees Celsius, defined as $\dfrac{1}{100}$ of the amount of heat between that needed to freeze or boil water. In this section, related quantities of radiation physics and dosimetry will be defined, as well as the units used to measure them.

The intensity of a beam of ionizing photons is characterized by the magnitude of charge (electrons or ionized atoms) generated in a certain amount (volume or mass) of air. Air is used as a reference material, similar to the use of mercury in a thermometer, and that the intensity of the beam is the same regardless of whether air is present. The traditional quantity is *exposure*, and the unit of exposure is the *roentgen* (R), which is the amount of x-ray or gamma ray radiation needed to liberate 1 electrostatic unit of charge of either sign (negative electrons or positive ionized atoms) in 1 cm³ of air at standard temperature and pressure (0° C at 760 mm Hg). Converting to coulombs (C) for charge and mass of air,

$$1\ R = 2.58 \times 10^{-4}\ C \text{ liberated in 1 kg of air}$$

Exposure is an intensive quantity that can be estimated at any point in space—that is, the exposure at a particular location (x,y,z) can be discussed, even if a cubic centimeter or kilogram of air cannot fit into that one point. Again, this is similar to temperature, which could be estimated at any point in space. Also, exposure is an integral quantity that is experienced over some period. Thus the exposure rate (e.g., in roentgens per hour) can be used to define the intensity of the photon beam at a particular point in time. Finally, exposure is defined only for photon (x-ray and gamma ray) irradiation and is not used to describe the intensity of beams such as electrons, protons, betas, alphas, or neutrons.

No International System of Units (SI units) for exposure exists, although the term *air kerma* is often used as an alternative. Kerma is the total amount of energy released by incident radiation per unit mass of the chosen material. The unit for kerma is the *gray* (Gy), which corresponds to 1 joule released in 1 kg of matter (in the case of air kerma, the matter is air). Thus air kerma characterizes the amount of energy released rather than the amount of ionization caused by the radiation beam. Although they are not the same, they are certainly related, and one can be calculated from the other.

1 Gy of air kerma = 1 R of exposure × 0.00869

Exposure can be directly estimated using an ionization chamber (which measures the amount of gas ionization) from which air kerma can be calculated.

Radiation absorbed dose is a quantity of the energy imparted per unit mass to a particular material. In the case of absorbed dose, the material of interest must be specified—for example, whether it is soft tissue or the detector material. Absorbed dose is also different from kerma, although the gray is the unit for both. Kerma is the energy released per unit mass, whereas absorbed dose is the energy imparted or absorbed. The traditional unit of dose is the *rad*, which is defined as 100 ergs imparted per gram. Thus 1 Gy = 100 rad. Radiation absorbed dose is an essential quantity in radiation physics and protection. In particular, adverse effects in biological tissues, in both culture and live organisms, have been shown to be related to the absorbed dose to the material.

Dose is energy imparted per unit mass. Therefore, if the hand is uniformly irradiated and the dose to one finger is 1 mGy, the dose to three fingers is also 1 mGy. The three fingers may have absorbed 3 times the energy as one finger, but they also weigh 3 times as much as one finger; thus the absorbed dose is the same.

If a material is exposed to a photon beam, it will receive a certain absorbed dose. The dose can be estimated if the absorptive properties of the material and the exposure (or air kerma) associated with the photon beam are known. Of course, the absorptive properties will vary depending on the materials and the energy of the photon beam. Figure 3-15 shows the f-factor, which is the ratio of the dose in a particular material divided by the absorbed dose in air for the same level of air kerma. For bone and photon energies less than 50 keV this ratio may be greater than 4 because of the higher probability for photoelectric effect for bone relative to air. However, the absorbing properties of soft tissue are similar to those of air per unit mass; therefore this ratio is always greater than 0.9 and is greater than 0.96 between 100 and 1000 keV. Thus, in the energy range of interest for nuclear medicine, soft tissue exposed to 1 R will receive an absorbed dose of approximately 1 rad.

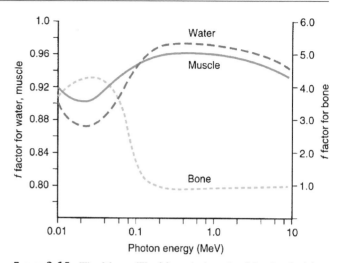

FIGURE 3-15. The f-factor. The f-factor is the ratio of the absorbed dose per gram to a certain material (e.g., water, muscle, or bone) and the absorbed dose per gram in air for the same air kerma (or exposure). Note that the f-factor for water and muscle is generally between 0.88 and 0.98 for all energies and the f-factor for bone is approximately 4 at low energies (below 0.1 MeV) at which the photoelectric effect is predominant and about 1 at higher energies at which Compton scatter is predominant. (Cherry SR, Sorenson JA, Phelps ME. *Physics in Nuclear Medicine.* 3rd ed. Philadelphia: WB Saunders; 2003:429.)

Different types of radiation have different levels of biological effectiveness. Specifically, radiation that causes dense ionization (many ionizations per track length) tend to be more damaging than those that are sparsely ionizing. In other words, radiations with high LET (in kiloelectron volts per centimeter; i.e., they deposit a lot of energy per unit track length) tend to be more effective at causing a subsequent radiation effect. The term *radiobiological effectiveness (RBE)* describes this phenomenon and is defined as the absorbed dose in low-energy x-rays (the reference radiation) to cause a specific biological effect divided by the dose in the radiation of interest to cause the same effect. As defined, x-ray and gamma rays have an RBE of 1 and other radiations that cause more effect have higher levels. In general, more massive charged particles such as protons and alpha particles have higher levels of both LET and RBE compared to x-rays, gamma rays, beta particles, and electrons.

The quantity, dose equivalent, takes into account the RBE over a wide range of detrimental biological effects. The SI and traditional units for dose equivalent are the Sievert (Sv) and the rem. Dose equivalent (DE) is calculated by multiplying the absorbed dose (D) by the quality factor associated with that radiation (Q).

$$DE = D \times Q$$

The quality factors for different radiations are listed in Table 3-3. It is not surprising that the quality factors for x-rays and gamma rays are the same as for electrons, because these photons transfer their energy to electrons via the photoelectric effect or Compton scattering, and it is the resultant energetic electron that does the large majority of the ionization.

To estimate the absorbed dose to human subjects from internally deposited radionuclides, the location of the

TABLE 3-3 Dosimetric Quality Factors

Radiation type	Quality factors
Gamma rays and x-rays	1
Electrons, beta particles	1
Neutrons	5-20
Protons	5
Alpha particles	20

nuclide within the body (which organs), how long it resided there, and the types and energies of the radiations that were emitted must be determined or estimated. From this, a certain model of the patient is assumed based on the size, shape, orientation, and location of each organ that either contains the radionuclide or is irradiated by it. The organs that contain the radionuclide are referred to as *source* organs, and those that are being irradiated are referred to as *target* organs. The internal distribution of the radionuclide is determined by the pharmaceutical to which the radionuclide is attached and the individual physiology of the human subject. Models have been developed and continue to be updated for standard sizes of man, woman, and child. Models also are available for women at different stages of gestation.

The absorbed dose to a particular target organ is the sum of the doses from all of the source organs for that radiopharmaceutical. The following equation was developed by the Medical Internal Radiation Dosimetry (MIRD) Committee of the Society of Nuclear Medicine:

$$D(r_T) = \sum_S \tilde{A}(r_S)\, S(r_T \leftarrow r_S)$$

where $D(r_T)$ is the radiation dose to a particular target organ, $\tilde{A}(r_S)$ is the time-integrated activity in a selected source organ and $S(r_T \leftarrow r_S)$ is the radionuclide-specific quantity representing the mean dose to the target organ per unit activity present in the source organ.

For a particular radiopharmaceutical, multiple source organs must be considered. The effective dose provides a manner to compare the potential for adverse health effects for nonuniform radiation exposures, such as those experienced from radiopharmaceuticals. It is a sum of the organ doses in which each organ is weighted by that organ's potential for adverse health effects.

$$ED = \sum D_T * H_T$$

where DT is the absorbed dose for each target organ and HT is the weight associated with that target organ.

SUGGESTED READING

Chandra R. *Nuclear Medicine Physics: The Basics*. 7th ed. Philadelphia: Williams & Wilkins; 2011.
Cherry SR, Sorenson JA, Phelps ME. *Physics in Nuclear Medicine*. 4th ed. Philadelphia: WB Saunders; 2012.
Eckerman KF, Endo A. *MIRD: Radionuclide Data and Decay Schemes*. 2nd ed. Reston, VA: Society of Nuclear Medicine; 2008.
Loevinger R, Budinger TF, Watson EE. *MIRD Primer for Absorbed Dose Calculations*. Reston, VA: Society of Nuclear Medicine; 1991, Revised ed.
Powsner RA, Powsner ER. *Essentials of Nuclear Medicine Physics*. 2nd ed. Malden, MA: Blackwell Science; 2006.
Saha GP. *Physics and Radiobiology of Nuclear Medicine*. 3rd ed. New York: Springer; 2006.

CHAPTER 4

Radiation Detection and Instrumentation

The passage of radiation such as x-rays and gamma rays through a given material leads to ionizations and excitations that can be used to quantify the amount of energy deposited. This property allows measurement of the level of intensity of a radiation beam or small amounts of radionuclides, including from within the patient. The appropriate choice of detection approach depends on the purpose. In some cases, the efficient detection of minute amounts of the radionuclide is essential, whereas in other cases the accurate determination of the energy or location of the radiation deposited is most important. A variety of approaches to radiation detection are used, including those that allow for in vivo imaging of radiopharmaceuticals.

CHARATERISTICS OF A RADIATION DETECTOR

Consider the model of a basic radiation detector, as shown in Figure 4-1. The detector acts as a transducer that converts radiation energy to electronic charge. Applying a voltage across the detector yields a measureable electronic current. Radiation detectors typically operate in either of two modes, *current mode* or *pulse mode*. Detectors that operate in current mode measure the average current generated within the detector over some characteristic integration time. This average current is typically proportional to the exposure rate to which the detector is subjected or the amount of radioactivity within the range of the detector. In pulse mode, each individual detection is processed with respect to the peak current (or pulse height) for that event. This pulse height is proportional to the energy deposited

in the detection event. The histogram of pulse heights is referred to as the *pulse height spectrum* or the *energy spectrum* because it also plots a histogram of the energy deposited within the detector.

Certain properties of radiation detectors characterize their operation. Some are applicable to all detectors, whereas others are used for detectors that operate in pulse mode. These characterizations are not only useful for describing the operation but can also give insight into the benefits and limitations of the particular detector.

The detection efficiency depends on several factors, including the intrinsic and extrinsic efficiency of the detector. The *intrinsic efficiency* is defined as the fraction of the incident radiation particles that interact with the detector. It depends on the type and energy of the radiation and the material and thickness of the detector. For photons, the intrinsic efficiency, D_I, is given to first order by:

$$D_I = (1 - e^{-\mu x})$$

where μ is the linear attenuation coefficient for the material of interest at the incident photon energy and x is the thickness of the detector. Thus the intrinsic efficiency can be improved by using a thicker detector or choosing a photon energy and detector material that optimizes the value of μ.

The *extrinsic efficiency* is the fraction of radiation particles emitted from the source that strike the detector. It depends on the size and shape of the detector and the distance of the source from the detector. If the detector is a considerable distance from the source (i.e., a distance that is >5 times the size of the detector), the extrinsic efficiency, D_E, is given by:

$$D_E = A/(4\pi d^2)$$

where A is the area of the detector and d is the distance from the source to the detector. This equation defines the *inverse square law*. For example, if the source-to-detector distance is doubled, the intensity of radiation beam is reduced by a factor of 4. The total detection efficiency is the product of the intrinsic and extrinsic efficiencies:

$$D_T = D_I \times D_E$$

In pulse mode, the pulse height is proportional to the energy deposited within the detector. However, the uncertainty in the energy estimation, referred to as the *energy resolution*, depends on the type of detector used and the energy of the incident radiation. For a photon radiation source of a particular energy, the feature associated with

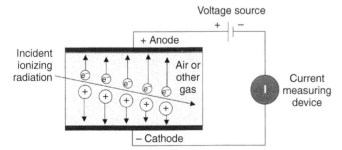

FIGURE 4-1. Block diagram of basic detector. The radiation detector basically acts as a transducer converting radiation energy deposited into electrical signal. In general, a voltage has to be supplied to collect the signal and a current or voltage measuring device is used to measure the signal. In some instances, the average current over a characteristic integration time is measured, which is referred to as *current mode*. In other cases, the voltage pulse of each detection event is analyzed, referred to as *pulse mode*. (From Cherry, Sorenson JA, Phelps ME. *Physics in Nuclear Medicine*. 3rd ed. Philadelphia: WB Saunders, 2003.)

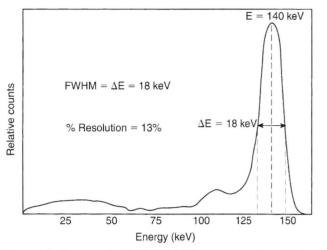

FIGURE 4-2. Spectrum for Tc-99m in air. The energy resolution is characterized by the width of the photopeak (the full width at half maximum [FWHM]) normalized by the photon energy. For the particular detector system illustrated, the FWHM is 18 keV. The energy resolution of the detector system for Tc-99m is 13% (100 × 18/140).

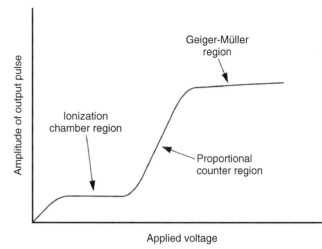

FIGURE 4-3. Amplitude of gas detector output signal as a function of applied voltage. This graph shows the relationship between the magnitude of the output signal from a gas detector (related to the amount of ionized charge collected) as a function of the voltage applied across the detector. There is no signal with no voltage applied. As the voltage is increased, the detector signal starts to increase until the *saturation voltage* is reached, the start of the plateau defining the *ionization chamber region*, where all of the initially liberated charge is collected. Further increasing the voltage leads to the *proportional counter region*, at which the liberated electrons attain sufficient energy to lead to further ionization within the gas. Finally, the *Geiger-Müller region* is reached, at which each detection yields a terminal event of similar magnitude (i.e., a "click"). (From Cherry, Sorenson JA, Phelps ME. *Physics in Nuclear Medicine*. 3rd ed. Philadelphia: WB Saunders, 2003.)

that energy is referred to as the *photopeak*, as shown in Figure 4-2. The width of the photopeak, as characterized by the full width at half of its maximum value (FWHM) normalized by the photon energy represented as a percentage, is used as a measure of the energy resolution of the detector.

When the detector is subjected to a radiation beam of low intensity, the count rate is proportional to the beam intensity. However, the amount of time it takes for the detector to process an event limits the maximum possible count rate. Two models describe the count rate limitations: *nonparalyzable* and *paralyzable*. In the nonparalyzable model, each event takes a certain amount of time to process, referred to as the *dead time*, which defines the maximum count rate at which the detector will saturate. For example, if the dead time is 4 μs, the count rate will saturate at 250,000 counts per second. With the paralyzable model, the detector count rate not only saturates but can "paralyze"—that is, lose counts at very high count rates.

■ TYPES OF RADIATION DETECTORS

The three basic types of radiation detectors used in nuclear medicine are *gas detectors*, *scintillators*, and *semiconductors*. These three operate on different principles and are typically used for different purposes.

Gas Detectors

A gas radiation detector is filled with a volume of gas that acts as the sensitive material of the detector. In some cases, it is air and in others it is an inert gas such as argon or xenon, depending on the particular detector. Electrodes are located at either end of the sensitive volume. The detector circuit also contains a variable voltage supply and a current detector. As radiation passes through the sensitive volume, it causes ionization in the gas. If a voltage is applied across the volume, the resulting ions (electrons and positive ions) will start to drift, causing a

measureable current in the circuit. The current will last until all of the charge that was liberated in the event is collected at the electrodes. The resulting current entity is referred to as a *pulse* and is associated with a particular detection event. As previously discussed, if only the average current is measured, this device operates in current mode. If the individual events are analyzed, the device is operating in pulse mode.

Figure 4-3 shows the relationship between the charge collected in the gas detector and the voltage applied across the gas volume. With no voltage, no electric field exists within the volume to cause the ions liberated in a detection event to drift, and thus no current is present and no charge is collected. As the voltage is increased, the ions start to drift and a current results. However, the electric field may not be sufficient to keep the electrons and positive ions from recombining and thus not all of the original liberated ions are collected. This portion of Figure 4-3 is referred to as the *recombination region*. As voltage is increased, the level is reached at which the strength of the electric field is sufficient for the collection of all of the liberated ions (no recombination). This level is referred to as the *saturation voltage*, and the resulting plateau in Figure 4-3 is the *ionization chamber* region. When operating in this region, the amount of charge collected is proportional to the amount of ionization caused in the detector and thereby to the energy deposited within the detector. Ionization detectors or chambers typically operate in current mode and are the detectors of choice for determining the radiation beam intensity level at a particular location. They can directly measure this intensity level in either exposure in roentgens (R) or air kerma in rad. Dose calibrators and the ionization meters used to monitor the output of an x-ray device or the exposure level from a patient who has received a radiopharmaceutical are examples of ionization chambers (or ion chambers) used in nuclear medicine.

If the voltage is increased further, the drifting electrons within the device can attain sufficient energy to cause further ionizations, leading to a cascade event. This can cause substantially more ionization than with an ionization chamber. The total ionization is proportional to the amount of ionization initially liberated; therefore these devices are referred to as *proportional counters* or *chambers*. Proportional counters, which usually operate in pulse mode, are not typically used in nuclear medicine. If the voltage is increased further, the drifting electrons attain the ability to cause a level of excitations and ionizations within the gas. The excitations can lead to the emission of ultraviolet radiation, which also can generate ionizations and further excitations. This leads to a terminal event in which the level of ionization starts to shield the initial event and the level of ionization finally stops. This is referred to as the *Geiger-Müller process*. In the Geiger-Müller device, every event leads to the same magnitude of response, irrespective of the energy or the type of the incident radiation. Thus the Geiger-Müller meter does not directly measure exposure, although it can be calibrated in a selected energy range in milliroentgens per hour. However, the estimate of exposure rate in other energy ranges may not be accurate. However, the Geiger Müller survey meter is excellent at detecting small levels of radioactive contamination and thus is often used to survey radiopharmaceutical packages that are delivered and work areas within the nuclear medicine clinic at the end of the day.

Gas detectors are used every day in nuclear medicine for assaying the amount of radiopharmaceutical to be administered and to survey packages and work areas for contamination. However, because of the low density of gas detectors, even when the gas is under pressure, the sensitivity of gas detectors in not high enough to be used for clinical counting and imaging applications.

Scintillation and Semiconductor Detectors

Some crystalline materials emit a large number of light photons upon the absorption of ionizing radiation. This process is referred to as *scintillation*, and these materials are referred to as *scintillators*. As radiation interacts within the scintillator, a large number of excitations and ionizations occur. On deexcitation, the number of light photons emitted is directly proportional to the amount of energy deposited within the scintillator. In some cases, a small impurity may be added to the crystal to enhance emission of light and minimize absorption of light within the crystal. Several essential properties of scintillating materials can be characterized, including density, effective Z number (number of atomic protons per atom), amount of light emitted per unit energy, and response time. The density and effective Z number are determining factors in the detection efficiency because they affect the linear attenuation coefficient of the scintillation material. The amount of emitted light affects both energy and, in the gamma camera, spatial resolution. Resolution is determined by the statistical variation of the collected light photons,

which depends on the number of emitted photons. Finally, the response time affects the temporal resolution of the scintillator. The most common scintillation crystalline material used in nuclear medicine is thallium-drifted sodium iodide (NaI).

Once the light is emitted in a scintillation detector, it must be collected and converted to an electrical signal. The most commonly used device for this purpose is the *photomultiplier tube* (PMT). Light photons from the scintillator enter through the photomultiplier entrance window and strike the *photocathode*, a certain fraction of which (approximately 20%) will lead to the emission of photoelectrons moving toward the first dynode. For each electron reaching the first dynode, approximately a million electrons will eventually reach the anode of the photomultiplier tube. Thus the photomultiplier tube provides high gain and low noise amplification at a reasonable cost. Other solid-state light detection approaches are now being introduced into nuclear medicine devices. In *avalanche photodiodes* (APDs), the impinging light photons lead to the liberation of electrons that are then drifted in the photodiode, yielding an electron avalanche. The gain of the APD is not as high as with the PMT (several hundred compared to about a million), but the detection efficiency is substantially higher (approximately 80%). A second solid-state approach is the *silicon photomultiplier tube* (SiPMT). This device consists of hundreds of very small APD channels that operate like small Geiger-Müller detectors—that is, each detection is a terminal event. The signal from the SiPMT is the number of channels that respond to a particular detection event in the scintillator. SiPMTs have moderate detection efficiency (approximately 50%) and operate at low voltages. One further advantage of APDs and SiPMTs compared to PMTs is that they can operate within a magnetic field. Thus the development of positron emission tomography/magnetic resonance (PET/MR) and single-photon emission computed tomography/magnetic resonance (SPECT/MR) scanners will most likely involve the use of either APDs or SiPMTs.

Solid-state technology is used to detect the light from a scintillation detector and also can be used to directly detect gamma rays. The detection of radiation within a *semiconductor detector* leads to a large number of electrons liberated, resulting in high energy resolution. The energy resolution of the lithium-drifted germanium (GeLi) semiconductor detector has approximately 1% energy resolution compared to the 10% energy resolution associated with a sodium iodide scintillation detector. However, thermal energy can lead to a measureable current in some semiconductor detectors such as GeLi, even in the absence of radiation, and thus these semiconductor detectors must be operated at cryogenic temperatures. On the other hand, semiconductor detectors such as cadmium telluride (CdTe) or cadmium zinc telluride (CZT) can operate at room temperature. CdTe and CZT do not have the excellent energy resolution of GeLi, but at approximately 5%, it is still significantly better than that of sodium iodide.

The pulse height spectrum corresponding to the detection of the 140-keV gamma rays from technetium-99m is illustrated in Figure 4-4. The photopeak corresponds to events where the entire energy of the incident photon is absorbed within the detector. These are the events of

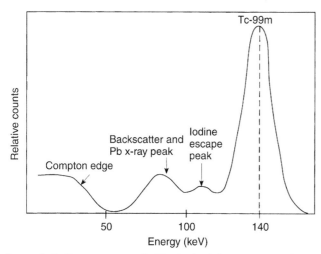

FIGURE 4-4. Energy spectrum for Tc-99m in air for a gamma scintillation camera with the collimator in place. Note the iodine escape peak at approximately 112 keV. The 180-degree backscatter peak at 90 keV merges with the characteristic x-ray peaks for lead (Pb). The Compton edge is at 50 keV.

primary interest in most counting experiments, and thus the *good* events are within an energy acceptance window about the photopeak. Other events correspond to photons scattered within the detector material and depositing energy, which can range from very low energy from a very-small-angle scatter to a maximum 180-degree scatter (in the spectrum referred to as the *Compton edge*). Events below the Compton edge correspond to these scattered events. In some cases, photons can undergo multiple scatters and possibly result in events between the Compton edge and the photopeak. Photons scattered within the patient and then detected may also result in events in this energy region. Finally, the pulse height spectrum will be blurred depending on the energy resolution of the detector. Thus, in Figure 4-4, the photopeak has approximately a 10% spread because of the energy resolution associated with NaI, rather than the narrow spike that might be expected from the emission of a monoenergetic gamma ray.

■ ANCILLARY EQUIPMENT

Besides the imaging equipment in the nuclear medicine clinic, other additional ancillary equipment may be necessary from either a medical or regulatory point of view or to otherwise enhance the operation of the clinic. This equipment will be reviewed, including the quality control required for proper operation.

Radiation Meters

As previously discussed, the two basic radiation meters commonly used in the nuclear medicine clinic are the Geiger-Müller (GM) meter and the ionization chamber. Both are gas detectors, although they operate differently. With the GM meter, all detections lead to a terminal event of the same magnitude—a "click." The device is excellent for detecting small amounts of contamination. It is routinely used to determine whether there is contamination on packages of radiopharmaceutical that are delivered

to the clinic and to test working surfaces and the hands and feet of workers for contamination. GM meters often are equipped with a test source of cesium-137, with a very small amount of radioactivity, that is affixed to the side of the meter. On calibration, the probe is placed against the source and the resulting exposure rate is recorded. The probe is tested daily using the source to ensure that the meter's reading is the same as at the time calibration. The GM meter should be calibrated on an annual basis.

The ionization chamber meter (ion chamber) operates in current mode and assesses the amount of ionization within an internal volume of gas (often air) and thus can directly measure exposure or air kerma rate. The ion chamber is used to evaluate the exposure rate at various locations within the clinic. For example, it could be used to measure the exposure rate in an uncontrolled area adjacent to the radiopharmaceutical hot laboratory. The ion chamber is also used to evaluate the exposure rate at a distance from a patient who has received radionuclide therapy (e.g., iodine-131 for thyroid cancer) to determine that the patient can be released without exposing the general public to unacceptable radiation levels. The ion chamber also should be annually calibrated.

Dose Calibrator

The dose calibrator is an ionization chamber used to assay the amount of activity in vials and syringes. This includes the assay of individual doses before administration to patients, as required by regulation. The dose calibrator operates over a very wide range of activities, from hundreds of kilobecquerels (10s of μCi) to tens of gigabecquerels (up to a curie). The device is also equipped with variable settings for each radionuclide to be measured, with typically about 10 buttons for ready selection of the commonly used radionuclides. In addition, often buttons for user-defined radionuclide selection can be set for the particular clinic. Others can be selected by entering the appropriate code for that radionuclide into the system.

The dose calibrator is used to assay the activity administered to the patient, and thus a comprehensive quality control program is necessary. Until 2003 a particular quality control program was specified by the U.S. Nuclear Regulatory Commission. Modification of the regulations since that time specify that the quality control program must meet the manufacturer's recommendations or national standards. Currently, the national standard continues to be almost universally followed. This program comprises four basic quality control tests: geometry, accuracy, linearity, and constancy.

The geometry protocol tests that the dose calibrator provides the same reading for the same amount of activity irrespective of the volume or orientation of the sample. A reading of a certain amount of activity in a 0.5-mL volume is obtained. The volume is then increased by augmenting the sample with amounts of nonradioactive water or saline and taking additional readings. The subsequent readings should not vary from the original readings by more than 10%. The geometry test is performed during acceptance testing and after a major repair or move of the equipment to another location.

For accuracy, calibrated sources (typically cobalt-57 and ^{137}Cs) are assayed; the resultant reading cannot vary by more than 10% from the calibrated activity decay corrected to the day of the test. The accuracy test should be performed during acceptance testing, annually thereafter, and after a major repair or move.

The linearity protocol tests that the dose calibrator operates appropriately over the wide activity range to which it is applied. The device is tested from 10 μCi (370 kBq) to a level higher than that routinely used in the clinic and perhaps as high as 1 Ci (37 GBq). The activity readings are varied by starting with a sample of radioactivity of Tc-99m at the highest value to be tested (e.g., tens of gigabequerels). The activity readings are then varied by either allowing the source to radioactively decay over several days or using a set of lead shields of varying thicknesses until a reading close to 370 kBq is obtained. Each reading should not vary by more than 10% from the line drawn through the calculated activity values. The linearity test should be performed during acceptance testing, quarterly thereafter, and after a major repair or move.

The constancy protocol tests the reproducibility of the readings as compared to a decay-corrected estimate for a reference reading obtained from the dose calibrator on a particular day. Today's constancy reading cannot vary from the decay-corrected reference reading by more than 10%. The constancy test varies from accuracy in that it evaluates the precision of the readings from day to day rather than accuracy. The constancy test should be performed on every day that the device is used to assay a dose to be administered to a patient.

Well Counter and Thyroid Probe

Two nonimaging devices are based on the scintillator, the well counter, and the thyroid probe that are routinely used in the nuclear medicine clinic. The well counter is used for both radiation protection and clinical protocols. The thyroid probe can provide clinical studies with a fraction of the equipment costs and space requirements of the use of nuclear imaging equipment. However, these devices also require comprehensive quality-control programs.

The well counter consists of a NaI crystal with a hole drilled into it allowing for test tubes, and other samples can be placed within the device for counting. The sample placed in the counter is practically surrounded by the detector, with a geometric efficiency in excess of 90%. Thus the well counter can measure very small amounts of radioactivity, on the order of a kilobecquerel. The well counter should not be confused with the dose calibrator, which is a gas-filled ionization chamber that can measure activities up to 37 GBq. The well counter is used to test for small amounts of removable radioactivity. It is used to test packages of radiopharmaceuticals to ensure that no radioactivity has been spilled on the outside of the package or leaked from the inside. The device also can be used to measure removable activity from working surfaces where radioactivity has been handled or from sealed sources such as calibration sources to ensure that the radioactivity is not leaking out.

The well counter can also be used for the assay of biological samples for radioactivity for a variety of clinical evaluations. For example, after the administration of Tc-99m diethylenetriamepentaacetic acid (DTPA), blood samples can be counted at several time points (e.g., at 1, 2, and 3 hours) to estimate the patient's glomerular filtration rate (GFR). The amount of radioactivity in a 0.2-mL blood sample will be very small, and thus the well counter is the appropriate instrument for these measurements. By making these measurements as well as the measurements of standards of known activity concentration (kilobecquerel per milliliter), the patient's GFR can be estimated. The thyroid probe consists of an NaI crystal on a stand with the associated counting electronics. The patient is administered a small amount of radioactive iodine. The probe is placed at a certain distance from the thyroid, and a count is obtained. In addition, a count is acquired of a known standard at the same distance. The thyroid uptake of iodine can be estimated from these measurements.

The quality control program for both the well counter and the thyroid probe include the energy calibration, the energy resolution, the sensitivity, and the chi square test. For the energy calibration, the energy window is set for the calibration source of a particular radionuclide—for example, the 662-keV peak of Cs-137. The amplifier gain is varied until the maximum count is found that corresponds with the alignment of the window with the 662-keV energy peak. In addition, the counts in a series of narrow energy windows across the peak can be measured to estimate the energy resolution. A standard window can be set, and the counts of a known calibration source can be counted and normalized by the number of nuclear transformations to estimate the sensitivity in counts per transformation (or counts per second per becquerel). Finally, the chi square test evaluates the operation of the counter by comparing the uncertainty of the count to that expected from the Poisson distribution.

■ NUCLEAR MEDICINE IMAGING

The Patient as a Radioactive Source

In nuclear medicine, the patient is administered a radiopharmaceutical that distributes according to a specific physiological or functional pathway. The patient is then imaged using external radiation detectors to determine the in vivo distribution and dynamics of the radiopharmaceutical through which the patient's physiology can be inferred, providing this essential information to the patient's doctor to aid in diagnosis, prognosis, staging, and treatment. The equipment used to acquire these data will be described in the sections ahead. Single photon emission computed tomography (SPECT) and positron emission tomography (PET) will be described in the next chapter. However, before examining how the instrumentation operates, it is instructive to understand the nature of the signal itself—that is, the radiation being emitted from within the patient.

The radiopharmaceutical is administered to the patient most commonly by intravenous injection, but also in some cases through other injection routes, such as intraarterial, intraperitoneal, or subdermal. In other cases, the radiopharmaceutical may be introduced through the gastrointestinal tract or through the breathing of a radioactive gas or aerosol. After administration, the path and rate of uptake depend on the particular radiopharmaceutical, the route of administration, and the patient's individual physiology. However, the characteristics and parameters associated with the radiopharmaceutical in vivo distribution and dynamics are of considerable clinical importance. In some cases, the enhanced uptake of the radiopharmaceutical in certain tissues (e.g., the uptake of fluorodeoxyglucose [FDG] in tumors) may be of most clinical importance, whereas in other cases it may be the lack of uptake (e.g., the absence of Tc-99m sestamibi in infarcted myocardium). In the first case, this would be referred to as a *hot spot* imaging task, and in the latter would be a *cold spot* task. In other situations, it may be rate of uptake *(wash in)* or clearance *(wash out)* that may be considered the essential characteristic of the study. In a Tc-99m mercaptoacetyltriglycine MAG3 renal study, fast wash in may indicate a well-perfused kidney and delayed clearance may indicate renal obstruction. In the Tc-99m DTPA counting protocol described previously, slow clearance of the radiopharmaceutical from the blood would indicate a reduced GFR. In some cases, the ability to discern uptake in a particular structure that is adjacent to other nonspecific uptake may require the ability to spatially resolve the two structures, whereas other tasks may not require such specific resolution. The choice of instrumentation, acquisition protocol, and data processing approach fundamentally depend on the clinical task at hand.

To characterize the rate, location, and magnitude of radiopharmaceutical uptake within the patient, the emitted radiation must be detected, in most cases, by detectors external to the patient's body. Some instruments are specially designed for internal use—for example, interoperative radiopharmaceutical imaging—but in most the cases, the imaging device is located outside the body while detecting radiation internally. This requirement limits the useful emitted radiations for nuclear medicine imaging to energetic photons—that is, gamma rays and x-rays. The amount of overlying tissue between the internally distributed radiopharmaceutical and the radiation detector may vary from several centimeters to as much as 20 to 30 cm. Alpha and beta particles will not be of use in most cases because their ranges in tissue are limited to a few millimeters and thus they will not exit the body and cannot be measured by external radiation detectors. Even x-rays and gamma rays must have energies in excess of 50 keV to penetrate 10 cm of tissue. On the other hand, once the radiation exits the patient, it is best that the radiation not be so energetic as to be difficult to detect with reasonable-size detectors. Thus the radiation types optimal for most nuclear medicine imaging applications are x-rays and gamma rays in the 50- to 600-keV energy range, depending on the equipment and collimation being used.

Consider a situation in which a radiopharmaceutical labeled with Tc-99m leads to a point source at some depth within the patient's body. The 140-keV gamma rays will be emitted isotropically from the point source. Therefore it would be advantageous to place the radiation detector close to the source or to place several detectors around the source to collect as many of the emitted photons as possible. In fact, acquiring data from several angles may allow the source to be better localized. Those emitted photons

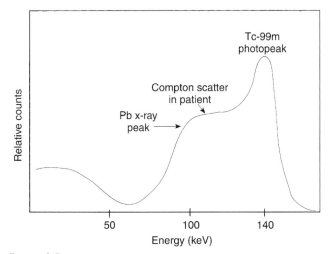

FIGURE 4-5. Energy spectrum from a gamma camera with the Tc-99m activity in the patient. Note the loss of definition of the lower edge of the Tc-99m photopeak. This spectrum illustrates the difficulty of discriminating Compton-scattered photons within the patient using pulse height analysis.

that exit the body without interaction and are subsequently detected will yield the highest quality spatial information. Conversely, those photons that scatter within the patient compromise spatial information. Photons that undergo very-small-angle scatter will perhaps not be of much consequence, but those that undergo scatter at larger angles will not be of much use. Noting that the Compton scattered photons have less energy than the incident photons, and that small-angle scatter leads to less energy loss than large-angle scatter, energy discrimination (i.e., only allowing photons to be counted within a narrow energy window about the photopeak energy) will lead to the elimination of a significant number of scattered photons from the nuclear medicine image. In contrast to the case of a point source, a more challenging clinical case with regard to scatter may be the imaging of a cold spot feature, such as an infarction in a myocardial perfusion scan or a renal scar in a Tc-99m DMSA scan. In these cases, scattered photons in the neighboring tissue may be displaced into the cold spot, leading to a loss in image contrast and an inability to properly discern the extent of the feature. It must also be kept in mind that in a true clinical case the distribution of the radiopharmaceutical is unknown and background levels in other tissues may compromise the situation. The pulse height spectrum from a patient is shown in Figure 4-5.

The Gamma Camera

In the earliest days of nuclear medicine, counting devices similar to the thyroid probe described in the previous section were used to evaluate the amount of activity in a particular tissue. For example, probes could be used to evaluate the iodine uptake of the thyroid gland. However, it was not long before clinicians realized that it would be helpful to not only know the total uptake of the radiopharmaceutical within the tissue of interest but also to be able to discern the spatial distribution of the uptake within the tissue. In the early 1950s, Benedict Cassan attached a

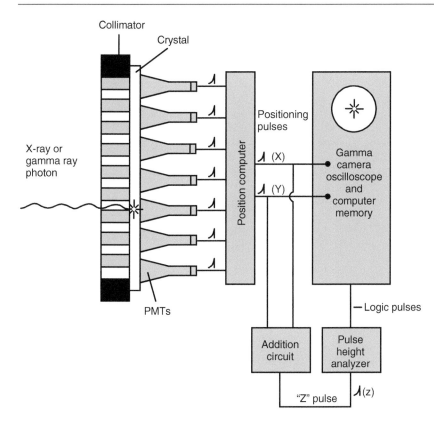

FIGURE 4-6. Schematic of gamma scintillation camera. The diagram shows a photon reaching the NaI crystal through the collimator and undergoing photoelectric absorption. The photomultiplier tubes *(PMTs)* are optically coupled to the NaI crystal. The electrical outputs from the respective PMTs are further processed through positioning circuitry to calculate *(x, y)* coordinates and through addition circuitry to calculate the deposited energy of the pulse. The energy signal passes through the pulse height analyzer. If the event is accepted, it is recorded spatially in the location determined by the *(x,y)* positioning pulses.

focused collimator to an NaI crystal and a mechanism for acquiring the counts from the patient at multiple locations in a raster fashion and plotting the spatial distribution of the counts. This device, the *rectilinear scanner*, provided nuclear medicine images of physiological function. As a result the term *scan*, as in a thyroid or bone scan, has remained in the nuclear medicine lexicon. However, these scans took a long time to acquire and did not allow for the acquisition of time-sequence or dynamic studies. Still, the rectilinear scanner continued to be used in nuclear medicine clinics through the late 1970s.

In the mid-1950s, Hal Anger developed his first prototype of the *gamma camera*, which allowed a section of the body to be imaged without a raster scan, opening the door for the possibility of both dynamic and physiologically gated studies. Further developments of the technology took place over the next 10 years, and the first commercial gamma camera was introduced in the mid-1960s. With further advances that have improved and stabilized the operation of the instrument, as well as the addition of tomographic capability, the gamma camera remains the most commonly used imaging device in the nuclear medicine clinic.

A block diagram of the gamma camera is shown in Figure 4-6. Gamma rays emitted from within the patient pass through the holes of an absorptive collimator to reach the NaI crystal. On interaction of the gamma ray with the NaI scintillating crystal, thousands of light photons are emitted, a portion of which are collected by an array of PMTs. By taking weighted sums of the PMT signals within the associated computer, the two-dimensional (2D) x and y location and the total energy of the detection event deposited is estimated. If the energy deposited is within

a prespecified energy window (e.g., within 10% of the photopeak energy), the event is accepted and the location of the event recorded. In this manner, the gamma camera image is constructed on an event-by-event basis, and a single nuclear medicine image may consist of hundreds of thousands of such events. Each component of the gamma camera will be described.

The detection material of the gamma camera is typically a single, thin large-area NaI scintillation crystal. Some smaller cameras rely on a 2D matrix of smaller crystals, but most rely on a single large crystal. In the most common gamma camera designs, the NaI crystal is about 30 cm × 50 cm in area and 9.5 mm thick. Some cameras designed for imaging only photons with energies below 150 keV may have thinner crystals. Others used more commonly for higher-energy photons may be thicker, but the 9.5-mm thickness provides a reasonable compromise because it detects more than 85% of the photons with energies of 140 keV or lower and stops about 28% of the 364-keV gamma rays emitted by I-131. NaI is hygroscopic and thus damaged by water. It is hermetically sealed and has a transparent light guide on the side adjacent to the PMT array and aluminum on the side closer to the collimator. The NaI crystal is the most fragile component of the gamma camera, being susceptible to both physical and thermal shock. When the collimator is not in place, the bare NaI crystal must be treated with extreme care. In addition, the environment in the room must be controlled so that the air temperature is maintained at a reasonable level (18-24° C) and is not subject to wide variations over a short period.

The PMT array consists of about 60 to 100 photomultiplier tubes that are each about 5 cm in diameter. The PMTs are usually hexagonal and arranged in a hexagonal close-packed array to collect as many light photons as possible. Although PMTs are used in practically all gamma cameras, some recent small camera designs are using avalanche photodiodes to collect the scintillation light. The signal from each PMT is input into the gamma camera host computer. First, the sum of all of the PMT signals is used to estimate the energy deposited in the detection event. In addition, each PMT has a weight associated with its position in both the x and y direction. For example, the PMTs on the left side of the camera may have a low weight and those on the right side of the camera would have a higher weight. For a particular detection event, if the weighted sum of the signal is low, the event would be on the left side, and if it were high, it would be on the right side of the camera. However, the weighted sum as described is dependent not only on the position of the event but also on the total amount of light collected, which is directly proportional to the energy deposited. Therefore the sum must be normalized by the energy estimate. This approach to determining the position of the detection event is often referred as *Anger logic*, in honor of the developer of the gamma camera, Hal Anger. This leads to an estimate of the detection event location to within 3 to 4 mm, which is referred to as the intrinsic spatial resolution of the camera.

However, distortions can occur in images with respect to both the energy and position estimates. Detection events directly over PMTs lead to the collection of slightly more light than the events between PMTs and therefore to a slightly higher pulse height. *Energy calibration* notes the shift in the pulse height spectrum as a function of position. Subsequently, an opposite shift is applied on an event-by-event basis, leading to improved energy resolution and greater energy stability. In addition, there is an inherent nonlinearity, with events being bunched over PMTs and spread out between PMTs. Analogous to energy calibration, *linearity calibration* determines the spatial shift from linearity as a function of position across the entire field of view. Again, these shifts in both energy and position are applied on an event-by-event basis, providing an image that is free of linear distortion. A very-high-count *uniformity calibration* map is acquired that characterizes the remaining nonuniformities inherent in the gamma camera acquisition process. These uniformity calibration maps are used to generate uniformity corrections that are applied during each acquisition.

Collimators

Although the NaI crystal, PMTs, and electronics can estimate the location of a detection event to within 3 to 4 mm, the directionality of the event is not known. Gamma rays from a point source could be detected anywhere across the field of view and the counts detected at a particular location in the NaI crystal could have also originated from practically anywhere within the patient. Thus collimation is required to determine the directionality of the detected event. Because gamma rays cannot be easily focused, absorptive collimation must be used—that is, all photons *not* heading in the desired direction will be absorbed by the collimator and those heading in the correct direction will be allowed to pass. Therefore absorptive collimation is

inherently very insensitive, because practically all of the emitted photons will be absorbed and only a very few will be accepted. In general, only 0.01% (i.e., 1 in 10,000) photons emitted from the radioactive source will be accepted by the collimator and incorporated into the image.

The simplest form is the *pinhole collimator* (Fig. 4-7). It consists of a single, small hole or aperture located a set distance (typically on the order of 20 cm) from the surface of the NaI crystal. Photons from one end of the source that pass through the aperture will be detected on the opposite side of the detector. In addition, objects that are closer to the aperture will be magnified compared to those farther away. If *b* is the distance from the aperture to the object and *f* is the distance from the aperture to the detector, the amount of magnification, M, is given by:

$$M = f/b$$

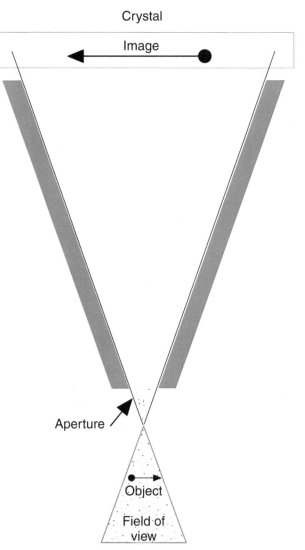

FIGURE 4-7. Pinhole collimator. The image is inverted. The image is magnified if the distance from the aperture to the object is smaller than the distance from the aperture to the gamma camera crystal. Spatial resolution improves and sensitivity decreases as the aperture diameter decreases. The sensitivity also decreases with the source-to-aperture distance, according to the inverse square law. In general, the pinhole collimator provides the best spatial resolution and the lowest sensitivity of any collimator used in nuclear medicine.

Magnification can be of significant value when imaging small objects using a camera with a large field of view. Magnification will minimize the effect of the intrinsic spatial resolution of the camera and thus enhance overall system resolution. The collimator spatial resolution of the pinhole, R_{PH}, is determined by the diameter or the aperture, d (typically 4-6 mm) and the distances from both the object and the NaI crystal to the aperture.

$$R_{PH} = d \times (f + b)/f$$

It must be kept in mind that spatial resolution is typically characterized by the size of an imaged point source and thus a large value corresponds to poor resolution and a very small value indicates excellent spatial resolution. A system with 1-mm spatial resolution will lead to an image with greater acuity than one with 5-mm spatial resolution. For this reason, the term *high resolution* can be ambiguous because it may be unclear whether the system referred to has very high resolution or a high R value (poor resolution). Based on the earlier formula, better spatial resolution is attained using a smaller aperture (small d value) with the source as close to the pinhole aperture as possible. In fact, all gamma camera collimators provide the best spatial resolution very close to the collimator and spatial resolution will degrade as the object is moved farther from the collimator. The geometric sensitivity of the pinhole collimator, G_{PH}, depends on the area of the pinhole (πd^2) compared to the squared distance of the source from the pinhole (b^2).

$$G_{PH} \approx 1/16 \, (d/b)^2$$

Thus the geometric collimator sensitivity is highest with a large aperture diameter and drops off as the inverse square of the distance from the source to the aperture—that is, it follows the inverse square law. A larger aperture diameter leads to better geometric sensitivity but poorer spatial resolution, whereas the converse is true for a smaller aperture diameter. As is true in some other instances in nuclear medicine imaging, a trade-off occurs between sensitivity and spatial resolution and improvement in one area may cause degradation of another. The choice of whether to lean toward high sensitivity or better resolution may depend on the clinical imaging task at hand, but often a compromise will lead to a reasonable value for both parameters. The pinhole collimator typically provides the best spatial resolution and the lowest sensitivity of all of the collimators commonly used in nuclear medicine. It is often used when imaging small organs (e.g., the thyroid gland) with a gamma camera with a large field of view or in special cases when a very-high-resolution spot view image is required, such as when trying to discern which bone in the foot may be demonstrating increased radiopharmaceutical uptake on a bone scan.

The *multihole collimator* provides substantially better geometric sensitivity compared to the pinhole collimator, because the object is viewed through many small holes rather than through a single hole. The most commonly used multihole collimators consist of a very large number of parallel holes with absorptive septa between the holes to restrict the emitted gamma rays from traversing from one hole to its neighboring hole. The holes are typically hexagonal and arranged in a hexagonal, close-packed array (Fig. 4-8). A typical low-energy, parallel-hole collimator may have hole diameters and lengths of about 1 and 20 mm, respectively, and septal thicknesses between holes of about 0.1 mm. No magnification occurs with a parallel-hole collimator. The collimator spatial resolution depends on the diameter (d) and the length (a) of the collimator holes and the distance from the source to collimator (b).

$$R_P = (d/a)(a + b)$$

A parallel-hole collimator with either small or long holes will provide the best spatial resolution (Fig. 4-8, *top*). Similarly to the pinhole collimator, the spatial resolution of the parallel-hole collimator is best at the surface of the collimator and degrades with distance from the collimator. The geometric sensitivity of the parallel-hole collimator also depends on the thickness of the septa between the holes (t) in addition to the hole diameter and length.

$$G_P \approx 1/16 \, (d/a)^2 \, d/(d + t)^2$$

The geometric sensitivity will be the highest for a collimator with the thinnest interhole septa. On the other hand, the septa must be thick enough to minimize *septal penetration* when a photon enters one hole, traverses the septa, and enters the neighboring hole. The septa are typically designed to be as thin as possible while limiting the amount of septal penetration to less than 5% of photons striking the septa. As a result, collimators designed for low-energy photons (under 200 keV) will require thinner septa than those designed for higher energies. Converse to collimator spatial resolution, the best geometric sensitivity is attained with a collimator with either large or short holes. Thus, again, a trade-off occurs between spatial resolution and geometric sensitivity. Because the geometric sensitivity is proportional to $(d/a)^2$ and the spatial resolution is proportional to (d/a), the geometric sensitivity of the collimator

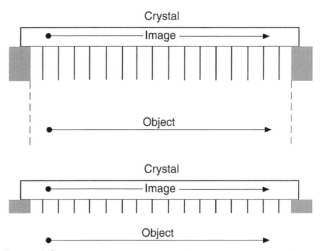

FIGURE 4-8. Multihole, parallel-hole collimator. The collimator shown at the *top* has longer holes designed to provide higher resolution. However, it would also have lower sensitivity than the collimator shown at the *bottom*. Septal thickness and thus energy rating are the same for both collimators.

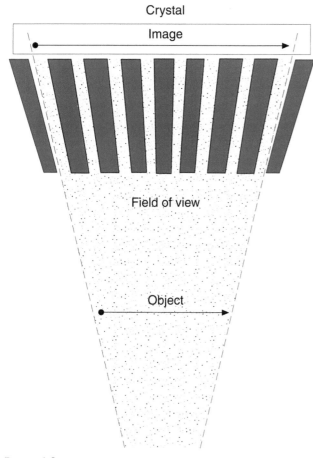

Crystal

Image

Field of view

Object

FIGURE 4-9. Converging-hole collimator. With this collimator, objects are magnified, which tends to minimize the blurring effects of the intrinsic spatial resolution and thus provide higher system spatial resolution. In addition, the sensitivity increases with distance as the collimator's focal distance is approached and thus it provides both improved spatial resolution and higher sensitivity, but with a decreased field of view.

is roughly proportional to the square of the spatial resolution.

$$G_P \propto R_P^2$$

Finally, it is notable that the geometric sensitivity of a parallel-hole collimator does not depend on the distance between the source and the collimator. The sensitivity is the same at the surface as it is at a distance removed from the surface. This fact may be counterintuitive because it might be expected that the sensitivity would drop off with distance as it does with the pinhole collimator. In fact, the sensitivity of a single hole of the collimator does go down with distance, but the degrading spatial resolution leads to the irradiation of more holes and these two facts cancel each other.

The *converging* multihole collimator provides both enhanced spatial resolution and improved sensitivity. With the converging collimator (Fig. 4-9), the direction of the holes is focused at a point some distance from the collimator surface. The distance from the collimator to the focal point is typically on the order of 50 cm and thus far beyond the boundaries of the patient. The focusing provides magnification similar to that with the pinhole collimator. As a result,

the spatial resolution is typically slightly better than that with a parallel collimator but not as good as that with a pinhole collimator. In addition, the geometric sensitivity of the converging collimator improves as the source approaches the focal point and thus the sensitivity improves at distances farther from the collimator. On the other hand, the field of view is slightly reduced at greater distances because of the increased magnification. The converging collimator is used in applications similar to those with the pinhole collimator—that is, for imaging smaller objects using a camera with a large field of view and to achieve a magnified image with slightly improved spatial resolution.

The extrinsic or system spatial resolution (R_E) depends on both the intrinsic and collimator geometric spatial resolution (R_I and R_C, respectively). To first order, the relationship between these is given by:

$$R_E = \sqrt{R_I^2 + R_C^2}$$

Based on this equation, the larger of the two values, the intrinsic or the collimator resolution, will dominate the system resolution. Except at distances very close to the collimator face, the collimator spatial resolution is substantially higher than the intrinsic resolution and thus the collimator spatial resolution is, in general, the more important factor. In cases involving magnification, the intrinsic spatial resolution, R_I, is modified by magnification, thus minimizing the effect of intrinsic spatial resolution on system spatial resolution.

$$R_E = \sqrt{\left(\frac{R_I}{M}\right)^2 + R_C^2}$$

The system spatial resolution and the collimator geometric sensitivity vary as a function of the distance from the radioactive source to the collimator (Fig. 4-10). The system spatial resolution of all of the collimators degrades with increasing distance from the collimator (Fig. 4-10). The pinhole provides the best spatial resolution, followed by the converging collimator and two types of parallel-hole collimators, the high-resolution and general-purpose collimators. On the other hand, the pinhole collimator has the poorest geometric sensitivity, which varies as the square of the distance (Fig. 4-10). For the two parallel-hole collimators, the sensitivity does not vary with distance, and the sensitivity of the converging collimator improves with distance.

Special Devices

The standard gamma camera can be used for various studies; however, some other nuclear medicine imaging devices are designed for very specific clinical applications. These often use novel approaches to either gamma ray or light detection. In some instances, they use a semiconductor detector such as CZT. In other cases, they may use avalanche photodiode light detection in conjunction with a scintillator. The most notable clinical planar imaging application for these types of devices is breast imaging.

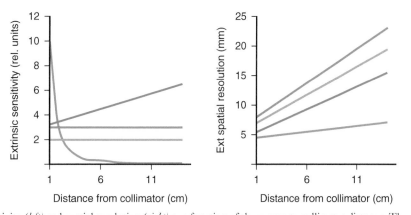

FIGURE 4-10. System sensitivity *(left)* and spatial resolution *(right)* as a function of the source-to-collimator distance. The system spatial resolution of all collimators degrades (increases in value) with distance. The pinhole collimator *(blue)* provides the best spatial resolution (lowest value) but the lowest sensitivity that varies according to the inverse square law. The converging collimator *(green)* provides very good spatial resolution with a sensitivity that increases with distance as the source approaches the focal distance of the collimator. The high-resolution parallel-hole collimator *(pink)* has good resolution and reasonable sensitivity. The general-purpose, parallel-hole collimator *(red)* has poorer spatial resolution than the high-resolution collimator but with a 50% increase in sensitivity. It is noted that the sensitivity of the two parallel-hole collimators do not vary with distance.

The compact size allows the device to stay close to the breast, resulting in high spatial resolution. In addition, the camera can be designed with limited dead space between the edge of the field of view and the patient, allowing imaging close to the chest wall. All of these characteristics result in improved imaging with this device relative to the standard gamma camera.

Gamma Camera Quality Control

To ensure proper operation of any medical device, including the gamma camera, it is essential that a comprehensive quality control program be applied. This involves acceptance testing of the device before its initial use and a program of routine tests and evaluations applied on a regular basis. It is essential that the performance be evaluated regularly to ensure that the images adequately demonstrate the in vivo distribution of the administered radiopharmaceutical and that any quantitation performed with the camera yields values that are accurate and precise.

Gamma camera quality control involves tests that are either quantitative or qualitative. For the quantitative tests, various parameters are used to measure characteristics of the gamma camera system. Some of these parameters are evaluated intrinsically (i.e., without a collimator, to characterize the optics and electronics of the system), and other parameters are evaluated extrinsically to include the collimator. If extrinsic tests are performed frequently (e.g., daily), they may be performed using the collimators most commonly used in the clinic. However, it may be best to perform the tests with all of the collimators used in the clinic at least annually. Certain parameters may be evaluated in different parts of the gamma camera's field of view. The *useful field of view (UFOV)* is the portion of the field of view the manufacturer has designated to be the proper extent for clinical imaging. Although the UFOV typically covers more than 95% of the total field of view, it may not extend to the very edge of the NaI crystal or collimator face. The *central field of view (CFOV)* is the central 50% of the area of the UFOV. The U.S. National Electronic

FIGURE 4-11. Uniformity (flood) phantom image.

Manufacturers Association, a trade association of electronic manufacturers, has defined parameters for gamma camera manufacturers to use to characterize the performance of their equipment. Although some of these parameters may be difficult to assess in the clinic, they still provide the basis for many of the quantitative measures used in the gamma camera quality control program.

The *uniformity* (or *flood*) test evaluates the consistency of response of the gamma camera to a uniform flux of radiation (Fig. 4-11). It should not be confused with the high-count uniformity calibration. The uniformity test can be applied either intrinsically or extrinsically. For the intrinsic test, the collimator is removed and exposed to the radiation from a point source of small activity (about 2 MBq) at a distance far enough to ensure uniform irradiation of the camera's field of view (at least 2 m). Extrinsic flood images are acquired with a large-area uniform source containing approximately 100 to 400 MBq. This may consist of a thin liquid source into which the radionuclide of choice (e.g., Tc-99m) is injected and thoroughly mixed. More commonly, a solid,

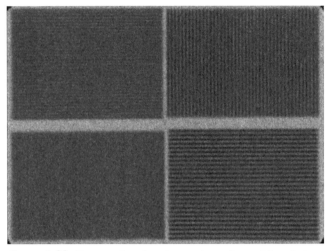

FIGURE **4-12.** Four-quadrant bar phantom image for spatial resolution.

sealed, large-area source of Co-57 (122-keV gamma ray, 270-day half-life) is used. For routine testing, 5 to 20 million counts are acquired and the images evaluated qualitatively for any notable nonuniformities. The daily flood should be acquired before administering the radiopharmaceutical to the first patient to ensure that the camera is working properly. Extrinsic floods for all collimators used with the camera may be acquired on an annual basis.

Gamma camera spatial resolution can be evaluated either intrinsically or extrinsically, qualitatively or quantitatively. In general, it may be evaluated quantitatively only during acceptance testing and perhaps during annual testing using very small point or line sources. The spatial resolution is characterized by width of the image of the small source. Typical values for intrinsic spatial resolution range from 3 to 4 mm. Extrinsic values depend on the particular collimator being evaluated and the distance at which the test was performed, but for collimators commonly used in the clinic, the extrinsic spatial resolution at 10 cm ranges from about 8 to 12 mm. In the clinic a qualitative assessment of extrinsic spatial resolution, typically a four-quadrant bar phantom (Fig. 4-12), is more commonly performed. Each quadrant of this phantom comprises alternating lead and spacing equal to the width of the bars of varying sizes (e.g., 2.0, 2.5, 3 0, and 3.5 mm). For extrinsic spatial resolution at the collimator surface, the phantom is placed on the collimator with the large-area uniformity source on top of it. The user reviews the resultant image and determines how many of the quadrants of the phantom can be discerned as separate bars. In general, the bars that can be discerned should be approximately 60% of the quantitative spatial resolution value. Thus, if the intrinsic spatial resolution is 3.5 mm, it should be possible to discern 2-mm bars of the four-quadrant bar phantom. The extrinsic spatial resolution at the surface of the most commonly used collimator in the clinic is qualitatively evaluated routinely on either a weekly or monthly basis. The number of quadrants that can be discerned should be compared to those determined during acceptance testing. The four-quadrant bar phantom image also can be used to qualitatively test spatial linearity by evaluate the straightness of the bars in the image.

Other performance parameters or characteristics that can be tested include the sensitivity, energy resolution, count rate performance, and multi-window registration. The sensitivity is most commonly evaluated extrinsically using a small-area source (e.g., 10 × 10 cm) of known activity (typically approximately 40-120 MBq of Tc-99m) placed on the collimator being evaluated, counted for 1 minute and reported as the counts per minute per unit activity. For parallel-hole collimators, the distance of the source to the collimator is inconsequential because the sensitivity does not vary with distance. For the pinhole or focusing collimators a standard distance such as 10 cm should be used. The sensitivity value will obviously depend on the collimator being evaluated, ranging from 5.0 to 8.5 cpm/kBq for typical high-resolution and general-purpose collimators. For the energy resolution, a pulse height (or energy) spectrum is acquired of a known radionuclide, typically Tc-99m, and the width of the photopeak is determined in a manner similar to that used for spatial resolution. A typical gamma camera will have an energy resolution of 9% to 11% at 140 keV. As discussed previously, radiation detectors take a certain amount of time to process each event and, if events are registered too quickly, some may be lost as a result of dead time or count rate losses. The count rate performance can be evaluated by using two sources of reasonably high activity to calculate the dead time value in microseconds or by varying the exposure rate to which the camera is exposed and recording the observed count rate. For modern cameras, the maximum observable count rate is typically between 200,000 and 400,000 counts per second (cps). Finally, the multi-window registration can be characterized. As previously discussed, the gamma camera position estimate obtained using Anger logic must be normalized by the energy deposited so that the position estimate does not vary as a function of photon energy. To test this, point sources of gallium-67, which emits photons of three different energies (90, 190, and 300 keV), are placed in several locations within the gamma camera field of view and the image location of each of the points sources are evaluated to make sure that they do not vary depending on which photopeak was imaged.

These parameters should be evaluated and compared to manufacturer specifications during acceptance testing. It is highly recommended that these tests be performed by a qualified nuclear medicine physicist. After acceptance testing, quality control tests will be run at various frequencies (daily, weekly, monthly, quarterly, or annually) and the evaluation may be qualitative rather than quantitative in these cases. Table 4-1 summarizes the recommended frequency for each of the described tests. These recommendations are for the typical gamma camera, and the most appropriate quality control program for a specific gamma camera depends on manufacturer recommendations and the clinical use and stability of performance for that particular camera.

The Nuclear Medicine Image

The x and y location of each accepted detection event is digitally stored within the acquisition host computer associated with the gamma camera. These data can be captured in two ways—matrix and list mode. In matrix mode, a specific matrix size (64 × 64, 128 × 128, 256 × 256, and so

TABLE **4-1** Gamma Camera Quality Control Summary

Parameter	Comment
DAILY	
Uniformity	Flood field; intrinsic (without collimator) or extrinsic (with collimator)
Window setting	Confirm energy window setting relative to photopeak for each radionuclide used with each patient
WEEKLY OR MONTHLY	
Spatial resolution	Requires a "resolution" phantom such as the four-quadrant bar
Linearity check	Qualitative assessment of bar pattern linearity
ANNUALLY	
System uniformity	High count flood with each collimator
Multi-window registration	For cameras with capability of imaging multiple energy windows simultaneously
Count rate performance	Vary counts using decay or absorber method
Energy resolution	Easiest in cameras with built in multi-channel analyzers
System sensitivity	Count rate performance per unit of activity for each collimator

on) is predetermined depending on the assumed spatial resolution of the imaging task. For tasks that involve higher spatial resolution, a larger matrix would be required. The chosen matrix size is mapped to the field of view, and each estimated (x,y) location is assigned to a particular picture element or *pixel* within the image matrix. The value of that pixel is then incremented by 1. In this manner, a 2D histogram of the event locations is generated, and, at the end of the acquisition, the value in a particular pixel is the total number of events assigned to that pixel during the data acquisition process. An example with a 6 × 6 matrix is shown in Figure 4-13. To display the image, the number of counts in a particular pixel are assigned a color or gray value according to a certain color scale lookup table on the computer monitor. An example might be that the pixel with the most counts is assigned the color white, pixels with no counts are assigned black, and all other pixels are assigned a shade of gray. Alternatively, the colors of the rainbow could be used, with violet indicating zero counts and red indicating the highest count. In addition, many other color tables could be used.

In many cases, more than one image is acquired during the imaging procedure. In some cases, a time-sequence of image frames, also known as a *dynamic study,* may be acquired. For example, a frame may be acquired every minute for 20 minutes. A multiphase study may be acquired, in which ten 30-second frames are followed by five 60-second frames, followed by five 120-second frames. In other instances, the data acquisition may be associated with a physiological gating signal such as the electrocardiogram (ECG) or a respiratory gate. In the cardiac example, counts from different parts of the heart cycle could be placed in different frames, resulting in frames across the heart cycle from the end of diastole to the end of systole

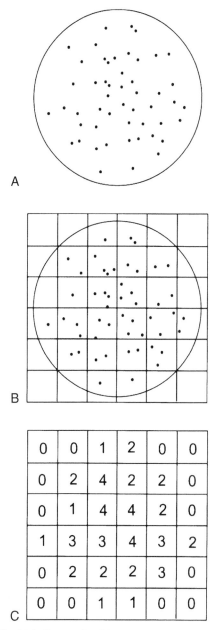

FIGURE 4-13. Digital image. Consider a nuclear medicine image acquired in matrix mode using a 6 × 6 matrix. **A,** The calculated positions based on Anger logic a number of events. **B,** A 6 × 6 matrix superimposed onto these events demonstrates into which of the pixels of the matrix each event would fit. **C,** The number of events (dots) in each pixel is recorded and assigned a particular shade of gray or color to create the digital matrix.

and back again. In matrix mode, these multiframe acquisitions would be obtained by establishing the desired number of the frames in the computer a priori. During the acquisition process, the appropriate pixel for each event would need to be determined, as well as the appropriate frame within the heart cycle.

In list mode, the (x,y) location of each event is stored using the highest level of digitization possible as a stream. In addition, timing and physiological gating marks may be stored periodically. For example, a timing mark may be stored every millisecond, as can the time of the R peak in the ECG (Fig. 4-14). After the acquisition is complete, the user can then select the desired matrix size and the

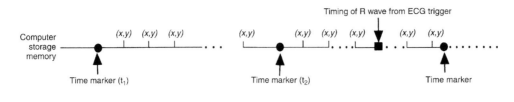

FIGURE 4-14. List mode data acquisition. In *list mode*, the (x,y) position of each detection event is determined at the highest available resolution and stored in sequence. In addition, time markers and physiological signals (such as the timing of the R wave from the electrocardiogram trigger) are periodically stored. Once the acquisition is completed, the desired matrix size, time-sequence, and physiological gate framing can be selected and a formatting program is run to provide the acquired data for viewing and analysis.

temporal or physiological framing rate a posteriori. Based on these criteria, a postacquisition program is run to format the data as defined. The user could then decide to reformat the data to a different set of parameters. In this way, list mode acquisition is very flexible because it does not require the user to define the acquisition matrix and framing a priori. On the other hand, it typically requires more computer storage and running the formatting program to view the data. For these reasons, matrix mode is most commonly used.

Each pixel in the planar nuclear medicine image can be considered its own detector, and thus the total counts in a pixel is governed by Poisson statistics similar to a well counter or a thyroid probe. Therefore the standard deviation of the pixel counts is simply estimated by the square root of the pixel counts. In addition, the sum of Poisson distributed values is also a Poisson distributed value. Therefore, if a region of interest is defined on a planar nuclear medicine image and the pixel values within that region are added, the result is also Poisson distributed. Nuclear medicine studies are often quantified by defining regions of interest (ROIs) over features of interest and subsequently comparing the counts. In some cases, the counts from different views of the patient can be combined to provide more accurate quantitation. For example, taking the geometric mean (square root of the product of the counts) of similar regions from opposite, conjugate views such as the anterior and posterior views, can provide an estimate that, to first order, does not depend on the depth of the activity within the body. Theoretically, this approach works for point sources, but also has been shown to work reasonably well for extended sources. The counts are determined from the ROIs drawn about each lung, right and left, on images acquired from both the anterior and posterior views of the patient. The geometric mean of the counts in each lung is calculated, and the differential function of each lung is estimated by dividing the counts for that lung by the sum of counts for both lungs.

In a dynamic study, the region of interest counts in each frame can be plotted as a function of time. The resulting plot is referred to as the time activity curve (TAC). In the case of relatively short-lived radionuclides, each value along the plot should be decay corrected to the beginning of the acquisition or the time of radiopharmaceutical administration. In the example of a Tc-99m MAG3 renal study, a TAC can be used to evaluate both renal perfusion and clearance of the agent.

▬ SUMMARY

Radiation detection and counting is the corner stone of nuclear medicine. Detectors of all types—gas detectors, scintillators, and semiconductors—are used every day in the nuclear medicine clinic. Some are used for ancillary purposes that support the clinic, such as those used in the context of radiation protection. Others are used to specifically acquire biological data for a particular clinical purpose. Most notably, the gamma camera is used to obtain images of the in vivo distribution of the administered radiopharmaceutical from which the patient's physiology or function can be inferred to further define the patient's medical picture. A rigorous quality control program must be maintained for all equipment used in the nuclear medicine clinic to ensure the integrity of the data obtained from the patient. The quality control program for the gamma camera includes acceptance testing and tests that need to be performed on a routine basis. The nuclear medicine image acquired with the gamma camera provides a snapshot of the patient's in vivo radiopharmaceutical distribution from a certain view and at a particular point in time. These images also can be acquired as a dynamic (time-sequence) study or in conjunction with a physiological gate such as the ECG. Regions of interest can be drawn about specific features to provide regional quantitation or TACs of dynamic processes. Nuclear medicine instrumentation continues to evolve, including the development of devices designed for a specific clinical task such as breast imaging. It is expected that this development will continue in the years ahead.

▬ SUGGESTED READING

Chandra R. *Nuclear Medicine Physics: The Basics.* 7th ed. Philadelphia: Williams & Wilkins; 2011.
Cherry SR, Sorenson JA, Phelps ME. *Physics in Nuclear Medicine.* 4th ed. Philadelphia: WB Saunders; 2012.
International Atomic Energy Agency. *IAEA Quality Control Atlas for Scintillation Camera Systems.* Publication 1141. Vienna, Austria: International Atomic Energy Agency; 2003.
International Atomic Energy Agency. *Nuclear Medicine Resources Manual.* Publication 1198. Vienna, Austria: International Atomic Energy Agency; 2006.
National Electrical Manufacturers Association. *Performance Measurements of Gamma Cameras:* NEMA NU 1-2007. Rosslyn, VA: National Electrical Manufacturers Association; 2007.
Powsner RA, Powsner ER. *Essentials of Nuclear Medicine Physics.* 2nd ed. Malden, MA: Blackwell Science; 2006.
Saha GP. *Physics and Radiobiology of Nuclear Medicine.* 3rd ed. New York: Springer; 2006.

Single-Photon Emission Computed Tomography, Positron Emission Tomography, and Hybrid Imaging

Conventional or planar radionuclide imaging suffers a major limitation in loss of object contrast as a result of background radioactivity. In the planar image, radioactivity underlying and overlying the object of interest is superimposed on that coming from the object. The fundamental goal of tomographic imaging systems is a more accurate portrayal of the three-dimensional (3D) distribution of radioactivity in the patient, with improved image contrast and definition of image detail. This is analogous to the way computed tomography (CT) provides better soft-tissue contrast than planar radiography. The Greek *tomo* means "to cut"; tomography may be thought of as a means of "cutting" the body into discrete image planes. Tomographic techniques have been developed for both single-photon and positron imaging, referred to as single-photon emission computed tomography (SPECT) and positron emission tomography (PET), respectively.

Restricted or limited-angle tomography keeps the plane of interest in focus while blurring the out-of-plane data in much the same way as conventional x-ray tomography. Various restricted-angle systems have been investigated, including multipinhole collimator systems, pseudocoded random coded-aperture collimator systems, and various rotating slant-hole collimator systems. Although clinical use has been limited, recent resurgent interest has been shown for specific imaging applications, including those designed for cardiac and breast imaging.

Tomographic approaches that acquire data over 180 or 360 degrees provide a more complete reconstruction of the object and therefore are more widely used. Rotating gamma camera SPECT systems offer the ability to perform true transaxial tomography. PET uses a method called *annihilation coincidence detection* to acquire data over 360 degrees without the use of absorptive collimation. The most important characteristic of these approaches is that only data arising in the image plane are used in the reconstruction of the tomographic image. This is an important characteristic leading to improved image contrast compared to methods using restricted-angle tomography. As will be discussed, the reconstruction of these data has historically been done with filtered backprojection. However, iterative techniques such as ordered subsets expectation maximization (OSEM) are increasingly used. This chapter will review the current approaches to the acquisition and reconstruction of SPECT and PET, including the use of hybrid imaging such as PET/CT and SPECT/CT, as well as the quality control necessary to ensure high-quality clinical results.

IMAGE RECONSTRUCTION

All tomographic modalities used in diagnostic imaging, including SPECT, PET, CT, and magnetic resonance imaging (MRI) acquire raw data in the form of *projection data* at a variety of angles about the patient. Although SPECT and PET use different approaches to acquiring these data, the nature of the data are essentially the same. Image reconstruction involves the processing of these data to generate a series of cross-sectional images through the object of interest.

Projection Data

The geometries associated with the acquisition of SPECT and PET are illustrated in Figure 5-1. In the simple SPECT example using a parallel-hole collimator, the data acquired at a particular location in the gamma camera crystal originated from a line passing through that point perpendicular to the surface of the sodium iodide (NaI) crystal face and is referred to in the figure as the *line of origin* (Fig. 5-1, *left*). Thus the data at this point can be seen to represent the sum of counts that originated along this line, or *ray*, referred to as a *ray sum*. These ray sum values across the patient are referred to as the projection data for this cross-sectional slice at this particular viewing angle. For PET, the ray sum represents the data collected along a particular line of response (LOR) connecting a pair of detectors involved in a coincidence detection event (Fig. 5-1, *right*).

For a SPECT acquisition, the projection image acquired at each angle consists of the stack of projections for all slices within the camera field of view at that angle. Figure 5-2, on the right, shows projections from a SPECT brain scan at five different viewing angles. For a particular slice (Fig. 5-2, *dashed white line*), a row of the projection data for each angle can be stacked such that the displacement along the projection is on the x-axis and the viewing angle is on the y-axis (Fig. 5-2, *right*). This plot is referred to as

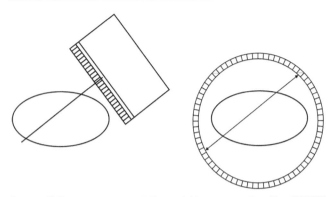

FIGURE 5-1. SPECT and PET acquisition geometries. For SPECT *(left)*, the gamma camera rotates about the patient, acquiring a projection image at each angle. Each projection image represents the projections of many slices acquired at that angle. For PET *(right)*, the patient is located within a ring of detectors. A positron annihilation event leads to two photons emitted in opposite directions. The detection of two events within a small timing acceptance window (5-12 ns) are considered to be from the same event and assumed to have originated along the line of response that connects the two detectors.

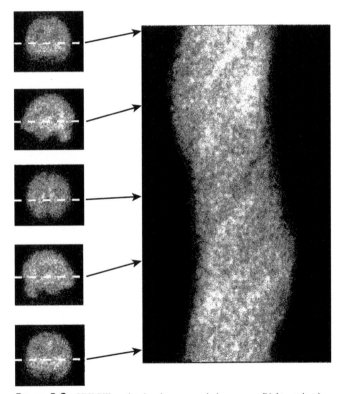

FIGURE 5-2. SPECT projection images and sinograms. *Right*, projection images of a SPECT brain scan at five different viewing angles. For a particular slice (indicated by the *dashed white line*), the projection data can be stacked to form the sinogram *(left)*. (From Henkin RE. *Nuclear Medicine.* St. Louis: Mosby; 2006, Fig. 15-7.)

the *sinogram* because the resulting plot of a point source resembles a sine wave plot turned on its side. A more complicated object such as a brain scan can be perceived as many such sine waves overlaid on top of each other for each point within the object. The sinogram represents the full set of projection data necessary to reconstruct a particular single slice. A separate slice is made in the sinogram for each cross-sectional slice through the object. The set of projection views and the set of sinograms are alternative means of displaying the projection data associated with a tomographic acquisition. Each projection view displays the projection data across all slices with a separate image for each angle, whereas the sinogram displays the projection data across all angles with a separate sinogram for each slice.

The geometry of PET acquisition (Fig. 5-1, *right*) involves the data acquired along a particular LOR connecting two detectors that may be involved in an annihilation coincidence detection event. These data thus represent the ray sum along this LOR. Data associated with a particular LOR is characterized in the sinogram by its distance from the center of the gantry (on the x-axis) and its angle of orientation (on the y-axis). In this manner, PET data acquisition directly into sinograms may be more straightforward than into projection views. In a PET detection event, the two detectors involved in the coincidence event are identified and the LOR is recorded. The location in the sinogram corresponding to that particular LOR is localized and its data incremented. After the collection of many such events, the projection data are represented by a set of sinograms for each PET slice. However, these data also can be displayed as projection views similar to those acquired in SPECT studies. This simple example illustrates the acquisition of PET data in *2D mode*, in which each cross-sectional slice basically is acquired separately. Most current PET scanners acquire data only in *3D mode*, in which LORs cut across the parallel cross-section slices. The corresponding projection data will include oblique views or sinograms through the object. With time-of-flight PET (discussed later in this chapter), it is necessary to record not only the LOR but also the time difference between the two detections involved in the annihilation coincidence detection event, which will also be incorporated into the reconstruction of these data.

Tomographic data can be acquired in a dynamic or gated approach. For example, a PET study can be acquired as a time-sequence of scans that might be simple or multiphase (e.g., ten 5-second frames, four 30-second frames, and five 60-second frames). In addition, the tomographic study can be acquired in association with a physiologic gate such as the electrocardiogram (ECG) or a respiratory signal. For example, myocardial perfusion SPECT is acquired in conjunction with the ECG. In dynamic or gated tomographic acquisitions, a full set of projection data acquired at each time or gate point is to be reconstructed separately.

Spatial Real and Frequency Space

Images, like time signals, can be considered as either a spatial variation of the signal or a sum of signals of varying frequencies. It is intuitive to consider images as a spatial variation in the signal, because some part of the image will be bright and others will be dark. In nuclear medicine, the bright and dark areas may correspond to regions of high and low radiopharmaceutical uptake, respectively. Conversely, it is not intuitive to consider an image to comprise signals of varying frequency, although this is in fact the case. On the other hand, we do naturally perceive audio

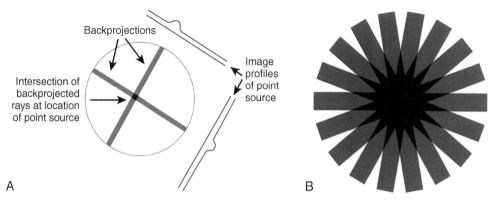

FIGURE 5-3. Simple backprojection. **A,** The counts in each position along the projection are backprojected across the reconstruction matrix because the algorithm has no knowledge as to the origin of the event. This process is referred to as *simple backprojection*. **B,** Simple backprojection leads to streak artifacts that render all but the simplest objects discernable.

signals in terms of frequencies. A choral performance comprises sopranos, altos, tenors, and basses, and the combination of these voices hopefully leads to a very pleasurable experience. On the other hand, we cannot perceive a presentation of the audio signal as a temporal variation of the signal and intuitively identify it as music. The music is fully described by either representation, and there may be cases in which either the temporal (i.e., real) or the frequency representation is the best approach for considering the audio data. The same is true for image data, except the variations are in space rather than time.

Image data may be best represented in either spatial (real) or frequency space. The mathematician Joseph Fourier noted in 1807 that any arbitrary signal can be generated by adding a large number of sine and cosine signals of varying frequencies and amplitudes. The plot of amplitude as a function of frequency is referred to as the *Fourier transform*, and it defines the components of the image at each frequency. The low frequencies provide the overall shape of the object, whereas the high frequencies help define the sharp edges and fine detail within the image. Audio signals can be manipulated by emphasizing certain frequencies (low or high); the same is true for images. Image noise is typically present in all frequencies; if the low frequencies are emphasized, the image may be less noisy but blurry, whereas emphasizing the high frequencies will accentuate both the edges of the objects and the noise. Such image manipulation is referred to as *filtering* because it allows certain spatial frequencies to be realized while removing others.

Filtered Backprojection

Since the initial development of CT 40 years ago, *filtered backprojection* has been the most common approach to reconstructing medical tomographic data, including SPECT, PET, and CT, although iterative techniques were introduced into the clinic for use with PET more than a decade ago. However, filtered backprojection is still used in SPECT and remains the most common method for CT. In backprojection, it is assumed that all of the data detected at a particular point along the projection originated from somewhere along the line emanating from this point. For SPECT using parallel-hole collimation, this would be the line of origin passing through the detection point and perpendicular to the NaI crystal surface. For PET, events would be assumed to have come from the LOR connecting the two detectors involved in the annihilation coincidence detection event. In general, backprojection makes no assumptions of where along the line the event occurred and thus the counts are spread evenly along the line. In other words, the counts are *backprojected* along the line of origin or LOR. All of the counts from every location along every projection are *backprojected* across the reconstructed image (Fig 5-3, *A*). The result is referred to as *simple backprojection*; it has substantial streak artifacts that, in all but the simplest objects, render the reconstructed image indiscernible (Fig. 5-3, *B*). These streaks are caused by uneven sampling of frequency space during the backprojection process, where low frequencies are sampled at a much higher rate than higher frequencies. To compensate for this, a filter is applied during the reconstruction that increases linearly with frequency called the *ramp filter* (Fig. 5-4). Applying backprojection in conjunction with such filtration is referred to as *filtered backprojection*. With a very large number of accurate, noiseless projections, filtered backprojection will yield an excellent, almost perfect reconstruction.

However, with true clinical data, the projections are noisy and thus the ramp filter will tend to accentuate the high-frequency noise in the data. Therefore a *windowing filter* is applied in addition to the ramp filter, to smoothly bring the filter back to zero at frequencies above the pertinent content in the study. Commonly used windowing functions include the Hamming and Butterworth filters (Fig. 5-4). With these filters, a cutoff frequency is defined, which is the point at which they return to zero with no higher frequencies being incorporated into the reconstructed image. Noting that low frequencies yield the overall shape and high frequencies yield the sharp edges and fine detail, the appearance of the resultant reconstructed image can be altered by varying the cutoff frequency. Selecting a cutoff frequency that is too low will yield a blurry reconstruction (Fig. 5-5, *A, far left*), and one that is too high will yield a noisy reconstruction (Fig. 5-5, *C, second from the right*). However, an appropriate choice for cutoff frequency will provide an image that is a fair compromise between noise and detail (Fig. 5-5, *B, second from left*). With an appropriate choice of cutoff frequency, filtered backprojection is a simple, fast, and robust approach to image reconstruction.

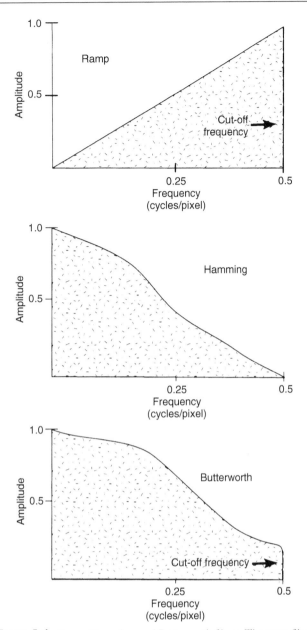

FIGURE 5-4. Ramp, Hamming, and Butterworth filters. The ramp filter is a "high-pass" filter designed to reduce background activity and the star artifact. Hamming and Butterworth filters are "low-pass" filters designed to reduce high-frequency noise.

Iterative Reconstruction

Iterative reconstruction provides an alternative to filtered backprojection that tends to be less noisy, have fewer streak artifacts, and often allows for the incorporation of certain physical factors associated with the data acquisition into the reconstruction process, leading to a more accurate result. In iterative reconstruction, an initial guess as to the 3D object that could have led to the set of acquired projections is estimated. In addition, a model of the imaging process is assumed that may incorporate assumptions regarding photon attenuation and Compton scatter. It may also include other assumptions regarding the data acquisition process such as estimates of the device's spatial resolution that vary with position within the field of view; for example, the variation of collimator spatial resolution as a function of the distance between the object and the collimator can be incorporated into the reconstruction process.

Based on this model and the current estimate of the object, a new set of projections are simulated that are then compared to the real, acquired set. Variations between the two sets, parameterized by either the ratio or difference between pixel values, are then backprojected and added to the current estimate of the object to generate a new estimate (Fig. 5-6). These steps are repeated, or *iterated*, until an acceptable version of the object is reached. The goodness of the current estimate is typically based on statistical criteria such as the maximum likelihood. In other words, the process generates an estimate of the object that has the highest statistical likelihood to have led to the set of acquired projection data. A commonly used approach for the reconstruction of SPECT and PET data is the *maximum likelihood expectation maximization* (MLEM) algorithm.

Iterative reconstruction often leads to a more accurate reconstruction of the data than that obtained through filtered backprojection. However, a large number of iterations, perhaps as many as 50, may be required to generate an acceptable estimation and each iteration may take about the same time as a single filtered backprojection; thus the iterative approach may take 50 times longer to reconstruct. One approach to reducing the number of iterations is to organize the projection data into a series of ordered subsets of evenly spaced projections and update the current estimate of the object after each subset rather than after the complete set of projections. If the data are organized into 15 subsets, in general, the data can be reconstructed about 15 times faster while generating a result of similar image

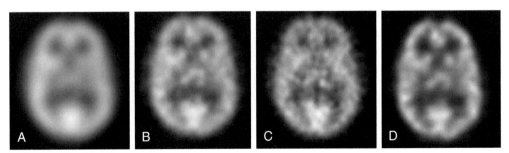

FIGURE 5-5. Effect of different filtration on reconstruction. **A,** SPECT study reconstructed with a cutoff frequency that is too smooth. The image is very blurry. **B,** SPECT study reconstructed with an appropriate cutoff frequency, with a moderate noise level and sharpness. **C,** SPECT study reconstructed with a cutoff frequency that is too sharp. The level of detail is good, but an excessive amount of image noise is present. **D,** SPECT study acquired with iterative reconstruction OSEM.

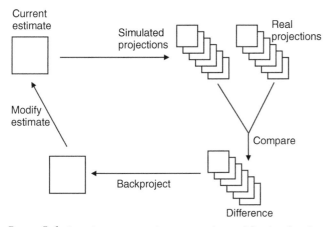

FIGURE 5-6. Iterative reconstruction process. A set of simulated projections is generated from an initial guess of the object. This is compared to the real projection data and the difference is backprojected and added to the initial guess. This process in iterated until the differences between the simulated and real projections is within an acceptable level.

quality. A similar result can be produced with 15 ordered subsets and 3 iterations, as would be obtained with 45 iterations using the complete set. The most common approach that uses ordered subsets in the clinic is referred to as OSEM. Figure 5-5, *D (far right)* shows an OSEM reconstruction compared to a filtered backprojection of the same object. The use of faster algorithms such as OSEM and the development of faster computers have allowed iterative reconstruction of SPECT and PET data in 5 minutes or less, which is considered acceptable for clinical work. With the development of even faster computers, iterative reconstruction may be routinely applied to the larger data sets associated with CT in the near future.

Attenuation Correction

A special problem of both SPECT and PET imaging is the attenuation of emissions in tissue. Photons emitted from deeper within the object are more likely to be absorbed in the overlying tissue than those emitted from the periphery. Therefore the signals from these tissues are *attenuated*. To obtain an image where the signal is not depth dependent, an *attenuation correction* must be performed to compensate for this effect. Good evidence indicates that studies that have not traditionally been attenuation corrected, such as myocardial perfusion imaging, benefit from proper attenuation correction. Two fundamentally different approaches are used for attenuation correction: analytic methods and those that incorporate transmission data into the process. Both are designed to create an image attenuation correction matrix, in which the value of each pixel represents the correction factor that should be applied to the acquired data. Some approaches are applied during reconstruction, whereas others are applied after reconstruction to the resultant images.

Analytic Attenuation Correction

For portions of the body consisting almost entirely of soft tissue, an assumption of near uniform attenuation can be made, and an analytic or mathematical approach such as the Chang algorithm can be used. The Chang algorithm is

a postreconstruction approach. After the object is reconstructed, an outline of the body part is defined on the computer for each tomographic slice. From this outline, the depth and therefore the appropriate correction factor for each pixel location inside the outline can be computed. A correction matrix is generated, and a multiplicative correction is applied on a pixel-by-pixel basis. The linear attenuation coefficient for Tc-99m in soft tissue is 0.15/cm. This applies only to "good" geometry—that is, a point source with no scatter. Thus a value for Tc-99m of approximately 0.12/cm is often used to compensate for scatter. At a depth of 7 cm in a liver SPECT study, almost 60% of the corresponding activity is attenuated. The observed count value would have to be multiplied by a factor of 2.5 ($0.4 \times 2.5 = 1$) to correct for attenuation. A similar analytic method has been developed for PET imaging, primarily of the brain.

Computed Tomography–Based Attenuation Correction

The major limitation of the analytic approach occurs when multiple types of tissue, each with a different attenuation coefficient, are in the field of view. This can be particularly problematic for cardiac imaging, in which the soft tissues of the heart are surrounded by the air-containing lungs and the bony structures of the thorax. To correct for nonuniform attenuation, a transmission scanning approach is incorporated into the attenuation correction. In essence, a CT scan of the thorax is obtained using an x-ray tube. Older SPECT and PET systems also have used radionuclide sources for this purpose. The technique is similar to the use of CT, except radioactive sources incorporated into the scanner are used rather than an x-ray tube. The data are much noisier and require segmentation into the different tissue types before the attenuation map can be created. Manufacturers are moving away from the radioactive source methodology.

A hybrid SPECT-CT or PET-CT scanner is used to acquire a CT over the same axial range as the SPECT or PET scan. The CT scan is acquired with a tube voltage of 80 to 120 kVp, leading to an effective energy of about 40 to 60 keV. The range of the tube current time product (milliamperes) is variable, depending on whether the CT scan is acquired for diagnostic purposes, for anatomical correlation, or for attenuation correction. Thus scans could be acquired with as little as 4 and as high as 400 mA. A lookup table is used to convert the Hounsfield units in the reconstructed CT scan to attenuation coefficients for the desired photon energy. The resulting attenuation map can then be applied as a post-reconstruction correction or incorporated in the reconstruction process.

Image Reformatting: Sagittal, Coronal, Oblique Views and Reprojection

A particular advantage of gamma camera rotational SPECT is that a volume of image data is collected simultaneously. PET data may be acquired in several steps, but the resultant reconstructed data are also a volume. The pixel size for SPECT is the same in the three axes; for PET, the axial sampling might be slightly different from that in the transverse plane. However, in either case, once the transaxial tomographic volume is reconstructed, it easily can be resorted into

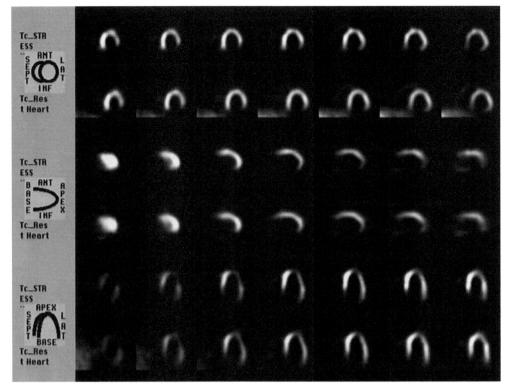

FIGURE 5-7. Cardiac SPECT images reformat data into multiple planes. The top two rows are short-axis views obtained perpendicular to the long axis of the left ventricle. The middle two rows are horizontal long-axis images, and the bottom two rows are vertical long-axis images. The patient has a large fixed perfusion defect involving the inferior wall of the left ventricle. The ability to reformat the data allows more precise and accurate localization of abnormalities.

other orthogonal planes. Thus the sagittal and coronal images can be directly generated from the reconstructed volume represented by the set of transaxial slices.

The data can be reformatted into planes oblique to the original transverse planes. This is particularly useful in cardiac imaging, in which the long axis of the heart does not coincide with any of the three major axes of the reconstructed data. It is desirable to reorient the data to obtain images that are perpendicular and parallel to the long axis of the left ventricle, which can be readily accomplished from the original volume data set. The computer operator defines the geometry of the long axis of the heart, and the data are reformatted to create cardiac long-axis and short-axis planes oblique to the transaxial slices (Fig. 5-7). The optimum angulation is highly variable across patients.

Another useful strategy is to view tomographic data as a sequence of planar images from different viewing angles in closed loop cine. In the early days of SPECT imaging, this was accomplished by viewing the closed loop cine of the raw projection data. This is still done in many cardiac imaging software packages for quality control. However, these data tend to be noisy, making it difficult to view small variations in intensity. Currently, a common approach is to reproject the transaxial images to generate a series of planar images that have the benefit of greatly reduced noise. The reprojection method often used is the *maximum intensity projection scan* (MIPS), created by reprojecting the hottest point along each particular ray for any given projection. These MIPS images emphasize areas of increased accumulation of radioactivity while providing an overall impression of the area of increased radioactivity in relation

to the normal structures in individual tomographic slices. In some cases the MIPS images are distance weighted to make activity that is farther from the viewer appear less intense, thereby enhancing the 3D effect.

■ SINGLE-PHOTON EMISSION COMPUTED TOMOGRAPHY

SPECT allows true 3D image acquisition, reconstruction, and display of radiopharmaceuticals routinely used in conventional nuclear medicine. Over the past 30 years, SPECT has developed, particularly in the field of nuclear cardiology, to the point at which SPECT has become the standard imaging method. In SPECT, a series of projection images are acquired about the patient. In most cases, these projection images are acquired by rotating the imaging device about the object but in other cases they may be acquired by viewing the object by multiple devices or through multiple pinhole apertures. These projection data are then reconstructed as described in the previous section, leading to the generation a series of slices through the object.

Instrumentation

The most common device used for SPECT is the rotating gamma camera, which consists of one or more gamma camera heads mounted onto a special rotating gantry. Nearly all gamma cameras marketed today incorporate SPECT capability. Early systems used a single gamma camera head, whereas modern systems more commonly have two

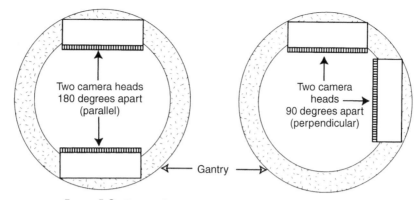

FIGURE 5-8. Two configurations for a dual-detector SPECT system.

detector heads. Dual head systems that allow flexibility in configuration between the heads are very popular. For body imaging, the heads are typically arrayed parallel to each other; for cardiac imaging they are often placed at right angles (Fig. 5-8). Some cameras are permanently configured in the 90-degree position for dedicated cardiac imaging. Multiple heads are desirable because they allow more data to be collected in a given period. Rotational SPECT is photon poor compared to x-ray CT, and thus SPECT imaging protocols commonly take 10 to 30 minutes for acquisition of a data set. Therefore it is desirable to obtain as many counts as possible while completing the imaging within a reasonable time to limit the effects of patient motion and to minimize pharmacokinetic changes during the imaging time. Rotational SPECT has highlighted the need to improve every aspect of gamma camera system performance. Flood field nonuniformities are translated as major artifacts in tomographic images because they distort the data obtained from each view or projection. Desirable planar characteristics of a camera to be used for SPECT are an intrinsic spatial resolution of 3.5 mm (as estimated by the full-width at half-maximum [FWHM]), linearity distortion of 1 mm or less, and corrected integral uniformity within 3%. All contemporary rotational SPECT systems have online energy and uniformity correction, as described in Chapter 4.

Dedicated Cardiac Single-Photon Emission Computed Tomography Systems
Recently, dedicated SPECT systems have been developed for cardiac imaging only. These cameras may use Anger logic for event positioning; however, they are distinctly different in that they are not large, single-crystal detectors as are found in the traditional gamma camera and many use solid-state detectors of cadmium zinc telluride (CZT) rather than NaI scintillating material. These detectors often use a pixelated design with detector elements approximately 2 × 2 mm. Because of their multicrystal design, the scintillation-based systems often use either position-sensitive photomultiplier tubes or photodiodes for light detection. The systems that use CZT have higher intrinsic efficiency and enhanced energy resolution (6% at 140 keV compared to 9%-11% compared to NaI). This allows for the reduction of Compton scatter in the images and may also enhance the ability to perform dual isotope acquisitions (e.g., technetium-99m and iodine-123).

Box 5-1. Image Acquisition Issues for Single-Photon Emission Computed Tomography

Collimator selection
Orbit
Matrix size
Angular increment: number of views
180- vs. 360-degree rotation
Time per view
Total examination time

Finally, the detectors in these systems have physical design characteristics that improve sensitivity. For instance, multiple detectors or pinhole apertures may be viewing the heart simultaneously. These improvements in sensitivity can be used to shorten the acquisition time or lower the quantity of injected radioactivity and thereby lower the patient's radiation dose. Each system has different design characteristics, acquisition procedures, and quality control methods. Although these devices are promising, their use remains quite limited; therefore the rest of this section will focus on the rotating camera.

Image Acquisition

Box 5-1 summarizes factors that must be considered in performing SPECT with a rotating gamma camera. In addition to the calibrations described earlier and standard gamma camera quality control, careful attention to each of these factors will result in the high-quality SPECT images.

Collimator Selection
Although collimator selection is generally limited to those supplied by the manufacturer, the specific choice depends on the clinical imaging task at hand. For a given septal thickness and hole diameter, collimators with longer channels provide better resolution but at a cost of lower sensitivity. However, even though SPECT is relatively photon poor, collimator selection should favor high resolution over high sensitivity when possible because high-resolution collimators provide improved image quality compared to high-sensitivity or general-purpose collimators, even with fewer counts. The use of multihead SPECT systems allows the operator to gain back some of the counts lost

when using high-resolution collimators by longer acquisition at each step or projection angle.

In addition to the parallel-hole collimators routinely used for planar and SPECT imaging, there are special focused collimator options specifically designed for SPECT imaging the brain and the heart. These typically are a type of converging collimator that permits more of the camera crystal to be used for radiation detection. These collimators cause magnification of the object and an increase in sensitivity proportional to the level of magnification. Thus, given a parallel-hole collimator and a focused collimator with the same spatial resolution, the focused collimator will have an improvement in sensitivity compared to the parallel-hole collimator. The use of focused collimators results in a geometric distortion that must be accounted for in the reconstruction.

Orbit

The orbit selected (circular or noncircular) depends on the organ of interest (Fig. 5-9). Almost all systems today offer both circular and noncircular orbits. The ideal orbit keeps the detector as close to the object of interest as possible during the acquisition since the best resolution is at the face of the collimator for parallel-hole collimators. For imaging the

trunk of the body, most cameras use noncircular orbit for this reason. Both circular and noncircular orbits may be used for imaging the brain depending on whether the operator is able to position the detectors to clear the shoulders. When using special focused collimators, the orbit is often determined automatically by the system that keeps the organ of interest in the focused area.

Angular Sampling, Matrix Size, Arc of Acquisition, and Rotation Motion

The choice of angular sampling and arc of acquisition depend on the clinical application and the collimator used. For body imaging applications, a full 360-degree acquisition arc is commonly used. Most SPECT data are acquired using a 128 × 128 image matrix with high-resolution collimators and Tc-99m radiopharmaceuticals. However, a 64 × 64 matrix may be used when the camera resolution is not as good or if the count density will be low because very little activity occurs in the patient at the time of imaging. Many SPECT/CT hybrid cameras in which a CT scan will be used for attenuation correction require that the emission data be acquired in a 128 × 128 matrix. If the 128 × 128 matrix is used, the angular sampling should be set to 3-degree increments. If the lower-resolution 64 × 64 matrix is used, the step size may be increased to 4- or 6-degree increments. These combinations of matrix size and angular sampling, along with the collimator selection, "balance" the resolution of the respective parameters. However, these parameters may be varied in some circumstances. For example, acquiring fewer steps may be acceptable for pediatric patients given their smaller size.

For cardiac imaging, a 180-degree acquisition arc is well accepted. Because the heart is located close to the anterior chest wall on the left side, the best data are obtained by imaging in a 180-degree arc that spans from the right anterior oblique to the left posterior oblique positions (Fig. 5-10). This acquisition paradigm is widely accepted in the clinical practice even when CT attenuation correction is applied to the data.

Another consideration is whether to use continuous or "step-and-shoot" data acquisition. Continuous acquisition has the advantage of not wasting time while the camera heads are moving from one angular position to the next.

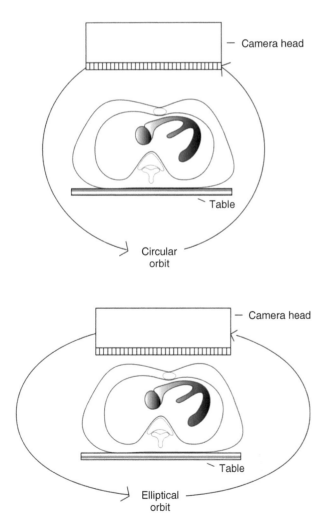

FIGURE 5-9. Circular orbit *(top)* and noncircular (elliptical in this case) orbit *(bottom)*.

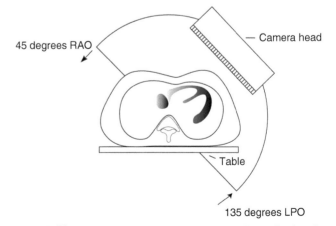

FIGURE 5-10. The 180-degree arc frequently used for cardiac imaging from right anterior oblique (RAO, 45 degrees) to left posterior oblique (LPO, 135 degrees).

However, the data are blurred by the motion artifact of the moving camera head. The resulting trade-off between sensitivity and resolution favor step-and-shoot acquisition for most clinical applications. Exceptions are applications with rapidly changing tracer distribution and when determination of overall tracer concentration is more important than spatial resolution.

Imaging Time and Patient Factors

In general, SPECT studies are count poor and thus it is beneficial to acquire the studies for as long as possible. Within accepted limits for dosimetry and radiation exposure, a larger administered dosage may allow for more available counts. Although clinically accepted limits for administered radioactivity should never be exceeded, the radiation risk versus benefit must take into account the likelihood of obtaining a diagnostic-quality image. The goal of obtaining higher counting statistics is meaningless if the patient moves, causing data between the different angular sampling views to be misregistered. Most clinical protocols limit the total imaging time to 20 to 40 minutes. Correspondingly, the time per projection is usually 20 to 40 seconds, but as much as 60 seconds may be needed for particularly count-poor studies with gallium-67 and indium-111.

Even when restricting the total SPECT acquisition time to less than 30 minutes, patient motion may still be an issue. Some camera manufacturers provide motion correction programs, but these work in only one dimension (vertical motion), not three dimensions. Patient compliance is improved by taking time during setup to position the patient comfortably. For scans of the head, the patient's arms can be in a natural position at the sides. For rotational SPECT studies of the heart, thorax, abdomen, or pelvis, the arms are typically raised out of the field of view so that they do not interfere with the path of photons toward the detector, which may increase the patient's discomfort. In all applications, it is important to keep the injection site out of the field of view to prevent artifacts resulting from residual or infiltrated activity (Fig. 5-11). Compliance also can be improved by positioning the patient for maximum comfort by placing support under the knees to reduce strain on the lower back. If the patient's arms are over the head, additional support for the arms may be needed to alleviate shoulder pain.

Corrections, Calibrations, and Quality Control

Before a rotating SPECT camera is used, it must be properly calibrated. The calibrations necessary for proper operation are uniformity, center of rotation, and pixel size. For cameras that have more than one detector, the heads must be matched so that when each head is at the same projection angle—for example, directly above the patient—it will record events that occur in the same location within the object, at the same (x, y) location in the acquired projection image. This is usually accomplished by imaging a set of sources at known locations and matching the pixel size and center of rotation for the two detectors. The head matching and pixel size adjustments may be performed by the field service engineer, with routine adjustments by the technologist. The technologist will usually perform the uniformity and center-of-rotation calibrations. Each

manufacturer will specify how and with what frequency these calibrations should be performed. The most common frequency is to perform these calibrations on a monthly basis. However, some manufacturers may recommend longer frequencies up to once per quarter.

Uniformity Calibration

All gamma cameras, regardless of how well tuned, will have residual nonuniformities. Minor variations in uniformity, not discernible in planar imaging, will result in significant *ring* or *bulls-eye* artifacts in a SPECT study (Fig. 5-12, *arrows*). The usual 5 to 10 million count uniformity image used for routine quality control is inadequate for uniformity calibration in SPECT imaging. For cameras with a large field of view and a 128 × 128 matrix, 100 to 200 million counts (roughly 10,000 counts per pixel) are required to achieve the desired pixel count that results in a relative standard deviation of 1%, which is necessary for artifact-free SPECT. Acquiring this number of counts requires a significant amount of time. The temptation to use very large amounts of radioactivity should be avoided because high count rates can also result in degraded performance of the gamma camera electronics and recording of spurious coincident events. Conservatively, the correction floods should be obtained at 20,000 to 30,000 counts per second. The uniformity calibration can be acquired either intrinsically using a point source or extrinsically with a flood source. The radioactivity in the flood source should have a uniformity of 1%. Although water-filled flood sources can be used for this calibration, they are difficult to mix and are subject to bulging. For this reason, sealed cobalt-57 sources are routinely used for acquiring the extrinsic uniformity calibration.

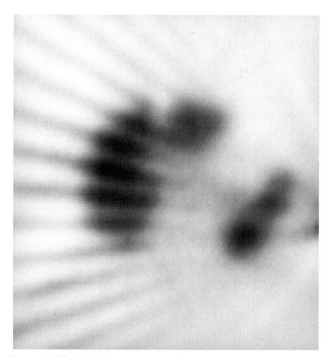

FIGURE 5-11. SPECT artifact caused by injection site activity in the field of view. Degraded SPECT image of the liver and spleen caused by including activity at the injection site in the imaging field of view. The starburst artifact is due to backprojection of the hot spot activity across the image. In this case, the degree of activity in the injection site could not be accommodated in the reconstruction algorithm.

Center of Rotation

The center of rotation calibration matches the axis of rotation to the center of the image matrix. When viewing the rotational display of the raw SPECT data, it is the point about which the raw data rotates. Most importantly, it is

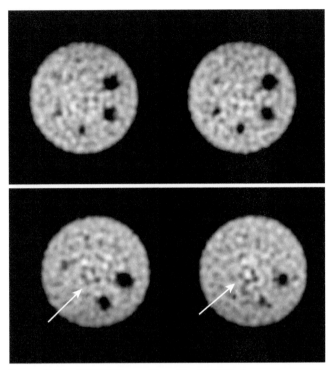

FIGURE 5-12. SPECT Ring artifacts. *Top,* SPECT phantom image with no ring artifact. *Bottom,* SPECT phantom image with significant ring artifacts (indicated by *arrows*) caused by inadequate uniformity calibration.

the alignment point for the reconstruction. A common practice is to acquire the center of rotation correction on the same schedule as the uniformity correction. Many multiple-detector systems also use these data to match the heads. Each manufacturer has a very specific protocol for the center of rotation and multihead registration that typically involves the acquisition of a series of images of a set of point or line sources of radioactivity.

Camera Quality Control

As previously discussed, rotational SPECT requires maximum performance of the gamma camera. Performance that may be considered acceptable for planar imaging can render a SPECT study unreadable. In addition to the calibrations discussed earlier, all routine daily, weekly, and annual quality control procedures for gamma cameras should be performed. Particular attention should be paid to variations in uniformity because small variations in the field uniformity may result in significant artifacts.

A cylindrical tomographic phantom should be imaged periodically. An example of a phantom is shown in Figure 5-13. Radioactivity can be added to this water-filled phantom to provide a uniform source that can be used to test for the presence of ring artifacts caused by inadequate uniformity calibration. In addition, other structures within the phantom can test SPECT system performance with respect to contrast and spatial resolution. In the example shown, solid Plexiglas rods of varying size and spacing as well as solid spheres of varying size are also imaged. These structures provide *cold* structures within the phantom— that is, areas of no activity. The phantom also may provide *hot* structures. It is customary to routinely acquire a SPECT study of such a phantom (e.g., quarterly) and compare the

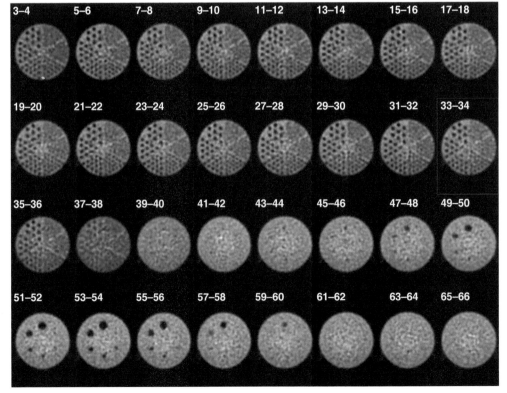

FIGURE 5-13. SPECT quality control phantom. A series of slices from a phantom acquisition.

results to a reference study to determine whether deterioration in SPECT performance has occurred.

Patient Data

An essential part of any imaging quality control program is the review of each patient's acquired data, and this is particularly true with SPECT. Excessive patient motion degrades the quality of SPECT scans because misregistration of the data in the different angular projections can lead to significant artifacts. Patient motion can be assessed in several ways. When the unprocessed projection images are viewed in a closed loop cine, excessive patient motion is readily detected as a flicker or discontinuity in the display. Some laboratories use radioactive marker sources placed on the patient to further assess motion. Another approach is to view a sinogram of a slice in the study. The borders of the sinogram should be smooth, and interslice changes in intensity should be small. Any discontinuity may indicate patient motion (Fig. 5-14). Only up-and-down motion can be readily corrected. Discontinuities in the sinogram also may indicate an instrument malfunction. In addition to patient motion, the sinogram is useful for evaluation of head misregistration. A lateral shift at the point in the sinogram where the data from the first head ends and the second head begins can indicate a problem with the head registration. A tomographic acquisition of a point source can help determine whether these shifts are due to head misregistration. Finally, the patient's reconstructed data should be carefully scrutinized for the presence of any irregularities or artifacts that may compromise the diagnostic quality of the study.

▬ POSITRON EMISSION TOMOGRAPHY

PET, and particularly PET/CT, is a rapidly growing area of nuclear medicine. PET is made possible by the unique fate of positrons. When positrons undergo annihilation by combining with negatively charged electrons, two 511-keV photons are emitted in opposite directions, 180 degrees apart. In contrast to SPECT imaging, which detects single events, in PET imaging, two detector elements on opposite sides of the object are used to detect paired annihilation photons. If the photons are detected at the same time (or "in coincidence"), the event is assumed to have occurred along the line connecting the two detectors involved (Fig. 5-15). Thus the direction of the photons can be determined without the use of absorptive collimation. This process is referred to as *annihilation coincidence detection* and is the hallmark of PET imaging.

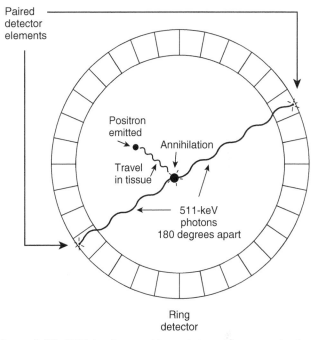

FIGURE 5-15. PET ring detector. After emission, positrons travel a short distance in tissue before the annihilation event. The 511-keV protons are given off 180 degrees apart.

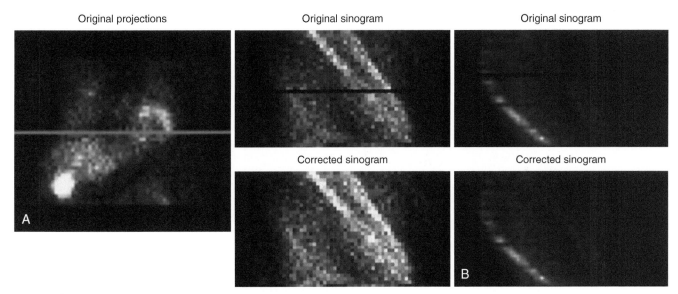

FIGURE 5-14. Patient quality control. **A,** Sinogram from a myocardial perfusion study. The sinogram corresponds to the level of the cursor in the image on the *left*. Note the regular progression in the data across the projection profiles, indicating stability and lack of unwanted movement of the heart from one projection view to the next. **B,** Sinogram illustrating multiple gaps in the sequential profile data. Compare these discontinuities with the regular progression of data in **A.** The discontinuities indicate unwanted motion of the object from one sampling position to the next.

Annihilation coincidence detection leads to at least a 100-fold increase in the sensitivity of PET relative to conventional nuclear medicine imaging and explains the higher image quality compared to SPECT. The counts occurring between a single pair of detectors can be considered a ray, and projections can thereby be generated and reconstructed, just as in SPECT. Although both filtered backprojection and iterative approaches such as OSEM can be used to reconstruct the data; the latter is more common for PET because of the greatly improved image quality.

Instrumentation

Instrumentation for PET has undergone several generations of development. Early systems had a single ring with multiple detectors and generated a single tomographic section at a time. Now, PET typically consists of many rings of multiple detectors that cover a 15- to 20-cm axial field of view. Each detector is typically paired with multiple other detectors on the opposite side of the detector ring. These detectors in coincidence are selected to encompass the field of view of the object or organ being imaged (Fig. 5-16). Multiple-ring systems allow a volume to be imaged simultaneously. Early systems typically had *septa* of absorptive material such as lead or tungsten inserted between the tomographic planes to reduce intraplane scatter and shield the detectors from crosstalk caused by activity outside of the plane of interest. These systems with interplane septa are referred to as *two-dimensional (2D)* systems because they limit the allowable coincidences to 2D transverse planes. Over time, the number of rings increased and the ability to remove the septa to acquire data across planes (i.e., 3D mode) became common. The 3D design greatly increases system sensitivity of the PET scanner and increases the number of Compton scattered and random events recorded. Most contemporary systems do not have septa between the planes and are referred to as *3D only systems*. This is made possible by

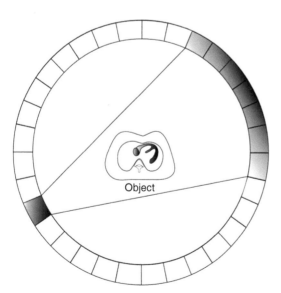

FIGURE 5-16. Pairing of detectors. In the PET tomograph, each detector is paired with multiple detectors on the opposite side of the ring to create an arc encompassing the object. This multiple-pairing strategy increases the sensitivity of the device.

improvements in scatter correction algorithms and a reduction in the number of random coincidence events detected because of newer, faster detector materials.

Detector Materials

When choosing the appropriate detector material for PET, the detection efficiency (related to the effective atomic number, Z, and mass density), resolution (spatial and energy, related to the number of scintillation light photons emitted per kiloelectron volt), and response time or decay time of the scintillator must be considered. The density and effective atomic number (Z) for NaI, the detector material commonly used in gamma cameras, are not optimal for detection of the 511-keV photons in PET imaging. Bismuth germinate oxide (BGO) is approximately twice as dense as NaI and has an effective Z of 74, compared to the effective Z of 50 for NaI, leading to its use in PET for the past 30 years. However, its drawbacks include significantly lower light output per kiloelectron volt (i.e., lower energy resolution) and longer light decay time. This longer light decay time necessitated the use of coincidence timing windows of 10 to 12 nanoseconds (ns). New detector materials, such as lutetium oxyorthosilicate (LSO), lutetium-yttrium oxyorthosilicate (LYSO), and gadolinium oxyorthosilicate (GSO) combine high density with better timing resolution and superior light yield. Timing windows have been reduced to about 5 to 6 ns, which in turn reduces the number of random events by approximately 50%. It also provides the opportunity for time-of-flight PET. The better light output allows for better energy discrimination and thus a reduction in the number of scatter events acquired. For these reasons, state-of-the-art PET scanners are incorporating either LSO or LYSO as the detection material.

Spatial Resolution

The spatial resolution of modern PET tomographs is excellent, primarily determined by the size of the detector modules. Resolution under clinical scanning conditions is superior in PET compared with SPECT. Resolution for clinical studies is in the 5- to 8-mm FWHM range with high-end contemporary PET scanners. Specialized devices designed for small animal imaging have about 1.5-mm spatial resolution.

The ultimate spatial resolution of PET is limited by two physical phenomena related to positrons and their annihilation. First, positrons are given off at different kinetic energies. Energetic positrons such as those emitted by oxygen-15, gallium-68, and rubidium-82 may travel several millimeters in tissue before undergoing annihilation (Fig. 5-15). Thus the location of the annihilation event is some distance from the actual location of the radionuclide. This travel in tissue degrades the ability to truly localize the biodistribution of the radioactive agent in the patient and results in images with poorer resolution, particularly for radionuclides with higher positron kinetic energies, such as Ga-68 and Rb-82, compared to F-18. The second phenomenon limiting resolution is the noncolinearity of the annihilation photons. If the positron–electron pair is still moving at the time of annihilation, the result is a small deviation from true colinearity along a single ray (Fig. 5-15), leading to a 1- to 2-mm spatial uncertainty in event localization for clinical whole-body PET scanners.

Image Acquisition

Annihilation Coincidence Detection

Special circuitry in the PET tomograph allows detection of two annihilation photons given off by a single positron annihilation event. The two events are considered to be from the same event if they are counted within a defined *coincidence timing window*. In current scanners, the coincidence window is on the order of 6 ns (although it may be as high as 12 ns in older, BGO-based scanners). Thus, when events are registered in paired detectors within 6 ns of each other, they are accepted as *true coincidence events* and recorded as occurring along the LOR that connects the two detectors. If a single recorded event is not matched by a paired event within the coincidence time window, the data are discarded. This approach effectively provides *electronic collimation* without the need for absorptive collimation. Therefore PET tomographs offer much higher sensitivity than gamma cameras. One complication in the coincidence approach occurs at higher count rates when two unrelated or random events are recorded within the coincidence timing window, leading to what is referred to as a *random coincidence*. Such random coincidences do not provide useful information with regard to localizing the radiopharmaceutical, thus, if no correction is applied, leading to a higher level of background signal that reduces the overall object contrast.

Data can be recorded in several ways, depending on whether the data are acquired in 2D or 3D format. PET data can be stored as sinograms (2D) or projections (3D). In either case, the counts in each pixel represent the coincidence events recorded along a particular LOR between a pair of detectors in coincidence. We know the coincidence event happened somewhere on the LOR but not specifically where along the LOR the event occurred. The sinogram or projection data are then reconstructed, most commonly using iterative reconstruction methods, although filtered back projection may sometimes be used.

Time of Flight

Time-of-flight PET uses the time difference in the arrival of the annihilation photons in the coincidence timing windows to estimate where on the LOR the event occurred. The estimated location of the event, Δd, is calculated from the time difference between the two events, Δt, using the formula: $\Delta d = (\Delta t \times c)/2$, where c is the speed of light. With the current detectors, such as LSO or LYSO, this methodology can be used to locate the annihilation event to within about 7 cm along the LOR, which can lead to a significant improvement in PET image quality, particularly in large patients. However, it has relatively little benefit when used for brain and pediatric imaging because of the smaller diameter of the object being imaged.

Corrections, Calibrations, and Quality Assurance

Uniformity Correction

A PET scanner has a very large number of detectors. A state-of-the-art scanner with 4-mm crystals and an 80-cm ring diameter can have as many as 32,000 crystals. As with any imaging system, variations occur in the response of the crystals to a uniform source of radiation. To correct for these variations, a high count uniformity calibration is acquired and a correction applied. This correction is analogous to the uniformity correction applied to SPECT cameras. However, it differs in that the detectors are stationary and therefore small variations in a given detector are not propagated over the complete 360 degrees of data. Thus, where uniformity variations in SPECT will result in ring artifacts, this is not the case in PET. As a result, the uniformity correction for PET is done much less frequently, perhaps quarterly.

Count-to-Activity Conversion Factor

The PET scanner records detected annihilation coincidence events as counts or, more correctly, counts per second per pixel. It is preferred to have these data in units of microcurie or becquerels per milliliter. Therefore a calibration scan is performed to determine a conversion factor to convert counts to activity. This is accomplished by imaging a uniform phantom with a known concentration of activity (becquerels per milliliter). The conversion factor is determined by calculating the ratio of activity concentration in the phantom to the counts per second per pixel in the image. This calibration factor is stored and later applied during image reconstruction so the resultant image is reported in units of activity concentration. This conversion factor is crucial when activity quantitation is applied, such as in determining the standard uptake value (SUV). The SUV is the ratio of the activity concentration in a pixel within the patient's PET study normalized by the administered activity and patient size (usually patient mass). If the radiopharmaceutical distributes uniformly within the patient, the SUV value will be 1. Inaccuracies in the count-to-activity calibration will result in inaccurate SUV values.

Daily Detector Quality Control

Each day, the detectors in a PET scanner are exposed to a uniform source of radioactivity to evaluate that each detector is working properly. Because of the large number of detectors, a small number of them may not be working. The data are presented to the user in a manner that allows evaluation of which detectors are not working as expected. Each manufacturer has a different method, but the end result is a report that indicates whether the system is working properly. Systems that are identified as not working properly will need corrective action.

Monthly Quantitative Accuracy Check

PET scans that are done for evaluation of different cancers are reconstructed, and the pixel values in some cases may be converted to SUV. It is common for physicians to report changes in these values from one scan to the next as indicative of progression or regression of disease. It is important that the SUV values generated by the scanner are consistent from scan to scan. Drift in the electronics of the scanner can result in discordance between the calibration factor and patient data. One method of verifying the SUV is to image a uniform distribution of known radioactivity concentration. The phantom is imaged using clinical scan parameters. The amount of activity in the phantom and the mass of the phantom are entered into the acquisition data as if it were a patient. When these data are reconstructed, the average SUV value in each reconstructed slice is determined. The resultant average SUV should be 1.0 ± 10%. Values outside this range would indicate that the scanner should be recalibrated. This test uses the methodology for calibrating the scanner as a check of the calibration. It has the advantage that, if necessary, the phantom is ready to be used for recalibration of the scanner.

Quarterly Quality Phantom Check

Another method for evaluating the performance of PET scanner is to image a cylindrical, tomographic quality control phantom. These phantoms are similar to those used in SPECT, but typically differ in that they often contain *hot* features in which the activity concentration is greater than that in the background for evaluating contrast (Fig. 5-17). They are usually imaged on a quarterly basis but could be imaged more frequently and combined with the quantitative accuracy value check. These phantoms typically allow for the evaluation of uniformity, resolution, contrast, and quantitative accuracy using one data acquisition. The hot features in the phantom are specified to have a certain target-to-background ratio (e.g., 2.5:1 or 4:1); the SUV of each is recorded. The targets may be spheres or cylinders of decreasing size. The resolution section typically consists of cold rods of decreasing size in a warm background, similar to those used in SPECT. The phantom is imaged using the clinical protocol. The SUV values in the hot features are compared to the expected value, and size of the smallest rods and targets are recorded. The background is evaluated for an average SUV of 1.0 ± 10%. Because of the complexity in filling this phantom, it is typically used less frequently than the uniform phantom for checking the quantitative accuracy of the scanner.

■ HYBRID POSITRON EMISSION COMPUTED TOMGRAPHY, SINGLE-PHOTON COMPUTED TOMOGRAPHY WITH COMPUTED TOMOGRAPHY, AND POSITRON EMISSION TOMOGRAPHY WITH MAGNETIC RESONANCE

Nuclear medicine images are excellent for looking at physiology but they are organ specific and generally low resolution. Thus it is sometimes difficult to accurately localize features seen on the emission tomography scans. The introduction of hybrid PET-CT and SPECT-CT allowing direct correlation of the functional information available from PET or SPECT with the anatomical information from CT has greatly enhanced the clinical utility of these modalities. The addition of CT to both PET and SPECT has been very useful in anatomically defining both pathological and normal anatomy in the emission images. For PET, areas of increased uptake can be more easily correlated with a metastatic lymph node or a region of brown fat. The same is true for a variety of SPECT procedures, such as parathyroid imaging and bone SPECT for back pain.

The PET-CT places the CT scanner in front of the PET scanner. In the case of SPECT, the CT scanner is behind or parallel with the SPECT scanner. On either system, the CT scan may be acquired either before or after the emission study, although the more common order is to acquire the CT first and then the emission study. The CT scan can then provide both the transmission scan for attenuation correction and anatomical correlation.

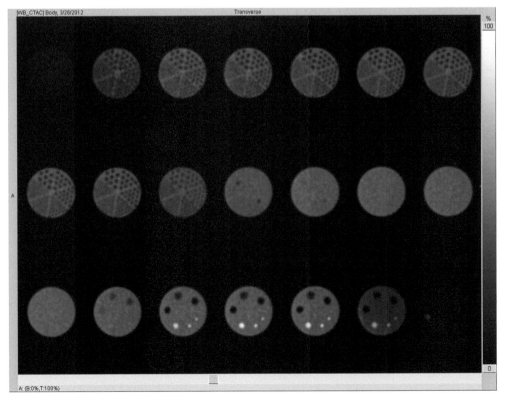

FIGURE 5-17. PET quality control phantom. A series of slices from a phantom acquisition.

The CT scanner incorporated into these devices may be a state-of-the-art CT scanner or, in some cases, particularly with SPECT-CT, it may be a CT scanner of less capability but still adequate for the imaging task at hand. The quality control of the CT scanner is the same as that necessary for a clinical CT scanner, and therefore beyond the scope of this chapter. However, a test object should be imaged periodically that can be seen with both modalities to ensure alignment of the two devices.

When the CT is used for attenuation correction of the emission scan, artifacts can be introduced when misregistration exists between the emission and transmission data sets. The CT scan is acquired much more quickly than the emission studies. This can result in different breathing patterns between the two scans that can make registration of the data in the area of the diaphragm difficult. Therefore it is important to review both the attenuation-corrected images and the non–attenuation-corrected images in conjunction with the CT scan to evaluate misregistration. In cardiac imaging, misregistration of the heart can result in false positive scans. This is true for both PET and SPECT.

In recent years, hybrid PET-MR scanners have been introduced by several vendors. In one case, the PET scanner is actually fitted within the MR device and the two scans can be acquired simultaneously. In other cases, the PET and MR scanners are adjacent to each other using a common bed that can service the two devices. Combined PET-MR acquisitions have the potential for interesting research applications; however, its clinical role is yet to be determined.

■ SUGGESTED READING

Chandra R. *Nuclear Medicine Physics: The Basics*. 7th ed. Philadelphia: Williams & Wilkins; 2011.

Cherry SR, Sorenson JA, Phelps ME. *Physics in Nuclear Medicine*. 3rd ed. Philadelphia: WB Saunders; 2003.

International Atomic Energy Association. *Planning a Clinical PET Centre*.Human Health Series No. 11. Pub. 1457 Vienna, Austria: International Atomic Energy Agency; 2010.

International Atomic Energy Association. *Quality Assurance for PET and PET/CT Systems*.Human Health Series. No. 1. Pub. 1393. Vienna, Austria: International Atomic Energy Agency; 2009.

International Atomic Energy Association. *Quality Assurance of SPECT Systems*.Human Health Series No. 6. Pub. 1394 Vienna, Austria: International Atomic Energy Agency; 2009.

International Atomic Energy Association. *Quality Control Atlas for Scintillation Camera Systems*. Pub. 1141. Vienna, Austria: International Atomic Energy Agency; 2003.

National Electrical Manufacturers Association. *Performance Measurements of Positron Emission Tomographs*. NEMA NU 2–2007 Rosslyn, VA: National Electrical Manufacturers Association; 2007.

Powsner RA, Powsner ER. *Essentials of Nuclear Medicine Physics*. 2nd ed. Malden, MA: Blackwell Science; 2006.

Part II
Clinical Nuclear Medicine

CHAPTER 6

Endocrine System

In the early days of nuclear medicine, endocrinologists were attracted to the field by the potential of radioiodine for diagnosis and therapy. Today, thyroid diagnosis and therapy continue to have an important role in the practice of nuclear medicine. The basic principles learned in those days provide the basis for much of current practice in clinical nuclear medicine.

Parathyroid scintigraphy has been used for a long time. However, it has gained increasing importance in recent years for the preoperative localization of hyperfunctioning parathyroid glands. The methodology for parathyroid scintigraphy continues to evolve.

■ THYROID SCINTIGRAPHY AND UPTAKE STUDIES

Radioactive iodine first became available in 1946. Its potential for the diagnosis and therapy of thyroid disease was quickly appreciated. Uptake tests in conjunction with various suppression and stimulation methods were used to study thyroid function. The advent of rectilinear scanners and then gamma cameras made thyroid scintigraphy possible. Radioiodine is still the primary therapy for Graves disease and standard therapy for well-differentiated thyroid cancer.

Thyroid Anatomy and Physiology

A basic understanding of iodine metabolism, thyroid physiology, and pathophysiology is important for interpretation of thyroid uptake and imaging studies.

Anatomy

The thyroid gland, located anterior to the trachea and below the thyroid cartilage, extends laterally, superiorly, and inferiorly (Fig. 6-1). The normal adult gland weighs 15 to 20 g. The lateral lobes measure approximately 4 to 5 cm from superior to inferior poles and are 1.5 to 2 cm wide. The isthmus, which connects the two lobes, shows considerable anatomic variability. The pyramidal lobe, a remnant of the thyroglossal duct, extends superiorly toward the hyoid bone.

Because of the thyroid's embryological development and descent from pharyngeal pouches, ectopic thyroid tissue can be found at distant sites, from the foramen cecum at the base of the tongue to the myocardium. Anatomically, the gland comprises many follicles of varying size. The epithelial follicular cells at the periphery of the follicle synthesize and secrete thyroid hormone into the follicular lumen, which contains colloid, where it is stored (Fig. 6-2).

Physiology

Iodine is essential for thyroid hormone synthesis. After oral ingestion, it is rapidly reduced to iodide in the proximal small intestine, where more than 90% is absorbed systemically within 60 minutes. It distributes in the blood as an extracellular ion similar to chloride and exits by thyroid extraction and urinary excretion.

Iodide Trapping and Organification

Thyroid follicular cells trap iodide by a high-energy sodium iodide symporter (thyroid pump). Iodine is concentrated intracellularly 25 to 500 times greater than plasma. Trapping, or uptake, can be blocked competitively by monovalent anions (e.g., potassium perchlorate). In the normal thyroid, organification promptly follows trapping. The iodide is oxidized to neutral iodine by thyroid peroxidase at the follicular cell–colloid interface and then binds to tyrosine residues on thyroglobulin. These monoiodinated and diiodinated tyrosines couple to form triiodothyronine (T_3) and thyroxine (T_4), which are stored in the colloid-filled follicular lumen (Fig. 6-2). Organification can be blocked by therapeutic drugs (e.g., propylthiouracil and methimazole).

Thyroid Hormone Storage and Release

Thyroid-stimulating hormone (TSH) initiates iodide uptake, organification, and release of thyroid hormone. Thyroid hormone is released by hydrolysis of thyroglobulin. Thyroglobulin does not enter the bloodstream, except during disease states (e.g., thyroiditis or thyroid cancer). The normal gland contains a 1-month supply of hormone. Therapeutic drugs that block hormone synthesis do not become fully effective in controlling thyrotoxicosis until intrathyroidal stores are depleted.

Thyroid–Pituitary Feedback

The thyroid–pituitary feedback mechanism is sensitive to circulating serum thyroid hormone levels and is the dominant method of adjusting TSH secretion (Fig. 6-3). When serum thyroid hormone levels are increased, serum TSH is suppressed; when serum thyroid hormone levels are low, serum TSH increases. The major hormone released by the thyroid is T_4, which is transported to peripheral tissues by thyroid-binding proteins and converted to the more metabolically active T_3 at peripheral tissue site of action.

Radiopharmaceuticals

Radioiodine Iodine-123 and Iodine-131

Because radioiodine is selectively trapped and organified by the thyroid and incorporated into thyroid hormone, it is an ideal physiological radiotracer, providing clinically pertinent information about thyroid function. Iodine-123 (I-123) and iodine-131 sodium iodide (I-131) are the two radiopharmaceuticals used clinically.

Because of iodine's rapid gastrointestinal absorption, uptake, and organification, radioiodine is detectable in the thyroid gland within minutes of oral ingestion and normally reaches the thyroid follicular lumen by 20 to 30 minutes. Normally, a progressive increase in thyroid uptake occurs over 24 hours (Fig. 6-4). The time delay between administration and imaging is dictated by the desire for background clearance and a high target-to-background ratio, not by slow gland accumulation. Although taken up by the salivary glands, stomach, and, to a lesser extent, choroid plexus, radioiodine is not concentrated nor retained in these organs. The kidneys and gastrointestinal tract serve as the excretory route.

Iodine I-131

Physics. I-131 undergoes beta-minus decay and emits a principle primary gamma photon of 364 kiloelecton volts (keV) (81% abundance) with an 8-day physical half-life

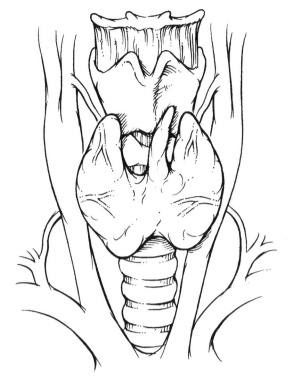

FIGURE 6-1. Thyroid anatomy. The anatomical relationship of the thyroid to the trachea, thyroid and cricoid cartilages, and vascular structures.

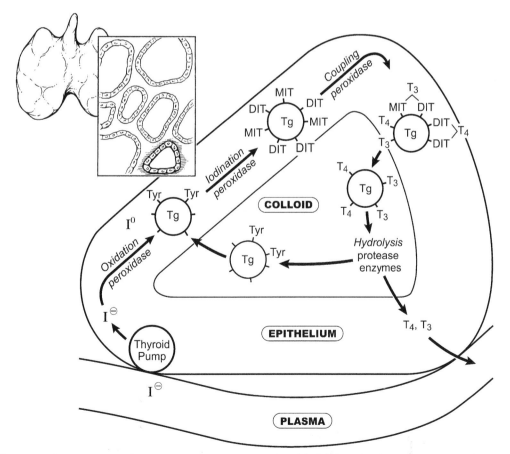

FIGURE 6-2. Iodine metabolism. The thyroid follicular cell epithelium extracts (traps) iodide from the plasma via the sodium iodide symporter (thyroid pump) and then organifies it. The iodide (I^-) is converted to neutral iodine (I^0), which is then incorporated into thyroglobulin-bound tyrosine molecules as monoiodotyrosine (MIT) or diiodotyrosine (DIT). Coupling of the iodotyrosines results in T_4 and T_3 hormone bound to the thyroglobulin, which is transported to and stored in the colloid until T_4 and T_3 are released into the plasma by proteolytic enzymes.

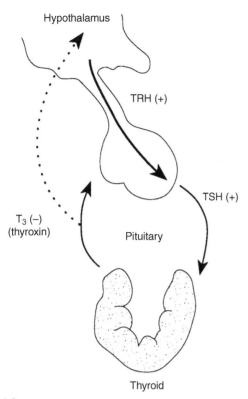

Figure 6-3. Thyroid–pituitary feedback. The normal thyroid is under the control of thyroid-stimulating hormone (TSH). The hypothalamic production of thyroid-releasing hormone (TRH) and the pituitary release of TSH are increased with low circulating levels of T_4 and T_3 and decreased with high circulating levels of thyroid hormone.

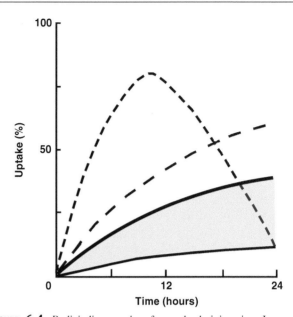

Figure 6-4. Radioiodine uptake after oral administration. In normal subjects the percent radioactive iodine thyroid uptake (%RAIU) increases progressively over 24 hours to values of 10% to 30% *(gray area)*. With Graves disease, the %RAIU rises at a more rapid rate to higher levels, often 50% to 80% and greater *(lower broken line)*. However, some patients with Graves disease have rapid iodine turnover within the thyroid with early, rapid, high uptake at 4 to 12 hours, but returning to a mildly elevated or even normal uptake by 24 hours *(top broken line)*.

(Table 6-1). The 364-keV photons are not optimal for gamma cameras. Count detection sensitivity for I-131 is poor; approximately half of the photons penetrate a ⅜-inch crystal without being detected. Other higher energy I-131 emissions penetrate the collimator septa and result in image degradation. High-energy beta particles of 0.606 megaelectron volt (MeV) (89% abundance) are also emitted from I-131 decay. They cannot be imaged but are valuable for therapy.

Dosimetry. The I-131 high-energy beta emissions and long physical half-life of gamma emissions result in a high radiation dose to the patient, particularly to the thyroid, approximately 1 rad/µCi administered (Table 6-2). This high radiation-absorbed patient dose severely limits the amount of activity that can be administered.

Iodine-123

Physics. I-123 decays by electron capture with a half-life of 13.2 hours. The principal gamma emission is a 159-keV photon (83.4% abundance), which is well suited for gamma camera imaging. I-123 emits a small percentage of higher energy emissions—440 to 625 keV (2.4%) and 625 to 784 keV (0.15%). No beta particle emissions occur (Table 6-1).

Dosimetry. In the past, I-123 was contaminated with long-lived impurities of I-124 and I-125, which increased percent-wise with time because of their long half-lives compared to I-123, increasing radiation exposure to the patient. Today, commercially available I-123 is 99.9% I-123.

Table 6-1 Physical Characteristics of Thyroid Radiopharmaceuticals

Characteristics	Tc-99m	I-123	I-131
Mode of decay	Isometric transition	Electron capture	Beta minus
Physical half-life ($T_{1/2}$)	6 hr	13.2 hr	8.1 days
Photon energy	140 keV	159 keV	364 keV
Abundance* (%)	89%	83%	81%
Beta emissions			606 keV

*Abundance is the percent likelihood that a certain photon emission will occur with each radioactive decay.

The normal thyroid receives a radiation dose of 1.5 to 2.6 rads from a 200-µCi dose of I-123 (Table 6-2). The much lower radiation dosimetry of I-123 compared to I-131 permits administration of 200 to 400 µCi of I-123 for routine thyroid scanning compared to 30 to 50 µCi of I-131, with considerably better image quality.

Technetium-99m Pertechnetate

Technetium-99m pertechnetate has been used as an alternative to I-123 for thyroid scintigraphy because of its ready availability from molybdenum99/Tc-99m generators and its low patient radiation dose.

Physics

The 140-keV photopeak of Tc-99m (89% abundance) is ideally suited for use with a gamma camera. It has a short 6-hour half-life and no particulate emissions (Table 6-1).

TABLE 6-2 Dosimetry of Thyroid Radiopharmaceuticals

Body area	Tc-99m pertechnetate rems/5 mCi, (mSv/185 MBq)	I-123 rems/200 µCi, (mSv/7.5 MBq)	I-131 rems/50 µCi, (mSv/1.85 MBq)
Thyroid	0.600	1.5-2.6*	39,000-65.000*
Bladder wall	0.430	0.070	0.150
Stomach	0.250	0.050	0.085
Small intestine	0.550	0.030	0.003
Red marrow	0.100	0.060	0.007
Testis	0.050	0.027	0.006
Ovaries	0.150	0.072	0.009
Total body	0.070	0.009	0.035
Total effective dose	0.009	0.163	0.400

*Lower estimate assumes a 15% radioactive iodine thyroid uptake (RAIU), and the higher estimate assumes a 25% RAIU

Pharmacokinetics

In contrast to oral administration of radioiodine, Tc-99m pertechnetate is administered intravenously. It is trapped by the thyroid by the same mechanism as iodine but is not organified nor incorporated into thyroid hormone. Thus it is not retained in the thyroid and imaging must be performed early, usually at peak uptake, 20 to 30 minutes after injection.

Dosimetry

The lack of particulate emissions and short 6-hour half-life result in relatively low radiation absorption by the thyroid (Table 6-2). The administered activity of Tc-99m pertechnetate (3-5 mCi) is considerably higher than that for I-123 for routine thyroid scans (200-400 µCi). The resulting large photon flux allows for high-quality images.

Choice of Radiopharmaceutical

I-123 has become the agent of choice for most adult thyroid imaging. Tc-99m pertechnetate is sometimes used in children because of its low radiation dosimetry and high count rate. Its disadvantage is that it is not organified and thus not ideal for nodule evaluation or uptake calculations. I-131 is not used for routine thyroid scans because of its very high dosimetry and poor image quality. A low dose (5-10 µCi) is sometimes used for an uptake calculation alone or in conjunction with Tc-99m pertechnetate thyroid imaging.

For thyroid cancer imaging, the long half-life of I-131 is an advantage, allowing time for whole-body washout and improved target-to-background ratio, increasing detectability of thyroid cancer metastases. Even for this indication, I-123 is replacing I-131 because of earlier patient imaging, similar accuracy, and lack of thyroid cell stunning. The high-energy I-131 beta emissions result in effective therapy for Graves disease, toxic nodules, and thyroid cancer.

TABLE 6-3 Drugs, Foods, and Radiographic Contrast Agents That Decrease or Increase the Percent Radioactive Iodine Thyroid Uptake

Decreased uptake	Duration of effect
Thyroid hormones	
Thyroxine (T₄)	4-6 wk
Triiodothyronine (T₃)	2 wk
Excess iodine (expanded iodine pool)	
Potassium iodide	2-4 wk
Mineral supplements, cough medicines, and vitamins	2-4 wk
Iodine food supplements	
Iodinated drugs (e.g., amiodarone)	Months
Iodinated skin ointments	2-4 wk
Congestive heart failure	
Renal failure	
Radiographic contrast media	
Water-soluble intravascular media	2-4 wk
Fat-soluble media (lymphography)	Months to years
Non–iodine-containing drugs	
Adrenocorticotropic hormone, adrenal steroids	Variable
Monovalent anions (perchlorate)	Variable
Penicillin	Variable
Antithyroid drugs	
Propylthiouracil (PTU)	3-5 days
Methimazole (Tapazole)	5-7 days
Goitrogenic foods	
Cabbage, turnips	
Prior radiation to neck	
Increased uptake	
Iodine deficiency	
Pregnancy	
Rebound after therapy withdrawal	
Antithyroid drugs	
Lithium	

Special Considerations and Precautions

Food and Medications Containing Iodine

Stable iodine in foods and medications can interfere with radionuclide thyroid studies (Table 6-3). Expansion of the iodine pool by parenteral administration or oral ingestion of iodine results in a reduced percent radioactive iodine thyroid uptake (%RAIU). Increasing amounts of iodine in the normal diet over the years (e.g., iodized salt) has resulted in lower normal values for the %RAIU. Numerous non–iodine-containing drugs also can affect thyroidal uptake.

Suppression of uptake by exogenous iodine may preclude successful imaging or accurate uptake measurements. As little as 1 mg of stable iodine can cause a marked reduction in uptake. Ten milligram can effectively block the gland (98% reduction). Radiographic contrast media are a common source of iodine that interferes with radioiodine thyroid studies. A food, drug, and imaging history should be obtained from patients before thyroid uptake and imaging studies.

Chronic renal failure impairs iodide clearance, expands the iodide pool, and thus lowers the %RAIU. Hypothyroidism reduces the glomerular filtration rate and slows urinary clearance of radioiodine from the body; hyperthyroidism increases the clearance rate.

Pregnancy

The fetal thyroid begins to concentrate radioiodine by 10 to 12 weeks of gestation. It crosses the placenta, and thus significant exposure of the fetal thyroid can occur after therapeutic doses to the mother, resulting in fetal hypothyroidism. A pregnancy test is mandatory before treating a patient with radioiodine I-131.

Nursing Mother

Radioiodine is excreted in human breast milk. Because of the long half-life of I-131, nursing should be discontinued after diagnostic or therapeutic studies with I-131 and not resumed. Breastfeeding may resume after 48 hours with I-123 and after 24 hours with Tc-99m pertechnetate.

Patient Information

Thyroid studies must be interpreted in light of the patient's clinical history, serum thyroid function studies, and findings at thyroid palpation.

Methodology for Thyroid Uptake Studies and Thyroid Scans

Clinical radioiodine thyroid uptake studies and thyroid scans are often performed together. However, they are usually acquired with different instrumentation and provide different, although complementary, information. Whereas scans are acquired with a gamma camera, a %RAIU study is usually acquired with a nonimaging gamma scintillation probe detector. Camera-based uptakes can be performed with Tc-99m pertechnetate scans and are routine with thyroid cancer scans.

Thyroid Uptake

Radioactive Iodine Percent Uptake

Both I-131 and I-123 can be used for calculation of the %RAIU. Indications for uptake determinations are few but are clinically important (Table 6-4).

Indications. The most common clinical indication for a %RAIU is the differential diagnosis of thyrotoxicosis. Diseases of the thyroid with autonomous function (e.g., Graves disease and toxic nodules) can be differentiated from diseases with intact pituitary–thyroid feedback (e.g., thyroiditis) (Table 6-5). Thus the %RAIU is elevated in Graves disease, the most common cause for thyrotoxicosis, but decreased in thyroiditis, the second most common cause (Box 6-1). The %RAIU is also used for calculation of an I-131 therapy dose for patients with Graves disease (Box 6-2).

TABLE 6-4 Clinical Indications for Thyroid Scintigraphy and Percent Radioactive Iodine Thyroid Uptake

Thyroid scans	Thyroid uptakes
Functional status (cold, hot) of thyroid nodule	Differential diagnosis of thyrotoxicosis
Detection of ectopic thyroid tissue (lingual thyroid)	Calculate Graves disease I-131 therapy dose
Differential diagnosis of mediastinal masses (substernal goiter)	Whole-body thyroid cancer scans
Thyroid cancer whole-body scan	Pre–I-131 therapy evaluation of disease extent
	Estimate I-131 therapeutic effectiveness
	Follow for recurrence

TABLE 6-5 Clinical Frequency of Various Causes for Thyrotoxicosis

Cause	Percentage
Grave Disease	70
Thyroiditis	20
Toxic multinodular goiter	5
Toxic adenoma	5
Others	<1

Box 6-1. **Differential Diagnosis of Thyrotoxicosis: Increased or Decreased Percent Radioactive Iodine Thyroid Uptake**

INCREASED UPTAKE
Graves disease
Multinodular toxic goiter
Hashitoxicosis
Hydatidiform mole, trophoblastic tumors, choriocarcinoma
Metastatic thyroid cancer

DECREASED UPTAKE
Subacute thyroiditis
   Granulomatous thyroiditis (de Quervain)
   Silent thyroiditis
   Postpartum thyroiditis
   Iodine-induced thyrotoxicosis (Jod-Basedow)
   Amiodarone-induced thyrotoxicosis
   Thyrotoxicosis factitia
   Struma ovarii (decreased in thyroid, increased in ovarian tumor)

Methodology. Medications that can interfere with the %RAIU should be discontinued for a time based on their half-lives (Table 6-3). Patients should have nothing by mouth for approximately 4 hours before radioiodine ingestion to ensure good absorption. I-123 and I-131 are usually administered in capsule form, although I-131 can be given as a liquid. The unit-dosed capsule formulation is convenient for handling and decreases potential airborne exposure of radioiodine to technologists and physicians.

Box 6-2. Calculation of Percent Radioactive Iodine Thyroid Uptake with Iodine-123 and Iodine-131

1. Preliminary measurements
   Place dose capsule in neck phantom and count for 1 minute.
   Count patient's neck and thigh (background) for 1 minute.
2. Administer oral dose capsule.
3. Uptake measurement at 4-6 hours and 24 hours:
   Count patient's neck for 1 minute.
   Count patient's thigh for 1 minute.
4. Calculation

$$\%RAIU = \frac{Neck\ (background\ corrected)\ counts/min}{Dose\ capsule\ (decay\ corrected\ and\ background\ corrected)\ counts/min} \times 100$$

If a scan is not needed, 5 to 10 µCi I-131 or 50 to 100 µCi I-123 is adequate for a %RAIU because of the gamma probe's high detection sensitivity compared to that of a gamma camera. If a scan is ordered, both can be performed with the I-123 scan dose (200-400 µCi). The %RAIU is usually performed at 24 hours after ingestion, although some acquire the %RAIU at 4 hours and others at both 4 and 24 hours.

A nonimaging gamma scintillation probe detector used for thyroid uptake studies has a 2-cm thick × 2-cm diameter sodium iodine crystal with an open, cone-shaped, single-hole lead collimator coupled to a photomultiplier tube and electronics (Figs. 6-5 and 6-6).

Room background activity is first determined. The radioiodine capsule with known calibrated activity is placed in a Lucite neck phantom, and counts are obtained with the detector placed at a standardized distance of 30 cm (Fig. 6-6). The radioiodine dose is then administered to the patient. At appropriate time intervals, the probe is placed 30 cm from the anterior surface of the patient's neck, so that the entire gland can be detected by the probe but most extrathyroidal activity is not. The patient's neck or thigh (background) is counted for background.

To calculate the %RAIU, counts are obtained for the patient's neck and thigh (for background). The percent radioiodine uptake is calculated according to the formula:

$$\%RAIU = \frac{Neck\ counts/min\ (background\ corrected)}{Administered\ dose\ capsule\ counts/min\ (background\ and\ decay\ corrected)} \times 100$$

In the past, a standard reference capsule similar in activity to the administered capsule was counted initially and at the uptake intervals and used to correct for decay. In today's uptake probe-computer systems, decay is automatically corrected.

Normal Values. The normal range for the %RAIU is approximately 4% to 15% at 4 to 6 hours and 10% to 30% at 24 hours. The early %RAIU at 4 to 6 hours serves two purposes. The early uptake confirms that %RAIU is indeed elevated without the need for the patient to return the next day. Some centers extrapolate the 24-hour uptake

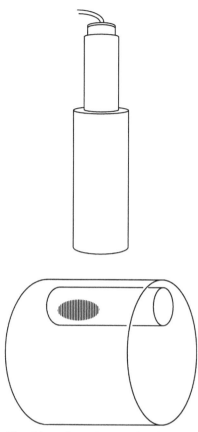

FIGURE 6-5. Thyroid uptake probe counting I-123 capsule in neck phantom. The neck phantom is solid Lucite plastic, except for the cylinder-like defect in which the capsule is placed. The nonimaging gamma detector is placed at a standard distance of 30 cm from the neck phantom and acquires emitted counts for 1 minute.

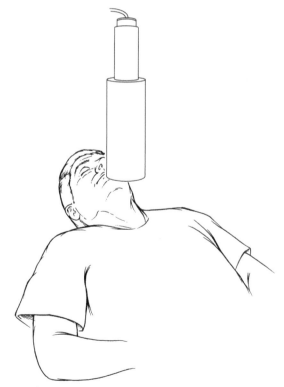

FIGURE 6-6. Thyroid uptake probe acquiring counts from patient's thyroid. The probe is positioned 30 cm from the patient's thyroid and acquires counts for 1 minute.

from the 4-hour value to plan the therapy I-131 dose. However, some patients have rapid thyroid iodine turnover. These patients may show a very high 4- to 6-hour %RAIU but much lower values at 24 hours, perhaps only mildly elevated (Fig. 6-4). Therefore the more accurate 24-hour measurement certainly needs to be used for therapy dose calculated from a 24-hour %RAIU whenever early values are markedly elevated.

Technetium-99m Pertechnetate Uptake

A Tc-99m pertechnetate uptake is not commonly performed. Advantages over a %RAIU are that the study can be completed within 20 to 30 minutes and radioiodine is not needed. The disadvantages include much lower accuracy than the %RAIU and a lack of widespread commercial software for Tc-99m pertechnetate calculation. In addition, the lack of organification prevents accurate measurement of the 24-hour %RAIU, standard practice for I-131 therapy dose calculation.

Methodology. A gamma camera imaging technique is used rather than a scintillation probe because of the high neck background. Before and after injection of the Tc-99m, the syringe is imaged (preinjection counts – postinjection residual counts = administered counts). Images are acquired on a computer. Regions of interest are drawn on a computer for the thyroid, thyroid background, and syringes. Areas of interest are normalized for pixel size, and thyroid and syringe counts are normalized for time of acquisition. Normal Tc-99m uptake is 0.3% to 4.5%.

Thyroid Scan

Thyroid scintigraphy depicts the entire gland in a single image and allows direct correlation of physical findings with abnormalities in the image. The combination of gamma camera and pinhole collimator makes possible multiple-view high-resolution images of the thyroid. Pinhole collimator magnification provides image resolution superior to parallel-hole collimators, approximately 5 mm compared to more than 1.5 cm with a parallel-hole collimator (Fig. 6-7).

The thyroid gland should be routinely examined by palpation at the time of imaging, to estimate gland size and confirm the presence and location of nodules. A radioactive marker source (122-keV cobalt-57 or Tc-99m) or lead can be used to correlate thyroid palpation findings with the scintigraphic image. Other imaging modalities performed before the scan (e.g., sonography, computed tomography [CT]) should always be reviewed.

Methodology

Iodine-123 and Technetium-99m Pertechnetate Scintigraphy. For an I-123 scan, the patient ingests 300 to 400 μCi orally. The scan is usually acquired 4 hours later. It may be more convenient to perform the scan at the same time as the 24-hour %RAIU. However, the low count rate at 24 hours requires longer acquisition time, which increases the likelihood of patient movement. Images can be acquired at 4 hours for a shorter time, and image quality is far superior. For a Tc-99m pertechnetate scan, 3 to 5 mCi is administered intravenously. Imaging begins 20 minutes after injection. Early imaging is required because Tc-99m is not organified and thus not retained within the thyroid.

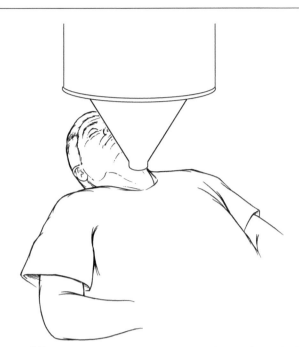

FIGURE 6-7. Pinhole collimator. The pinhole collimator is attached to the front of the gamma camera and positioned close to the thyroid to permit optimal magnification. If positioned farther away, the resulting image would be smaller.

For both radiopharmaceuticals, a large field-of-view gamma camera is equipped with a pinhole collimator that has an interchangeable lead pinhole insert of 3- to 6-mm in internal diameter placed in its distal aspect. Smaller diameter inserts provide higher resolution but lower sensitivity for count detection. A 4-mm insert is commonly used.

A 15% to 20% photopeak window is centered at 159 keV for I-123 and at 140 keV for Tc-99m. Imaging protocols for the two radiopharmaceuticals are otherwise similar and described in more detail in Box 6-3. The patient is positioned supine with the neck hyperextended and the plane of the thyroid gland roughly parallel to the crystal face of the camera. The gland should fill approximately two thirds of the field of view. This is achieved by placing the collimator 6 to 8 cm from the surface of the neck. Collimator magnification increases as the pinhole approaches the neck.

On one image, a radioactive marker (Tc-99m, Co-57) or computer cursor is routinely placed at the sternal notch and right side. For this image, the collimator could be placed at a greater distance to the neck, resulting in a smaller thyroid image (Fig. 6-8). In some clinics, a line source marker or two point sources 4 or 5 cm apart are placed on the neck lateral to the thyroid lobes and parallel to their long axis to estimate the size of the thyroid and nodules.

Images are routinely obtained in the anterior, right anterior oblique, and left anterior oblique views. Each image is acquired for approximately 100,000 counts or 5 to 7 minutes. It is preferable for the patient to remain in one position while the camera and collimator are moved to the different projections, thus making images more reproducible between patient and resulting in less image distortion and patient motion.

Additional images using a radioactive marker can help determine whether a palpable nodule takes up the radiopharmaceutical—that is, a hot or cold nodule. Care should be taken to avoid the pinhole collimator *parallax effect*, which is a change in the relationship between a near and distant object when viewed from different angles, resulting in misinterpretation of location of a nodule or suspected substernal goiter. To minimize this effect, the region of interest and marker should be positioned in the center of the field of view. For a suspected substernal goiter, an additional parallel-hole collimator with a suprasternal marker may be preferable.

Iodide Iodine-131 Scintigraphy. Because of the high radiation dose to the thyroid from I-131, clinical indications are limited to thyroid cancer scintigraphy where the thyroid has been surgically removed. Thyroid cancer protocols are described in a later section.

In the past, I-131 was also used to confirm the thyroid origin of a mediastinal mass (i.e., a suspected substernal goiter); however, today I-123 is preferable and standard.

Normal and Abnormal Thyroid Scintigraphy

A systematic interpretation of the thyroid scan requires assessment of thyroid size and configuration and identification of focal abnormalities. Gland size can be estimated but has limitations because of the scan's two-dimensional nature and the magnification produced by pinhole collimation. Image appearance and surface radiomarkers can provide some indication of size; however, gland palpation is more reliable. Thyroid scans should be interpreted in light of patient history, thyroid function studies, thyroid palpation examination, sonography, and %RAIU.

The normal scintigraphic appearance of the thyroid varies among patients. The gland has a butterfly shape, with

---

Box 6-3. Iodine-123 and Technetium-99m Pertechnetate Thyroid Imaging: Protocol Summary

PATIENT PREPARATION
Discontinue medications that interfere with thyroid uptake (Table 6-3)
Nothing by mouth for 4 hours before study

RADIOPHARMACEUTICAL
Iodine I-123, 100-400 µCi, orally in capsule form
Tc-99m pertechnetate, 3-5 mCi (111-185 MBq), intravenously

TIME OF IMAGING
Iodine I-123, 4-6 hours after dose administration
Tc-99m pertechnetate, 20 minutes after radiopharmaceutical injection

IMAGING PROCEDURE
Use gamma camera with a pinhole collimator.
Energy window:
    Tc-99m pertechnetate: 15-20% energy window centered at 140 keV
    I-123: 20% window centered at 159 keV
Position the supine patient with the chin up and neck extended.
Acquire initial anterior view for 75,000 counts or 5 minutes with collimator placed to include right side and suprasternal notch markers.
Place the collimator closer so that the thyroid fills about approximately two thirds of the field of view.
Acquire anterior, left anterior oblique, and right anterior oblique images for 100,000 counts or 7 minutes.

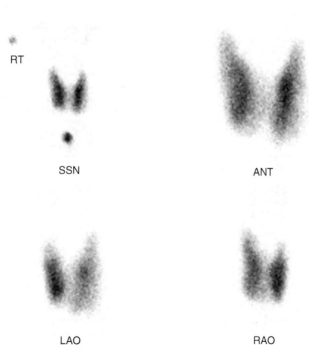

FIGURE 6-8. Normal I-123 thyroid scan. The *left upper* image is acquired with the collimator distanced further from the neck than the other three images, permitting a larger field of view and clear view of the suprasternal notch *(SSN)* and the right side *(RT)* hot markers. The anterior *(ANT)*, left anterior oblique *(LAO)*, and right anterior oblique *(RAO)* views are acquired with the pinhole close enough to the patient's neck that the image fills two thirds of the field of view. The right lobe is best viewed on the RAO view and the left lobe on the LAO image because those lobes are closest to the collimator and best magnified.

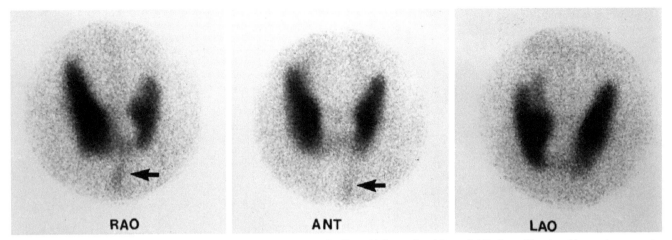

FIGURE 6-9. Esophageal activity. Anterior *(ANT)*, right anterior oblique *(RAO)*, and left anterior oblique *(LAO)* views. The thyroid scan shows esophageal activity below the thyroid to the left of midline *(arrows)*. Intensity is set high to best visualize esophageal activity. No esophageal activity is seen in the LAO view, the last view acquired. The activity spontaneously transited distally. When in doubt, the patient is asked to drink water to wash activity distally.

usually thin lateral lobes extending along each side of the thyroid cartilage (Fig. 6-8). The right lobe is often larger than the left. Visualization of the isthmus varies considerably among patients. The thin pyramidal lobe is normally not seen; it ascends anteriorly and superiorly from the isthmus or either lobe but more often the left lobe.

The normal gland has homogeneous uptake throughout. Increased intensity may be seen in the middle or medial aspects of the lateral lobes in the anterior view because of the gland's central thickness. Anterior oblique views show a more uniform appearance.

Higher background is seen on Tc-99m pertechnetate scans compared to I-123 scans. Salivary glands are routinely seen with Tc-99m pertechnetate, imaged at 20 to 30 minutes. However, they are not often seen with I-123 imaged at 4 hours because the background activity has washed out.

With thyroid enlargement the lobes appear plump. Relatively hot and cold regions should be noted. These do not necessarily represent nodules, which are diagnosed by palpation or anatomical imaging. Radionuclide markers can aid in confirming that the palpated nodule correlates with the scintigraphic finding.

Esophageal activity may be seen with either radiotracer. It is frequently not midline, but displaced by the trachea and cervical spine when the neck is hyperextended in the imaging position. Often it is seen just left of midline and relatively posterior. It can usually be confirmed by having the patient swallow water to clear the esophagus (Fig. 6-9).

Clinical Utility of the Percent Radioactive Iodine Thyroid Uptake and Thyroid Scan

The %RAIU does not define thyroid function per se—that is, euthyroid, hyperthyroid, or hypothyroid (Table 6-6) as these are clinical diagnoses. With normal pituitary feedback, the uptake depends on pituitary TSH stimulation. Increased uptake can be seen in patients not only with hyperthyroidism but also with hypothyroidism or euthyroidism—for example, iodine deficiency, dyshormonogenesis (organification defect), and chronic autoimmune

thyroiditis (Table 6-6). In these patients, feedback is normal, and the increased uptake is a normal physiological response to a hypofunctioning gland. Tc-99m and radioiodine uptakes may show different results (e.g., in patients with organification block). Thus the %RAIU must be interpreted in light of the clinical indication and laboratory results.

Thyrotoxicosis

Thyrotoxicosis is defined as hypermetabolism caused by a high level of circulating thyroid hormone. The term *hyperthyroidism* best describes thyrotoxicosis resulting from a hyperfunctioning thyroid gland—for example, Graves disease or toxic nodular goiter. Examples of thyrotoxicosis not caused by a hyperfunctioning thyroid gland are subacute thyroiditis and thyroiditis factitia (Box 6-4).

Clinical Diagnosis

The symptoms of thyrotoxicosis are those of increased metabolism—for example, heat intolerance, hyperhidrosis, anxiety, weight loss, tachycardia, and palpitations. These symptoms are nonspecific, and the diagnosis requires confirmation with serum thyroid function studies. A suppressed serum TSH less than 0.1 mU/L is diagnostic of thyrotoxicosis. This results from negative feedback on the pituitary by the elevated serum thyroid hormones. The only exception to a suppressed TSH without thyrotoxicosis is a rare hypothalamic or pituitary cause.

Differential Diagnosis

The clinical history and physical examination sometimes can suggest the cause of thyrotoxicosis—for example, a recent upper respiratory infection and tender thyroid gland with subacute thyroiditis or exophthalmos and pretibial edema, classic for Graves disease. A protracted course suggests Graves over thyroiditis. In some patients, the clinical question is Graves disease versus toxic multinodular goiter and in others Graves disease versus subacute thyroiditis. (Table 6-4).

Graves Disease. Approximately 75% of patients with thyrotoxicosis have Graves disease as the cause. Graves is

TABLE **6-6** Relationship of Thyroid Uptake to Thyroid Function

Thyroid function	Thyroid Uptake		
	Increased	Normal	Decreased
Thyrotoxicosis	Graves disease Hashitoxicosis	Antithyroid drugs Propylthiouracil Methimazole	Expanded iodide pool Subacute thyroiditis, thyrotoxic phase Thyrotoxicosis factitia Antithyroid drugs Struma ovarii
Euthyroid	Rebound after antithyroid drug withdrawal Recovery from subacute thyroiditis Compensated dyshormonogenesis		Decompensated dyshormonogenesis
Hypothyroid	Decompensated dyshormonogenesis Hashimoto disease	Hashimoto disease After I-131 therapy Subacute thyroiditis, recovery phase decompensated dyshormonogenesis	Hypothyroidism: primary or secondary

Box 6-4. Classification of Thyrotoxicosis Based on Thyroid Gland Function

THYROID GLAND HYPERFUNCTION
A. Abnormal thyroid stimulator
   1. Graves disease
   2. Trophoblastic tumor
      a. Hydatiform mole, choriocarcinoma (uterus or testes)
B. Intrinsic thyroid autonomy
   1. Toxic single adenoma
   2. Toxic multinodular goiter
C. Excess production of thyroid-stimulating hormone (rare)

NO THYROID GLAND HYPERFUNCTION
A. Disorders of hormone storage
   1. Subacute thyroiditis
B. Extrathyroid source of hormone
   1. Thyrotoxicosis factitia
   2. "Hamburger toxicosis" (epidemic caused by thyroid gland–contaminated hamburger meat)
   3. Ectopic thyroid tissue
      a. Struma ovarii
      b. Functioning follicular carcinoma

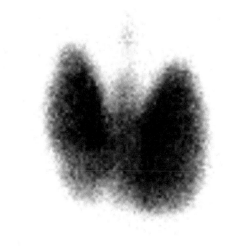

FIGURE **6-10.** Graves disease. The patient is thyrotoxic. The anterior view shows both thyroid lobes to be plump with convex borders and evidence of a pyramidal lobe arising from the isthmus. The thyroid to background ratio is high. The percent radioactive iodine thyroid uptake was 63%.

an autoimmune disease causing a *thyrotropin receptor antibody*, which stimulates thyroid follicular cells, resulting in the production of excess thyroid hormone. Thyroid gland function is autonomous, independent of TSH feedback. It is most commonly seen in middle-aged women but also occurs in children, the elderly, and men.

Patients with Graves disease typically have a diffusely enlarged thyroid gland (goiter), which is firm and nontender. An elevated %RAIU, usually in the range of 50% to 80%, confirms the diagnosis and excludes most other causes of thyrotoxicosis, which have a suppressed uptake. Thyroid scan shows a high thyroid-to-background ratio (Fig. 6-10). The scan can help differentiate a diffuse toxic goiter (Graves) from a toxic multinodular goiter (Fig. 6-11). Experienced endocrinologists can often distinguish the two on examination and sonography and refer patients for only %RAIU

without scan. In some cases, Graves disease can be superimposed on a nontoxic multinodular goiter and the scan is usually diagnostic.

Multinodular Toxic Goiter (Plummer Disease). Patients are often elderly and present with tachyarrhythmias, weight loss, depression, anxiety, and insomnia. The hypermetabolism may exacerbate other medical problems, and thus the disease requires prompt therapy. The %RAIU is often only moderately elevated or may be in the high normal range. The thyroid scan shows high uptake within hyperfunctioning nodules but suppression of the extranodular nonautonomous tissue (Fig. 6-11). A nontoxic multinodular goiter may have hot or warm nodules, but the extranodular tissue is not suppressed (Fig. 6-12).

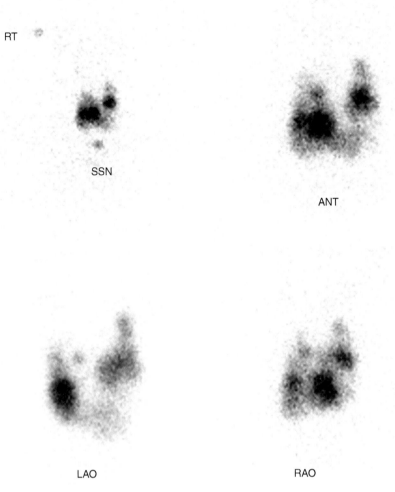

FIGURE 6-11. Toxic multinodular goiter. Thyrotoxic patient who had multiple thyroid nodules seen on ultrasonography. The thyroid scan shows multiple areas of increased uptake consistent with hot nodules in both lobes and suppression of the remaining normal functioning thyroid. *ANT,* Anterior; *LAO,* left anterior oblique; *RAO,* right anterior oblique; *RT,* right; *SSN,* suprasternal notch.

Single Autonomously Functioning Thyroid Nodule. Most thyroid nodules are either nonfunctioning (cold) or functioning normally. However, toxic nodules occur in approximately 5% of patients with a palpable nodule. Once an autonomous nodule grows to a size of 2.5 to 3.0 cm, it may produce the clinical manifestations of thyrotoxicosis. Although the %RAIU may be elevated, it is often in the normal range. The thyroid scan shows uptake in the nodule but suppression of the remainder of the gland and low background (Fig. 6-13).

Hashitoxicosis. Hashimoto disease is an uncommon cause of thyrotoxicosis. It typically presents in middle-aged women as goiter and *hypo*thyroidism. Histopathologically, lymphocytic infiltration is characteristic. The gland is diffusely and symmetrically enlarged, nontender, firm, and usually without nodules. Serum antithyroglobulin and antimicrosomal antibodies are elevated. Scintigraphic findings are variable. Uptake may be inhomogeneous throughout the gland, or focal cold areas without a palpable nodule may be present.

Approximately 3% to 5% of patients with Hashimoto disease develop thyrotoxicosis, or hashitoxicosis, at some point during the course of the disease. During the thyrotoxic

phase, the %RAIU is increased and the scan shows diffuse increased uptake, similar to Graves disease. This is thought to be an overlap syndrome with Graves and is treated with radioactive iodine.

Subacute Thyroiditis. The most common cause for thyrotoxicosis associated with a decreased %RAIU is subacute thyroiditis. This has various causes. *Granulomatous thyroiditis* (de Quervain) is typically preceded by several days of upper respiratory illness and tender thyroid. *Silent thyroiditis,* usually occurring in the elderly, is not associated with respiratory symptoms or thyroid tenderness and is not a granulomatous process, but probably viral. Patients often have arrhythmia and a normal-sized thyroid. *Postpartum thyroiditis* occurs within weeks or months of delivery, with positive antithyroid antibodies.

During the initial stage of subacute thyroiditis, thyrotoxicosis predominates, caused by release of thyroid hormone as a result of inflammation and increased membrane permeability. The elevated serum thyroid hormone suppresses TSH. This is the stage at which patients are usually referred for a scan and uptake to differentiate it from Graves disease.

As the inflammation resolves and the thyroid gland hormone is depleted, thyroid hormone levels decrease and

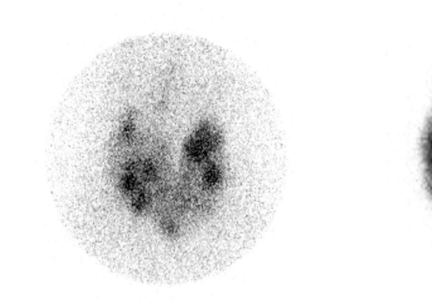

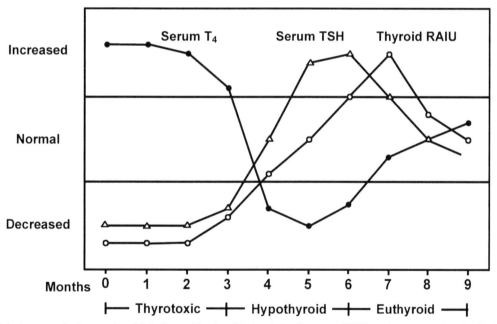

FIGURE 6-12. Nontoxic multinodular goiter. The patient is euthyroid with an enlarged gland on examination and multiple thyroid nodules by ultrasonography. The scan (anterior view) shows multiple areas of focally increased uptake, which correspond to palpable nodules. The extrathyroidal tissue is not suppressed, and the background is relatively high.

FIGURE 6-13. Toxic (hot) thyroid nodule. The patient presented with thyrotoxic symptoms. Thyroid palpation detected a 3-cm right thyroid nodule. Thyroid function studies revealed an elevated T_4 and suppressed TSH (<0.05 mIU/L). The I-123 scan shows intense uptake in the nodule; however, the remainder of the gland suppressed.

FIGURE 6-14. Clinical course of subacute thyroiditis. Serum T_4, thyroid-stimulating hormone (TSH), and percent radioactive iodine thyroid uptake (%RAIU) from initial presentation to resolution 9 months later. When the patient is thyrotoxic on initial examination, the T_4 is elevated and TSH and %RAIU suppressed. After the stored thyroid hormone has been released secondary to inflammation and then metabolized, the patient becomes hypothyroid as a result of the inflamed, poorly functioning thyroid. TSH and %RAIU rise. With time, the thyroid regains function and the patient usually becomes euthyroid, with normalized T_4, TSH, and %RAIU.

may fall into the hypothyroid range, causing a rise in serum TSH. The %RAIU depends on the stage of the disease and the damaged thyroid's ability to respond to endogenous TSH stimulation. Hypothyroidism resolves over weeks or months, and the TSH and %RAIU return to normal (Fig. 6-14).

The decreased uptake that occurs initially with subacute thyroiditis during the thyrotoxic stage is the result of an intact pituitary feedback mechanism, not damage and dysfunction of the gland. Uptake is suppressed in the entire gland (Fig. 6-15), although the disease is often patchy or regional. During recovery the appearance is variable,

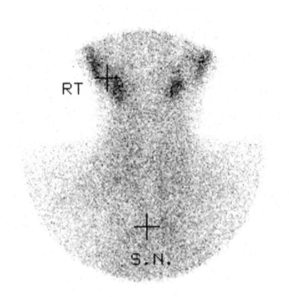

FIGURE **6-15.** Subacute thyroiditis. The patient presented with recent onset of thyrotoxicosis. The thyroid was tender and slightly enlarged. The technetium-99m thyroid scan shows suppressed thyroid uptake. *RT,* Right side; *S.N.,* suprasternal notch.

depending on the severity and distribution of the thyroid damage. The scintigram may show inhomogeneity of uptake or regional or focal areas of hypofunction.

Iodine-Induced Thyrotoxicosis (Jod-Basedow Phenomenon). In the past, this condition occurred with the introduction of iodized salt into the diet in iodine-deficient areas (goiter belts). Today it is most commonly seen in patients who have received iodinated contrast media with CT. The iodine induces thyroiditis and thyrotoxicosis, and the %RAIU is suppressed. Less commonly, the iodine load causes activation of subclinical Graves disease or toxic multinodular goiter; %RAIU is elevated.

Amiodarone-Induced Thyrotoxicosis. Amiodarone, an antiarrhythmic therapeutic drug, contains 75 mg iodine per tablet. It has a physiological half-life of more than 3 months, but its effect may last longer. Hyperthyroidism or hypothyroidism occurs in up to 10% of patients on the drug. Two types of thyrotoxicosis are seen. In type 1, which is iodine induced (Jod-Basedow) in patients with preexisting nodular goiter or subclinical Graves disease, the %RAIU is elevated. Type 2, which is more common, results in a destructive thyroiditis, and the %RAIU is near zero.

Thyrotoxicosis Factitia. Thyrotoxicosis factitia is not rare. In some cases, thyroid hormone has been prescribed by a physician. In other cases, it is surreptitiously taken by a patient for weight loss or other reasons. Often the patients are health care workers.

Infrequent Causes for Thyrotoxicosis. A pituitary adenoma secreting TSH is a rare cause of thyrotoxicosis. An even rarer condition is resistance of the pituitary to thyroid hormone feedback. In both cases, TSH is elevated.

Hydatidiform mole, trophoblastic tumors, and choriocarcinoma may produce symptoms of hyperthyroidism. Human chorionic gonadotropin is a weak TSH-like agonist. Serum TSH is suppressed, and the %RAIU is elevated. Hyperthyroidism secondary to metastatic thyroid cancer is quite rare, most commonly occurring with follicular carcinoma.

Approximately 1% to 2% of benign ovarian teratomas have functioning thyroid tissue as a major component (struma ovarii), and in rare instances this tumor produces sufficient thyroid hormone to cause thyrotoxicosis. The diagnosis is suspected in a patient with a concomitant pelvic mass. Neck thyroid uptake is suppressed. The ectopic pelvic thyroid tissue can be visualized with a thyroid scan.

Pharmacological Diagnostic Interventional Tests with Percent Radioactive Iodine Thyroid Uptake

In the past, the %RAIU was used in conjunction with various pharmacological interventions for diagnosis. Although the interventions nicely delineate underlying pathophysiological processes, they are rarely required today because of advancements in diagnostic methods. An understanding and appreciation of thyroid disease pathophysiology is enhanced by a brief review of these tests.

Triiodothryronine Suppression Test

The T_3 suppression test was used to diagnose borderline Graves disease by demonstrating autonomous function. After a baseline 24-hour %RAIU, the patient receives 25 mcg of T_3 four times per day for 8 days. The %RAIU is repeated beginning on day 7. A normal response is a fall in the %RAIU to less than 50% of baseline and less than 10% overall. Autonomously functioning glands will not suppress. Sensitive serum TSH values have made this test unnecessary.

Thyroid-Stimulating Hormone Stimulation Test

The TSH stimulation test distinguishes primary from secondary (pituitary) hypothyroidism. Failure to respond to exogenous TSH is indicative of primary hypothyroidism. Patients with secondary hypothyroidism have increased %RAIU after TSH stimulation. A baseline 24-hour %RAIU is first determined. TSH is then administered, and the %RAIU is repeated the next day. In patients with hypopituitarism the uptake doubles, whereas those with primary hypothyroidism show no response.

Perchlorate Discharge Test

The perchlorate discharge test demonstrates dissociation of trapping and organification seen with congenital enzyme deficiencies, in chronic thyroiditis, and during propylthiouracil therapy. After administering radioiodine, the %RAIU is measured at 1 and 2 hours. Potassium perchlorate is given orally, and the measurement is repeated an hour later. A washout greater than 10% suggests an organification defect.

Clinical Indications for Thyroid Scintigraphy

Patients are referred for thyroid scintigraphy less frequently today than in the past primarily because of the use of percutaneous aspiration biopsy of thyroid nodules. Scintigraphy can still provide valuable clinical information for some patients.

Thyroid Nodules

Differentiating a benign versus malignant nodule is a common clinical problem. Thyroid nodules are common, and the incidence of benign and malignant nodules increases with age. They occur more often in women than men. Concern for malignancy is increased in a young person, a man, or a patient with recent nodule growth. The presence of multiple nodules decreases the likelihood of malignancy. A nodule in a patient with Graves disease requires investigation.

Radiation to the head and neck or mediastinum has been associated with an increased incidence of thyroid nodules and thyroid cancer. Several decades ago, external radiation therapy was used to shrink asymptomatic enlarged thymus glands and treat enlarged tonsils, adenoids, and acne. Patients received radiation in the range of 10 to 50 rem, a radiation dose that has been associated with an increased incidence of thyroid cancer. Radiation exposure at Hiroshima, Nagasaki, and Chernobyl also resulted in an increased incidence of thyroid nodules and cancer.

Radiation exposure up to 1500 rem increases the incidence of thyroid nodules and cancer. The mean latency period is approximately 5 years. For radiation greater than 1500 rem, the risk decreases, presumably because of tissue destruction. High radiation doses used for therapy of malignant tumors may cause hypothyroidism.

Ultrasonography

Nodules can be confirmed by sonography when suspected on physical examination, and sonography can be used to determine whether a nodule is solid or cystic. Purely cystic lesions are benign; however, cancer cannot be excluded if the cyst has a soft tissue component or cystic degeneration. Additional nodules may be detected. Sonography often is used to guide biopsy.

Fine Needle Aspiration Biopsy

With palpable nodules, fine needle aspiration biopsy can be performed in the endocrinologist's office and is often done without prior scintigraphy or sonographic guidance. Nonpalpable nodules require sonography for biopsy. Biopsy accuracy is high, although subject to some sampling error. On occasion, a benign follicular adenoma cannot be distinguished histopathologically from follicular cancer. In these cases, a thyroid scan can help. Thyroid cancer is hypofunctional (cold), whereas a follicular adenomas function and have uptake.

Thyroid Scintigraphy

The thyroid scan provides functional, not anatomical, information. It does not diagnose nodules per se, because a hot or cold region on the scan may be due to various pathological conditions other than a nodule—for example, thyroiditis, scarring, necrosis, hemorrhage, and hyperplasia. A nodule must be confirmed by thyroid palpation or anatomical imaging, usually ultrasonography.

Thyroid scintigraphy can determine the functional status of a nodule and thus guide further diagnosis procedures (Table 6-7). On scintigrams, nodules are classified as *cold* (Fig. 6-16) (hypofunctioning compared to adjacent normal tissue), *hot* (Fig. 6-13) (hyperfunctioning with suppression of the extranodular gland), *warm* (Fig. 6-17)

TABLE 6-7 Likelihood of Thyroid Cancer in Nodule Based on Thyroid Scintigraphy

Nodule	Likelihood of thyroid cancer (%)
Cold	15-20
Indeterminate	15-20
Multinodular	5
Hot	<1

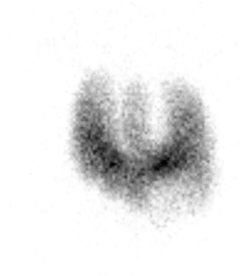

FIGURE 6-16. Cold nodule. Focal decrease in iodine-123 uptake in the left lobe of the thyroid that corresponded to a palpable nodule. This patient has Graves disease. Note the prominent pyramidal lobe and apparent enlarged thyroid lobes.

(increased uptake compared to adjacent tissue but without suppression of the extranodular tissue), or *indeterminate* (palpable or seen on anatomical imaging but not visualized on scintigraphy).

Cold Nodule

Approximately 85% to 90% of thyroid nodules are cold (hypofunctional) on thyroid scans. The incidence of cancer in a cold thyroid nodule is 15% to 20%, although it is reported to be as high as 40% in surgical series and as low as 5% in general medical series. Thus most cold nodules have a benign cause—for example, simple cysts, colloid nodules, thyroiditis, hemorrhage, necrosis, or infiltrative disorders (e.g., amyloid or hemochromatosis) (Box 6-5). The incidence of malignancy in cold nodules in multinodular goiters is lower than in glands with a single nodule, probably less than 5%. Dominant nodules—for example, those that are distinctly larger than the other nodules in a multinodular goiter or those that are enlarging—require further evaluation.

Hot Nodule

Radioiodine uptake in a nodule denotes function. A functioning nodule is very unlikely to be malignant. Less than

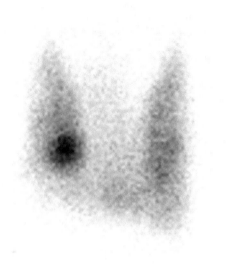

Figure 6-17. Warm nodule in euthyroid patient. Patient presented with a palpable 1.5-cm nodule. Increased uptake is seen in the inferior aspect of the right lobe of the thyroid. The extranodular gland does not appear to be suppressed. The patient had normal thyroid function tests. The warm nodule may be autonomous, but it is not a toxic nodule. Compare to Figure 6-13.

1% of hot nodules are reported to harbor malignancy. The term *hot nodule* specifies not only that it has high uptake but also that suppression of adjacent extranodular tissue is present (Fig. 6-13). Without suppression, this should be referred to as a *warm nodule* (Fig. 6-17).

Hot nodules are autonomous hyperfunctioning follicular adenomas. Warm nodules may be caused by autonomous adenomas; however, they are not producing enough thyroid hormone to cause thyrotoxicosis (TSH is not suppressed) and thus not "toxic." A warm nodule may also be caused by nonautonomous hyperplastic tissue or even normal functioning tissue surrounded by poorly functioning thyroid. A toxic follicular adenoma cannot be suppressed with thyroid hormone.

Hot nodules greater than 2.5 to 3.0 cm often produce overt thyrotoxicosis. Some patients with smaller nodules and less hormone production may have subclinical hyperthyroidism, with a suppressed serum TSH but normal T_4. Serum T_3 may be elevated (T_3 thyrotoxicosis). A small autonomous nodule may be followed clinically because it can progress, regress, undergo involution, or stabilize. Increasingly, autonomous nodules are treated at an early stage because of the low incidence of regression and adverse consequences associated with subclinical hyperthyroidism, (e.g., bone mineral loss).

Radioiodine I-131 is the usual therapy for toxic nodules because the radiation is delivered selectively to the hyperfunctioning tissue while sparing suppressed extranodular tissues. This results in a low incidence of posttherapy hypothyroidism. After successful treatment, the suppressed tissue regains function. On occasion, surgery may be performed for patients with local symptoms or cosmetic concerns.

Box 6-5. Differential Diagnosis for Thyroid Nodules

COLD NODULES (NONFUNCTIONING)
Benign
  Colloid nodule
  Simple cyst
  Hemorrhagic cyst
  Adenoma
  Thyroiditis
  Abscess
  Parathyroid cyst or adenoma
Malignant
  Papillary
  Follicular
    Hurthle cell
  Anaplastic
  Medullary
  Lymphoma
  Metastatic carcinoma
    Lung
    Breast
    Melanoma
    Gastrointestinal
    Renal

HOT NODULES (AUTONOMOUS FUNCTION)
Toxic follicular adenomas

WARM NODULES
  Nontoxic hyperfunctioning adenomas
  Hyperplastic thyroid tissue

Indeterminate Nodule

When a palpable or sonographically detected nodule greater than 1 cm cannot be differentiated by thyroid scan as definitely hot or cold compared to surrounding normal thyroid, it is referred to as an *indeterminate nodule*. This may occur with a posterior nodule that has normal thyroid uptake superimposed anterior to it, making it appear to have normal uptake. Nodules less than 1 cm may be too small to be detected by scintigraphy. For management purposes, an indeterminate nodule has the same significance as a cold nodule.

Discordant Nodule

Some apparently hot or warm nodules on Tc-99m scans appear cold on radioiodine scans (Fig. 6-18). This occurs in only 5% of patients. Because some thyroid cancers maintain trapping but not organification, a single hot nodule identified on Tc-99m imaging should not be considered a functioning nodule until confirmed by I-123 scan. Of discordant nodules, 20% are malignant. The discordant nodule is a disadvantage to the use of Tc-99m pertechnetate for evaluation of thyroid nodules.

Colloid Nodular Goiter

Before the addition of iodine supplements to salt and food, goiter was endemic in the northern United States around the Great Lakes and still occurs in some parts of the world. These endemic goiters are composed of colloid nodules that are usually benign. The pathogenesis of iodine-deficient

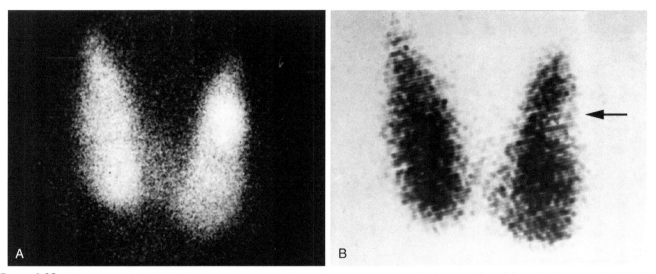

FIGURE 6-18. Discordant nodule. **A,** Tc-99m pertechnetate scan shows relatively increased uptake in a palpable nodule in the *left upper* pole. **B,** In the corresponding radioiodine scan the nodule *(arrow)* is cold. Thus the nodule can trap but not organify iodine. This discordance requires further workup to exclude malignancy.

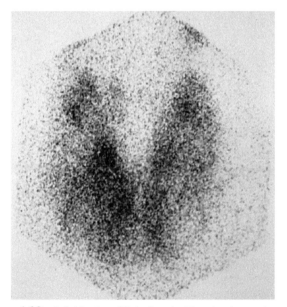

FIGURE 6-19. Colloid goiter. Clinically palpable goiter in a patient who grew up in a Michigan goiter belt. Inhomogeneous tracer distribution with multiple focal cold areas. The patient was mildly hypothyroid.

nodule formation is hyperplasia followed by the formation of functioning nodules that undergo hemorrhage and necrosis replaced by lakes of colloid. Repetition of this process over time leads to glandular enlargement, with nonfunctioning colloid nodules as the dominant histopathological feature. The typical scintigraphic appearance is inhomogeneous uptake with cold areas of various sizes (Fig. 6-19).

Substernal Goiter

Substernal goiters are usually extensions of the thyroid into the mediastinum. Most show continuity with the cervical portion of the gland, although some have only a fibrous band connecting the substernal and cervical thyroid tissues. Many are asymptomatic and incidentally detected on CT as an anterior upper mediastinal mass. As they enlarge, they may cause symptoms of dyspnea,

stridor, or dysphagia. Scintigraphy can confirm the thyroid origin of the mass.

Uptake in substernal goiters is often lower than thyroid bed activity. Tc-99m pertechnetate is not ideally suited for this purpose because of its high mediastinal blood pool activity, although the study can sometimes be diagnostic (Fig. 6-20). I-131 has been used because it can be imaged at 24 to 48 hours and thus will have high target-to-background ratio (Fig. 6-21). Currently, I-123 is usually the first radiopharmaceutical of choice with images obtained at 4 hours. Single-photon emission computed tomography (SPECT), but particularly SPECT with CT (SPECT/CT) can be confirmatory (Fig. 6-22).

Ectopic Thyroid Tissue

Because the thyroglossal duct extends from the foramen cecum at the base of the tongue to the thyroid, lingual or upper cervical thyroid tissue can present in the neonate or child as a midline mass. It is often accompanied by hypothyroidism. Ectopic thyroid tissue may occur in the mediastinum or even in the pelvis (struma ovarii).

The typical appearance of a lingual thyroid is a focal or nodular accumulation at the base of the tongue and absence of tracer uptake in the expected cervical location (Fig. 6-23). Lingual thyroids often function poorly. Lateral thyroid rests also may be hypofunctional. However, rests can function, hyperfunction, or be the focus of thyroid cancer. Ectopic thyroid tissue should be considered metastatic until proved otherwise.

Reidel Struma

Reidel struma is an uncommon form of thyroiditis in which all or part of the gland is replaced by fibrous tissue. No uptake is seen in the region of fibrous tissue.

Therapy of Thyrotoxicosis with Radioiodine I-131

Radioiodine has been used with great success for many decades for the treatment of Graves disease and toxic single and multiple nodular thyroid disease (Box 6-6).

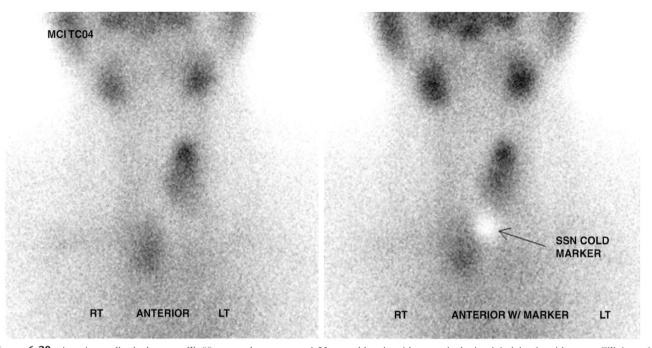

MCI TC04

SSN COLD
MARKER

RT   ANTERIOR   LT

RT   ANTERIOR W/ MARKER   LT

FIGURE 6-20. Anterior mediastinal mass on Tc-99m pertechnetate scan. A 52-year-old euthryoid woman had prior right lobe thyroidectomy. CT showed a right paratracheal mass. The Tc-99m scan shows considerable background and normal salivary gland uptake. In addition to uptake in the left thyroid lobe, uptake is seen to the right and inferior of the suprasternal notch marker (SSN), consistent with a substernal goiter.

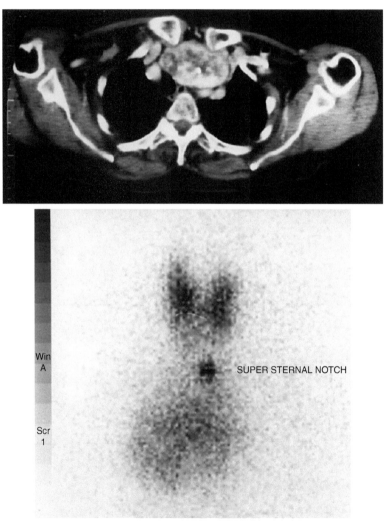

Win
A

Scr
1

SUPER STERNAL NOTCH

FIGURE 6-21. Substernal goiter on I-131 scan. The contrast CT image *(left)* shows the presence of an anterior mediastinal mass. I-131 thyroid scan *(right)* has uptake in a normal-appearing thyroid and a large substernal goiter that corresponds to the mediastinal mass seen on CT. A radioactive marker denotes the suprasternal notch.

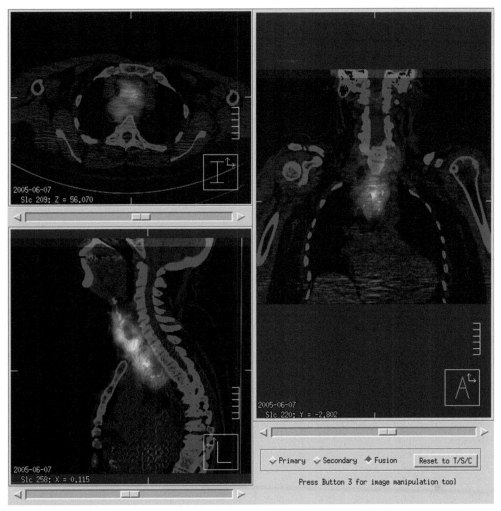

FIGURE 6-22. Substernal goiter with I-123 hybrid SPECT/CT. The I-123 thyroid scan is fused with the CT scan in selected transverse, sagittal, and coronal views. This patient had a multinodular toxic goiter with substernal extension.

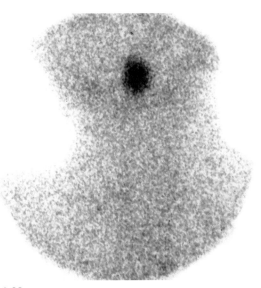

FIGURE 6-23. Lingual thyroid. Hypothyroid infant with neck mass. Thyroid scan (anterior view) shows prominent uptake within the midline neck mass. There is no thyroid uptake in the region of thyroid bed.

Box 6-6. **Indications for Iodine-131 Therapy**

INDICATED
Graves disease (diffuse toxic goiter)
Plummer disease (toxic nodules)
Functioning thyroid cancer (metastatic)

NOT INDICATED
Thyrotoxicosis factitia
Subacute thyroiditis
"Silent" thyroiditis (atypical, subacute, lymphocytic, transient, postpartum)
Struma ovarii
Thyroid hormone resistance (biochemical or clinical manifestations)
Secondary hyperthyroidism (pituitary tumor, ectopic thyroid-stimulating hormone, trophoblastic tumors [human chorionic gonadotropin])
Thyrotoxicosis associated with Hashimoto disease (hashitoxicosis)
Jod-Basedow phenomenon (iodine-induced hyperthyroidism)

Graves Disease

Patients with newly diagnosed Graves disease are often initially treated with beta-blockers for symptomatic relief and more specific therapy with thiourea antithyroid drugs (e.g., propylthiouracil [PTU] and methimazole [Tapazole]), which block organification and reduce thyroid hormone production. These drugs "cool" the patient down and render the patient euthyroid, providing time to consider further therapeutic options. Patients may be instructed to take these drugs for 6 to 12 months. However, the drugs have a high incidence of adverse effects (50%), the most serious being liver dysfunction and agranulocytosis. Thus they are rarely prescribed for longer than a year. Thyroidectomy is an uncommon therapy and associated with significant risk. Most patients ultimately receive radioiodine I-131 therapy. Increasingly patients are being treated with I-131 soon after diagnosis.

The exophthalmos of Graves disease is not controlled by thiourea antithyroid drugs or I-131 therapy. Some evidence even suggests that exacerbation of exophthalmos may occur with I-131 therapy; thus corticosteroids may be administered concomitantly.

Most patients with Graves disease are effectively treated with one therapeutic dose of I-131. The patient usually notes symptomatic improvement within 3 weeks of therapy; however, the full therapeutic effect takes 3 to 6 months because stored hormone must first be released. Radioiodine therapy may not initially be effective in up to 10% of patients. They require repeat treatment, usually with a higher administered dose.

Pregnancy must be excluded before I-131 therapy is administered. Women should be counseled to avoid pregnancy for 3 to 6 months after therapy in the event that retreatment is necessary.

Many decades of experience with therapeutic I-131 have shown it to be safe and effective. Endocrinologists have become comfortable with treating patients, even children, with I-131 because of its high efficacy and low incidence of acute or chronic adverse effects.

Most patients treated with I-131 ultimately develop hypothyroidism and require replacement hormone therapy. This may occur as early as several months after therapy or may take decades. With a larger administered dose, the likelihood increases for early onset of hypothyroidism. With a lower administered dose, the likelihood of disease recurrence is higher.

Occasional patients develop radiation thyroiditis after I-131 therapy, causing local neck pain, tenderness, or swelling. Very rarely, this can result in thyroid storm. It is important to recognize this serious complication, which may require hospitalization and steroid therapy. Patients in a very toxic state and those treated with higher amounts of radioactivity are at greater risk. Beta-blockers used before and after therapy can minimize this risk.

Evidence over many decades of I-131 therapy has not shown a statistically significant increase in the frequency of secondary cancers, infertility, or congenital defects in children of patients receiving I-131 therapy for Graves disease.

Iodine-131 Dose Selection

Various approaches have been used for selecting an I-131 dose for therapy in patients with Graves disease. One method is to prescribe standard I-131 dose in the range of 8 to 15 mCi. This often works. However, factors such as the size of the gland and %RAIU may result in very different radiation doses to the thyroid across patients. Large glands require a relatively higher therapeutic dose, and patients with a high %RAIU need a lower dose. Some radiotherapists adjust this dose based on these two factors.

Another common approach is to use a standard formula that takes gland size, the %RAIU, and the proposed administered I-131 dose per gram of thyroid tissue into consideration:

$$\text{I-131 administered dose} = \frac{\text{Gram size of thyroid gland} \times 100-180\ \mu\text{Ci/g}}{24\text{-hour }\%\text{RAIU}}$$

This approach calculates an individual therapy dose for each patient with Graves disease. See example (Box 6-7). An estimation of the gram weight of the gland is required. A normal gland weighs 15 to 20 g. Patients with Graves disease typically have glands in the range of 40 to 80 g but sometimes considerably larger. Considerable interphysician variability exists in estimation of gland size by palpation; however, an experienced physician is able to reproducibly estimate gland size. The size of larger glands is often underestimated.

Another variable in this calculation is the microcurie per gram dose. In the past, referring physicians often requested low I-131 doses to minimize the radiation to the patient (e.g., 60-80 µCi/g tissue). Today, referring physicians are more comfortable with the safety of higher doses (120-180 µCi/g tissue) and often prefer the higher likelihood of success with a single therapeutic dose. Early-onset hypothyroidism is also often preferred by some physicians because they feel it is inevitable and prompt replacement therapy can be instituted.

Patients with rapid radioiodine turnover in the gland (e.g., high 4-hour but normal or near-normal 24-hour %RAIU) have a shorter I-131 thyroid residence time. Thus a higher I-131 dose than would be calculated using the standard 24-hour %RAIU should be considered.

Toxic Nodular Disease

Toxic nodules are more resistant to therapy with radioiodine than Graves disease. The reason is unclear, but it may be that I-131 thyroid residence time in the nodule(s) is reduced, leading to a lower retained dose. The administered I-131 therapeutic dose is often increased by 50% over what would be prescribed for Graves disease. An empirical dose of 20 to 25 mCi is also often used. Because extranodular tissue is suppressed and spared from radiation, normal function usually resumes after successful therapy.

Thyroid Cancer

Well-differentiated thyroid cancer originates from thyroid follicular epithelium and retains biological characteristics of healthy thyroid tissue, including expression of the sodium iodide symporter, which is responsible for radioiodine uptake. The prognosis with appropriate treatment is generally good, with an estimated 10-year survival rate of 85%. Even with distant metastases, the 10-year survival is 25% to 40%. However, the lifetime recurrence rate is 10% to 30%, so long-term follow-up is required and subsequent therapy is necessary for many patients.

Box 6-7. Example Calculation of Iodine-131
Therapeutic Dose for Graves Hyperthyroidism

INPUT DATA
Gland weight: 60 g
24-hour uptake: 80%
Desired dose to be retained in thyroid (selected to
deliver 8,000-10,000 rads to thyroid): 100 µCi/g

CALCULATIONS

$$\text{Required dose } (\mu Ci) = \frac{60 \text{ g} \times 100 \text{ }\mu Ci/g}{0.80} = 7500$$

$$\text{Dose (mCi)} = \frac{7500}{1000} = 7.5 \text{ mCi}$$

Papillary thyroid carcinoma is the most common histopathological type of differentiated thyroid malignancy (70%). Pure follicular cell carcinoma occurs less frequently (25%). Papillary thyroid cancer spreads via regional lymphatic vessels, whereas follicular thyroid carcinoma is more likely to disseminate hematogenously, resulting in distant metastases and a worse prognosis. Hürthle cell and tall cell variants of papillary cancer behave similarly to the follicular cell and have a poorer prognosis. Medullary carcinomas and anaplastic carcinomas do not concentrate radioiodine and are not detected with radioiodine scintigraphy or effectively treated with I-131 therapy.

The primary treatment for newly diagnosed thyroid cancer is surgery. In uncomplicated cases, near-total thyroidectomy is the standard operation. Patients with cervical or mediastinal metastases require more extensive lymph neck dissection. Effective radioiodine I-131 therapy requires removal of the uninvolved normal thyroid and as much of the thyroid cancer as possible.

After total thyroidectomy, the serum thyroglobulin level should not be detectable; therefore serum thyroglobulin becomes a specific thyroid cancer marker. Its sensitivity for detection of residual or recurrent cancer is enhanced when it is stimulated by serum TSH.

Whole-Body Thyroid Cancer Scintigraphy

Well-differentiated thyroid cancer cells maintain physiological function; however, they are hypofunctional compared to normal thyroid tissue and thus take up radioiodine to a lesser degree. This is the reason that thyroid cancer nodules appear cold on thyroid scans. However, after thyroidectomy with TSH stimulation, either by hormone withdrawal or exogenous stimulation with recombinant TSH (Thyrogen), thyroid cancer imaging with radioiodine becomes feasible.

Patient Preparation

After Thyroidectomy. Whole-body thyroid scans are acquired 6 weeks after surgery. Two methods of preparation have been used: (1) The patient is not prescribed thyroid hormone replacement postoperatively, and thus the serum TSH progressively rises as the patient becomes increasingly hypothyroid. The patient's serum TSH level should be greater than 30 U/mL before radioiodine is administered, to ensure good uptake. (2) Alternatively, patients are placed on replacement thyroid hormone and are pretreated with recombinant TSH (Thyrogen) (see later discussion).

Follow-Up Whole-Body Scan. Two methods are used in follow-up scans. One is similar to that described earlier. The patient discontinues the long-acting thyroid hormone T$_4$ analog levothyroxine (Synthroid) for 4 to 6 weeks, until the TSH level is greater than 30 U/mL. To minimize hypothyroid symptoms, some patients are prescribed a shorter half-life T$_3$ thyroid hormone analog, triiodothyronine (Cytomel). However, this drug must be discontinued 2 weeks before radioiodine administration to ensure an adequate rise in the serum TSH.

Rrecombinant Thyroid-Stimulating Hormone (Thyrogen) as an Alternative to Thyroid Hormone Withdrawal. Symptoms of hypothyroidism can be quite debilitating for many patients, particularly those with other medical problems. Thyrogen, a recombinant form of TSH (rTSH), is administered on 2 consecutive days as an intramuscular injection of 0.9 mg. A serum TSH level is usually obtained. On the third day, radioiodine is administered. Imaging is performed on day 5 for I-131 and day 4 for I-123.

Hypothyroidism causes a decrease in the glomerular filtration rate (GFR) and radioiodine clearance. Recombinant TSH does not affect GFR, which has been suggested as a cause for differing sensitivities between Thyrogen and synthroid withdrawal scans. To expose thyroid cancer cells to similar extracellular radioiodine and maximize opportunity for uptake, a larger administered dose is required using recombinant TSH.

Methodology for Whole-Body Thyroid Cancer Scintigraphy

Iodine-131 Whole-Body Scan. In the past, 5 mCi or more of I-131 was the commonly administered dose for whole-body diagnostic thyroid cancer scans. Because of reports of thyroid "stunning" after this diagnostic dose (i.e., reduced uptake of the subsequent therapeutic dose), the recommended I-131 diagnostic dose is now less than 5 mCi, commonly 2 to 3 mCi.

Box 6-8 presents a summary of the protocol. A large field-of-view gamma camera equipped with a high-energy parallel-hole collimator is used, with a 20% to 30% window centered at 364 keV. Whole-body imaging is acquired 48 hours after oral administration. Whole-body views allow detection of thyroid metastases at distant sites—for example, in bones of the skull, humeri, spine, and femurs and in the liver and brain.

Scans performed after I-131 therapy are obtained in a similar manner, except that the scan is acquired approximately 7 days after therapy.

Iodine-123 Whole-Body Scan. Increasingly, I-123 is replacing I-131 for diagnostic whole-body thyroid cancer scans. Stunning is not an issue with I-123, image quality is superior, and the study is completed 24 hours after dose administration, rather than 48 hours. I-123 might be expected to detect fewer tumors than I-131 because of the earlier imaging period with less time for background clearance. However, investigations have shown similar ability to detect metastases, possibly because of the higher photon flux with I-123.

Box 6-9 presents a summary of the protocol. The orally administered dose of I-123 is typically 1.5 to 3 mCi. A

medium-energy parallel-hole collimator is preferable
because of the concomitant high-energy photons emitted
by I-123, although a low-energy collimator can be used. A
20% window is placed around the 159-keV photopeak.
Whole-body imaging and high-count spot images of the
head, neck, and chest are obtained. SPECT and SPECT/
CT are increasingly used for anatomical localization.

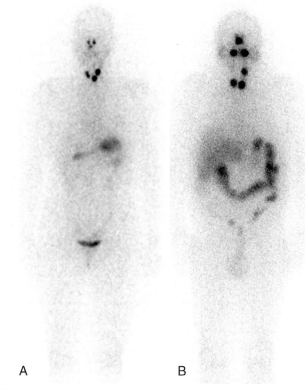

A   B

FIGURE 6-24. Whole-body I-123 thyroid cancer scan and after I-131 ablation therapy scan. **A,** Pretherapy I-123 scan. The postthyroidectomy, pre–I-
131 ablation therapy scan shows abnormal uptake limited to three focal areas
in the thyroid bed. No local or distant metastases are present. Stomach and
urinary clearance are normal. **B,** Posttherapy I-131 scan. Seven days after
I-131 therapy, the scan shows no significant change, with the exception of
liver uptake resulting from metabolism of I-131–labeled thyroid hormone.

*Interpretation of the Whole-Body Thyroid Cancer
Scan.* Scans performed after thyroidectomy but before
therapy often show residual focal thyroid uptake in the
neck, typically with a %RAIU uptake of less than 2%. Surgeons frequently cannot remove all of the thyroid tissue,
either because of the volume of tissue or caution to not
damage the parathyroids. This normal uptake cannot be
differentiated from residual tumor on scintigraphy. Uptake
is normally seen in the nasal area, oropharynx and salivary
glands, and stomach and intestines, the latter as a result of
gastric uptake, secretion, and transit (Fig 6-24). Uptake is
commonly seen in normal breasts and must not be confused
with lung uptake. Genitourinary clearance is also seen.

Posttherapy Scans. Scintigraphy is routinely performed 7 days after therapy. Approximately 10% of patients
show abnormal uptake on the posttherapy scan not seen on
the pretherapy scan, which may alter subsequent therapy
(Fig. 6-25). Some differences exist between the routine 24-
to 48-hour radioiodine scan and the 7-day posttherapy scan.
Only on the posttherapy scan is liver uptake seen; minimal
if any intestinal and urinary activity is seen. SPECT with
CT can greatly improve localization (Fig. 6-26).

Star Artifact. The high therapeutic dose can result in
intense uptake in the thyroid bed (Fig. 6-27). The uptake
typically has six points of the star caused by septal penetration of the hexagonal collimator holes.

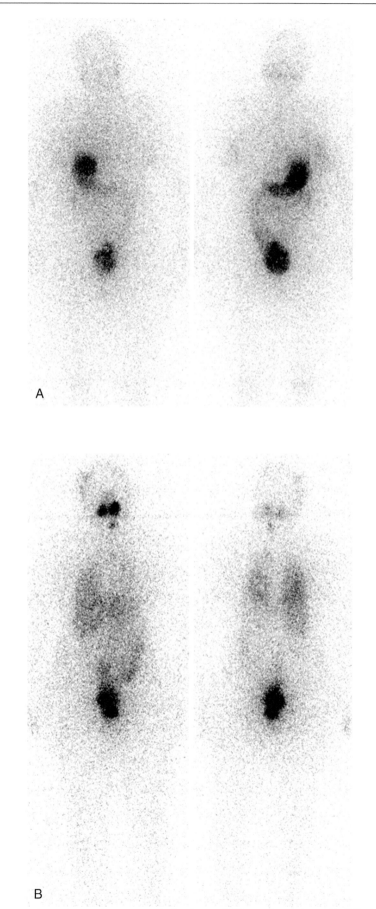

FIGURE 6-25. Lung metastases seen only on the posttherapy scan. **A,** Pretherapy I-123 scan in a patient with follicular cell thyroid cancer is negative, showing only gastric, intestinal, and bladder radiotracer. **B,** Posttherapy I-131 scan shows diffuse lung uptake consistent with miliary metastases throughout the lung.

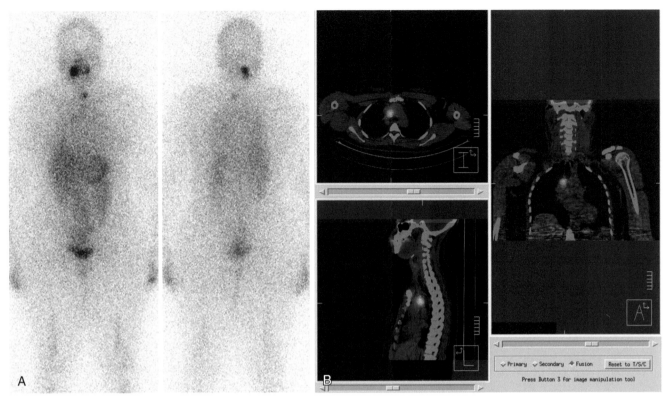

FIGURE 6-26. Added value of SPECT/CT for metastatic thyroid cancer. **A,** Whole-body posttherapy I-131 scan for 48-year-old woman with thyroid cancer. Lymph node dissection of the neck revealed positive nodes. The scan shows uptake in the upper mediastinum. **B,** SPECT/CT three-view fused images precisely localize the uptake to pretracheal nodes.

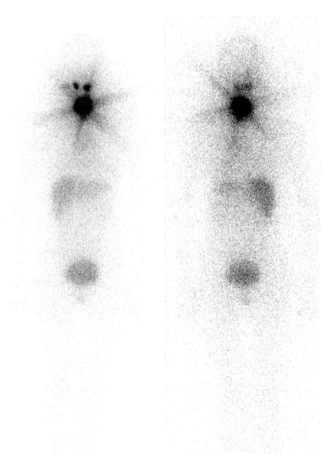

FIGURE 6-27. Star artifact. Whole-body thyroid cancer scan obtained 7 days after high-dose I-131 therapy. The intense uptake in the thyroid bed results in a star artifact caused by septal penetration of the high-energy photons.

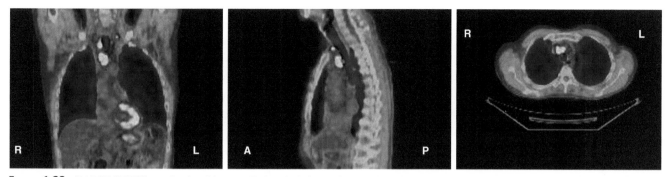

FIGURE 6-28. F-18 FDG PET scan for thyroid cancer. Patient had elevated serum thyroglobulin but negative I-123 whole-body scan. Multiple hypermetabolic lymph nodes from levels II to IV in the right neck and levels III to IV in the left neck, right paratracheal region, and left hilum consistent with thyroid cancer metastases.

Whole Body Percent Radioactive Iodine Thyroid Uptake. Quantification of uptake after thyroidectomy is an indicator of the adequacy of surgery, and follow-up scan uptakes allow evaluation of therapeutic effectiveness or recurrence. The whole-body scan is used to quantify uptake, not the probe detector used for routine thyroid scans. A radioiodine standard with calibrator-measured activity is also imaged. Regions of interest are drawn for the thyroid, background, and standard. The uptake is calculated at the time of whole-body imaging.

F-18 Fluorodeoxyglucose. Whole-body imaging with F-18 fluorodeoxyglucose (FDG) positron emission tomography (PET)/CT is used in patients with elevated serum thyroglobulin but negative I-131 whole-body scan. In these patients, the tumor has dedifferentiated into a higher grade tumor, increasing the likelihood of FDG uptake (Fig. 6-28). Localization of the tumor allows for surgical resection and evaluation of response to therapy. F-18 FDG PET is not routinely used for initial detection of metastatic disease in well-differentiated thyroid cancer because it does not have high sensitivity (~70%) in that setting.

On whole-body FDG PET/CT performed for oncological staging or surveillance of nonthyroid tumors, F-18 FDG uptake is sometimes seen in the thyroid. Diffuse gland uptake is usually caused by chronic thyroiditis (Hashimoto disease) and less frequently subacute thyroiditis and Graves disease. However, focal increased FDG thyroid uptake is of concern because the incidence of primary thyroid malignancy is 30% to 50% in these patients.

Radioactive Iodine Thyroid Ablation and Cancer Therapy

Postsurgical I-131 ablation of normal thyroid remnants permits using the serum thyroglobulin as a tumor marker. Residual functioning thyroid tissue would inhibit TSH and radioiodine uptake. I-131 ablation may also help treat microscopic disease.

Radioiodine I-131 therapy is indicated for locoregional neck, mediastinal, and distant thyroid cancer metastases. Thyroid cancer metastases have a predilection for the mediastinum, lung, and bone. Brain and liver metastases are less common and prognostically worse. I-131 therapy is

not useful for treating patients with anaplastic, poorly differentiated, or medullary thyroid cancer.

Patients are initially treated with I-131 6 weeks after thyroid surgery. A diagnostic radioiodine scan is often obtained before therapy to determine the extent of disease; however, in patients at low risk this may not be necessary.

Patients with low risk and no known metastases are commonly treated with 30 to 50 mCi to ablate normal remaining thyroid tissue. Those with regional metastases typically receive 50 to 100 mCi and patients with distant metastases 100 to 200 mCi. A low-iodine diet before therapy is recommended to increase uptake. This works by reducing the iodine pool. A follow-up whole-body scan is performed 1 week after therapy using the therapeutic I-131 dose gamma emissions.

All patients are prescribed thyroid hormone, not just as replacement therapy but also to suppress TSH, which otherwise can stimulate tumor growth. Patients are followed after therapy with unstimulated serum thyroglobulin levels, often at 6-month intervals. A diagnostic radioiodine scan is usually performed 1 year after therapy, at which time a TSH stimulated (withdrawal or recombinant TSH) serum thyroglobulin level is obtained. If the patient has persistent or recurrent disease, retreatment is indicated. If disease free, the patient is followed with serum thyroglobulin levels; whole-body scans would be repeated at 2- to 5-year intervals.

Therapy Adverse Effects

Side effects soon after radioiodine I-131 therapy may include nausea and vomiting and sialoadenitis. This problem may be minimized with oral hydration and sour candy. Late complications are related to the total dose received. Chronic sialadenitis and xerostomia are not rare. Infertility is very uncommon. Pulmonary fibrosis and bone marrow aplasia occur in patients with high tumor burden and repeated I-131 therapy. Concern for bone marrow suppression and leukemia increase as the total therapy dose approaches 500 to 1000 mCi.

The Nuclear Regulatory Commission (NRC) patient release regulations (10 CFR 20 and 35) are based on the likely exposure to others. The regulations state that no person should receive more than 5 millisieverts (0.5 rem) from exposure to a released I-131 therapy patient. Agreement States generally follow NRC guidelines, and hospitals vary as to their own release requirements, never less stringent than the NRC regulations. At many centers, patients are treated primarily on an outpatient basis. For very-high-dose therapy (>200 mCi) or for reason of radiation safety for family members, patients may be treated as inpatients.

Radiation safety instructions should be discussed with the patient and family. Patient-specific information regarding limiting close contact and preventing exposure to others should be provided (Boxes 6-10 and 6-11). Physicians and technologists who administer the therapy dose are required to have a thyroid bioassay (uptake counts) within a week of dose administration to confirm that they did not receive an internal dose during patient administration.

■ PARATHYROID SCINTIGRAPHY

Parathyroid scintigraphy has become an important part of the routine preoperative evaluation of patients with the clinical diagnosis of hyperparathyroidism. The clinical diagnosis is made in patients who have elevated serum calcium, reduced serum phosphorus, and elevated parathormone levels. The purpose of the parathyroid scan is to localize the hyperfunctioning parathyroid gland or glands before surgery, making possible minimally invasive surgery.

Anatomy and Embryology

Normally patients have four parathyroid glands, two superior and two inferior, measuring around 6 × 3 mm and weighing 35 to 40 mg each. A fifth supernumerary gland occurs in up to 10% of individuals. The *inferior* glands arise embryologically from the third brachial pouch and migrate caudally with the thymus. Their normal location is somewhat variable, with 60% located immediately posterior and lateral to the thyroid lower poles and 40% in the cervical portion of the thymus gland (Fig. 6-29). The *superior* glands arise from the fourth brachial pouch and migrate with the thyroid. Seventy-five percent are posterior to the midpoles and 25% posterior to the upper poles of the thyroid. The distinction between superior and inferior glands has surgical implications because the inferior glands are anterior to and the superior glands posterior to the recurrent laryngeal nerve. Resection of the superior glands poses a potential risk for nerve damage.

The term *ectopic* refers to glands that have descended to an unusual location. They can be found cephalad at the carotid bifurcation, inferior in the mediastinum and pericardium, anterior to the thyroid, and posterior in the superior mediastinum in the tracheoesophageal groove and paraesophageal region (Fig 6-30).

Pathophysiology of Hyperparathyroidism

Parathormone (PTH) is an 84–amino acid polypeptide hormone synthesized, stored, and secreted by the chief cells of the parathyroid glands. PTH regulates calcium and phosphorus homeostasis by its action on bone, small intestine, and kidneys. Increased synthesis and release of PTH from a single gland or multiple parathyroid glands characterizes hyperparathyroidism.

Primary hyperparathyroidism is caused by autonomous hyperfunction of a parathyroid adenoma. These adenomas are caused by somatic mutations with clonal expansion of the mutated cells; primary hyperplasia is a polyclonal proliferation. More than 85% of patients have a single adenoma, fewer than 5% have two adenomas, and fewer than 10% have four-gland hyperplasia (Table 6-8).

Patients with multiple endocrine neoplasia syndrome often have hyperparathyroidism with multigland hyperplasia as one of its manifestations. Fewer than 1% of patients with hyperparathyroidism have parathyroid carcinoma. They often present with severe elevations in serum calcium, a palpable neck mass, bone pain, fractures, and renal colic.

Secondary hyperparathyroidism occurs in patients with severe renal disease. They have low serum calcium and elevated serum phosphorus levels. Stimulation of PTH is a compensatory physiological mechanism that occurs in all

NORMAL PARATHYROID GLAND LOCATIONS

SUPERIOR GLANDS

INFERIOR GLANDS

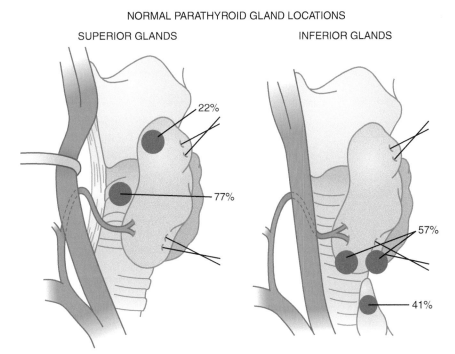

FIGURE 6-29. Normal parathyroid gland locations. The superior pair of glands *(closed circles)* usually lie within the fascial covering of the posterior aspect of the thyroid gland outside the capsule. Intrathyroidal locations are rare. Most are adjacent to the thyroid or cricothyroid cartilage. Superior glands are located just posterior to the superior pole or midpole of the thyroid *(left)*. Inferior glands *(closed circles)* are located immediately posterior or lateral to the inferior pole of the thyroid or in the thyrothymic ligament *(right)*.

ECTOPIC GLAND
LOCATION

SUPERIOR
GLANDS

INFERIOR
GLANDS

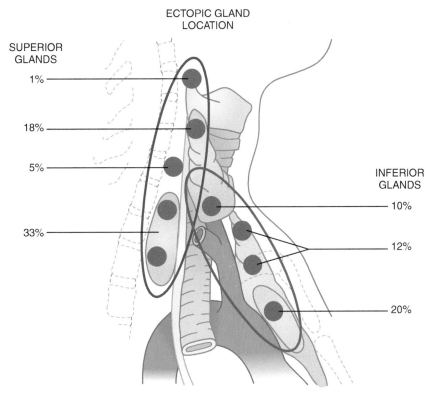

FIGURE 6-30. Ectopic gland locations. Because of abnormal embryological descent, ectopic glands can be found as cephalad as the carotid bifurcation, as inferior as the region of the pericardium, anterior to the thyroid, posterior in the tracheoesophageal groove, and in the superior mediastinum. In the anterior-posterior plane, inferior glands descend anteriorly and superior glands descend more posteriorly.

TABLE 6-8 Causes of Hyperparathyroidism

Cause adenoma	Percentage
Adenoma	85
Hyperplasia	10
Ectopic	<5
Carcinoma	<1

patients with renal failure. Despite the elevated serum PTH, the serum calcium remains below normal levels. Surgery is not indicated

Tertiary hyperparathyroidism presents as hypercalcemia in patients with renal failure. One or more parathyroid glands become autonomous and no longer responsive to serum PTH. Surgical resection is indicated.

Clinical Presentation

In the past, patients with hyperparathyroidism presented with nephrolithiasis, osteitis fibrosa cystica, osteoporosis, pathological fractures, gastrointestinal and neuropsychiatric symptoms, and brown tumors. Today, most patients are asymptomatic at diagnosis. Hypercalcemia and hypophosphatemia are detected during routine blood screening.

Diagnosis

An elevated PTH level in a patient with hypercalcemia is diagnostic of hyperparathyroidism. Other causes for hypercalcemia include malignancy, vitamin D intoxication, sarcoidosis, and thiazide diuretics. However, these patients have reduced serum PTH levels because of a physiological feedback mechanism. Patients with hypoparathyroidism have osteopenia.

Treatment

Surgical resection is curative. In the recent past, the standard operation was bilateral neck exploration with localization of each parathyroid gland by the surgeon and removal of the offending adenoma. Hyperplasia required removal of 3.5 glands, sometimes with placement of one gland elsewhere—for example, in the arm to ensure a functioning parathyroid gland. The need for preoperative imaging was controversial because expert surgeons reported a greater than 90% detection rate.

Today, minimally invasive unilateral surgery using a small incision is the operation of choice because it results in reduced operation time and fewer complications. This approach requires imaging for preoperative localization. During surgery, some surgeons use a specialized small gamma probe to help localize the hyperfunctioning gland(s). An intraoperative reduction in the serum PTH level by 50% after gland surgical removal confirms successful surgery.

Postoperative recurrence rates are approximately 5%. Common reasons for surgical failure include (1) an ectopic location of the tumor in the neck or in the mediastinum, (2) failure to recognize hyperplasia, or (3) the presence of an undiscovered fifth gland. Reexploration has increased morbidity and a poorer success rate than the primary procedure.

Preoperative Noninvasive Imaging

The radionuclide method has superior detection accuracy compared to ultrasonography, CT, and magnetic resonance imaging for the preoperative localization of the hyperfunctioning parathyroid. However, these other imaging modalities are often ordered for anatomical correlation and confirmation. The anatomical imaging methods are fairly insensitive for detecting ectopic and mediastinal glands.

Radiopharmaceuticals

In the 1980s, thallium-201 was used for parathyroid scintigraphy, in conjunction with Tc-99m pertechnetate thyroid imaging. In the 1990s, Tc-99m sestamibi became the standard radiopharmaceutical, with or without thyroid imaging. Detection and localization are superior to Tl-201, probably because of the superior Tc-99m imaging characteristics.

Technetium-99m Sestamibi
Mechanism of Uptake
Tc-99m sestamibi (Cardiolite) is most commonly used as a myocardial perfusion imaging agent. Chemically, it is a lipophilic cation member of the isonitrile family (hexakis 2-methoxyisobutyl isonitrile). Localization is related to the parathyroid adenoma's high cellularity and vascularity. The radiotracer localizes and is retained in the region of mitochondria. The large number of mitochondria in oxyphil cells in parathyroid adenomas is thought responsible for its avid uptake and slow release. Normal functioning parathyroid glands are not visualized. Tc-99m tetrofosmin (Myoview) has a similar mechanism of uptake and localization and is reported useful for parathyroid imaging; however, published data are considerably more limited.

Pharmacokinetics
After intravenous injection, peak accumulation of Tc-99m sestamibi occurs in a hyperfunctioning parathyroid gland at 3 to 5 minutes. It has a variable clearance half-time of approximately 60 minutes. Similar rapid uptake occurs in the thyroid; however, it usually washes out more rapidly than it does in the parathyroid. This is the rationale for two-phase parathyroid scintigraphy.

Methodologies
Tc-99m sestamibi, 20 to 25 mCi, is injected intravenously. Imaging begins 10 to 15 minutes later. Generally, two different acquisition methodologies have been used.

Combined Thyroid and Parathyroid Imaging. The combined thyroid and parathyroid imaging protocol is similar to that used for Tl-201/Tc-99m pertechnetate subtraction imaging. Tc-99m sestamibi is injected, and images are acquired 10 minutes later. I-123 is then injected, and images are acquired at 20 minutes. Images are visually compared for different distribution. Digital subtraction of the I-123 thyroid image from the Tc-99m sestambi image is performed, resulting in an image only of the hyperfunctioning parathyroid gland (Fig. 6-31). Subtraction methodology requires some experience. Technical errors occur as a result of patient movement, image misalignment, and subtraction artifacts.

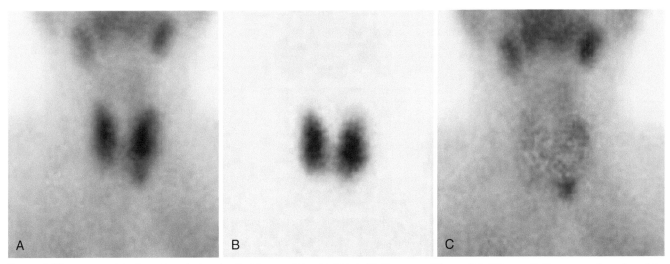

FIGURE 6-31. Parathyroid subtraction scintigraphy. Tc-99 sestamibi and I-123. **A,** Tc-99m sestamibi scan. **B,** I-123 scan. **C,** Computer subtraction of the I-123 scan from the Tc-99m sestamibi scan reveals uptake only in the parathyroid, consistent with an adenoma.

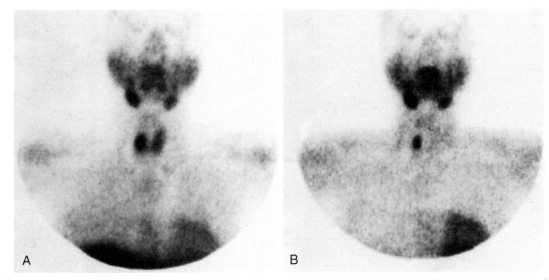

FIGURE 6-32. Tc-99m sestamibi parathyroid scan, delayed planar imaging method. Patient has hypercalcemia and increased parathormone. **A,** Early planar imaging at 15 minutes with Tc-99m sestamibi reveals somewhat asymmetrical activity with slightly more uptake on the right in the region of the thyroid gland. **B,** Delayed imaging at 2 hours demonstrates washout of thyroid activity, and focal uptake on the right is retained, consistent with a parathyroid adenoma.

Two-Phase Imaging Parathyroid Imaging. Initial images are obtained 10 to 15 minutes after Tc-99m sestambi injection. A second set of images is obtained at 2 to 3 hours. Because of more rapid washout of the thyroid, the delayed images often show only the hyperfunctioning parathyroid (Fig. 6-32). However, in up to 30% of patients this characteristic differential washout pattern is not seen. Either both the thyroid and the parathyroid wash out at the same rate or often both wash out so rapidly that little tracer remains on delayed imaging.

Many variations and combinations of these two methods are in clinical use at different imaging centers. The imaging methods used include planar imaging, SPECT, and SPECT/CT.

Planar Imaging. Planar two-dimensional imaging has long been the methodology most commonly used (Fig. 6-32). The two options are a parallel-hole collimator that permits simultaneous imaging of the neck and mediastinum or a combination of magnified pinhole imaging for the neck and parallel-hole collimator imaging of the thorax. Anterior images are acquired, sometimes with additional right anterior oblique and left anterior oblique views. The disadvantages of planar imaging are the overlapping of thyroid and parathyroid uptake and its limited two-dimensional information—that is, right and left, and superior and inferior localization, but not anterior and posterior.

Single-Photon Emission Computed Tomography. SPECT is increasingly used because of the improved target-to-background ratio compared to planar imaging and it reduces overlapping activity, improves detectability, and, most importantly, localizes the hyperfunctioning gland(s) in three-dimensions (Fig. 6-33). Anatomical localization, like planar imaging, depends on its position relative to the thyroid.

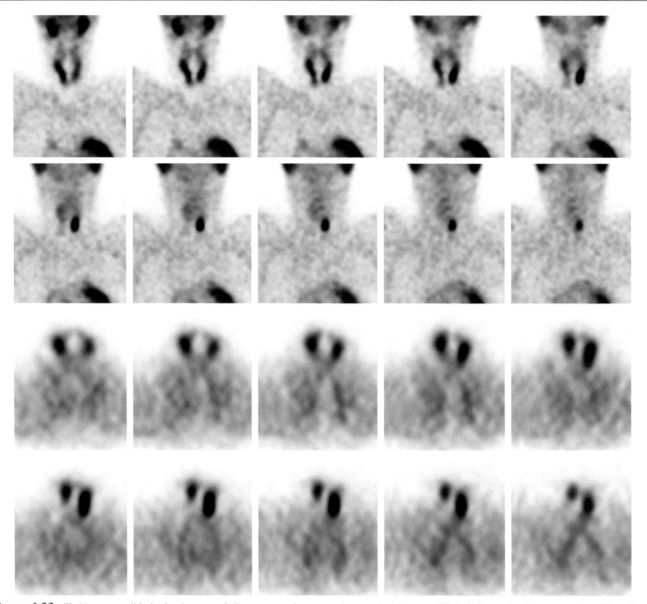

FIGURE 6-33. Tc-99m sestamibi single-photon emission computed tomography parathyroid scan. Clinical diagnosis of hyperparathyroidism. Scan ordered for localization. Sequential coronal *(top two)* and transverse *(bottom two)*, each with early images above and delayed images below. The coronal images show that the adenoma is inferior to the thyroid on the left side. The transverse images show that the parathyroid is rather posterior on the left side, suggesting a superior parathyroid adenoma.

Single-Photon Emission Computed Tomography with Computed Tomography. Hybrid SPECT/CT systems are increasingly used because they combine the functional information from SPECT Tc-99m sestamibi and the anatomical information from CT (Figs. 6-34 through 6-36).

Image Interpretation

Initial images at 10 to 15 minutes after injection typically show prominent thyroid uptake, unless the patient has had a thyroidectomy or is on thyroid hormone suppression. On scintigraphy a parathyroid uptake is typically focal and often distinct from thyroid uptake, even when superimposed; in other cases, it is adjacent to or distant from the thyroid. On delayed 2-hour imaging, much of the thyroid uptake has washed out and the hyperfunctioning parathyroid gland is a focus of residual activity. With rapid washout of the thyroid and parathyroid, the false negative rate is increased; however, the diagnosis often can be made based on the characteristic pattern on early images.

Although a parathyroid adenoma located in the region of the inferior thyroid lobe is often an inferior parathyroid adenoma, superior glands may descend to that region, as well. Inferior parathyroid glands are usually located immediately adjacent to the posterior aspect of the thyroid, while superior glands tend to be more posterior and clearly separated from the thyroid. Although sometimes distinguishable with oblique static image, SPECT and SPECT/CT can better make this distinction (Figs. 6-34 through 6-36).

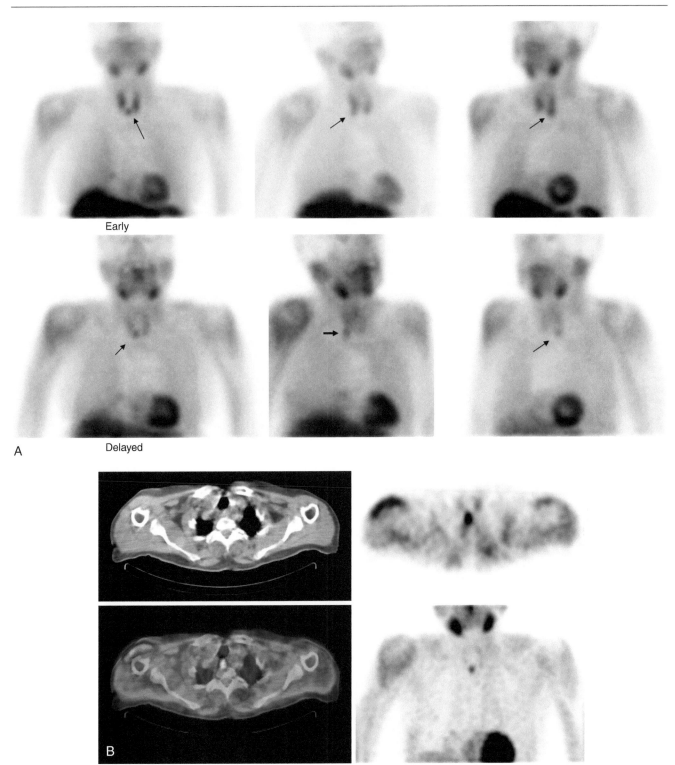

FIGURE 6-34. Retrosternal localization with SPECT/CT. **A,** Early and delayed images. Anterior *(left)*, right anterior oblique (RAO) *(middle)*, left anterior oblique (LAO) *(right)*. In the anterior view, a suspicious adenoma is noted midline just below the two thyroid lobes. On the RAO and LAO views the adenoma appears to be in the lower right lobe and lower left lobe, respectively. **B,** The fused SPECT/CT images *(left lower)* show that the parathyroid adenoma is retrotracheal.

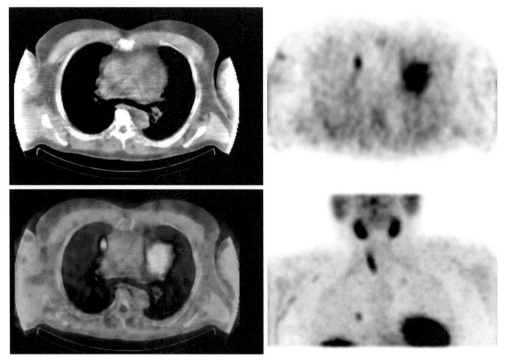

FIGURE 6-35. Pericardial localization with SPECT/CT. The maximal intensity projection *(right lower)* view shows focal uptake in the right mediastinum in a patient with prior parathyroid surgery and left thyroidectomy who now has recurrent hypercalcemia. The fused SPECT/CT image shows localization in the region of the right pericardium.

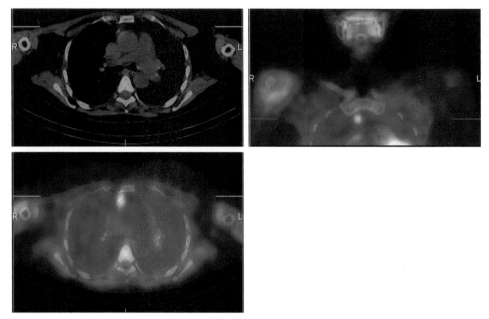

FIGURE 6-36. SPECT/CT with 16-slice CT. CT *(upper left)*, fused transverse *(lower left)*, and fused coronal *(right)* images. The parathyroid adenoma is clearly localized—anterior to the aorta, immediately behind the sternum.

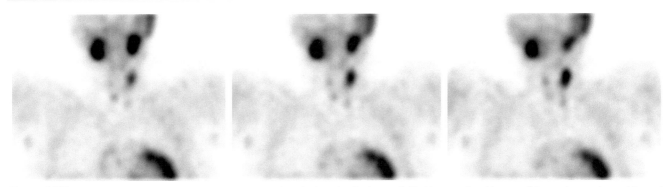

FIGURE 6-37. Tertiary hyperparathyroidism with four hyperfunctioning glands detected. Tc-99m parathyroid sestamibi scan in a patient with renal failure with elevated calcium. SPECT/CT sequential coronals show four abnormal foci, the left superior parathyroid gland being the largest, but also the left inferior, right superior, and right inferior glands detected.

Accuracy

Sensitivity for detection of parathyroid adenomas larger than 300 mg approaches 90%. The most common cause for a false negative study is small size. Sensitivity for detection of second adenomas or four-gland hyperplasia is lower than for single adenomas (~50%-60%). Localization of autonomous tertiary hyperfunctioning adenomas is generally good (Fig. 6-37). The most common cause for a false positive parathyroid study is a thyroid follicular adenoma. Thyroid cancer and even metastatic tumors may appear similar.

Little data directly comparing the dual-isotope method combining thyroid and parathyroid imaging with the early and delayed image method have been published. However, review of the data suggests similar accuracy. Some investigations have reported better accuracy for adenoma localization with SPECT compared with planar imaging. However, no study has shown SPECT to be statistically superior. A large investigation directly comparing early and delayed planar imaging, SPECT, and SPECT/CT found that early SPECT/CT in conjunction with any delayed imaging method was statistically superior to dual-phase planar or SPECT.

SUGGESTED READING

Chapman EM. History of the discovery and early use of radioactive iodine. *JAMA.* 1983;250(15):2042-2044.

Cooper DS, Doherty GM, Haugen BR, et al. 2009 revised American Thyroid Association management guidelines for patients with thyroid nodules and differentiated thyroid cancer. *Thyroid.* 2009;19(11):1167-1214.

Coover LR, Silberstein EB, Kuhn PJ, et al. Therapeutic ^{131}I in outpatients: a simplified method conforming to the Code of Federal Regulations, title 10, part 35.75. *J Nucl Med.* 2000;41(11):1868-1875.

Gelfand MJ. Meta-iodobenzylguanidine in children. *Semin Nucl Med.* 1993;23(3):231-242.

Intenzo CM, dePapp AE, Jabbour S, et al. Scintigraphic manifestations of thyrotoxicosis. *Radiographics.* 2003;23(4):857-869.

Lavely WC, Goetz S, Friedman KP, et al. Comparison of SPECT/CT, SPECT, and planar imaging with single-and dual-phase (99m)Tc-sestamibi parathyroid scintigraphy. *J Nucl Med.* 2007;48(7):1084-1089.

Nichols KJ, Tomas MB, Tronco GG, et al. Preoperative parathyroid scintigraphic lesion localization: accuracy of various types of readings. *Radiology.* 2008;248(1):221-232.

Robbins RJ, Larson SM. The value of positron emission tomography (PET) in the management of patients with thyroid cancer. *Best Pract Res Clin Endocrinol Metab.* 2008;22(6):1047-1059.

Shankar LK, Yamamoto AJ, Alavi A, Mandel SJ. Comparison of I-123 scintigraphy at 5 and 24 hours in patients with differentiated thyroid cancer. *J Nucl Med.* 2002;43(1):72-76.

Taillefer R, Boucher Y, Potvin C, Lambert R. Detection and localization of parathyroid adenomas in patients with hyperparathyroidism using a single radionuclide imaging procedure with technetium-99m sestamibi (double-phase study). *J Nucl Med.* 1992;33(10):1801-1807.

CHAPTER 7

Skeletal Scintigraphy

▬ BONE SCAN

The skeleton is an active, constantly changing organ. It is made up of inorganic calcium hydroxyapatite crystal, $Ca_{10}(PO_4)_6(OH)_2$, and an organic matrix of collagen and blood vessels. Bone responds to injury and disease with increased turnover and attempts at self-repair. This physiological process can be imaged with a variety of radiotracers that localize to areas of bone formation.

The nuclear medicine bone scan is a versatile tool because of its high sensitivity for tumors, infection, and trauma, as well as its ability to image the entire skeleton at a reasonable cost. Therefore skeletal scintigraphy remains popular despite technological advances in magnetic resonance imaging (MRI), computed tomography (CT), and positron emission tomography (PET). Because of the low specificity of bone scan, it is essential to know the patient's history, understand when radiographic correlation is necessary, and know how to use it. In addition, the development of single-photon emission computed tomography (SPECT) and SPECT/CT has improved sensitivity and specificity.

Radiopharmaceuticals

An ideal radiopharmaceutical for skeletal scintigraphy must be inexpensive, stable, rapidly localized to bone, and quickly cleared from the background soft tissues, and it must have favorable imaging and dosimetry characteristics. The combination of technetium-99m, desirable for gamma camera imaging, with members of the phosphate family met these parameters in Tc-99m hydroxymethylene diphosphonate (Tc-99m HMDP or HDP) and Tc-99m methylene diphosphonate (Tc-99m MDP). Although some differences exist, and Tc-99m MDP is more commonly used, both are excellent agents, showing extensive skeletal detail (Fig. 7-1).

Preparation

Tc-99m MDP can be prepared from a simple kit. Tc-99m, in the form of sodium pertechnetate ($NaTcO_4$), is injected into a vial containing MDP, stabilizers, and stannous ion. Stannous tin acts as a reducing agent, allowing the Tc-99m to form a chelate bond with the MDP carrier molecule.

Incomplete labeling may occur if air is introduced into the vial causing stannous ion hydrolysis (from Sn II into Sn IV). Insufficient stannous ion results in free technetium pertechnetate ("free tech"), causing image degradation with increased background soft tissue activity and uptake in the thyroid, stomach, and salivary glands. Excess alumina from the technetium generator eluate may lead to colloid formation, which can accumulate in the reticuloendothelial system of organs, such as the liver. Tc-99m MDP should be used within 2 to 3 hours of preparation or radiopharmaceutical breakdown may also yield technetium pertechnetate.

Uptake and Pharmacokinetics

After intravenous injection, Tc-99m MDP rapidly distributes into the extracellular fluid and is quickly taken up into bone. Accumulation of Tc-99m MDP does relate to the amount of blood flow to a region, but uptake is primarily controlled by the amount of osteogenic activity, being much higher in areas of active bone formation or repair compared with mature bone (Fig. 7-2). Tc-99m MDP binding occurs by chemisorption in the hydroxyapatite mineral component of the osseous matrix. Uptake in areas of amorphous calcium phosphate may account for Tc-99m MDP uptake in sites outside the bone, such as dystrophic soft tissue ossification. Decreased activity is seen in areas of reduced or absent blood flow or infarction. Diminished uptake or cold areas are also seen in regions of severe destruction occurring in some very aggressive metastases (Fig. 7-3).

Approximately 50% of the dose is localized to the bone, with the remainder excreted by the kidneys. Although peak bone uptake occurs approximately 1 hour after injection, the highest target-to-background ratios are seen after 6 to 12 hours. Images are typically taken at 2 to 4 hours to balance the need for background clearance with the relatively

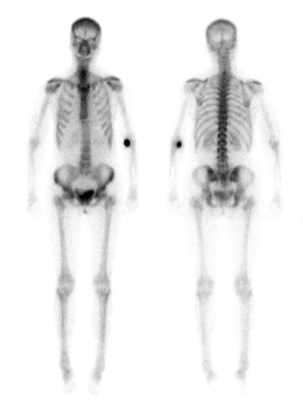

FIGURE 7-1. Normal Tc-99m MDP whole-body bone scan. A high level of anatomical detail can be visualized. Some areas of increased uptake are normally seen in the adult, including activity in the joints. A small dose infiltration is present in the left antecubital fossa.

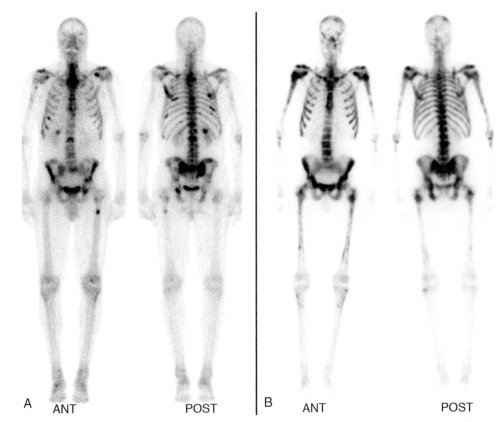

FIGURE 7-2. Prostate cancer metastatic disease. **A,** Numerous foci of increased activity, largely in the axial skeleton, are typical as the bones respond to metastases. **B,** Two years later, with disease progression diffuse increased uptake is seen in the spine, pelvis, and ribs, with multiple new lesions in the skull and proximal long bones. In some areas, such as the pelvis, bones appear intense but almost normal, in a pattern referred to as a *superscan* or a *beautiful bone scan*, corresponding to the near now confluent sclerotic lesions that had progressed on CT.

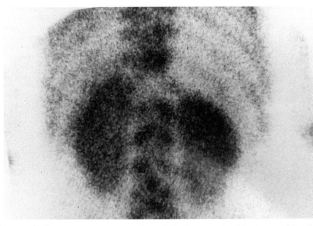

FIGURE 7-3. Complete destruction of the L1 vertebral body, resulting in a photon-deficient (or cold) lesion.

TABLE 7-1 Radiation Dosimetry of Technetium-99m Methylene Diphosphonate*

Age	Administered activity	Organ receive highest dose	Effective dose
Adult	20-30 mCi (740-1110 MBq)	Bone surface: 0.23 rad/mCi (0.063 mGy/ MBq)	0.021 rem/mCi (0.0057 mSv/ MBq)
Child (5 yr old)	0.2-0.3 mCi/ kg (7-11 MBq/kg)	Bone surface: 0.81 rad/mCi (0.22 mGy/ MBq)	0.092 rem/mCi (0.025 mSv/ MBq)

Data from Radiation dose to patients from radiopharmaceuticals (addendum 3 to ICRP publication 53): ICRP publication 106. *Ann ICRP.* 2008;38:1-197.

*Assumes voiding interval of 3.5 hr.

short 6-hour half-life of Tc-99m and patient convenience. The half-life of Tc-99m effectively limits imaging to within approximately 24 hours of injection.

Dosimetry

Estimates of absorbed radiation doses are listed in Table 7-1. The radiation dose to the bladder wall, ovaries, and testes depends on the frequency of voiding. The dosimetry provided assumes a 2-hour voiding cycle. Significantly higher doses result if voiding is infrequent.

Radiopharmaceuticals are administered to pregnant women only if clearly needed on a risk-versus-benefit basis. Tc-99m is excreted in breast milk, so breastfeeding should be stopped for 24 hours.

Imaging Protocol

A sample protocol is listed in Box 7-1. Several modifications are possible. Although many diagnostic questions can be answered with routine delayed imaging, the three-phase

BOX 7-1. Whole-Body Survey and Single-Photon Emission Computed Tomography Skeletal Scintigraphy: Protocol Summary

PATIENT PREPARATION

Patient should be well hydrated.

Patient voids immediately before study and frequently for next several hours.

Patient should remove metal objects (jewelry, coins, keys) before imaging.

RADIOPHARMACEUTICAL ADMINISTRATION

Select injection site to avoid possible sites of pathology.

Adult dose: 20 mCi (740 MBq), intravenously

Pediatric dose: Webster's rule:

Adult dose × [(age + 1)/(age + 7)].

Minimum dose 1.08 mCi (40 MBq)

TIME OF IMAGING

Begin imaging 2-4 hours after tracer administration.

PROCEDURE

Capture anterior and posterior images of whole skeleton.

Whole-body scan (table rate ≈ 10 cm/min)

Multiple spot views

300k-500k counts/image entire body or time a 500k posterior chest view and image remaining views for that amount of time

Detail spot areas of concern (1000k counts/image)

SINGLE-PHOTON EMISSION COMPUTED TOMOGRAPHY

Attenuation correction with computed tomography or external rods optional.

Acquisition: Contoured orbit, 128 × 128 matrix, 6-degree intervals, 15-30 sec/stop.

Reconstruction: Filtered back projection, Butterworth filter; cutoff 0.4, power 7 or iterative reconstruction.

*Selection of single-photon emission computed tomography acquisition and reconstruction parameters depends greatly on available equipment and software.

BOX 7-2. Three-Phase Skeletal Scintigraphy: Protocol Summary

PREPARATION

Position gamma camera immediately over area of concern.

RADIOPHARMACEUTICAL ADMINISTRATION

Administer intravenous bolus of Tc-99m methylene diphosphonate using standard dosage.

FLOW PHASE

Obtain dynamic 2- to 5-second images for 60 seconds after bolus injection.

BLOOD POOL AND TISSUE PHASE

Obtain immediate static images for time (5 minutes) or counts (300k).

SKELETAL PHASE

Delayed 300k-1000k images at 2 to 4 hours.

bone scan is helpful in addressing several problems. The most frequent indication for three-phase imaging is to assess possible osteomyelitis. However, it is also beneficial in the evaluation of the painful joint prosthesis, trauma, bone graft status, and complex regional pain syndrome (reflex sympathetic dystrophy). Dynamic scanning technique is summarized in Box 7-2.

If dynamic three-phase scanning is to be performed, a bolus of Tc-99m MDP is injected intravenously with the area in question under the camera. The injection site should be chosen to avoid any suspected pathological condition. For example, if comparison with the opposite hand may be needed at any time, injection in a site such as the foot should be considered. The first phase consists of serial 2- to 5-second dynamic images acquired for 60 seconds. Then blood pool or soft tissue second-phase images are

obtained of the region and secondary areas of interest, such as in patients with arthritis or multiple stress injuries. Delayed images constitute the third phase of a three-phase bone scan. Alternatively, delayed images are done alone for routine studies, such as the assessment of metastatic disease. The patient should be well hydrated, and after injection the patient must be instructed to drink several cups of fluid to improve background clearance. Frequent voiding reduces radiation dose. Care must be used because urinary contamination frequently causes confusion or masks potential lesion sites. Although a delay of 2 hours may yield images of sufficient quality in younger patients, waiting 3 or 4 hours after injection is often necessary in the elderly and in those with poor renal function. Images delayed further, at 24 hours, which is a fourth phase, may be needed to clear soft tissue activity in the most severe cases.

Using a low-energy, high-resolution collimator, delayed planar images can be obtained by whole-body scan or spot views. The whole-body scan allows rapid, seamless coverage as the camera moves over the patient at a predetermined rate. Spot views, on the other hand, can provide greater detail because of higher resolution and can better define pathological conditions by using different camera positions. In most centers, a whole-body scan is performed with high count spot views reserved for symptomatic areas or additional views of suspicious-appearing regions (Fig. 7-4).

Other modifications include magnified pinhole collimator views, commonly used in cases of osteonecrosis of the hips and trauma to the carpal bones. Pinhole images also may be needed in children to better visualize the joints. Three-dimensional assessment of the bones with SPECT allows for high-contrast images that can be formatted in transaxial, sagittal, and coronal planes. SPECT images fused to CT or acquired on a SPECT/CT scanner are sometimes much easier to interpret. Compared with planar images, SPECT shows improved contrast of cold and hot lesions, more precise localization, and better resolution (Fig. 7-5). The ability to precisely localize a lesion on

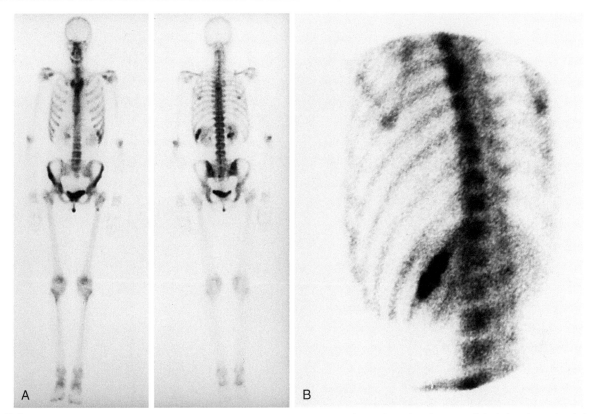

FIGURE 7-4. A, Anterior and posterior whole-body images of a patient with breast carcinoma have the advantage of depicting the entire skeleton in a single view. Note the abnormal uptake in one of the left lower posterior ribs. **B,** High count density spot view of left posterior ribs from the same patient. The location and appearance of the lesion are better delineated by the spot view. Tracking along the rib is classic for a metastatic lesion.

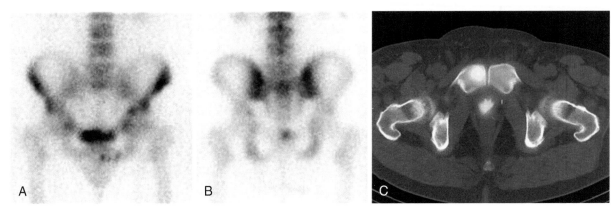

FIGURE 7-5. Planar anterior **(A)** and posterior **(B)** spot views of the pelvis show what appears to be radiotracer in urinary bladder and probable skin contamination on the genitalia. **C,** SPECT/CT reveals that one of the areas actually corresponds to a metastasis in the right superior pubic ramus.

SPECT can improve specificity, such as separating uptake in the vertebral facets from arthritis or vertebral pedicle from metastasis.

Normal and Altered Distribution

The normal bone scan varies dramatically with the age of the patient. Most notably, the growing skeleton will concentrate radiotracer at all active growth plates (Fig. 7-6). These areas are often the critical sites in child abuse, primary bone tumors, and osteomyelitis. Therefore it is essential that children are immobilized and positioned

symmetrically during acquisition. By adulthood, growth plate activity diminishes and disappears.

Numerous normal or expected variants exist depending on age and history. Some bones, such the sacroiliac joints normally appear to have intense uptake. Other areas are more intense because of proximity to the camera, such as the iliac wings or a lordotic spine. The sternum often has residual ossification centers, and the normal sternomanubrial joint may have mild increased uptake. The skull is highly variable in appearance and may show increased uptake in the frontal bone from benign hyperostosis frontalis interna. The costochondral junction is a common site

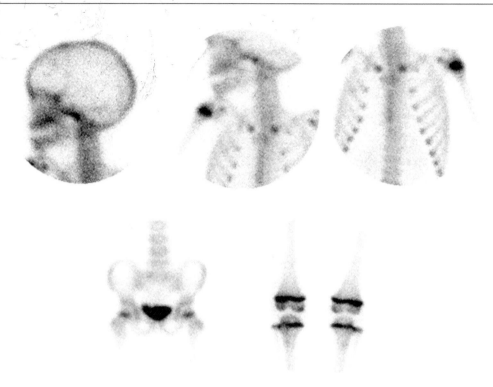

FIGURE 7-6. Normal radiotracer distribution in the immature skeleton. An anterior whole-body image shows increased uptake in the growth centers. Uptake is seen in the anterior rib ends, sternal ossification centers, and major joints.

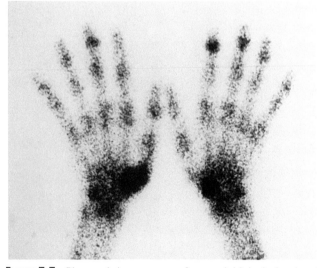

FIGURE 7-7. Characteristic appearance of osteoarthritis in the hands and wrists. Uptake is increased in multiple distal interphalangeal joints and is particularly intense at the base of the first left metacarpal, a common place for osteoarthritis.

of benign uptake and is an unlikely location for solitary metastasis.

Osteoarthritic changes are routinely seen and usually identified by classic locations. These include the medial compartment of the knee, hand, and wrist (especially at the base of the first metacarpal), shoulder, and bones of the feet (Fig. 7-7). The patella may show increased uptake as a result of chondromalacia and degenerative change. Arthritis is frequently bilateral and occurs on

both sides of the joint. Asymmetry has been noted in the shoulders, with sternoclavicular activity apparently affected by handedness and use. Of note, Florine-18 fluorodeoxyglucose (FDG) PET rarely shows intense uptake in arthritis.

Caution must be exercised when assessing uptake in the spine. In addition to the potential need for SPECT, radiographic correlation with CT is frequently needed to identify degenerative processes causing abnormal uptake, such as facet hypertrophy, disk space narrowing, and osteophyte formation. Osteoporosis may result in classic insufficiency vertebral compression fractures (Fig. 7-8). Abnormal uptake in osteoporotic compression fractures may be seen before radiographic changes and may not resolve in the elderly. The H-shaped insufficiency fracture occurring in the sacrum (Fig. 7-9) is seen more readily on bone scan than with other modalities such as CT and even MRI.

The effects of trauma are frequently seen on bone scan. In the ribs, vertically aligned focal uptake in several or successive ribs is classic for trauma (Fig. 7-10). Metastatic lesions, on the other hand, tend to track along the bone, as shown in Figure 7-4. When fractures are present, history or callous formation on CT may suggest benign uptake from a healing traumatic fracture. Uptake in a fracture associated with a poorly defined lytic lesion or aggressive periosteal change favors pathological fracture. However, the cause of a fracture may be difficult to determine without follow-up. Radiographs are often sufficient for comparison, particularly when looking at lesions in the extremities. However, CT is often preferred, being more sensitive for bone lesions than radiographs. MRI

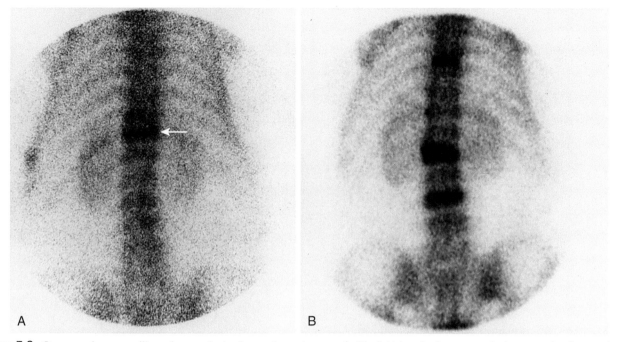

FIGURE 7-8. Osteoporosis on surveillance images obtained several months apart. **A,** The initial study shows a vertebral compression fracture *(arrow)* caused by osteoporosis involving the lower thoracic spine. **B,** The subsequent study shows healing with normalization of uptake in the initial abnormality. Three new compression fractures are seen in the thoracic and lumbar spine.

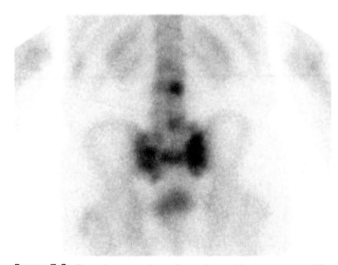

FIGURE 7-9. Posterior spot view of a patient with osteoporosis. The patient has a characteristic H-type pattern of a sacral insufficiency fracture with a horizontal band of increased uptake across the body of the sacrum and bilaterally increased uptake in the sacral alae.

may add valuable information when characterizing a lesion and the surrounding soft tissues in musculoskeletal pathology.

Analysis of the soft tissues is essential. Increased or decreased activity in the kidneys and bladder must be explained (Box 7-3). Soft tissues such as breast or abdomen attenuate intensity of the underlying bones. Abnormal uptake outside of bone must be differentiated from true bone lesions (Fig. 7-11). Evidence of surgery and abnormal soft tissue uptake may be present from the

tumor (Figs. 7-12 and 7-13). In the right lower chest and upper abdomen, abnormal soft tissue activity must be identified and localized to breast, malignant pleural effusion, or liver. When the liver is involved, correlation with CT and radiopharmaceutical quality control tests may be needed to differentiate uptake in metastases from dose preparation artifact resulting in colloid formation.

▬ CLINICAL USES OF SKELETAL SCINTIGRAPHY

Metastatic Disease

A significant fraction of patients with known malignancy develop osseous metastasis. Patients may present with bone pain (50%-80%) and elevated alkaline phosphatase (77%), but these findings are nonspecific. The evaluation of osseous metastatic disease is the most common use of skeletal scintigraphy. Determining whether a bone scan is appropriate depends on factors such as tumor and stage, history of pain, and radiographic abnormalities.

More than 90% of osseous metastases distribute to the red marrow, which is found in the axial skeleton and the proximal portions of the humeri and femurs in adults (Fig. 7-2, *A*). As the tumor enlarges, the cortex becomes involved. Tc-99m MDP binds to areas of attempted repair, not the tumor itself. Even a 5% bone turnover can be detected by bone scan, whereas radiographs require a minimum mineral loss of 50% before a lesion is visualized. MRI is often more sensitive than bone scan because signal changes in the marrow from the tumor can be

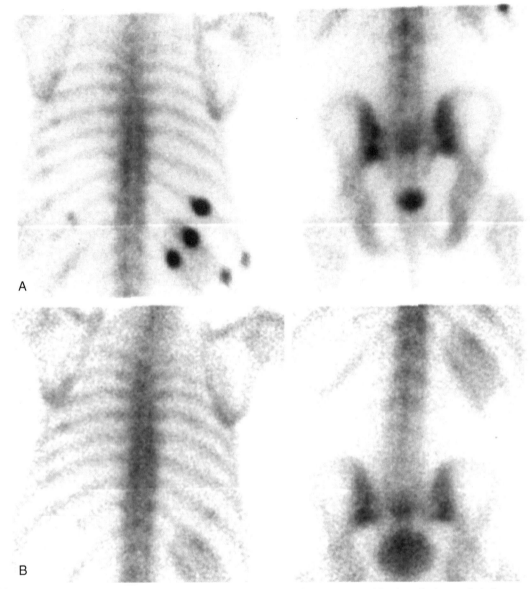

FIGURE 7-10. Typical appearance of traumatic rib fractures. **A,** Posterior views of the chest reveal focal uptake in a vertical alignment in the right lower ribs and a recent left nephrectomy with resection of some lower left ribs. **B,** A follow-up study 18 months later shows resolution of the right rib uptake as the fractures healed.

Box 7-3. Reported Causes of Bilaterally Increased and Decreased Renal Visualization on Skeletal Scintigrams

INCREASED UPTAKE	DECREASED UPTAKE
Nephrotoxic antibiotics	Renal failure
Urinary tract obstruction	Superscan
	Metastatic disease
Chemotherapy (doxorubicin, vincristine, cyclophosphamide)	Metabolic bone disease
	Paget disease
	Osteomalacia
	Hyperparathyroidism
Nephrocalcinosis	Myelofibrosis
Hypercalcemia	Nephrectomy
Radiation nephritis	Prolonged delays in imaging
Acute tubular necrosis	
Thalassemia	

visualized directly. However, whole-body MRI is not widely available and generally not practical at this time.

Bone scan is said to be 95% sensitive, but this sensitivity depends on several factors, such as tumor type. Predominantly osteoblastic sites are easily seen as areas of increased activity. Lesions that are mostly osteoclastic or lytic are more difficult to detect because they will appear cold or isointense. Sensitivity is highest for prostate cancer, which is mainly osteoblastic. The detection of breast and lung cancer is also very high, although these tumors are more mixed in their lesion pattern. The sensitivity of bone scan is low for tumors that are predominantly lytic, such as multiple myeloma and renal cell carcinoma, as well as those contained in the marrow, such as lymphoma. F-18 FDG PET often can detect involvement from cancers in the marrow or in lesions that are more aggressive and lytic. In some tumors, particularly those with mixed lytic and blastic lesions, the Tc-99m MDP bone scan and F-18 FDG

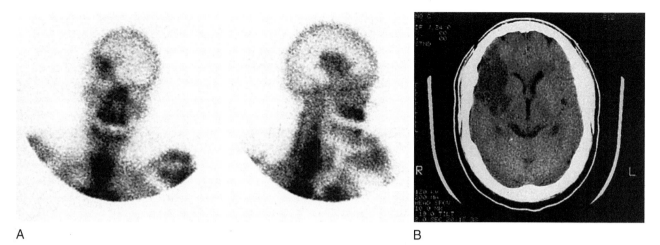

FIGURE 7-11. A, Tc-99m MDP uptake in a right parietal stroke. **B,** CT confirms the cause of the uptake is intracranial and not in the skull.

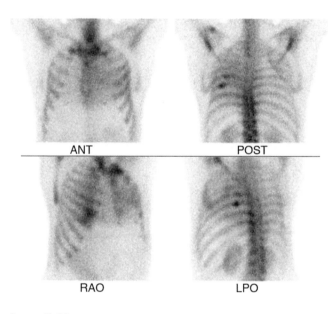

ANT POST

RAO LPO

FIGURE 7-12. Bone scan following chemoradiation for non–small cell lung cancer demonstrates mild hazy uptake outside of the skeleton in an area of pleural thickening and residual tumor in the left upper thorax. In addition, decreased uptake is seen in the T-spine corresponding to the radiation port. Two probably posttraumatic rib lesions on the *left* show focal increased uptake.

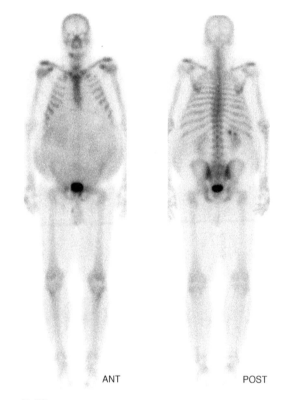

ANT POST

FIGURE 7-13. Abnormal mild uptake in the distended abdomen is characteristic of malignant ascites.

PET may be complimentary tests, each detecting different lesions. The use of F-18 sodium fluoride (NaF) PET is also being investigated for the assessment of bone metastasis.

Scintigraphic Patterns in Metastatic Disease

Multiple Lesions

The scintigraphic patterns encountered in skeletal metastatic disease are summarized in Box 7-4. Multiple focal lesions distributed randomly in the skeleton provide a high degree of clinical certainty in the diagnosis of metastases. However, other causes also can show multiple areas of uptake (Box 7-5). Often, different features and patterns can help identify these causes. For example, Paget disease may be differentiated from metastasis by a coarse expansion of the bone.

Solitary Lesions

The chance that a solitary lesion is due to malignancy varies by location (Table 7-2). Uptake in a rib in a patient with known malignancy has a 10% to 20% chance of being malignant, whereas uptake in the central skeleton has a much higher likelihood of being malignant from metastases. Primary bone tumors, such as osteosarcoma, must be suspected, especially in younger patients with long-bone involvement. Common benign causes for a solitary lesion include arthritis and trauma. Some benign bone lesions such as enchondroma, osteoma, fibrous dysplasia, osteomyelitis, and monostotic Paget disease can also cause solitary abnormalities. Rarely, a benign bone island may accumulate some Tc-99m MDP.

Box 7-4. Scintigraphic Patterns in Metastatic Disease

Solitary focal lesions
Multiple focal lesions
Diffuse involvement ("superscan")
Photon-deficient lesions (cold lesions)
Normal (false negative)
Flare phenomenon (follow-up studies)
Soft tissue lesions (tracer uptake in tumor)

Box 7-5. Differential Diagnosis of Multiple Focal Lesions (Listed in Order of Decreasing Likelihood)

Metastatic disease
Arthritis
Trauma, osteoporotic insufficiency fractures
Paget disease
Other metabolic bone disease
Osteomyelitis
Numerous other conditions (fibrous dysplasia, multiple enchondromas, infarction)

TABLE 7-2 Metastatic Disease Presenting as a Solitary Focus in Patients with Known Cancer

Site	Percentage
Spine and pelvis	60-70
Skull	40-50
Rib	10-20
Sternum (in breast carcinoma)	75

Box 7-6. Differential Diagnosis for Superscan Pattern

COMMON
Metastases (prostate, breast)
Renal osteodystrophy
Delayed images

LESS COMMON
Severe hyperparathyroidism (rare primary)
Osteomalacia
Paget disease

Superscan
A potentially problematic scintigraphic pattern is the "superscan" or "beautiful bone scan." The differential diagnosis of the superscan pattern is provided in Box 7-6. In some patients with prostate cancer and breast cancer, the entire axial skeleton is involved. Uptake may be sufficiently uniform to appear deceptively normal (Fig. 7-2, *B*). Classically, absent or faint visualization of the kidneys is seen with a superscan. Confusion from a superscan is a less common interpretive problem than in the past because of improved technology and image quality, and it should be possible to discriminate diffuse metastasis. Reviewing the available radiographs on each patient will help prevent mistakes.

Box 7-7. Differential Diagnosis of a Cold Defect

Metal artifact (pacemaker, prosthesis)
Radiation changes
Barium in bowel
Vascular
  Early avascular necrosis
  Early infarct
Multiple myeloma
Osseous metastasis
  Renal cell carcinoma
  Thyroid carcinoma
  Anaplastic tumors
  Neuroblastoma
  Breast and lung carcinoma
Tumor marrow involvement
  Lymphoma
  Leukemia
Benign tumors, cysts

Flare Phenomenon
Another potentially perplexing pattern is seen in some bone scans done on patients undergoing cyclical chemotherapy. When a patient has a good response to chemotherapy, the bone scan may paradoxically worsen, with a flare of increased activity (Fig. 7-14). To add to the confusion, these patients may experience increased pain. If these lesions are followed over 2 to 6 months, CT shows increased sclerosis from an osteoblastic response as the bone begins to heal. This is the same time frame at which the bone scan typically shows increased uptake. Activity should regress by 4 to 6 months after the flare. This phenomenon reinforces the fact that tracer uptake is not in the tumor but rather in the surrounding bone.

Cold Lesions
Lesions that are aggressive, purely lytic, or completely replaced by tumor may show decreased uptake (Fig. 7-3). A list of possible causes for cold defects is provided in Box 7-7. These cold, or photon-deficient, areas may be difficult to spot because of overlying or adjacent uptake (Fig. 7-15). Other causes for decreased uptake such as metal attenuation artifact, radiation ports, compromised blood flow early in a pediatric septic joint, or very early infarct or avascular necrosis should be considered in the differential.

Imaging Findings in Specific Tumors

Prostate Carcinoma
Skeletal scintigraphy is very sensitive in the detection of metastatic disease from prostate cancer. Until the introduction of the prostate-specific antigen (PSA) blood test, bone scan was considered the most sensitive technique for detecting osseous metastasis. Serum alkaline phosphatase measurement detects only half the cases detected by scintigraphy. Radiographs may be normal 30% of the time.

The likelihood of an abnormal scintigram correlates with clinical stage, Gleason score, and PSA level. In early stage I disease, scintigrams demonstrate metastasis less

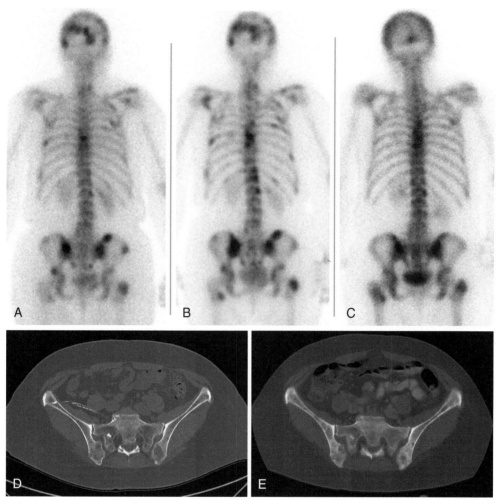

FIGURE 7-14. Flare phenomena on bone scan (**A** to **C**). **A,** Metastatic lesions in a patient with breast cancer appear to progress during therapy on (**B**) bone scan 4 months later. However, marked improvement is seen (**C**) on a scan after 6 months. Pelvic CT images (**D,E**) obtained at the time of the first bone scan (**D**) show lytic lesions initially but fairly diffuse sclerosis on a follow-up CT (**E**) performed after the third bone scan, corresponding to treatment response.

than 5% of the time. The incidence increases to 10% in stage II and 20% in stage III disease. In patients with PSA levels less than 10 ng/mL, bone metastases are rarely found (<1% of the time). Scintigraphy is still indicated to evaluate symptomatic patients and suspicious areas seen radiographically. With increasing PSA levels, the chance of detecting metastatic disease increases.

Breast Carcinoma

Despite increased screening with mammography, a large number of patients with breast cancer are initially diagnosed with advanced disease. Autopsy studies have shown osseous metastases in 50% to 80% of patients with breast carcinoma. Like prostate cancer, stage of disease correlates with the incidence of osseous metastases on bone scan—0.5% in stage I, 2% to 3% in stage II, 8% in stage III, and 13% in stage IV. Bone scans are not generally performed in patients with stage I or II disease.

Skeletal scintigraphy is highly sensitive in breast cancer. Patients may show local invasion of the ribs or sternum or disseminated disease. Although activity in the sternum is most often benign, a high incidence of metastatic disease is seen in patients with breast cancer (>75%-80%). Abnormal

soft tissue activity can be seen from tumor or surgery in the breast, in disease that is metastatic the liver (Fig. 7-16), and in malignant pleural effusions. F-18 FDG PET complements bone scan, detecting lytic lesions and those in marrow, but showing lower sensitivity for blastic lesions.

Lung Carcinoma

Although up to 50% of patients dying from a primary lung cancer have osseous metastasis at autopsy, no complete agreement exists on when to use skeletal scintigraphy. Staging is generally done with CT, surgery (including mediastinoscopy and video-assisted thoracoscopic surgery), and increasingly F-18 FDG PET. Skeletal scintigraphy is useful in a patient who develops pain during or after treatment.

Interesting patterns of disease may occur on scintigrams in lung cancer. Because these tumors can easily invade the vasculature, arterial metastases are more common. These tumor emboli can reach the distal extremities. Thus appendicular involvement is more common with aggressive lung cancer than cancer of the breast or prostate. Also, increased cortical activity, prominent in the extremities, can be seen in lung cancer as a result of hypertrophic osteoarthropathy (Figs. 7-17 and 7-18).

Neuroblastoma

Neuroblastoma has a neural crest origin and is the most common solid tumor to metastasize to bone in children (Fig. 7-19). Tc-99m MDP scintigraphy is twice as sensitive as radiographs on a lesion-by-lesion basis. MRI is better than bone scan for determining lesion extent. Iodine-131 or iodine-123 meta-iodo-benzyl-guanidine (MIBG) scan is more sensitive than bone scan for metastases, although the combination of both gives the highest sensitivity.

Lesions are typically multifocal and occur in the metaphyses. However, involvement in the skull, vertebrae, ribs, and pelvis is also common. Early involvement may be symmetrical and therefore difficult to diagnose on the bone scan because of the normal intense activity in the ends of growing bones. A unique characteristic of neuroblastoma is the avidity of Tc-99m diphosphonates for the primary tumor. Approximately 30% to 50% of primary tumors are demonstrated scintigraphically. Occasionally, neuroblastomas are discovered in children undergoing radionuclide imaging to evaluate another condition. Particular attention should be paid to the abdomen.

Other Tumors

Numerous other tumors metastasize to bone. The sensitivity for renal cell carcinoma is low and best assessed on skeletal survey or by MRI. Likewise, thyroid cancer is rarely detected on skeletal scintigraphy and is better evaluated with I-131 or, if noniodine avid, F-18 FDG PET. Gastrointestinal tract and gynecological cancers do not commonly metastasize to bone early in their courses. As a result of longer survival and control of local and regional metastases that usually cause death, bone metastases can manifest.

Primary Tumors

Malignant Tumors
Sarcomas of the Bone

Osteosarcoma is the most common primary skeletal malignancy after multiple myeloma and is particularly common at the ends of long bones in children. Rarely, it occurs as a multifocal process and occasionally can occur as an extraosseous tumor. Metastases frequently develop in the lungs, although in approximately 15% they can occur in the bones before being detected in the lungs. After osteosarcoma, the most common primary bone tumor in children is Ewing sarcoma. Approximately 25% of tumors arise in soft tissues rather than bone. At diagnosis, 25% have metastases. Metastatic lesions involve the lungs in 50%, bones in 25%, and marrow in 20%. Chondrosarcoma tends to be more common in adults and ranks third among all primary bone neoplasms after multiple myeloma and osteosarcoma. Chondrosarcoma can present in several ways and may originate as either a primary tumor or a secondary tumor from degeneration of a benign lesion.

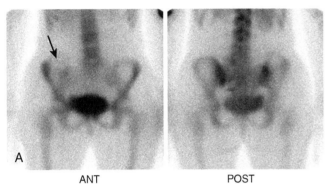

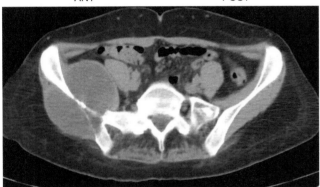

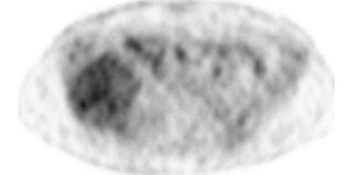

FIGURE 7-15. **A,** Bone scan images show a barely perceptible cold lesion in the right ileum *(arrow)* corresponding to a large soft tissue mass involving bone on **(B)** F-18 FDG PET-CT.

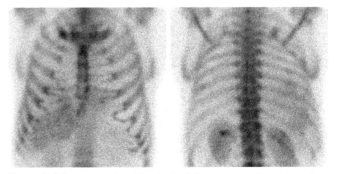

FIGURE 7-16. Increased activity in the right upper quadrant in a patient with breast cancer corresponded to liver metastases on CT.

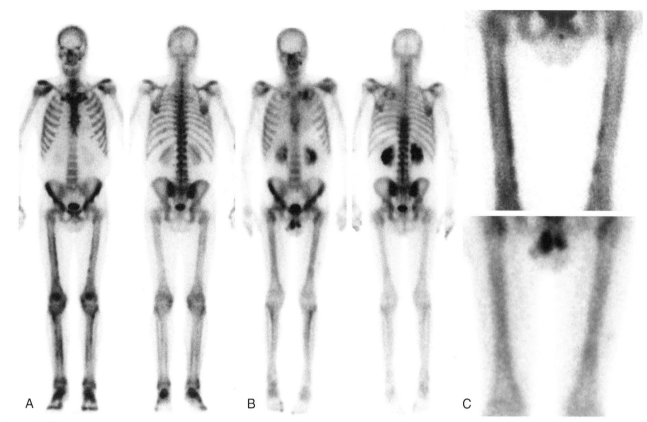

FIGURE 7-17. Hypertrophic osteoarthropathy in a patient with bronchogenic lung carcinoma. **A,** Whole-body scintigrams reveal classic uptake in the periosteal region of the long bones. (**B**) Follow-up 9 months later shows increased activity in a treated left apical lung mass. Radiation therapy changes of decreased uptake in the upper thoracic spine are seen. With successful treatment, the findings of hypertrophic osteoarthropathy have resolved. **C,** Spot views of the femurs more clearly show the abnormal uptake *(left)* that later resolves *(right)*.

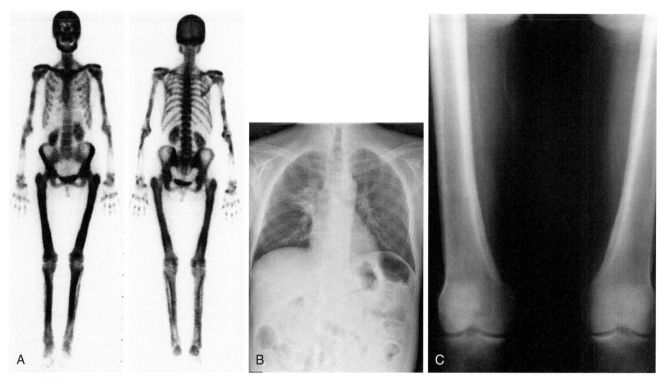

FIGURE 7-18. Florid hypertrophic osteoarthropathy. **A,** Bones of the upper and lower extremities are diffusely involved, as are the clavicles, mandible, and skull. Although the pattern may be confusing, the patient did not have skeletal metastatic disease. Involvement of the extremities is one clue. **B,** Chest radiograph reveals a bronchogenic carcinoma in the right upper lobe just above the right hilum. (**C**) Radiograph of the femurs shows characteristic periosteal new bone bilaterally on both the medial and lateral aspects of the femoral shaft.

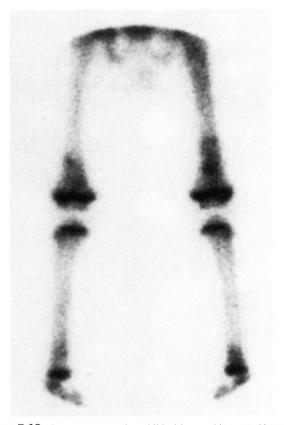

FIGURE 7-19. Bone metastases in a child with neuroblastoma. Abnormal tracer localization is present in both femurs and distal tibial metaphyses, more extensive on the left than the right.

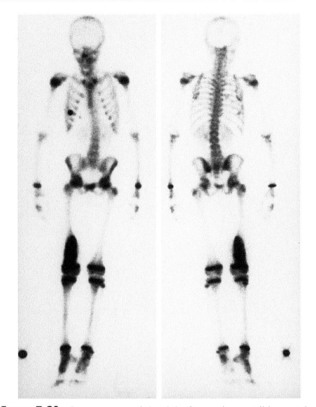

FIGURE 7-20. Osteosarcoma of the right femur shows striking uptake. The increased blood flow induced by the tumor results in increased tracer delivery to the entire limb can add to difficulty using the scintigram to determine the tumor margins. (Note: activity over the right ribs is a marker.)

Primary bone tumors such as osteosarcoma, Ewing sarcoma, and chondrosarcoma have avid uptake of the bone-seeking radiopharmaceuticals (Fig. 7-20). Bone scan tends to overestimate the extent of tumor but can identify skip lesions in osteosarcoma or involvement of other bones. In addition, both thallium-201 and Tc-99m sestamibi have been used for sarcoma imaging. They may help determine if the primary tumor is high or low grade, can serve as a baseline to evaluate response to therapy, and may show better definition of tumor margin. However, MRI is the primary modality for osteosarcoma evaluation (Fig. 7-21), providing detailed anatomical information and allowing assessment of soft tissue involvement. CT is generally used for surveillance of lung metastases. In addition to the detection of osseous metastases, the occasional polyostotic tumor would be missed without a whole-body survey of some kind (Fig. 7-22). Increasingly, however, that role also may be filled by FDG PET-CT, which has also shown promise in the assessment of therapeutic response.

Multiple Myeloma

The most common primary bone tumor in adults is multiple myeloma. It is a tumor of the marrow and typically involves the vertebrae, pelvis, ribs, and skull. Radiographs may show only osteopenia or a permeative pattern that can be confused with metastatic disease. Although bone scan will show 46% to 65% of the lesions as areas of decreased and sometimes increased uptake, this is lower than the 75% to 91% sensitivity of radiographs. This likely relates

to the lack of reactive bone formation in response to the lesions. MRI has a positive predictive value of 88%, and when F-18 FDG PET is additionally performed, this further increases to nearly 100%.

Leukemia and Lymphoma

Bone scan plays a very limited role in the evaluation of leukemia. Patients with leukemia imaged with Tc-99m MDP may show focal increased uptake in areas of marrow infiltration. In blast crisis, diffusely increased uptake that is greater at the ends of the long bones may be present.

Hodgkin disease will involve the skeleton approximately one third of the time, and bone scan may show focal or diffuse uptake of Tc-99m MDP. Skeletal scintigraphy is less useful in non-Hodgkin lymphoma. In general, lymphoma is best evaluated with F-18 FDG PET and CT.

Histiocytosis

The sensitivity of bone scan varies with the spectrum of disease in histiocytosis. Although uptake is reliably seen in eosinophilic granuloma, detection of histiocytosis is limited, with lesions seen from one third to two thirds of the time. Frequently, decreased uptake is shown.

Benign Bone Tumors

Usually, benign bone tumors are characterized by their radiographic appearance. The role of skeletal scintigraphy is very limited, although understanding is critical because benign tumors may be encountered during imaging for

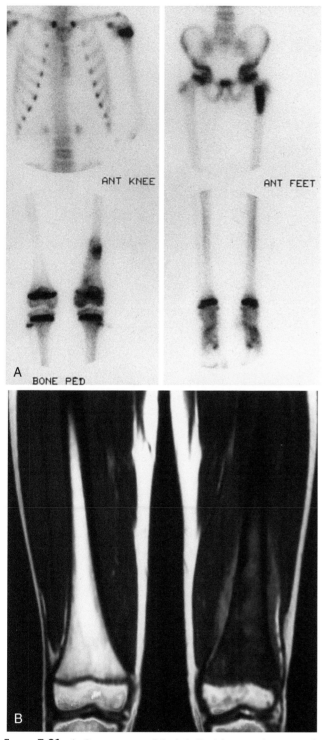

FIGURE 7-21. A, Osteosarcoma of the left distal femur and a metastatic lesion in the left proximal femur. **B,** Coronal T1-weighted MRI reveals superior anatomical information about the osseous and soft tissue extent of the tumor. However, it missed the second lesion that was out of the field of view.

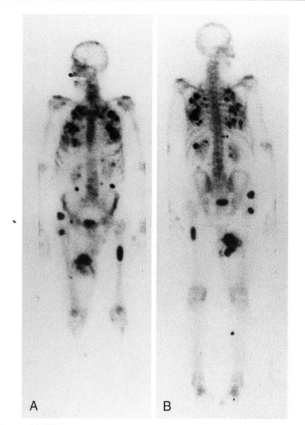

FIGURE 7-22. A and **B,** Extraosseous osteosarcoma arising in the right medial thigh with widely disseminated skeletal, soft tissue, and pulmonary metastases. This study is a dramatic example of the ability of skeletal scintigraphy to survey the entire body.

other reasons. Some benign tumors have intense uptake similar to that in malignant tumors. These include osteoid osteomas, giant cell tumors, and fibrous dysplasia. Other tumors may show a characteristic pattern such as a peripheral rim of activity around a cold central area in aneurismal bone cyst. Benign bone tumors are variable in appearance; selected benign bone tumors are listed in Table 7-3.

Osteoid osteoma classically presents in adolescents and young adults as severe pain at night. Commonly occurring in the proximal femur and spine, they may be difficult to detect with conventional radiography. The diagnosis on radiographs can be made if a central lucent nidus is seen surrounded by sclerosis (Fig. 7-23). Skeletal scintigraphy is very sensitive, and the lesion will show increased uptake (Fig. 7-24). SPECT adds to this sensitivity and is particularly useful in the spine. Surgeons can use an intraoperative probe to localize the lesion with its increased activity. However, CT has largely eliminated the need for the bone scan.

Bone islands rarely accumulate Tc-99m MDP, so bone scan may be useful in assessing an atypical bone island on radiographs. If the sclerotic lesion on radiograph does not show increased activity, it is unlikely to be malignant.

Osteochondromas, common cartilage-containing benign tumors, may show variable uptake that diminishes as the skeleton matures. Rarely, osteochondromas will show malignant transformation, usually into a chondrosarcoma. This degeneration occurs less than 1% of the time in a solitary lesion and less than 5% of the time in hereditary multiple osteochondromatosis (hereditary multiple exostoses). Although bone scan can exclude malignancy if no increased uptake is seen, the presence of increased activity does not differentiate benign from malignant lesions. Any new uptake in a lesion that previously had none is suspicious. Osteochondromas are usually best evaluated with CT and MRI.

Enchondromas usually present as a cystic lesion in the hands or a sclerotic area reminiscent of a bone infarct

TABLE 7-3 Benign Bone Lesions on Skeletal Scintigraphy

Degree of uptake	Malignancy potential	Comments
INTENSE UPTAKE		
Aneurysmal bone cyst	No	Donut sign pattern
Chondroblastoma	Almost always benign	Positive bone scan does not diagnose malignancy
Giant cell tumor	10%	
Fibrous dysplasia	<1%	
Osteoma	No	Gardner syndrome
Osteoid osteoma	No	Osteoblastoma >2 cm
ISOINTENSE/MILD UPTAKE		
Bone island	No	
Enchondroma	Solitary: <20% long bones	
	Multiple enchondromatosis: <50%	
Nonossifying fibroma	No	
VARIABLE UPTAKE		
Osteochondroma	<1%	
HEREDITARY MULTIPLE EXOSTOSES		
Hemangioma	No	Prominent trabeculae on CT diagnostic
Eosinophilic granuloma	No; least aggressive histiocytosis group	Monostotic/polyostotic
LOW UPTAKE		
Unicameral bone cyst	No	

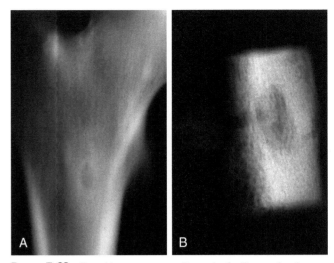

FIGURE 7-23. Osteoid osteoma on radiograph. **A,** Conventional tomogram of the right proximal femur reveals a characteristic radiolucent nidus surrounded by sclerotic bone. **B,** Specimen radiograph confirms the complete excision of the nidus.

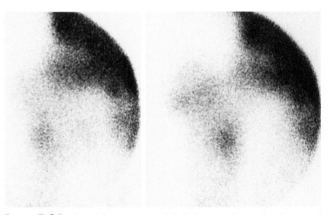

FIGURE 7-24. Osteoid osteoma on pinhole images. Internal and external rotation pinhole spot views of the proximal femur in a patient with suspected osteoid osteoma. An area of abnormally increased uptake demonstrated just lateral to the lesser trochanter confirms the clinical suspicion.

elsewhere. They are benign but can degenerate into a malignant tumor. This degeneration is more common in multiple enchondromatosis (Ollier disease). Bone scan may help identify multiple lesions, but the role is otherwise very limited.

Fibrous Dysplasia

Numerous bone dysplasias demonstrate increased skeletal tracer uptake. Fibrous dysplasia is the most commonly encountered of these and may be monostotic or polyostotic (Fig. 7-25). The degree of increased tracer uptake is typically high, rivaling that seen in Paget disease. Distinguishing features are the younger patient age and different patterns of involvement. When Paget disease involves a long bone, it invariably extends to at least one end of the bone, whereas fibrous dysplasia frequently does not involve the epiphysis. Other dysplasias associated with increased tracer uptake are listed in Box 7-8.

Metabolic Bone Disease

Paget Disease

Paget disease may be included in the metabolic bone disease category, although mechanisms causing this disorder are not entirely understood. Typically a chronic disease of the elderly, abnormal bone remodeling is seen in three phases: the early resorptive, mixed middle, and final sclerotic phases. The diagnosis usually can be made by radiographs, which reveal coarsened, expanded bones. Although CT and MRI can be used to assess complications, a bone scan is useful to evaluate the extent of disease. Additionally, the patterns of Paget disease must be recognized when it is found incidentally.

The scintigraphic appearance is striking, with intensely increased tracer localization (Figs. 7-26 and 7-27). Increased uptake is seen in all phases of the disease. The bone expansion demonstrated radiographically is not well assessed by scintigraphy, owing to the lower resolution of the technique and the "blooming" appearance of very intense areas of uptake, but it is certainly suggested on the images. The pelvis is the most commonly involved site, followed by the spine, skull, femur, scapula, tibia, and humerus. In osteoporosis circumscripta, a characteristic rim of increased uptake borders the lesion.

Hyperparathryoidism and Renal Osteodystrophy

Some metabolic conditions, such as osteomalacia, hyperparathyroidism, renal osteodystrophy, and hypervitaminosis

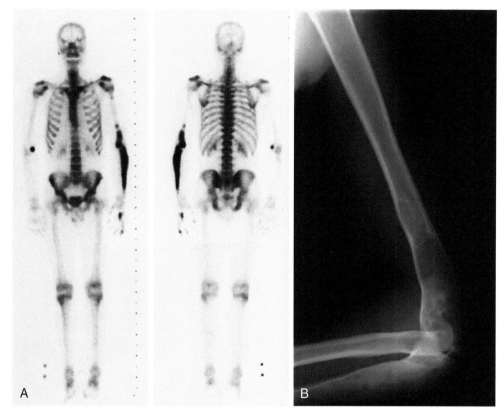

FIGURE 7-25. Fibrous dysplasia. **A,** Uptake is markedly increased in the distal humerus, most of the forearm, and focal areas in the hand. **B,** Corresponding radiograph of the left elbow reveals characteristic expansile lesions of fibrous dysplasia.

Box 7-8. Bone Dysplasias Associated with Increased Skeletal Tracer Uptake

Fibrous dysplasia
Osteogenesis imperfecta
Osteopetrosis
Progressive diaphyseal dysplasia (Engelmann disease)
Hereditary multiple diaphyseal sclerosis (Ribbing disease)
Melorheostosis

D, can cause patterns of increased scintigraphic uptake (Table 7-4). Although the patterns associated with these must be recognized to avoid confusion with pathological conditions such as metastatic disease, bone scan has no role in the diagnosis and management of these processes.

Inadequate osseous mineralization from deficiencies in vitamin D, calcium, or phosphate results in osteomalacia. Radiographically, bones have a washed-out, chalky appearance with decreased trabeculae. Although adults are affected, findings in the growing skeleton, known as rickets, are most striking. Changes at the growth plates (fraying, widening, cupping) of the proximal humerus, distal femur, distal tibia, and distal forearm and findings such as beading at the costochondral junctions are common. Bone scan shows a generalized increased uptake in the axial skeleton, including the skull and mandible. Uptake in the sternum is

often increased in a "tie" pattern with lines at the segmental junctions. Pseudofractures, beading of the costochondral junctions, and real fractures are common (Fig. 7-28).

Hyperparathyroidism may be primary, as from a parathyroid adenoma secreting parathormone (PTH), secondary as a response to the hypocalcemia of chronic renal disease, or tertiary when PTH is secreted by autonomously functioning tissue. Resulting bone turn over leads to generalized tracer uptake that may be seen throughout the body (Box 7-9). Uptake in the skull, mandible, sternum, periarticular regions, and costochondral beading may occur (Fig. 7-29). These same findings may be seen to a varying degree in secondary hyperparathyroidism and osteomalacia. The bone scan in long-standing renal osteodystrophy often has the most extreme appearance. In fact, severely increased skeleton-to-soft tissue ratio and poor renal visualization may create an appearance similar to that of a superscan seen in metastatic disease (Fig 7-30). Patients with uncomplicated primary hyperparathyroidism usually have normal bone scans.

Extraskeletal uptake is not uncommon from an increased serum calcium-to-phosphate ratio. In hyperparathyroidism, especially with renal disease, a classic pattern of soft tissue uptake is seen in the lungs, stomach, and kidneys as a result of imbalances in calcium and phosphate (Fig. 7-31).

Skeletal Trauma

Although bone scan is highly sensitive for fracture (Fig. 7-32), radiographs, CT, and MRI are usually used when acute

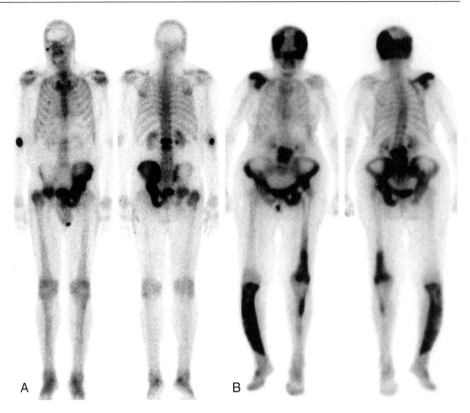

FIGURE 7-26. Multifocal Paget disease. **A,** Abnormal uptake in the left hemipelvis, upper lumbar spine, and, to a lesser extent, right hip in a patient with Paget disease. When Paget disease involves the axial bones, it must be differentiated from metastatic disease by the location and bone expansion. Radiographic correlation will show the typical coarsened trabeculae. **B,** When the sites are more numerous, the diagnosis is obvious based on the typical distribution of lesions.

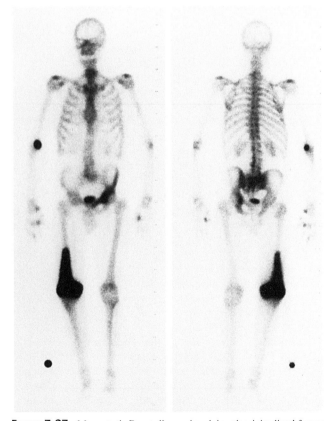

FIGURE 7-27. Monostotic Paget disease involving the right distal femur. The uptake is extremely intense, with the appearance of bony expansion. The observation about expansion must be made with caution because of the extreme intensity of uptake and "blooming" of the recorded activity. Also note involvement of the ischium.

fractures are suspected. MRI is not only sensitive but also provides information on surrounding soft tissues. When patients cannot undergo MRI, when MRI findings are negative, or when a precise area of concern is not known, a bone scan may be used to detect occult fracture.

Acute fractures generally result in a three-phase positive scintigram, with chronic or partially healed fractures typically positive only on delayed images. Approximately 80% of fractures can be visualized by 24 hours after trauma. Ninety-five percent of fractures are positive after 3 days, and in patients under the age of 65, essentially all fractures are positive by this time. Advanced age and debilitation are factors contributing to delayed visualization of fractures. The maximum degree of fracture uptake occurs 7 or more days after trauma, and delayed imaging in this time frame is recommended in difficult or equivocal cases. Occasionally, decreased uptake is seen acutely as a result of compromised vascular supply (Fig. 7-33).

The time a fracture takes to return to normal on the bone scan depends on location, stability, and the degree of damage to the skeleton. Approximately 60% to 80% of nondisplaced uncomplicated fractures revert to normal in 1 year, and more than 95% revert in 3 years (Table 7-5). However, in many instances, displaced fractures remained positive indefinitely. Structural deformity and posttraumatic arthritis were the most common reasons for prolonged positive studies. Patients undergoing metastatic skeletal survey should be routinely asked about prior trauma.

Iatrogenic Trauma

Iatrogenic trauma to either the skeleton or soft tissues may result in abnormal uptake on the bone scan, so

TABLE 7-4 Metabolic Bone Disorders

OSTEOPOROSIS

Primary (idiopathic)

Senile, postmenopausal

Secondary

Disuse	
Drugs	Corticosteroids, chemotherapy, anticonvulsants
Endocrine	Hyperthyroidism, primary hyperparathyroidism, Cushing disease, hypogonadism

OSTEOMALACIA

Vitamin D	Vitamin D deficiency, hereditary disorders of vitamin D metabolism
Decreased calcium	Calcium malabsorption, inadequate intake, calcitonin secreting tumors
Phosphate loss	Renal tubular disease, hemodialysis, transplant
Other	Liver disease, phenytoin, prematurity

HYPERPARATHYROIDISM

Primary	Parathyroid adenoma, parathyroid hyperplasia
Secondary	Chronic renal insufficiency, phosphate metabolism abnormalities, parathyroid hyperplasia
Tertiary	Autonomous parathyroid glands from long standing secondary hyperparathyroidism
Renal Osteodystrophy	Chronic renal failure
Hypoparathyroidism	Iatrogenic loss/damage parathyroid glands during thyroidectomy; pseudohypoparathyroidism genetic end-organ resistance

METAL TOXICITIES

Aluminum-induced bone disease

Fluorosis

Heavy metal poisoning

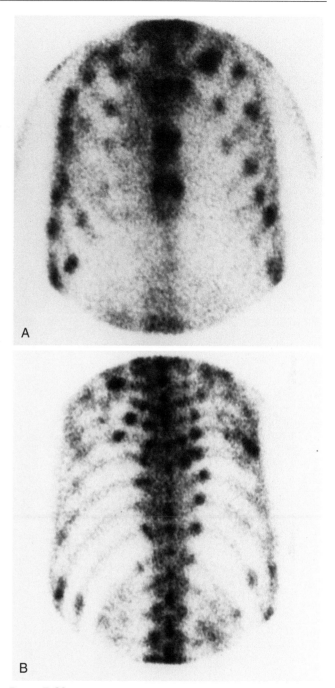

A

B

FIGURE 7-28. Osteomalacia. Anterior (**A**) and posterior (**B**) views. The patient was referred to rule out metastatic disease. The unusually large number of rib lesions raised the suspicion of metabolic bone disease rather than metastases.

accurate history is often key. Craniotomy typically leaves a rim pattern at the surgical margin that may persist for months postoperatively. Rib retraction during thoracotomy can elicit periosteal reaction and increased uptake without actual resection of bone being involved. Bone resections are recognized as photon-deficient areas, although small laminectomies are usually not appreciated scintigraphically.

Areas of the skeleton receiving therapeutic levels of external beam ionizing radiation characteristically demonstrate geometrical decreased uptake within 6 months to 1 year after therapy (Figs. 7-12 and 7-17). The mechanism is probably decreased osteogenesis and decreased blood flow to postirradiated bone.

Child Abuse

The generally high sensitivity of skeletal scintigraphy would seem to make it an ideal survey test in cases of

Box 7-9. Distribution of Increased Skeletal Uptake in Hyperparathyroidism

Diffuse axial	Costochondral
Periarticular	junctions
Skull	Sternum
Mandible, fascial	Lungs
bones	Stomach

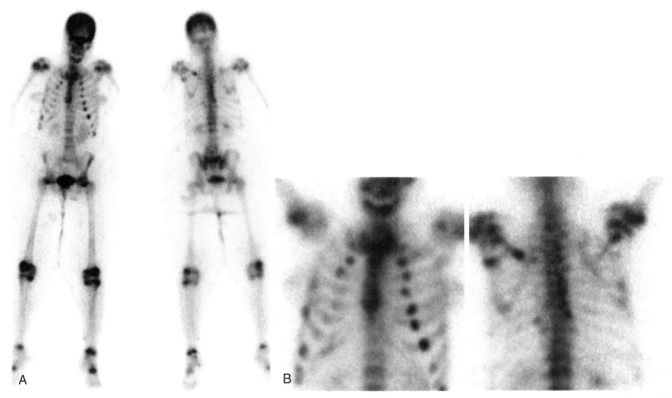

FIGURE 7-29. Renal osteodystrophy. Whole-body **(A)** and spot images **(B)** of a patient with long-standing renal failure show classic skeletal changes of severe renal osteodystrophy. Abnormal activity is seen in the face and skull and the distal ends of the long bones. The rib tip activity has been called the rachitic "rosary bead" configuration. Focal uptake in the left scapula was a fracture although brown tumors can have a similar appearance.

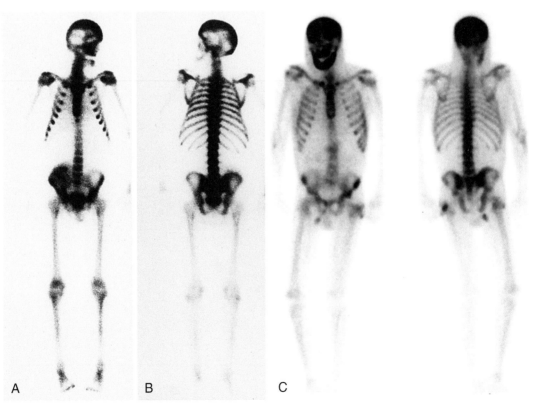

FIGURE 7-30. Renal osteodystrophy. **A** and **B,** The absence of soft tissue uptake with a superscan appearance even more striking than seen in metastatic disease. The prominent rib end activity may help differentiate the two causes. The native kidneys failed, and a renal transplant is noted in the right iliac fossa. **C,** Increased activity in the skull and sternum may be especially prominent. Note the increased axial skeletal uptake and paucity of soft tissue background activity.

suspected child abuse. However, in practice, radiographic skeletal survey is more sensitive than bone scintigraphy because of its ability to demonstrate old fractures that have healed, subtle fractures along growth plates with their normally high levels of uptake, and calvarial fractures in young children that may be difficult to see on bone scan. Scintigraphy is often reserved for cases of suspected child abuse when radiographs are unrevealing. In these cases, symmetrical positioning of the patient is critical.

Complex Regional Pain Syndrome

Complex regional pain syndrome, previously known as reflex sympathetic dystrophy, is an exaggerated response to injury and immobilization with sensory, motor, and autonomic features. Although presentation is variable, patients typically have pain, edema, and muscle wasting in an affected extremity.

Scintigraphic findings are variable depending on the stage of disease. The classic pattern of unilaterally increased flow and blood pool activity with increased periarticular uptake on delayed images is seen less than 50% of the time but provides the highest diagnostic accuracy. Early disease (up to 5-6 months) usually shows increased blood flow (Fig 7-34), but blood flow may be normal or decreased later in the course of the disease. The periarticular uptake on delayed images is found in most cases (>95%), although specificity is lower if this finding is seen without the increased blood flow. Infection and arthritis

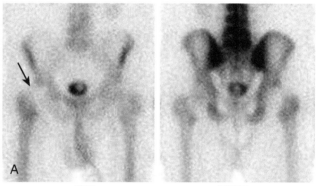
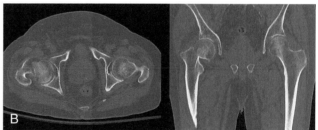

ANT POST

FIGURE 7-33. Planar images of the pelvis (**A**) in an elderly man with hip pain after a fall in the hospital show decreased uptake in the right femoral head and neck *(arrow)* corresponding to a displaced femoral neck fracture in osteoporotic bone on CT (**B**).

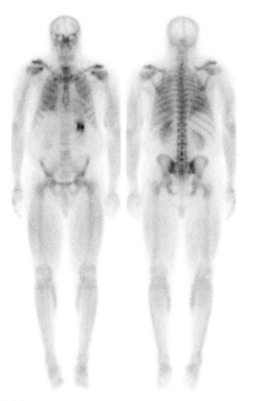

FIGURE 7-31. Tertiary hyperparathyroidism. Whole-body views show diffusely increased uptake in the lungs, stomach, and heart.

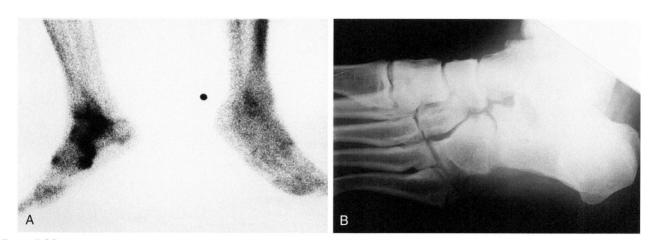

FIGURE 7-32. Trauma to the distal extremity. **A,** Skeletal scintigram of a patient who had sustained direct trauma to the right foot and ankle reveals multiple focal areas of abnormal tracer accumulation from fracture. **B,** The radiograph illustrates fractures of the base of the fifth metatarsal and lateral cuneiform.

TABLE 7-5 Skeletal Scintigraphy in Trauma: Time Course From Fracture to Return to Normal

Fracture type and site		Percent of normal	
Nonmanipulated closed fractures		1 year	3 years
Vertebra		59	97
Long bone		64	95
Rib		79	100
ALL FRACTURES*	**<1 YEAR**	**2-5 YEARS**	**>5 YEARS**
All sites	30	62	84

Data from Matin P. The appearance of bone scans following fractures, including immediate and long term studies, *J Nucl Med.* 1979;20(12):1227-1231.

*Modified from Kim HR, Thrall JH, Keyes JW Jr. Skeletal scintigraphy following incidental trauma, *Radiology.* 1979;130(2):447-451.

could cause false positive results. Some variants have been found, including cold areas or decreased uptake in some adults. Children often have normal or decreased uptake.

Stress Fractures

A significant change in activity level or a repetitive activity may lead to injury to the bone (Fig 7-35). If the process causing injury is allowed to continue to the point of overt fracture, healing predictably takes several months or more, compared with the several weeks required for healing of an early stress reaction (Table 7-6). Therefore prompt diagnosis and appropriate change in activity are critical. Exquisitely sensitive, skeletal scintigraphy reveals characteristic intense uptake at the fracture site ranging from the earlier oval or fusiform uptake to activity traversing the bone in outright fracture (Fig. 7-36). Stress injury is not uncommonly multifocal; thus additional sites of involvement may be detected.

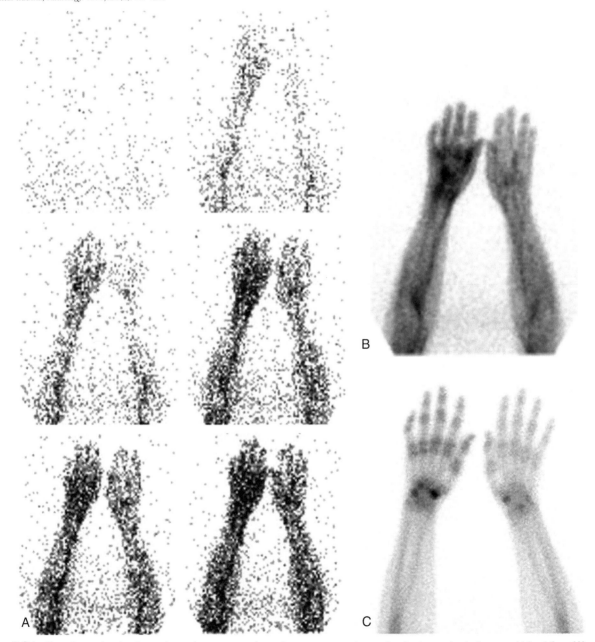

FIGURE 7-34. Complex regional pain syndrome in a young patient after trauma months previously shows clearly increased blood flow **(A)** and blood pool **(B)** activity in the left arm, with mild periarticular uptake on the delayed image **(C)** in the left hand on a three-phase bone scan. Activity varies but may be much more asymmetric on delayed images.

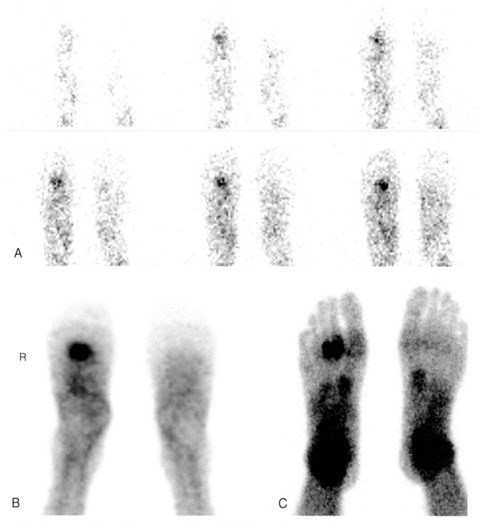

FIGURE 7-35. Three-phase bone scan images in a runner with marked focal pain in the right foot show focal increased flow **(A)**, blood pool **(B)**, and delayed bone localization to the second and third proximal right metatarsals traversing the bone consistent with acute stress fracture. Bone scan may be positive well before radiographs. *R*, Right.

TABLE 7-6 Sequence of Findings in Stress Reaction

	Clinical findings	X-ray	Scintigram
Normal (resorption = replacement)	−	−	−
Accelerated remodeling (resorption > replacement)	+/−	−	+
Fatigue (resorption >> replacement)	+	+/−	+++
Exhaustion (resorption >>> replacement)	++	+	++++
Cortical fracture	++++	++++	++++

Data from Roub LW, et al: Bone stress: a radionuclide imaging perspective, *Radiology*. 1979;132(2):431-438.

Spondylolysis occurs in the lumbar spine in the pars articularis, often seen as a result of repetitive trauma in young athletes. Most commonly the abnormality occurs at L4-5. In some instances, all examinations, including radiographs, MRI, and planar bone scan, may be normal, but a SPECT study may reveal the pathologic condition (Fig. 7-37).

Shin Splints

The term *shin splints* is applied generically to describe stress-related leg soreness along the medial or posteromedial aspect of the tibia. In nuclear medicine, the term is now used to describe a specific combination of clinical and scintigraphic findings. Increased tracer uptake is seen on the scintigram, typically involving a large portion of the middle to distal tibia (Fig. 7-38). Most cases are bilateral, although not necessarily symmetrical. The radionuclide uptake is superficial, only mild to moderate in intensity, and lacks a focal aspect seen with true stress fractures. Hyperemia is limited, unlike in stress fractures, which show intense hyperemia.

A phenomenon perhaps related to shin splints is activity-induced enthesopathy. In athletes, repeated microtears with subsequent healing reaction can result in increased tracer uptake at the site of tendon or ligament attachment. Osteitis pubis, plantar fasciitis, Achilles tendonitis, and some cases of pulled hamstring muscles are examples. A periosteal reaction develops at the site of stress, sometimes resulting in increased skeletal tracer localization.

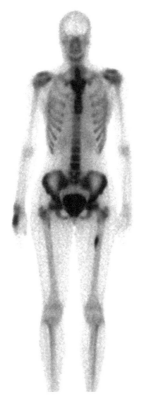

FIGURE 7-36. Whole-body bone scan images in a runner with leg pain reveal a fusiform, superficial lesion in the left medial femur from stress injury.

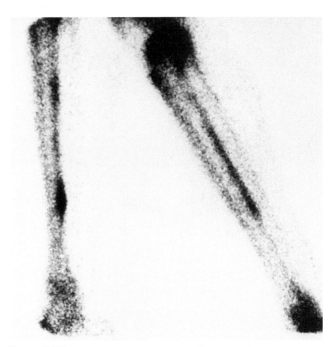

FIGURE 7-38. Shin splint. Lateral views of a patient demonstrating the classic finding of increased tracer uptake along the posterior and medial aspects of the tibia on the left *(left side of image)*. A similar pattern can be seen on the *right,* but with the addition of a focal area distally, which could indicate stress fracture.

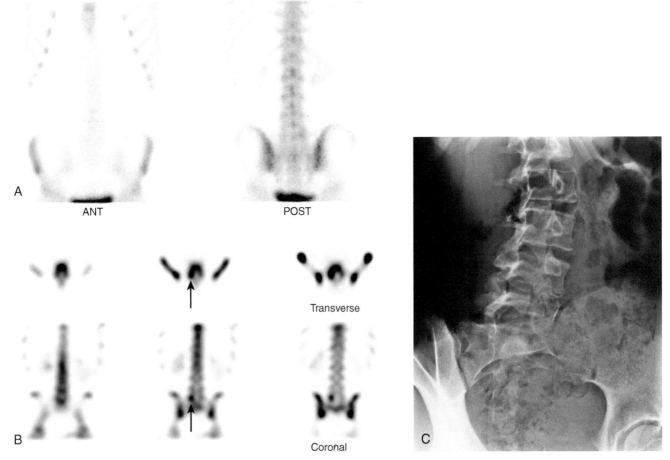

FIGURE 7-37. Spondylolysis. **(A)** Planar bone scan images are normal in a 20-year-old gymnast with severe low back pain and negative radiographs and MRI. **(B)** However, transverse and coronal SPECT images show focal abnormal activity in the right posterior elements of L5-S1 *(arrow)* consistent with spondylolysis. **(C)** Oblique LS spine radiograph from a different patient shows a pars interarticularis defect at L5.

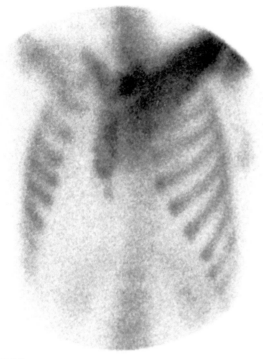

FIGURE 7-39. Rhabdomyolysis. Marked pectoral muscle uptake on bone scan after injury from repetitive strenuous weight lifting.

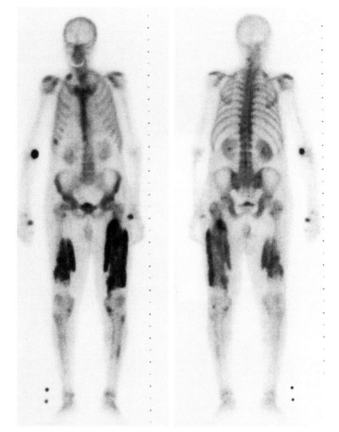

FIGURE 7-40. Myositis ossificans. Anterior and posterior whole-body scintigrams with extensive myositis ossificans involvement in the legs.

Rhabdomyolysis

Another athletic injury that is seen in this day of marathons and triathlons is rhabdomyolysis. The localization of skeletal tracers in exercise-damaged skeletal muscle is probably similar to the localization in damaged myocardium. Calcium buildup in damaged tissue provides a site for radionuclide deposition when combined with phosphate.

The scintigraphic pattern reflects the muscle groups undergoing injury (Fig 7-39). In marathon runners, the most striking uptake is usually in the muscles of the thigh. Rhabdomyolysis induced by renal failure is generally diffuse. The time course of scintigraphic abnormality appears to be similar to that for acute myocardial infarction. The greatest degree of uptake is seen at 24 to 48 hours after injury. The changes resolve by 1 week.

Heterotopic Bone Formation

Heterotopic bone formation can occur in the muscle as a result of numerous conditions. It is most often a direct result of trauma to the muscle in myositis ossificans (Fig. 7-40). However, it also can be a serious problem in paralyzed muscles and prolonged immobilization. The bone scan in these patients will reveal increased Tc-99m MDP deposition in the muscles on delayed images. Often, the blood flow and immediate blood pool images show more intense activity than the delayed images. Increased soft tissue uptake on a bone scan typically occurs long before any radiographic change. If patients are treated in these early stages, they may avoid more severe and lasting complications, such as severely contracted and ossified muscles at the hips in paraplegia.

BOX 7-10. Causes of Aseptic Bone Necrosis

Trauma (accidental, iatrogenic)
Drug therapy (steroids)
Hypercoagulable states
Hemoglobinopathies (sickle cell disease and
 variants)
After radiation therapy (orthovoltage)
Caisson disease
Osteochondrosis (pediatric age group;
 Legg-Calvé-Perthes disease)
Polycythemia
Leukemia
Gaucher disease
Alcoholism
Pancreatitis
Idiopathic

■ BONE INFARCTION AND OSTEONECROSIS

Necrosis of the bone has numerous causes (Box 7-10). Because this is an evolving process, the appearance on skeletal scintigraphy depends greatly on the time frame in which imaging is performed. With acute interruption of the blood supply, newly infarcted bone appears scintigraphically cold or photon deficient. In the postinfarction or healing phase, osteogenesis and tracer uptake at the margin of the infarcted area are increased. Skeletal scintigrams can show intensely increased tracer uptake during the healing period.

Legg-Calvé-Perthes Disease

Legg-Calvé-Perthes disease most commonly affects children between the ages of 5 and 9 years with predominance in boys (4:1-5:1). It is a form of osteochondrosis and results in avascular necrosis of the capital femoral epiphysis. The mechanism of injury is unknown except that the vascular supply of the femoral head is thought to be especially vulnerable in the most commonly affected age group.

The best scintigraphic technique for detecting the abnormality in the femoral head is to use some form of magnification and to image in the frogleg lateral projection. Classically, early in the course of the disease before healing has occurred, a discrete photon-deficient area can be seen in the upper outer portion of the capital femoral epiphysis with a lentiform configuration (Fig. 7-41). Areas of photon deficiency are well demonstrated by SPECT imaging.

As healing occurs, increased uptake is first seen at the margin of the photon-deficient area and gradually the scintigram demonstrates filling in of activity. In severe cases, the femoral head never reverts to normal. Increased tracer uptake is seen for a prolonged period—many months or longer.

Currently, MRI is the imaging modality of choice for the evaluation of Legg-Calvé-Perthes disease and other causes of osteonecrosis. MRI has comparable or higher sensitivity and specificity to nuclear scintigraphy and provides a range of additional information, including evaluation of articular cartilage, detection of acetabular labral tears, and visualization of metaphyseal cysts that are indicators of prognosis.

Steroid-Induced Osteonecrosis

Skeletal scintigraphy rarely shows photon-deficient areas in steroid-induced osteonecrosis. The vast majority of cases show increased radiotracer uptake. Although the pathogenesis of steroid-induced osteonecrosis is still being debated, it is a chronic process manifested by microfractures and repair. The net effect most often seen scintigraphically is increased tracer localization.

Sickle Cell Anemia

Skeletal scintigrams in patients with sickle cell anemia have characteristic features that suggest the diagnosis (Fig. 7-42). An expanded marrow space results in increased uptake of tracer in the calvarium, periarticular locations in the long bones, and even the distal extremities. The overall skeleton-to-background ratio is usually good and is accentuated by the increased appendicular uptake. In many patients, the kidneys appear somewhat larger than normal, which may be related to a defect in the ability to concentrate urine. Avid accumulation of skeletal tracer is sometimes seen in the spleen, presumably because of prior splenic infarction and calcification.

Infarctions in bone and bone marrow result in both acute and long-standing changes. If the involvement is primarily in the marrow space, the skeletal scintigram may not reveal the extent of the lesion because it does not involve the cortex where Tc-99m MDP binds. While the image may be normal acutely, the scan typically demonstrates increased uptake within a few days as healing begins (Fig. 7-43).

Bone marrow scans using Tc-99m sulfur colloid are able to show infarcts immediately, with affected areas failing to accumulate tracer and appearing cold. The marrow defects from prior bone marrow infarctions persist, unlike on MRI, which can generally distinguish acute from chronic changes. The correlation between the marrow scan and the bone scan is considered when the need to differentiate acute osteomyelitis from infarct arises. If the marrow shows a defect in the region of increased bone scan activity, it is consistent with infarct. If the marrow shows no change, any increased activity on the bone scan in an acute situation is most likely osteomyelitis.

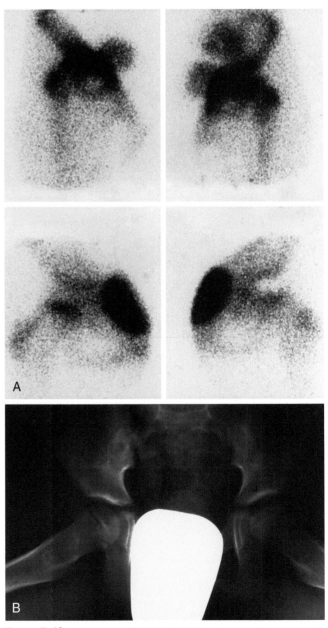

FIGURE 7-41. Legg-Calvé-Perthes disease. **A,** *(top row)* Scintigrams by standard parallel-hole collimator fail to reveal the abnormality. Pinhole images of the same patient *(bottom row)* reveal the characteristic lentiform area of decreased uptake on the left. **B,** Corresponding radiograph obtained months later reveals deformity of the left femoral epiphysis with flattening, increased density and increased distance between the epiphysis and the acetabulum.

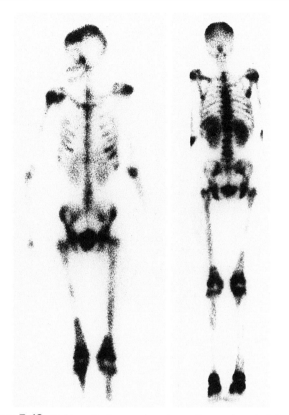

FIGURE 7-42. Sickle cell disease. Anterior and posterior whole-body views. Calvarial uptake is increased with relative thinning at the midline. Prominent skeleton to soft tissue uptake is seen. The kidneys appear large, and the spleen shows intense uptake. Uptake in the knees and ankles is greater than expected for an adult subject. The photon-deficient areas in the right femur are due to bone and bone marrow infarction.

▬ OSTEOMYELITIS

Acute hematogenous osteomyelitis typically begins by seeding of the infectious organism in the marrow space. The untreated process extends through Volkmann canals horizontally and in the haversian canal system axially. In children, *Staphylococcus aureus* is the most common organism and is probably responsible for 50% or more of cases (Fig. 7-44). The skeletal infection is commonly associated with another staphylococcal infection, often of the skin. Enteric bacteria and *Streptococcus* are also important pathogens.

Osteomyelitis in adults may occur by hematogenous spread or by direct extension in an area of cellulitis. The

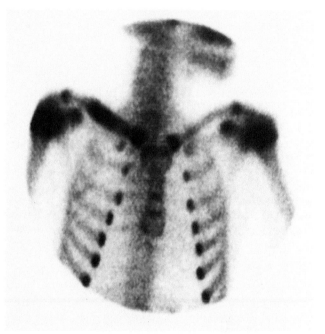

FIGURE 7-44. Osteomyelitis of the right clavicle. Anterior scintigram in a child showing that the uptake on the right is markedly greater than in the left clavicle.

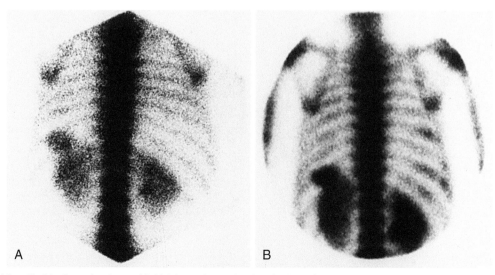

A   B

FIGURE 7-43. Sickle cell crisis. Posterior views with high intensity obtained at the time of onset of acute chest pain (**A**) and several days later (**B**) from a patient with sickle cell anemia. The initial image reveals no abnormality in the ribs. The follow-up image demonstrates increased uptake, particularly in the right ribs, associated with healing of the infarctions. Note the uptake in the spleen on both images. Typically, once the spleen is visualized scintigraphically, it remains positive.

foot is a common site of direct extension in patients with diabetes, whereas the spine is commonly involved by the hematogenous route. In adults without diabetes, the axial skeleton is more commonly involved than the appendicular skeleton. When vertebrae are involved, the organisms may be carried through the perispinous venous plexus, producing involvement at multiple levels. Infection may extend from the vertebral end plates into the disk space causing diskitis.

Numerous studies in the literature document the superior sensitivity of skeletal scintigraphy compared with conventional radiography in the diagnosis of acute hematogenous osteomyelitis. Although MRI with gadolinium enhancement is very sensitive, bone scans are still frequently used, especially in complex cases or when multiple sites must be visualized. With its increased specificity over bone scan, radiolabeled white blood cells are also important in the evaluation of infected bone.

Scintigraphic Findings

Dynamic (or three-phase) imaging is a special technique used in the differential diagnosis of cellulitis and osteomyelitis (Box 7-2). The key diagnostic criteria of osteomyelitis are shown in Box 7-11, and bone scan is invariably positive by the time symptoms develop. Typical osteomyelitis appears positive on all three phases of the study. Early or arterial hyperemia with focally, and possibly diffusely, increased radiotracer uptake on blood pool images is seen. Progressive focal accumulation then occurs in the involved bone on delayed images (Fig. 7-45). Cellulitis, on the other hand, typically demonstrates delayed or venous phase hyperemia (occurring later in the dynamic perfusion images) and increased blood pool activity but no uptake localizing to bone on delayed images. This differentiation is important, especially in patients with diabetes, in whom both processes frequently occur, because of the prolonged therapy needed for osteomyelitis.

Although the technique has been shown useful and sensitive, bone scan is not specific. The same sequence of image findings seen in osteomyelitis can be seen in neuropathic joint disease, gout, fractures (including stress fractures), and rheumatoid arthritis, among other conditions

---

Box 7-11. Three-Phase Skeletal Scintigraphy: Interpretive Criteria

Osteomyelitis: *Arterial* hyperemia, progressive focal skeletal uptake with relative soft tissue clearance; in children a focal cold area may be seen if osteomyelitis is associated with infarction.

Cellulitis: *Venous* (delayed) hyperemia, persistent soft tissue activity; no focal skeletal uptake (may have mild to moderate diffusely increased uptake).

Septic joint: Periarticular increased activity on dynamic and blood pool phases that persists on delayed images; less commonly the joint structures appear cold if pressure in the joint causes decreased flow or infarction.

(Box 7-12). Improved specificity can be achieved by comparing the three-phase bone scan to radiographs.

The use of Tc-99m hexamethylpropyleneamine oxime (HMPAO) or indium-111 radiolabeled white blood cells (WBCs) also can increase specificity and can even be used without prior bone scan. WBCs will normally localize where marrow is present, but significantly higher levels of activity above background occur with most acute bone infections. In some cases, such as the severe destruction seen in a neuropathic or Charcot joint (Fig. 7-46, *A*), non-specific increased activity is seen on both bone scan and WBC scan.

As in any situation in which marrow distribution is altered, comparison between the WBC scan and a Tc-99m sulfur colloid marrow scan may help identify abnormal accumulation resulting from infection (Fig. 7-46, *B*). Freshly made Tc-99m sulfur colloid 10 mCi (370 MBq) is injected, and images are generally acquired for 10 minutes per view. If done along with In-111 WBCs, sulfur colloid images can be done as part of a 2-day protocol. However, if Tc-99m HMPAO WBCs are used, activity from whichever scan is done first often persists at 48 hours, so a delay of 72 hours between cases is preferred.

The detection of vertebral osteomyelitis also may be a challenge. Diskitis is often diagnosed on MRI (Fig 7-47). Bone scan typically shows disk space narrowing and increased uptake around the joint from osteomyelitis of the adjacent vertebral bodies, but this is not specific (Fig. 7-48). It is even more confusing in cases in which the changes on bone scintigraphy could be due to fracture or surgery. In the spine, diagnosis with WBC scans is limited by low sensitivity, with infections frequently appearing cold or normal. It is often possible to identify sites of vertebral osteomyelitis by performing a gallium-67 scan after a bone scan. Areas with more intense uptake on Ga-67 are more specific and are consistent with osteomyelitis.

In some patients, especially children, increased pressure in the marrow space or thrombosis of blood vessels results in paradoxically decreased tracer uptake and a cold or photon-deficient lesion. A septic hip in a child also can result in decreased activity by compromising the blood supply to the femoral head, potentially resulting in avascular.

False-negative scintigraphic studies are unusual but have been reported, more commonly in infants under the age of 1 year. Other causes of false-negative examinations are imaging very early in the course of disease and failure to recognize the significance of photon-deficient areas.

Prosthesis Evaluation

Numerous attempts have been made to use skeletal scintigraphy for the evaluation of pain after total joint replacement or implantation of other metallic prostheses. The distinction between component loosening and infection is critical in guiding management.

Diffuse or more focal uptake is expected for several months after surgery. Activity persisting after a year is generally abnormal for a cemented prosthesis but may last longer when uncemented. Any area of worsening uptake on serial concerns must be evaluated. However, assessing the pattern of activity around the joint is not a reliable method

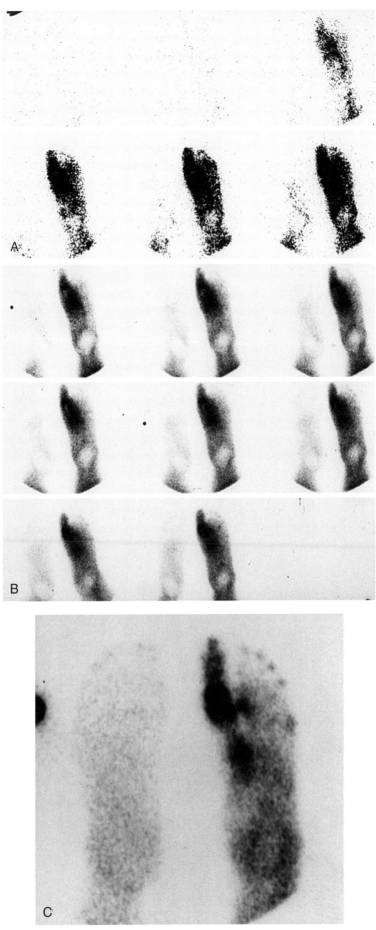

Figure 7-45. Osteomyelitis on three-phase study. **A,** Sequential dynamic images in a middle-aged man with diabetes and osteomyelitis. Note the intense arterial phase hyperemia. **B,** Blood pool images already show localization in skeletal structures. **C,** Delayed static images reveal intense focal accumulation in multiple areas of the great toe and distal first and second metatarsals.

to discriminate between aseptic loosening and infection (Fig. 7-49). The differential diagnosis between loosened prosthesis and infection is better made with tracers such as radiolabeled WBCs.

Detection of an infected prosthesis with In-111 or Tc-99m HMPAO–labeled WBCs offers the highest sensitivity and specificity. This tracer localizes in areas of infection and not in areas of remodeling or reactive bone. Use of labeled WBCs has three pitfalls. First, false-negative studies may occur in low-grade chronic osteomyelitis. Some increased sensitivity is seen with Ga-67 when a false negative is encountered because of chronic infection. Second, cellulitis can be difficult to distinguish from septic arthritis. Third, false-positive studies can result from normal radiolabeled white cell uptake in bone marrow around a prosthesis as a result of remodeling and altered marrow distribution from the surgery. WBC and sulfur colloid marrow scanning are combined to avoid this pitfall. Infection is diagnosed only in marrow-bearing areas that show a combination of increased radiolabeled WBC uptake and absence of Tc-99m sulfur colloid uptake.

▬ FLOURINE-18 SODIUM FLUORIDE POSITRON EMISSION TOMOGRAPHY

F-18 sodium fluoride (NaF) was originally approved as a bone scan agent by the U.S. Food and Drug Administration (FDA) in 1972 but was listed as a discontinued drug in 1984. Although it is possible to reapply for an Investigational New Drug (IND) based on the original approval, the agent can be produced and distributed by authorized user prescription under state pharmacy laws. With the widespread availability of dedicated PET cameras and growing concerns over Tc-99m shortages and molybdenum generator unavailability, F-18 NaF has reemerged after decades. The rapid soft tissue clearance, high target-to-background ratio, and superior of resolution of PET are particularly appealing (Fig 7-50).

Pharmacokinetics and Dosimetry

Protocols are still being refined. Patient preparation is similar to routine bone scan, with patients being well hydrated. Doses ranging from 5 to 10 mCi (185-370 MBq) have been suggested in adults, although doses as low as 3 mCi may be

Box 7-12. Lesions That Can Mimic Osteomyelitis on Three-Phase Skeletal Scintigraphy

Osteoarthritis
Gout
Fracture
Stress fracture
Osteonecrosis (healing)
Charcot's joint
Osteotomy
Complex regional pain syndrome
(reflex sympathetic dystrophy)

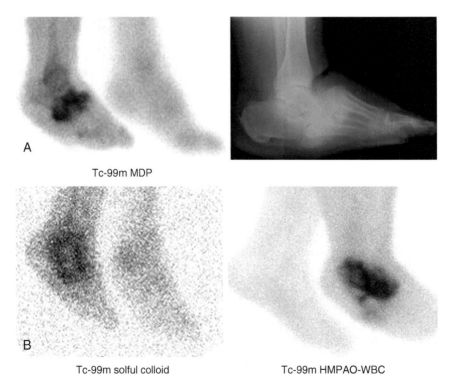

Tc-99m MDP

Tc-99m solful colloid

Tc-99m HMPAO-WBC

Figure 7-46. Charcot joint. **A,** Marked bone scan uptake corresponds to destruction on radiographs in a patient with diabetes and a plantar ulcer. **B,** Tc-99m sulfur colloid marrow images *(left)* do not completely match Tc-99m HMPAO WBC images *(right)*, particularly centrally and just inferiorly, suggesting osteomyelitis. Patchy uptake along the plantar foot was in the region of an ulcer, likely resulting from cellulitis, although separation from bone is difficult.

adequate. In children, 0.06 mCi/kg (2.22 MBq/kg) with a range of 0.5 to 5 mCi (18.5-185 MBq) may be used.

Uptake in bone occurs as an initial association with the bone and then incorporation into bone as fluorohydroxyapatite over hours to days. Although the half-life of F-18 is short at 110 minutes, it is sufficient because of the rapid clearance from soft tissues. Even a 30-minute delay may be sufficient for visualization; however, most centers image 60 minutes after injection. A delay of 90 to 120 minutes may be optimal for the extremities.

Dosimetry is reported in Table 7-7. F-18 has an effective dose of 0.089 rem/mCi (0.024 mSv/MBq) compared to an effective dose of 0.021 rem/mCi (0.0057 mSv/MBq) for

Tc-99m MDP. Therefore it would be desirable to use doses at the lower end of the suggested F-18 NaF range so that radiation dose is comparable for the two agents. In addition, because excretion into urine is sensitive to urine flow, good hydration is even more critical than with Tc-99m MDP.

Findings

Many small studies have shown F-18 NaF PET-CT to have better sensitivity and specificity than Tc-99m MDP. Higher bone uptake and improved resolution are useful for assessing osseous metastases, but interpretive difficulties can occur. Unlike with F-18 FDG PET, many benign

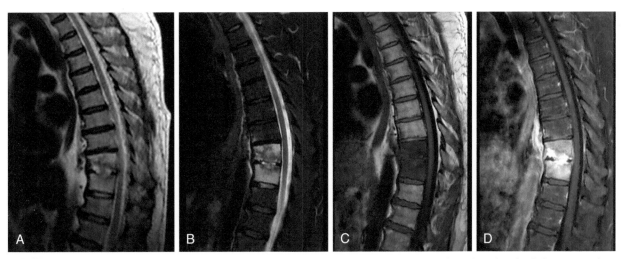

FIGURE 7-47. MRI of the spine in vertebral osteomyelitis with diskitis at T11-T12 shows marrow edema irregular enhancing inflammatory changes in the disk space, but no paraspinal mass or extension is evident on **(A)** T2, **(B)** short tau inversion recovery (STIR), **(C)** T1 precontrast, or **(D)** gadolinium-enhanced T1 images.

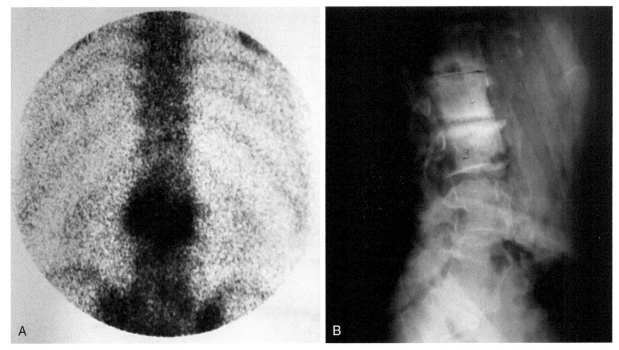

FIGURE 7-48. Osteomyelitis of the spine. **A,** Posterior spot view of an adult show intensely increased uptake in the midlumbar region, involving more than one vertebral level. **B,** Corresponding radiograph shows destructive and sclerotic changes involving the L2 vertebral body and adjacent portions of L1 and L3. The process has involved the intervertebral disks with loss of height in the disk space.

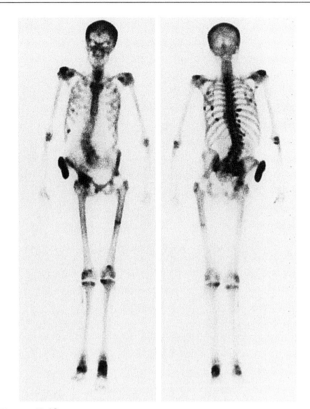

Figure 7-49. Loose hip prosthesis. Anterior and posterior images in a patient with severe scoliosis and skeletal metastases from breast carcinoma. Uptake is increased at the tip of the left prosthesis and subtly increased in the region of the trochanters, especially the greater trochanter from loosening. Uptake is intensely increased in the right femoral head because of degenerative arthritic changes.

lesions, such as arthritis, may show intense activity (Fig 7-51). This is a potentially more critical problem in cases in which small lesions that appear to be benign bone islands show increased uptake. Although this agent is an obvious alternative to Tc-99m MDP, many factors, such as the effects of therapy on uptake and length of time healing lesions remain positive, need to be examined.

BONE MINERAL MEASUREMENT

Multiple methods have been developed for quantitative measurement of bone mineral mass. These procedures have progressed from the use of radioactive sources such as gadolinium-153 to more rapid x-ray techniques, including

TABLE 7-7 Radiation Dosimetry of Florine-18 Sodium Fluoride*

	Adult	Child (5 yr old)
Administered Activity	5-10 mCi (185-370 MBq)	0.06 mCi/kg (185-370 MBq/kg)
Organ Receive Highest Dose	Bladder: 0.81 rad/mCi (0.22 mGy/MBq)	2.3 rad/mCi (0.61 mGy/MBq)
Effective Dose	0.089 rem/mCi (0.024 mSv/MBq)	0.32 rem/mCi (0.086 mSv/MBq)

Data from Radiation dose to patients from radiopharmaceuticals (addendum 3 to ICRP publication 53): ICRP publication 106. *Ann ICRP.* 2008;38:1-197.
*Assumes voiding interval 3.5 hr.

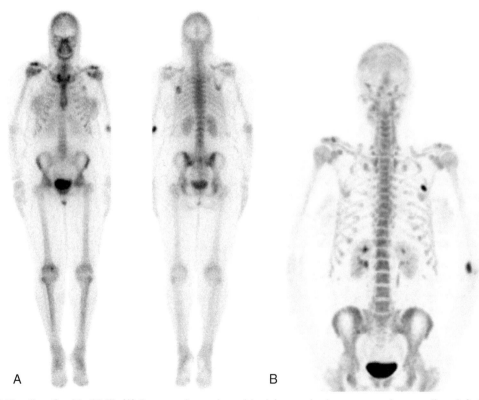

A   B

Figure 7-50. F-18 sodium fluoride (NaF). **(A)** Bone scan in a patient with triple-negative breast cancer shows a solitary left rib lesion clearly seen on F-18 NaF PET. **B,** Maximal intensity projection images (MIP) suspicious for metastasis with no fracture on CT. Focal activity in the right antecubital fossa was not related to the injection site. This area localized to the elbow from arthritis, demonstrating the lack of specificity often seen with NaF.

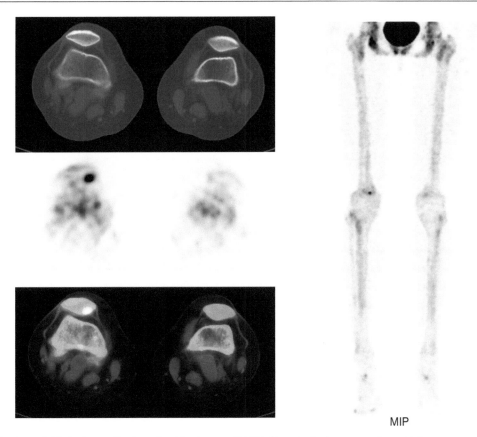

MIP

FIGURE 7-51. Benign arthritis in the patella shows focal but intense F-18 NaF uptake in the same patient with breast cancer shown in Figure 7-50. In addition to being an unusual location for tumor involvement, the activity remained unchanged on serial examinations and is consistent with arthritis, which can be very avid, unlike F-18 FDG PET.

CT. Advances also include moving from single- to dual-energy techniques.

Dual-energy techniques are especially important for areas such as the spine and hips, where soft tissues can have considerable impact. By comparing a lower energy beam or photon that is attenuated by bone and soft tissue with a higher energy source that is affected only by bone (or metal), it is possible to calculate the differential absorption, allowing more accurate assessment of bone density without impact from the surrounding soft tissues. Dual energy x-ray absorptiometry (DXA) was used as the basis for the World Health Organization (WHO) criteria for categorizing osteopenia and osteoporosis.

Quantitative CT (QCT) can measure cortical and trabecular bone separately. Dual-energy QCT has the additional advantage over single-energy QCT of allowing correction for fat in the marrow space. Both techniques are quite flexible with respect to body part examined. QCT is an important research tool but is too expensive for population screening.

Several ultrasound devices are now approved by the FDA for measurement of bone mass. Sound is transmitted faster in dense bone than in osteopenic bone, and the devices are calibrated against other methods to correlate with bone mass. Application of the technique is limited to peripheral structures such as the calcaneus. The low cost, small size, and ease of use of ultrasound devices make them attractive for population screening, although they may not be as accurate. These devices remain under investigation.

Fracture risk markedly increases when bone mineral density is less than 1 g/cm^2. Bone mineral measurements establish baseline diagnostic measurements in the evaluation of patients with suspected osteopenia and osteoporosis and can follow the course of therapy. Primary osteoporosis has been divided into two subtypes. Type I, or postmenopausal, osteoporosis is related to decreased estrogen secretion after menopause. Type II or senile osteoporosis is presumably due to age-related impaired bone metabolism. Risk factors for osteoporosis include female sex, Caucasian or Asian race, smoking, chronic alcohol intake, and a positive family history. Early menopause, long-term treatment with corticosteroids, and some nutritional disorders, including malabsorption, are also risk factors. Obesity is protective.

The WHO classification system for bone mass, based on DXA measurements of the spine and femoral neck, compares an individual's measurements with the mean and standard deviation (SD) for a control population. Results are reported as a T-score or a Z-score. A Z-score reflects comparison with age-matched controls. The T-score, which is based on comparison with a young control population representing comparison with peak bone mass, is used to determine if osteoporosis is present. Normal T-scores include all values greater than 0 down to T-scores above –1.0, because this is within 1 SD of the young control population. Osteopenia is taken as 1 to 2.5 SD below the control mean (or a T-score between –1.0 and –2.5). Osteoporosis is defined as 2.5 SD or more below the control mean (or a T-score <–2.5).

The use of bone mineral density has been accelerated by the availability of new drugs such as alendronate, a bisphosphonate that localizes in bone and promotes mineralization. Estrogen is also widely used in postmenopausal women but is not uniformly well tolerated, and concerns remain about its effects on other diseases such as breast cancer.

▰ SUGGESTED READING

Connolly LP, Strauss J, Connolly SA. Role of skeletal scintigraphy in evaluating sports injuries in adolescents and young adults. *Nucl Med Ann.* 2003:171-209.

Fournier RS, Holder LE. Reflex sympathetic dystrophy: diagnostic controversies. *Semin Nucl Med.* 1998;28(1):116-123.

Freeman LM, Blaufox MD. Metabolic bone disease. *Semin Nucl Med.* 1997;27:195-305.

Gemmel F, Van den Wyngaert H, Love C, et al. Prosthetic joint infections: radionuclide state of the art imaging. *Eur J Nucl Med Mol Imaging.* 2012;39(5):892-909.

Iagaru A, Mittra E, Yaghoubi SS, et al. Novel strategy for cocktail ^{18}F-fluoride and ^{18}F-FDG PET/CT scan for the evaluation of malignancy: results of the pilot-phase study. *J Nucl Med.* 2009;50(4):501-505.

Palestro CJ, Love C, Tronco GG, Tomas MB, Rini JN. Combined labeled leukocyte and technetium-99m sulfur colloid bone marrow imaging for diagnosing musculoskeletal infection. *Radiographics.* 2006;26(3):859-870.

Rajiah P, Ilaslan H, Sundaram M. Imaging of primary malignant bone tumors (nonhematological). *Radiol Clin North Am.* 2011;49(6):1135-1161.

Segall G, Delbeke D, Stabin MG, et al. SNM practice guideline for sodium ^{18}F-fluoride PET/CT bone scans 1.0. *J Nucl Med.* 2010;51(11):1813-1820.

Stacey GS, Kapur A. Mimics of bone and soft tissue neoplasms. *Radiol Clin North Am.* 2011;49(6):1261-1286.

Stauss J, Hahn K, Mann M, De Palma D. Guidelines for paediatric bone scanning with Tc-99m-labelled radiopharmaceuticals and F-18 fluoride. *Eur J Nucl Med Mol Imaging.* 2010;37(8):1621-1628.

Treves ST. *Pediatric Nuclear Medicine.* 3rd ed. New York: Springer; 2007.

Zuckier LS, Freeman LM. Nonosseous, nonurologic uptake on bone scintigraphy: atlas and analysis. *Semin Nucl Med.* 2010;40(4):242-256.

CHAPTER 8

Hepatobiliary System

Hepatic, biliary, and splenic scintigraphy have had an important role in radionuclide imaging since the 1960s. Many of the radiopharmaceuticals, methodologies, and indications have changed; however, modern scintigraphy provides unique physiological and diagnostic information not available from anatomical imaging. The various radiopharmaceuticals used today have functional mechanisms of uptake, distribution, and localization that take advantage of the complex anatomy and physiology of the liver and spleen (Table 8-1 and Fig. 8-1).

CHOLESCINTIGRAPHY

Cholescintigraphy is used routinely for the diagnosis of various acute and chronic hepatobiliary diseases, including acute cholecystitis, biliary obstruction, bile leak, and acalculous chronic gallbladder disease (Box 8-1).

Radiopharmaceuticals

Technetium-99m–labeled hepatobiliary radiopharmaceuticals became available in the early 1980s; because of their superior image and diagnostic quality they replaced iodine-123 rose bengal.

Three hepatobiliary radiopharmaceuticals have been approved by the U.S. Food and Drug Administration (FDA) for clinical use in the United States (Fig. 8-2). The first was Tc-99m dimethyl iminodiacetic acid (IDA), which was referred to as hepatic IDA (HIDA). Although it is no longer used, HIDA has become a generic term for all Tc-99m IDA radiopharmaceuticals. The two agents in clinical use today in the United States are shown in Table 8-2.

Chemistry

Tc-99m serves as a bridging atom between two IDA ligand molecules (Fig. 8-2). Both IDA molecules bind to an acetanilide analog of lidocaine. The latter determines the radiopharmaceutical's biological and pharmacokinetic properties.

Minor structural changes in the phenyl ring (N substitutions) result in significant alterations in the pharmacokinetics of IDA radiopharmaceuticals (Table 8-3). Many Tc-99m HIDA analogs with different aromatic ring chemical substitutions have been investigated, with generic names of BIDA, DIDA, EIDA, PIPIDA, and so forth; however, most were found to have less uptake and slower clearance than the approved commercially available agents.

Kit Preparation

Tc-99m HIDA radiopharmaceuticals are commercially available as kits containing the non-labeled HIDA analog and stannous chloride in lyophilized form. With the addition of Tc-99m pertechnetate to the vial, a Tc-99m–HIDA complex is formed. It is stable for at least 6 hours.

Radiopharmaceutical Physiology and Pharmacokinetics

HIDA radiopharmaceuticals are organic anions excreted by the liver in a manner similar to that of bilirubin. After intravenous injection, they are tightly bound to protein in the blood, minimizing renal clearance. Extraction occurs

TABLE 8-1 Liver and Spleen Radiopharmaceuticals, Mechanisms, and Clinical Indications

Radiopharmaceutical	Mechanism of uptake	Indication
Tc-99m mebrofenin, disofenin	Hepatocyte uptake	Cholescintigraphy
Tc-99m red blood cells	Blood pool distribution	Liver hemangioma, spleen
Tc-99m sulfur colloid	Kupffer cell uptake	Focal nodular hyperplasia
Tc-99m MAA	Blood flow, capillary occlusion	Hepatic arterial perfusion
Xe-133	Lipid soluble	Focal fatty tumor uptake
Gallium-67 citrate	Iron binding	Tumor/abscess imaging
F-18 FDG	Glucose metabolism	Tumor imaging
Y-90 microspheres	Blood flow, capillary occlusion	Liver tumor radiotherapy

FDG, Fluorodeoxyglucose; *MAA,* macroaggregated albumin.

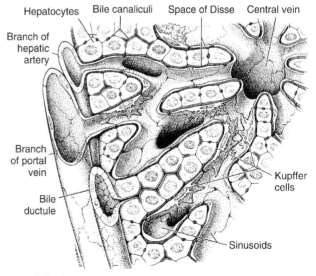

FIGURE 8-1. Anatomy of a liver lobule. Plates of hepatocytes and Kupffer cells are distributed radially around the central vein. Branches of the portal vein and hepatic artery located at the periphery of the lobule deliver blood to the sinusoids. Blood leaves through the central vein (proximal branch of hepatic veins). Peripherally located bile ducts drain bile canaliculi that course between hepatocytes.

via a high-capacity, carrier-mediated, anionic clearance mechanism. HIDA is transported into bile canaliculi by an active membrane transport system. Unlike bilirubin, the Tc-99m IDA compounds are excreted in their original radiochemical form without conjugation or metabolism. Because Tc-99m HIDA travels the same pathway as bilirubin, it is subject to competitive inhibition by high serum bilirubin levels.

Hepatic dysfunction causes altered HIDA pharmacokinetics—that is, delayed uptake, secretion, and clearance. The kidneys serve as the alternative route of excretion, clearing only a small percentage of the dose

(Table 8-3). With hepatic dysfunction, urinary excretion increases.

After extraction by hepatocytes, HIDA is excreted into the biliary canaliculi and follows biliary flow into the larger ducts (Fig. 8-3). Approximately two thirds enters the gallbladder via the cystic duct, and the remainder travels

Box 8-1. Cholescintigraphy: Clinical Indications

Acute cholecystitis
Acute acalculous cholecystitis
Biliary obstruction
Biliary atresia
Sphincter of Oddi dysfunction
Biliary leak
Chronic acalculous gallbladder disease
Biliary diversion assessment
Biliary stent function
Enterogastric bile reflux
Focal nodular hyperplasia
Hepatocellular carcinoma

TABLE 8-2 Technetium-99m Hepatobiliary Agent Names

Chemical	FDA	Commercial
Tc-99m diisopropyl IDA (DISIDA)	Disofenin	Hepatolite
Tc-99m bromotriethyl IDA	Mebrofenin	Choletec

FDA, U.S. Food and Drug Administration.

TABLE 8-3 Normal Pharmacokinetics of Technetium-99m Hepatobiliary Iminodiacetic Acid Radiopharmaceuticals

Agent	Hepatic uptake (%)	Clearance half-time (min)	2-hr renal excretion (%)
Tc-99m disofenin (DISIDA)	88	19	<9
Tc-99m mebrofenin (BrIDA)	98	17	<1

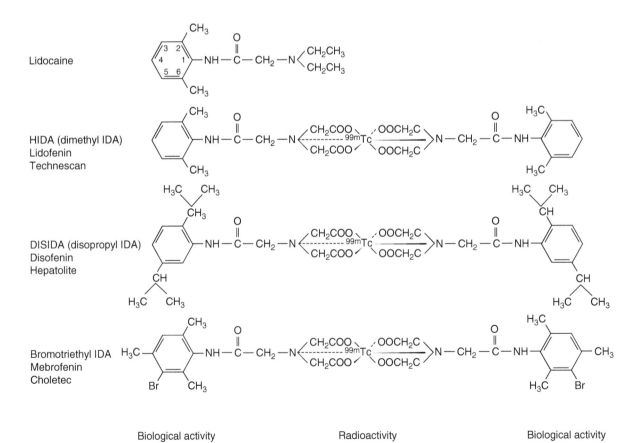

FIGURE 8-2. Chemical structure of Tc-99m HIDA radiopharmaceuticals, analogs of lidocaine *(top)*. Tc-99m is located centrally, bridging two ligand molecules. Iminodiacetate (NCH₂COO) attaches to Tc-99m and the acetanilide analog (IDA) of lidocaine. The lidocaine analog carries the biological activity. Substitutions on aromatic rings differentiate the various Tc-99m IDAs and determine their pharmacokinetics. Lidofenin was the first Tc-99m IDA approved for clinical use, but is no longer available. Disofenin and mebrofenin are in clinical use.

through the common hepatic and common bile duct via the sphincter of Oddi into the second portion of the duodenum. The distribution is determined by the patency of the biliary ducts, sphincter of Oddi tone, and intraluminal pressures.

Because of their high extraction efficiency, today's HIDA radiopharmaceuticals provide diagnostic images in patients with bilirubin levels as high as 20 to 30 mg/dL (Table 8-3). Mebrofenin has somewhat greater hepatic extraction and resistance to displacement by bilirubin than disofenin and thus is preferable in patients with poor liver function.

Dosimetry

The large intestine receives the highest radiation dose, approximately 2 rads (cGy), followed by the gallbladder with 0.6 rads (cGy). The total effective dose is 0.32 rem (cGy) (Table 8-4).

Patient Preparation

Patients should not be permitted to eat for 3 to 4 hours before the study. Ingested food stimulates endogenous release of cholecystokinin (CCK) from the proximal small bowel, causing gallbladder contraction that may prevent radiotracer entry.

If a patient has been fasting for more than 24 hours, the gallbladder will have had no stimulus to contract and will

contain viscous bile, which can prevent radiotracer entry. In this situation, the patient should be administered sincalide (Kinevac; CCK) before the study to empty the gallbladder. Tc-99m HIDA should be administered at least 30 minutes after cessation of the sincalide infusion to allow time for gallbladder relaxation.

All opiate drugs should be withheld at least 3 half-lives or approximately 6 hours before starting the study because they can contract the sphincter of Oddi, producing a functional partial biliary obstruction, which is indistinguishable from a true obstruction.

Pertinent Clinical History Before Initiating the Study

Questions should include: What is the clinical question being asked by the referring physician? Are the symptoms acute or chronic? Has sonography or other imaging been performed? What were the results? Has the patient had biliary surgery? If the patient had a biliary diversion procedure, what is the anatomy? Are there intraabdominal tubes or drains? If so, where are they placed and which tubing drains each? Should the drains be open or clamped during the study to answer the clinical diagnostic question? Did the patient's most recent meal contain fat that would cause gallbladder contraction?

Methodology

A standard protocol for cholescintigraphy is described in Box 8-2. Acquisition of 1-minute frames for 60 minutes is standard. An initial 60-second flow study may be acquired (1-3 seconds/frame). Right lateral and left anterior oblique

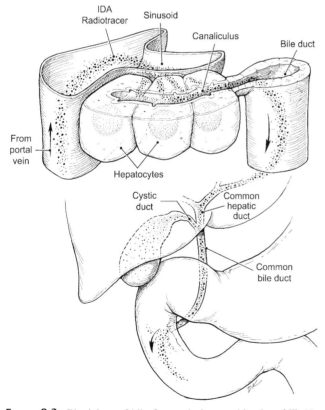

FIGURE 8-3. Physiology of bile flow and pharmacokinetics of Tc-99m IDA. Bilirubin is transported in the blood bound to albumin, distributes via the sinusoids, dissociates from albumin in the space of Disse, and then is extracted by the hepatocyte, secreted into the bile canaliculi, and cleared through the biliary tract into the bowel. Hepatic uptake and clearance of Tc-99m IDA are similar to that of bilirubin except that it is not conjugated or metabolized.

TABLE 8-4 Dosimetry: Technetium-99m Mebrofenin, Tehnetium-99m Red Blood Cells, Technetium-99m Sulfur Colloid

Dose	Tc-99m mebrofenin rem/5 mCi (cGy/185 MBq)	Tc-99m RBC rem/25 mCi (cGy/925 MBq)	Tc-99m sulfur colloid rem/5 mCi (cGy/185 MBq)
TARGET ORGAN			
Heart wall		1.35	
Blood		0.86	
Liver	0.19	0.65	1.70
Gallbladder	0.60		
Spleen		1.03	1.10
Large intestine	1.90		
Bone marrow			0.14
Kidneys		0.63	
Urinary bladder	0.46	1.28	
Ovaries	0.41	0.43	0.03
Testes	0.03		0.01
Total body	0.08	0.38	0.10
Effective dose	0.32	0.65	0.17

views are acquired at 60 minutes to confirm or exclude gallbladder filling, which can be uncertain because of overlap of biliary ducts and duodenum. Delayed imaging, morphine sulfate, and CCK are optional and will be discussed later.

Normal Cholescintigraphy

Blood Flow
The spleen and kidneys are seen during the early arterial phase. Because of the liver's predominantly venous blood

---

Box 8-2. Cholescintigraphy: Protocol Summary

PATIENT PREPARATION

Patient should have nothing by mouth (NPO) for 4 hours before study.

If fasting longer than 24 hours, infuse sincalide 0.02 μg/kg over 60 minutes. Wait 30 minutes after sincalide infusion complete to infuse the radiopharmaceutical.

RADIOPHARMACEUTICAL

Tc-99m (mebrofenin, disofenin) 5 mCi, as intravenous injection

Adults: bilirubin <2 mg/dL-5.0 mCi (185 MBq)

2-10 mg/dL-7.5 mCi (278 MBq)

>10 mg/dL-10 mCi (370 MBq)

Children: 200 μCi/kg or 7.4 MBq/kg (minimum dose 1 mCi or 37 MBq)

INSTRUMENTATION

Camera: large-field-of-view gamma camera

Collimator: Low energy parallel hole

Window: 15%-20% over 140-keV photopeak

PATIENT POSITIONING

Supine; upper abdomen in field of view.

COMPUTER SETUP

1-second frames × 60, and then 1-minute frames × 59

IMAGING PROTOCOL

1. Inject Tc-99m HIDA intravenously and start computer.
2. At 60 minutes, acquire right lateral and left anterior oblique images.
3. If the gallbladder has not filled and acute cholecystitis is suspected, either obtain delayed images up to 3 to 4 hours or inject morphine sulfate.
   A. If liver activity has washed out, Tc-99m HIDA reinject (2 mCi) before morphine infusion.
   B. Morphine infusion: inject intravenously 0.04 mg/kg over 1 minute (if good biliary duct clearance and biliary-to-bowel transit is seen). Acquire 1-minute frames for an additional 30 minutes.
4. Perform delayed imaging at 2 and 4 hours:
   A. If morphine sulfate is not administered and gallbladder has not filled.
   B. For other indications (hepatic insufficiency, partial common duct obstruction, suspected biliary leak).

---

flow (75% portal vein, 25% hepatic artery), the liver is normally seen during the venous phase (Fig. 8-4, *A*). Early hepatic flow may be seen with arterialization of the liver's blood supply—for example, in cirrhosis or generalized tumor involvement.

Increased blood flow to the gallbladder fossa may be seen with severe acute cholecystitis or an intrahepatic abscess or malignant mass.

Liver Morphology and Hepatic Function
During the early hepatic phase, liver size can be approximated and intrahepatic lesions seen. Most masses will have decreased uptake, with the exception of focal nodular hyperplasia. Liver function can be judged by noting how rapidly the cardiac blood pool clears. With normal hepatic function, HIDA clears within 5 to 10 minutes (Fig. 8-4, *B*). Delayed clearance suggests hepatic dysfunction (Fig. 8-5).

Gallbladder Filling
The gallbladder normally starts to fill by 10 minutes and is clearly seen by 30 to 40 minutes. Visualization later than 60 minutes is considered delayed (Fig. 8-6). Right lateral and left anterior oblique views can help confirm or exclude gallbladder filling (Fig. 8-7). In the right lateral projection, the gallbladder is seen anterior and to the viewer's right. In the left anterior oblique view, the gallbladder, an anterior structure, moves toward the patient's right; the common duct and duodenum, more posterior structures, move to the patient's left. Upright imaging and ingestion of water can be used to clear duodenal activity. Size and shape of the gallbladder are quite variable.

Biliary Clearance
The smaller peripheral biliary ducts are not usually visualized unless enlarged. Normal left and right hepatic bile ducts, common hepatic duct, and common bile duct are typically seen (Fig. 8-4). The left hepatic ducts may appear more prominent than the right because of the anterior position of the left lobe and close proximity to the detector.

Prominence of biliary ducts suggests dilation, although duct size is not accurately assessed with cholescintigraphy. The strength of scintigraphy is to confirm or exclude functional patency. The common bile duct is normally seen by 20 minutes, with substantial clearance into the small bowel by 60 minutes and typically greater than 50% of peak activity. Biliary duct-to-bowel transit usually occurs by 60 minutes, but may be delayed and must be differentiated from obstruction.

Pharmacological Interventions

Morphine Sulfate
Morphine, an opiate drug, is commonly used to aid in the diagnosis of acute cholecystitis. When morphine is given intravenously as a low dose and slow push (0.04 mg/kg), the sphincter of Oddi constricts and intrabiliary pressure increases. Unless the cystic duct is obstructed, good gallbladder visualization occurs by 30 minutes after injection (Fig. 8-8).

Cholecystokinin

CCK is a polypeptide hormone released by mucosal cells of the proximal small bowel in response to fat and protein. The terminal octapeptide is the physiologically active portion of the hormone. Interaction of CCK with receptors in the gallbladder wall and sphincter of Oddi cause gallbladder contraction and sphincter relaxation. The bile stored in the gallbladder is discharged into the small intestines. Bile acids assist in intestinal fat absorption.

Imaging Gallbladder Contraction

Fatty meals and various formulations of CCK have been used to image gallbladder contraction since the days of oral cholecystography. Fatty meals have limitations. An underlying assumption is that gastric emptying is normal. Delayed gastric emptying results in delayed endogenous stimulation of CCK and subsequent delayed and reduced gallbladder contraction during the standard imaging time. Normal values depend on the size and type of fatty meal. Only limited data are available on normal values for specific meals.

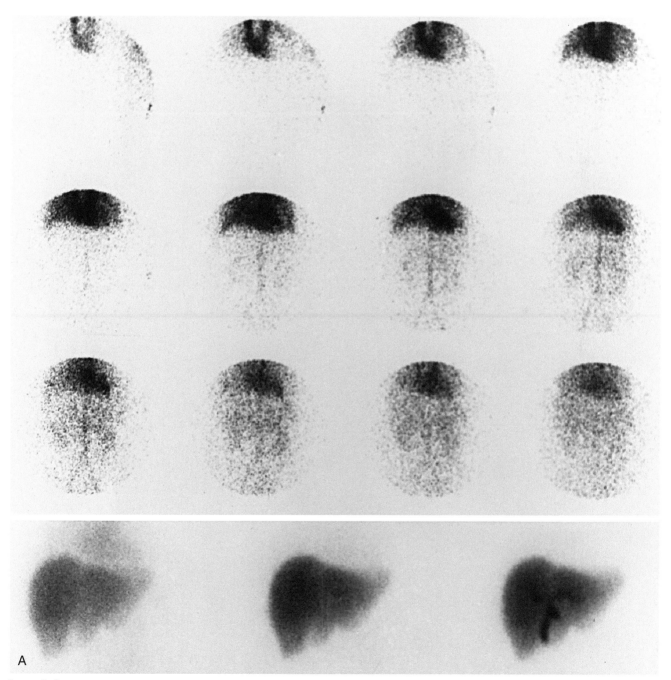

FIGURE 8-4. Normal technetium-99m HIDA studies. **A,** *Top three rows,* Two-second blood flow images. Blood flow to the liver is delayed compared with that of the spleen and kidneys because of the liver's predominantly portal venous blood flow. *Bottom,* Heart blood pool seen on immediate image clears over next two frames at 5 and 10 minutes, consistent with good hepatic function.

Continued

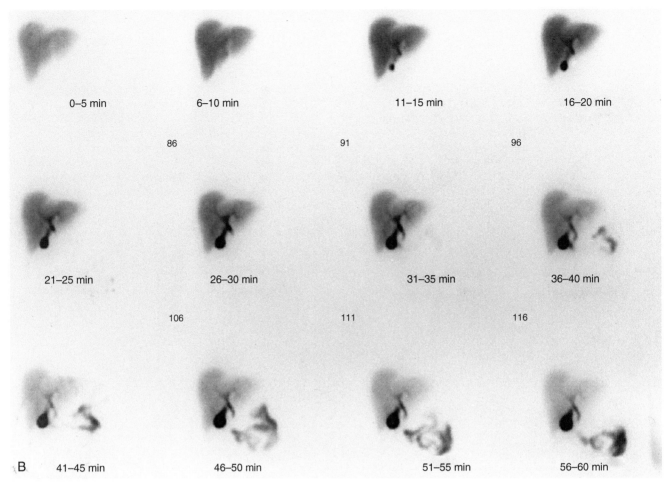

FIGURE 8-4, cont'd. B, Five-minute summed images for 60 minutes in a different patient. Right, left, and common hepatic ducts are seen by 15 to 20 minutes and the common bile duct by 30 minutes. Biliary-to-bowel clearance is noted at 36 minutes. The gallbladder is visualized early.

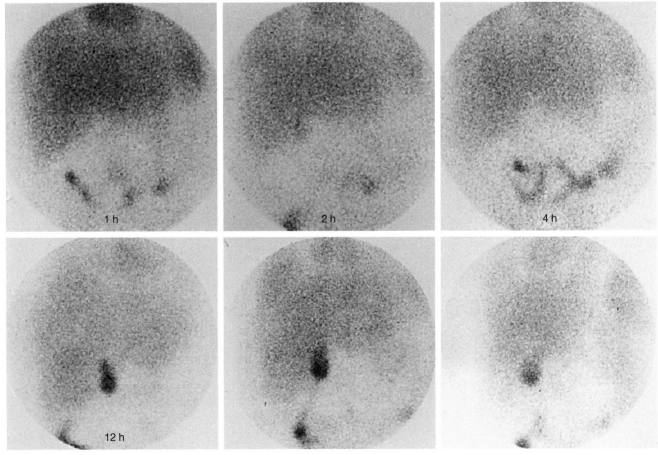

FIGURE 8-5. Severe hepatic dysfunction. Slow blood pool clearance and poor liver-to-background ratio. Gallbladder is not visualized until 12 hours. Last two images are right and left anterior oblique views respectively.

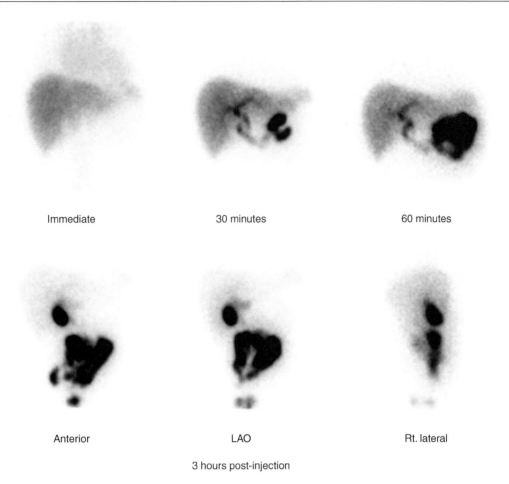

Immediate   30 minutes   60 minutes

Anterior   LAO   Rt. lateral

3 hours post-injection

FIGURE 8-6. Delayed gallbladder visualization. *Above:* Immediate, 30- and 60-minute images show no gallbladder visualization. Delayed images obtained at 3 hours shows gallbladder filling in three views, anterior, left anterior oblique, and right lateral. The right lateral shows the gallbladder anteriorly (to the right) and the left anterior oblique shows the gallbladder lateral to the small bowel (moved to the left).

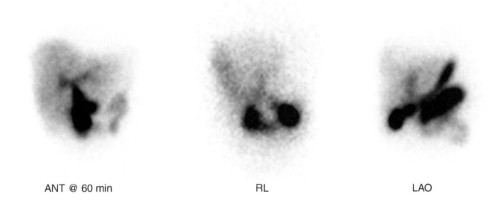

ANT @ 60 min   RL   LAO

FIGURE 8-7. Overlying gallbladder, common duct, and duodenal activity at 60 minutes. Right lateral *(RL)* and left anterior oblique *(LAO)* views confirm gallbladder filling. *ANT,* Anterior.

Sincalide is the only commercial form of CCK available in the United States. It is an analog of the terminal octapeptide of CCK. Clinical indications are listed in Box 8-3. It is used to empty the gallbladder before cholescintigraphy in patients who have fasted for more than 24 hours and after the gallbladder has been visualized to quantify a gallbladder ejection fraction (GBEF) in those suspected of acalculous gallbladder disease.

When sincalide is infused before cholescintigraphy, Tc-99m HIDA should not be injected until 30 minutes

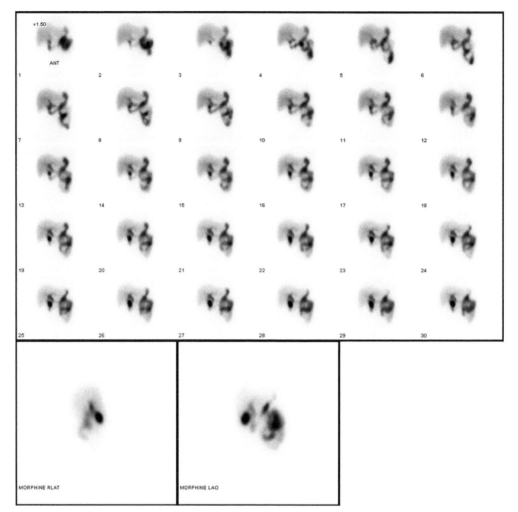

FIGURE 8-8. Morphine-augmented cholescintigraphy. Gallbladder was not seen during the initial 60-minute study (not shown). Morphine is administered intravenously *(frame 1)*. Over 30 minutes, the gallbladder visualizes, confirmed by right lateral *(RL)* and left anterior oblique *(LAO)* views, excluding acute cholecystitis. *ANT,* Anterior.

Box 8-3. Clinical Indications for Sincalide Infusion

BEFORE HIDA EXAMINATION
Empty gallbladder in patient fasting longer than 24 hours.
Diagnose sphincter of Oddi dysfunction.

AFTER HIDA EXAMINATION
Differentiate common duct obstruction from functional causes.
Exclude acute acalculous cholecystitis if gallbladder fills.
Diagnose chronic acalculous gallbladder disease.

---

after cessation of infusion, to allow time for gallbladder relaxation. HIDA pharmacokinetics may be altered by pretreatment with sincalide, manifested by delayed biliary-to-bowel transit. Because of its short half-life (3 minutes) in serum, CCK can be infused before the HIDA study and after it. The infusion method should be the same for all indications.

Common Clinical Applications

Acute Cholecystitis
The most frequent indication for Tc-99m HIDA cholescintigraphy is to confirm or exclude clinically suspected acute cholecystitis (Box 8-1).

Pathophysiology
Obstruction of the cystic duct by a stone is the cause of acute cholecystitis in more than 95% of patients. Following obstruction, a series of sequential histopathological inflammatory changes ensues, beginning with venous and lymphatic obstruction, and then edema of the gallbladder mucosa, followed by white blood cell infiltration, hemorrhage, ulceration, necrosis, and, if untreated, gangrene and perforation (Box 8-4).

Clinical Presentation
Acute cholecystitis presents with colicky right upper quadrant abdominal pain, nausea, and vomiting. Physical examination reveals right upper quadrant tenderness. Laboratory studies show leukocytosis. Liver function tests are usually normal. Even for patients with classic symptoms and

findings, a confirmatory imaging study is required for the diagnosis before surgery.

Ultrasonography

Most patients with acute cholecystitis have gallstones, which can usually be seen on sonography; however, the presence of stones is not specific for acute cholecystitis. Asymptomatic gallstones are common and often unrelated to the cause of the presenting abdominal pain.

Many of the sonographic findings seen with acute cholecystitis are not specific. Thickening of the gallbladder wall and pericholecystic fluid occur with other acute and chronic diseases. A more specific indication of acute inflammation is intramural lucency. The sonographic Murphy sign (localized tenderness in the region of the gallbladder) in experienced hands is reported to have high accuracy. However, the finding is operator-dependent and not always reliable. The combination of gallstones, intramural lucency, and sonographic Murphy sign makes the diagnosis of acute cholecystitis likely. However, most patients with acute cholecystitis do not have all of these findings and the diagnosis is less certain.

Cholescintigraphy and ultrasonography provide complementary functional and anatomical information. Ultrasonography may reveal other factors that may be causing the patient's symptoms—for example, common duct dilation of biliary obstruction, pancreatic or liver tumors, renal stones, pulmonary consolidation, or pleural effusion.

Cholescintigraphy

Cholescintigraphy demonstrates the underlying pathophysiology of acute cholecystitis—nonfilling of the gallbladder consistent with cystic duct obstruction. Nonfilling of the gallbladder by 60 minutes after Tc-99m HIDA injection is abnormal; however, it is not diagnostic of acute cholecystitis. Nonfilling at 3 to 4 hours is diagnostic. The most common reason for delayed gallbladder filling (>60 minutes) is chronic cholecystitis (Fig. 8-6).

The accuracy of cholescintigraphy for the diagnosis of acute cholecystitis using the delayed imaging method has been extensively investigated (Table 8-5). Its sensitivity (nonfilling of the gallbladder in those with the disease) is greater than 95% to 98% and specificity (filling of the gallbladder in those who do not have the disease) is greater than 90%. Studies directly comparing cholescintigraphy with ultrasonography have found cholescintigraphy clearly superior for the diagnosis of acute cholecystitis (Table 8-5).

In spite of its high specificity, false positive cholescintigraphic studies occur. However, these can be minimized by anticipating situations in which they might occur (Box

TABLE 8-5 Accuracy for Diagnosis of Acute Cholecystitis: Cholescintigraphy vs. Ultrasonography

Study author and date	Patients	Sensitivity/specificity (%)	
		Cholescintigraphy	Ultrasonography
Stadalnik, 1978	120	100/100	70/93
Weissmann, 1979	90	98/100	
Freitas, 1980	186	97/87	
Suarez, 1980	62	98/100	
Szalabick, 1980	271	100/98	
Weissmann, 1981	296	95/99	
Zeman, 1981	200	98/82	67/82
Worthen, 1981	113	95/100	67/100
Mauro, 1982	95	100/94	
Rails, 1982	59	86/84	86/90
Freitas 1982	195	98/90	60/81
Samuels, 1983	194	97/93	97/64
Overall	**1988**	**97/94**	**77/83**

8-5) and using state-of-the-art methodology. Ensuring that patients have fasted 3 to 4 hours before the study is mandatory. Those fasting longer than 24 hours or receiving hyperalimentation should be administered CCK before the study to contract the gallbladder, which likely is full of viscous bile. Patients with hepatic dysfunction have delayed pharmacokinetics—that is, delayed uptake and clearance of the radiotracer and unpredictable gallbladder filling. Delayed imaging up to 24 hours may be necessary to confirm or exclude gallbladder filling (Fig. 8-5).

Patients with chronic cholecystitis may have false positive findings in a study for acute cholecystitis, because they may have a fibrotic obstructed duct or more likely a functional obstruction resulting from a gallbladder filled with viscous bile. In the latter patients, CCK may not empty the gallbladder because it is hypofunctional. Very ill hospitalized patients with a concurrent serious illness may have false positive scintigraphy results for acute cholecystitis. The reason for this is unclear.

False negative study results (gallbladder filling in a patient with acute cholecystitis) are rare. One cause is the cystic duct sign—that is, dilation proximal to the cystic duct obstruction that may be misinterpreted as a gallbladder (Fig. 8-9).

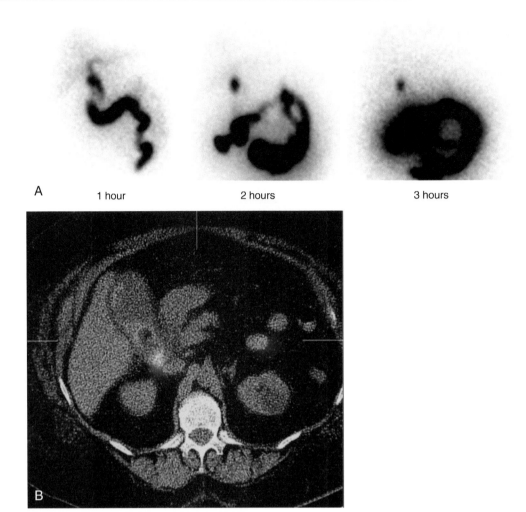

FIGURE 8-9. Cystic duct sign on planar and SPECT/CT. **A,** Images at 1, 2, and 3 hours show focal accumulation of activity medial to the usual position of the gallbladder, which remains mostly unchanged over this time. **B,** SPECT/CT fused selected transverse image (10-minute acquisition time) shows that the focal activity is in the cystic duct, obstructed by a hypodense stone immediately proximal to it.

Morphine Augmentation. An imaging study lasting 3 to 4 hours is not ideal for an acutely ill patient who requires prompt diagnosis and surgery. Morphine is often used an as alternative to the delayed imaging method. Morphine increases intraluminal biliary pressure by constricting the sphincter of Oddi, thus causing preferential bile flow to and through the cystic duct, if patent. Its accuracy is similar to that of the delayed imaging method (Table 8-6).

If the gallbladder does not fill by 60 minutes, morphine 0.04 mg/kg is infused. With cystic duct patency, the gallbladder begins to fill within 5 to 10 minutes after infusion and is complete by 20 to 30 minutes. If no gallbladder filling is seen by 30 minutes, acute cholecystitis is confirmed. Thus the entire Tc-99m IDA study requires only 90 minutes (Fig. 8-8).

Morphine should not be administered if scintigraphic findings at 60 minutes are suggestive of biliary obstruction—for example, delayed clearance from the common duct (<50%) or delayed transit into the small bowel. Morphine produces a functional partial common duct obstruction that cannot be differentiated by scintigraphy from a pathological obstruction caused by stone or stricture. If

TABLE 8-6 Accuracy of Morphine-Augmented Cholescintigraphy

Study author and date	Patients	Sensitivity (%)	Specificity (%)
Choy, 1984	59	96	100
Keslar, 1987	31	100	83
Vasquez, 1987	40	100	85
Fig, 1990	51	94	69*
Flancbaum, 1994	75	99	91
Fink-Bennett, 1991	51	95	99
Kistler, 1991	32	93	78*
Overall	**339**	**96**	**86**

*High percentage of patients with concurrent illness and chronic cholecystitis.

normal biliary-to-bowel clearance is not seen, 3- to 4-hour delayed images should be obtained.

Rim Sign. The *rim sign*, increased hepatic uptake adjacent to the gallbladder fossa, is an ancillary diagnostic scintigraphic finding of acute cholecystitis. With cholescintigraphy,

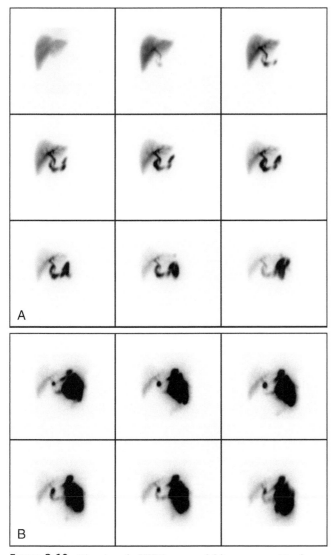

TABLE 8-7 Acute Acalculous Cholecystitis: Accuracy of Cholescintigraphy

Study author and date	Patients	Sensitivity (%)	Specificity (%)
Shuman, 1984	19	68	
Weissmann, 1983	15	93	
Mirvis, 1986	19	90	61
Swayne, 1986	49	93	
Ramanna, 1984	11	100	
Flancbaum, 1995	16	75	100
Prevot, 1999	14	64	100
Mariat, 2000	12	67	100
Overall	**155**	**81**	**90**

FIGURE 8-10. Rim sign. **A,** HIDA sequential images over 60 minutes show no gallbladder filling but good biliary-to-bowel transit. Increased activity in a curvilinear pattern along the inferior right hepatic lobe (rim sign) persists from beginning to 60 minutes. **B,** Sequential images for 30 minutes after morphine injection show no gallbladder filling, but persistence of the rim sign. Surgery confirmed severe acute cholecystitis.

25% to 35% of patients with acute cholecystitis have this finding (Fig. 8-10). It can be seen throughout the study, but is best seen as the radiotracer clears from the liver. The rim sign clears slower than normal liver and thus becomes more obvious.

The rim sign is caused by liver inflammation adjacent to the gallbladder fossa. With severe acute cholecystitis, gallbladder inflammation spreads to adjacent normal liver, resulting in increased blood flow and Tc-99m HIDA delivery to the region. The high liver HIDA extraction efficiency results in increased uptake. It has slower clearance compared to adjacent noninflamed liver because of inflammatory edema.

The importance of the rim sign is twofold. First, it is a very specific scintigraphic finding for acute cholecystitis. It increases confidence in interpretation that nonfilling of the gallbladder is indeed caused by acute cholescystitis (true positive) in a patient at increased risk for a false positive study results (Box 8-5)—for example, a sick hospitalized patient with concurrent serious illness.

The rim sign identifies patients with acute cholecystitis who have more severe disease and are therefore at increased risk for complications, such as gallbladder perforation and gangrene. Even without these complications, patients with the rim sign tend to be sicker and at a later stage of the pathophysiological spectrum of disease—for example, with hemorrhage and necrosis rather than edema and white blood cell infiltration (Box 8-4).

Acute Acalculous Cholecystitis

The acalculous form of acute cholecystitis is uncommon; however, it can be a life-threatening disease. It presents in seriously ill hospitalized patients, often in the intensive care unit (Box 8-6). Because of its high mortality (30%) and morbidity (55%), early diagnosis is imperative, although in the case of concomitant serious illness, diagnosis is often delayed.

In the majority of patients, acute acalculous cholecystitis is initiated by cystic duct obstruction, not by cholelithiais, but rather by inflammatory debris, inspissated bile, and local edema, aggravated by dehydration. Some patients do not have cystic duct obstruction, but rather direct inflammation of the gallbladder wall caused by systemic infection, ischemia, or toxemia.

The sensitivity of cholescintigraphy for diagnosis of acute acalculous cholescintigraphy is lower than for the calculous form of the disease, approximately 80%, compared to 95% to 98% for acute calculous cholecystitis (Table 8-7).

If a false-negative study result (filling of the gallbladder) is suspected in a patient with a high clinical suspicion for acute acalculous cholecystitis, sincalide infusion may be helpful. An acutely inflamed gallbladder does not contract normally. Good contraction excludes the diagnosis. Poor contraction in the proper clinical setting is suggestive, but not diagnostic. The patient may have an underlying chronic cholecystitis or be on medications or have a disease process (Boxes 8-7 and 8-8) that inhibits gallbladder emptying.

In unclear cases, a radiolabeled leukocyte study can confirm the diagnosis. Indium-111 leukocytes have the advantage of not being cleared through the biliary tract like Tc-99m hexamethylpropyleneamine oxime (HMPAO) leukocytes. However, early HMPAO imaging at 1 to 2 hours before biliary clearance may avoid this problem. Although the standard imaging time for In-111 leukocytes is at 24 hours, imaging at 4 hours can be diagnostic if gallbladder uptake is seen.

Chronic Cholecystitis
Calculous Chronic Cholecystitis
Patients with chronic cholecystitis present with symptoms of recurrent biliary colic. The clinical diagnosis is often confirmed by detection of gallstones on ultrasonography. Cholecystectomy is the standard therapy. On

---

Box 8-7. Drugs Known to Inhibit Gallbladder Contraction

Opiates
Atropine
Nifedipine (calcium channel blocking agent)
Indomethacin
Progesterone
Oral contraceptives
Octreotide
Theophylline
Isoproterenol
Benzodiazepine
Phentolamine (alpha-adrenergic blocking agent)
Nicotine
Alcohol

Box 8-8. Diseases or Conditions Associated with Poor Gallbladder Contraction

Diabetes mellitus
Sickle cell disease
Irritable bowel syndrome
Truncal vagotomy
Pancreatic insufficiency
Crohn disease
Celiac disease
Achalasia
Dyspeptic syndrome
Obesity
Cirrhosis
Pregnancy

---

histopathology, the gallbladder has evidence of chronic inflammation.

Cholescintigraphy is not commonly ordered for patients with chronic calculous cholecystitis. If ordered, it would likely be a normal study. Abnormal findings, including nonfilling of the gallbladder, delayed filling, or delayed biliary-to-bowel transit, which are not specific or diagnostic, may be seen in less than 5% of patients. Most will have poor gallbladder contraction if stimulated with a fatty meal or cholecystokinin. However, patients with asymptomatic cholelithiasis have normal gallbladder contraction.

Acalculous Chronic Gallbladder Disease
The acalculous variety of chronic cholecystitis occurs in approximately 10% of patients with symptomatic chronic gallbladder disease. It is clinically and histopathologically indistinguishable from chronic calculous cholecystitis, except that there are no gallstones. This entity has been referred to by various names, including gallbladder dyskinesia, gallbladder spasm, cystic duct syndrome, functional gallbladder disease, and chronic acalculous gallbladder disease (Box 8-9). Although varying somewhat in reported descriptions, they all present with recurrent biliary colic, have poor gallbladder contraction, and are usually cured with cholecystectomy.

Numerous investigations have reported that sincalide cholescintigraphy can confirm the clinically suspected diagnosis of chronic acalculous gallbladder disease. A poor GBEF with sincalide infusion can predict postcholecystectomy symptomatic relief and histopathological evidence of chronic gallbladder inflammation; a normal GBEF excludes the disease (Fig. 8-11). Publications report that a low GBEF has a positive predictive value of more than 90%.

Sincalide cholescintigraphy should be performed on an outpatient basis after a negative clinical workup, including negative ultrasonography. The study should not be performed when the patient is acutely ill or hospitalized, because other diseases and numerous therapeutic drugs can adversely affect gallbladder function (Boxes 8-7 and 8-8).

Sincalide Infusion Methodology. The usual total sincalide infusion dose has been 0.02 µg/kg, although this has been given over different infusion lengths, including 3, 15, 30, and 60 minutes. The 3-minute infusion method with

---

Box 8-9. Synonyms for Recurrent Pain Syndromes of Biliary Origin

CHRONIC ACALCULOUS GALLBLADDER DISEASE
Chronic acalculous cholecystitis
Gallbladder dyskinesia
Gallbladder spasm
Cystic duct syndrome
Functional gallbladder disease

SPHINCTER OF ODDI DYSFUNCTION
Papillary stenosis
Biliary spasm
Biliary dyskinesia

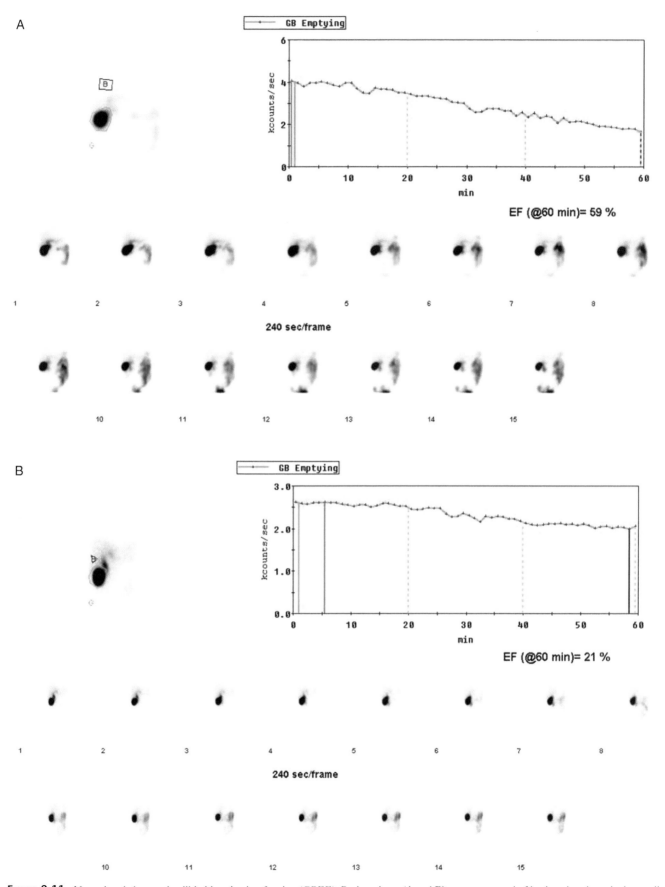

FIGURE 8-11. Normal and abnormal gallbladder ejection fraction (GBEF). Both patients (**A** and **B**) were suspected of having chronic acalculous gall-bladder disease. Both had a 60-minute infusion of sincalide after gallbladder visualization. A region of interest was drawn for the gallbladder and background. **A,** Good gallbladder contraction, GBEF 59%. **B,** Poor gallbladder contraction, GBEF 21%. (Abnormal <38%). The patient in **B** had a cholecystectomy with relief of his symptoms.

calculation of a GBEF at 20 to 30 minutes was commonly used in the past; however, it is no longer recommended. It causes abdominal cramping or nausea in 50% of subjects, may lead to a false positive result, and normal values have never been established because of the wide range of GBEFs in normal subjects (0-100%).

A misconception is that reproduction of the patient's pain with sincalide infusion is diagnostic of acalculous chronic gallbladder disease. This is not true. A side effect of sincalide is that it stimulates intestinal motility, which can cause cramping abdominal pain the drug is infused too rapidly (Box 8-8). Symptoms are not seen with 30- to 60-minute infusions.

A multicenter comparison trial found that a 60-minute infusion of 0.02 μg/kg has the least variability in normal subjects compared to 15- and 30-minute infusions and the best defined normal value (lower range of normal is 38%) (Box 8-8). A published consensus paper written by experts in gastroenterology, surgery, primary care, and nuclear medicine has recommended that the 60-minute infusion method become the standard.

Biliary Obstruction
Biliary obstruction has multiple causes. Cancerous and non-cancerous causes usually present differently (Table 8-8). Malignancy (e.g., pancreatic or biliary duct cancer) usually causes painless obstructive jaundice, whereas choledocholithiasis produces severe acute or recurrent abdominal pain.

High-Grade Biliary Obstruction
Pathophysiology. With high-grade obstruction, the sequence of pathophysiological events progresses in a predictable manner (Box 8-10), although the time course may vary depending on the rapidity of onset, the degree of obstruction, and the cause. Obstruction causes increased intraductal pressure and high back-pressure, reducing bile flow and causing biliary duct dilation. If unchecked, hepatocellular damage and ultimately biliary cirrhosis occur.

Patients with high-grade biliary obstruction often present with abdominal pain, jaundice, and elevated alkaline phosphatase and direct serum bilirubin. Increased serum alkaline phosphatase occurs early in the natural history, whereas hyperbilirubinemia is a late manifestation.

The diagnosis is often confirmed by anatomical imaging—for example, ultrasonography or magnetic resonance cholangiopancreatography (MRCP), showing biliary duct dilation. Anatomical imaging also may detect an obstructing mass. Obstructing biliary stones are not always seen on anatomical imaging.

Biliary duct dilation is diagnostic only of obstruction in patients who have not had prior obstruction or biliary surgery, because the ducts may remain dilated postoperatively.

Box 8-10. High-Grade Biliary Obstruction: Sequential Pathophysiology

1. Obstruction of hepatic or common bile duct
2. Increased intrabiliary pressure
3. Significantly decreased bile flow
4. Ductal dilation
5. Biliary cirrhosis

Cholescintigraphy can determine whether the dilated biliary ducts are patent or again obstructed. Ductal dilation often does not become evident until 24 to 72 hours after obstruction. Cholescintigraphy can diagnose obstruction before dilation occurs because it depicts the underlying pathophysiology—that is, severely reduced or no bile flow.

Partial Biliary Obstruction
The most common cause for partial obstruction is choledocholithiasis. Liver function tests and serum bilirubin may be normal. Biliary ducts often are not dilated with a partial or intermittent low-grade obstruction, probably because of the lower intraductal pressure. In some cases, ductal dilation may be restricted by edema and scarring.

Imaging Diagnosis
Ultrasonography is often the first imaging study ordered. Without dilation, the study may be normal. Rapid T2-weighted MRCP scans viewed in the coronal plane mimic the appearance of contrast cholangiography. It is superior to sonography for detecting stones that do not result in ductal dilation. However, small symptomatic stones may not be detected. MRCP does not evaluate bile flow.

Cholescintigraphy can help determine if the patient's symptoms are biliary in origin when anatomical imaging is unrewarding and if a more invasive workup is considered—for example, percutaneous cholangiography or endoscopic retrograde cholangiopancreatography (ERCP). Discordance between anatomical and functional imaging with cholescintigraphy is not uncommon. Functional abnormalities precede morphologically evident disease. When there is no ductal dilation, scintigraphy may show evidence of partial biliary obstruction manifested by delayed bile flow. In patients without obstruction but dilated ducts from prior obstruction, cholescintigraphy can exclude recurrent obstruction by demonstrating normal bile flow.

Cholescintigraphic Diagnostic Patterns
High-Grade Obstruction. Recent onset of obstruction demonstrates a characteristic pattern of good hepatic function, manifested as rapid Tc-99m HIDA uptake and blood pool clearance, with no rapid excretion into the biliary tree (i.e., a persistent hepatogram) (Fig. 8-12). Imaging delayed up to 24 hours is often unchanged. With less severe high-grade obstruction, delayed excretion into biliary ducts may be seen on delayed imaging. In patients with good hepatic function, delayed imaging is not necessary for diagnosis. In patients with poor hepatic function, delayed imaging is needed to differentiate obstruction from primary hepatic dysfunction (Fig. 8-13). The lack of biliary clearance by 24 hours is consistent with obstruction.
Partial Biliary Obstruction. The cholescintigraphic findings are different in partial or low-grade biliary obstruction from those in high-grade obstruction. With partial obstruction, prompt hepatic uptake and secretion into biliary ducts occurs. The diagnostic scintigraphic finding is delayed clearance from biliary ducts—that is, activity decreasing in the common duct by less than 50% from the peak (Fig. 8-14). Delayed transit into the intestinal tract (delayed biliary-to-bowel transit) is often, but not invariably, seen (Box 8-11). Transit into the bowel by 60 minutes occurs in many patients with partial biliary obstruction.

Most important is to judge whether good common duct clearance has occurred. Delayed images at 2 hours or sincalide infusion should be performed to confirm or exclude partial obstruction (Figs. 8-15 and 8-16).

Patients may have delayed biliary-to-bowel transit for reasons other than obstruction (Box 8-12). It occurs in patients who have received sincalide before the study to empty the gallbladder. As its prokinetic effect dissipates, the gallbladder relaxes and the resulting negative intraluminal

gallbladder pressure causes bile to flow preferentially toward the gallbladder rather than through the common duct and sphincter of Oddi. Delayed transit also can be seen in patients with chronic cholecystitis and some normal patients with a hypertonic sphincter of Oddi, considered a normal variation (Fig. 8-17). Delayed imaging or sincalide can exclude a pathological cause.

Opiate drugs produce a functional partial biliary obstruction. Thus opiates should be withheld for at least several

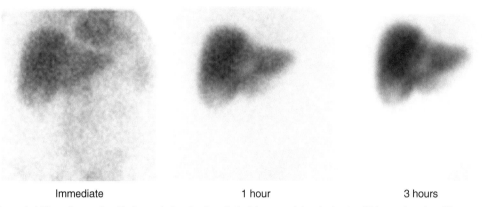

Immediate   1 hour   3 hours

FIGURE 8-12. High-grade biliary obstruction. Patient admitted to hospital with acute abdominal pain of 8 hours duration. Ultrasonography did not show biliary dilation. Cholescintigraphy with immediate *(left)*, 1 hour *(middle)*, and 3 hour images *(right)*. Cardiac blood pool cleared by 10 minutes. This persistent hepatogram is classic for a high-grade biliary obstruction. At surgery, a stone was found to be obstructing the common duct.

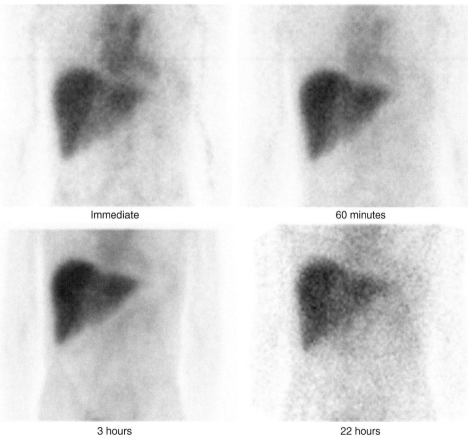

Immediate   60 minutes

3 hours   22 hours

FIGURE 8-13. Biliary obstruction vs. hepatic dysfunction. Patient has recurrent pancreatitis, elevated serum alkaline phosphatase and bilirubin. *Upper left:* Immediate image. *Upper right:* 60 minutes shows persistent blood pool and no biliary secretion. *Lower left:* 3 hours, essentially unchanged from 1 hour. *Lower right:* 22 hours, no biliary secretion, most consistent with obstruction.

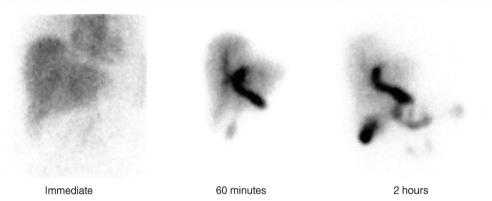

Immediate   60 minutes   2 hours

Figure 8-14. Partial biliary obstruction. Patient with recurrent upper abdominal pain over 6 months. Cholescintigraphy immediately after injection *(left)*, at 60 minutes *(middle)*, and at 2 hours *(right)* delayed image. Cardiac blood pool cleared by 5 minutes. The common duct has retained activity at 1 hour, which worsens at 2 hours consistent with partial biliary obstruction. The delayed gallbladder visualization (faint at 1 hour, filled by 2 hours) suggests a concomitant chronic cholecystitis.

Box 8-11. Scintigraphic Diagnosis of Partial Biliary Obstruction

Poor biliary duct clearance (<50% of peak common duct activity at 60 minutes)

Delayed or reduced biliary-to-bowel transit

No further biliary duct clearance on delayed imaging at 120 vs. 60 minutes

No biliary duct clearance with sincalide infusion between 60 and 120 minutes

---

half-lives before cholescintigraphy. In urgent cases, naloxone (Narcan) has been used to reverse the effect of opiate drugs before cholescintigraphy.

Accuracy. The sensitivity and specificity of cholescintigraphy for high-grade obstruction is high, approaching 100%. Cholestatic jaundice, as seen in drug hepatotoxicity (erythromycin, chlorpromazine), may have similar scintigraphic findings; however, the clinical presentation is quite different. For low-grade, partial, or intermittent obstruction, the sensitivity and specificity have been reported to be 95% and 85%, respectively.

Choledochal Cyst

Choledochal cysts are not true cysts, but rather congenital dilations of biliary ducts. They usually involve the common hepatic duct or common bile duct, but may occur anywhere in the biliary system, usually in an extrahepatic or occasionally intrahepatic (Caroli disease) location, and are sometimes multifocal (Fig. 8-18).

Choledochal cysts present in young children as biliary obstruction, pancreatitis, or cholangitis. They may be asymptomatic and detected incidentally, or they may be first detected in adulthood. Ultrasonography or computed tomography (CT) may detect a saccular or fusiform cystic structure; however, it may be unclear whether the cystic structure connects with the biliary tract. Cholescintigraphy can confirm or exclude the diagnosis. Choledochal cysts fill slowly and have prolonged retention. Even nonobstructed cysts have slow clearance. Delayed imaging is often required (Fig. 8-19). A high-grade obstruction will show no biliary secretion or filling because of the high back-pressure.

Biliary Atresia

Biliary atresia is characterized by a progressive inflammatory sclerosis and obliteration of extrahepatic and intrahepatic biliary ducts. It presents during the neonatal period with cholestatic jaundice, acholic stools, and hepatomegally. Without treatment, the disease leads to hepatic fibrosis, cirrhosis, liver failure, and death within 2 to 3 years. The cause is unknown.

Early diagnosis is critical because surgery must usually be performed within the first 60 days of life to prevent irreversible liver failure ensues. Treatment involves surgery, a palliative hepatoportoenterostomy (Kasai procedure), and ultimately liver transplantation.

The disease must be differentiated from neonatal hepatitis, which is caused by various genetic, infectious, and metabolic causes—for example, Alagille syndrome (arteriohepatic dysplasia), alpha-1-antitrypsin deficiency, and cystic fibrosis.

Cholescintigraphy

Preparation. Patients are routinely pretreated with phenobarbital 5 mg/kg per day for 5 days to activate liver excretory enzymes and increase bile flow, to increase the specificity of the test. The usual administered dose of Tc-99m IDA is 200 micro Ci/kg (minimum dose of 1 mCi).

Cholescintigraphy has been used for decades to differentiate biliary atresia from neonatal hepatitis. The atretic bile ducts produce a picture of high-grade biliary obstruction (Fig. 8-20), with good blood pool clearance, but no biliary secretion or clearance, and a persistent hepatogram. The obstructive pattern is caused by the high biliary duct backpressure, preventing secretion into biliary ducts or gallbladder. Neonatal hepatitis shows hepatic dysfunction, delayed blood pool clearance, but usually biliary clearance by 24 hours after Tc-99m HIDA injection (Fig. 8-21). Gallbladder filling excludes biliary atresia.

The sensitivity for detection of biliary atresia with cholescintigraphy is very high, approaching 100%; however, the specificity is lower, approximately 75% to 80%. False positive study results (no biliary-to-bowel transit, but not ultimately biliary atresia) occur in patients with severe parenchymal liver disease. When a false positive study result is clinically suspected, a repeat study in several days to a week may be helpful. Single-photon emission

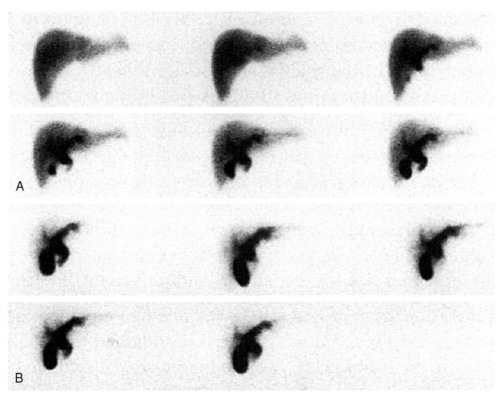

FIGURE 8-15. Partial common bile duct obstruction response to sincalide. **A,** Increasing biliary secretion over time. The common duct appears prominent. No biliary-to-bowel transit is seen at 60 minutes. **B,** Sincalide infusion. No gallbladder contraction and no significant biliary-to- bowel transit. This is consistent with partial common bile duct obstruction.

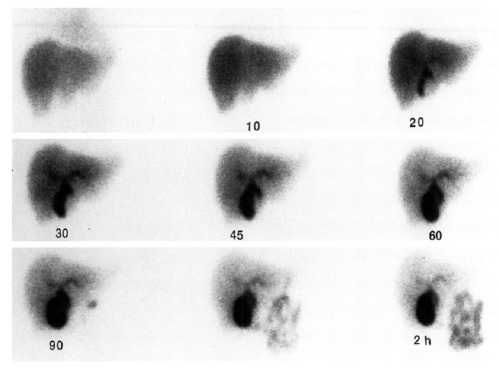

FIGURE 8-16. Delayed biliary-to-bowel transit caused by sincalide administered before the study. The gallbladder fills by 30 minutes, the common duct is seen at 60 minutes, but there is no bowel clearance. Delayed imaging shows intestinal clearance first seen at 90 minutes and reduced activity in the common duct by 2 hours.

computed tomography (SPECT) and SPECT/CT can improve specificity (Fig 8-22).

Chronic Acalculous Cholecystitis. An increasingly common indication for cholescintigraphy is to confirm the clinical diagnosis of acalculous chronic gallbladder disease.

Box 8-12. Causes of Delayed Biliary-to-Bowel Transit

Biliary obstruction
Sincalide administration before cholescintigraphy
Opiate drugs
Chronic cholecystitis
Normal variation (hypertonic sphincter of Oddi)

When a patient complains of recurrent biliary colic and gallstones are detected on ultrasonography, the patient is referred for cholecystectomy, which is usually curative. The acalculous form of the disease occurs in about 10% of patients with chronic cholecystitis. Symptoms are similar and the gallbladder histopathology is the same, but no stones are present. Thus diagnosis is more challenging.

Multiple studies have found that sincalide cholescintigraphy with calculation of GBEF can accurately confirm or exclude the diagnosis of acalculous chronic gallbladder disease. An abnormally low GBEF predicts a good response to cholecystectomy.

When sincalide is not available, a fatty meal can be used as an alternative to evaluate gallbladder contraction.

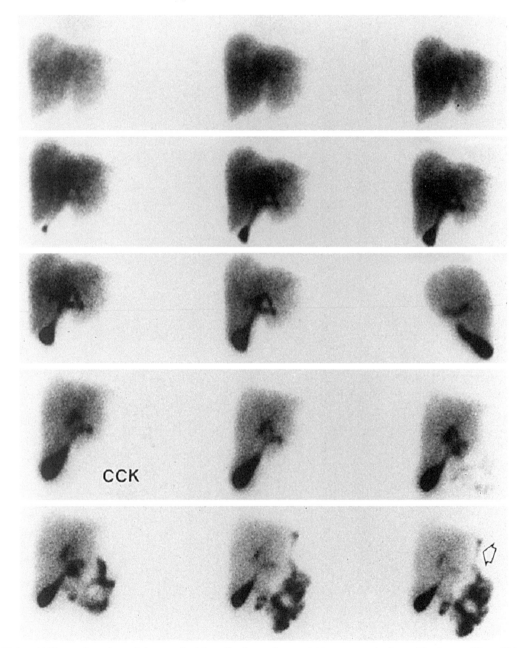

FIGURE 8-17. Delayed biliary-to-bowel transit in normal subject. *Top 3 rows,* Sequential images acquired over 60 minutes. The gallbladder fills, biliary ducts are visualized, but no biliary-to-bowel transit by 60 minutes. *Bottom 2 rows,* Sincalide infusion. Gallbladder contracts (gallbladder ejection fraction, 51%), and biliary-to-bowel transit occurs as a result of relaxation of sphincter of Oddi. *Arrowhead,* Mild enterogastric reflux. Interpreted as "hypertonic sphincter of Oddi." *CCK,* Cholecystokinin.

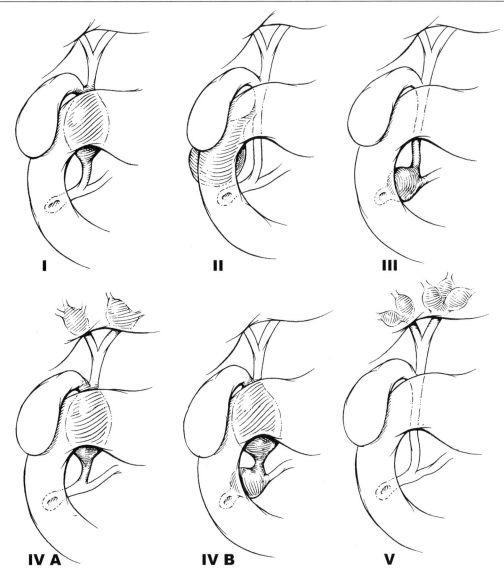

FIGURE 8-18. Classification of choledochal cysts. Type I: Cystic dilation of an extrahepatic duct (most common). Type II: Sac or diverticulum opening from the common bile duct. Type III: choledochocele, located within the duodenal wall. Type IV A: Involving intrahepatic and extrahepatic biliary ducts. Type IV B: Dilation of multiple segments confined to extrahepatic biliary ducts. Type V: Multiple intrahepatic ducts (Caroli disease).

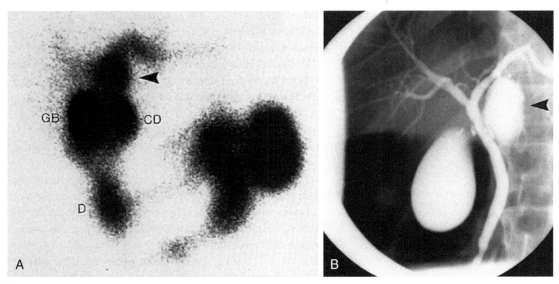

FIGURE 8-19. Choledochal cyst. A 25-year-old patient with abdominal pain. Sonography detected a cystic structure adjacent to the common hepatic duct without definite connection to the biliary system. **A,** Tc-99 IDA images acquired at 90 minutes after the liver had cleared show filling of choledochal cyst in the region of the common hepatic duct *(arrowhead)*. *CD,* Common duct; *D,* duodenum; *GB,* gallbladder. **B,** Cholangiogram confirmed the diagnosis.

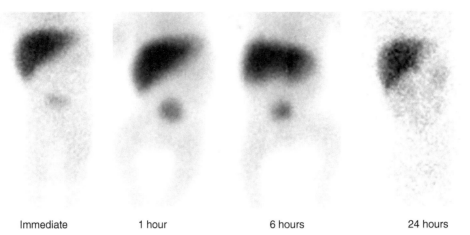

Immediate   1 hour   6 hours   24 hours

FIGURE 8-20. Biliary atresia. A 13-week-old child with jaundice, pretreated with phenobarbital for 5 days. No biliary excretion occurred over 24 hours. Bladder clearance is seen. Biliary atresia was confirmed at cholangiography, and subsequently a Kasai procedure was performed.

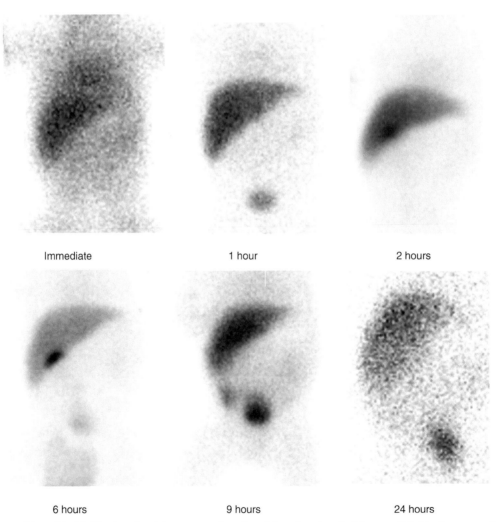

Immediate   1 hour   2 hours

6 hours   9 hours   24 hours

FIGURE 8-21. Neonatal hepatitis. No blood pool at 1 hour, suggestive of good liver function. At 2 hours gallbladder is suggested. By 6 hours, good gallbladder filling is seen. At 9 hours, bowel clearance is seen, and the gallbladder has emptied. By 24 hours, image quality is reduced, with possibly some mild bowel activity at hepatic flexure. The patient was clinically followed with progressive improvement in liver function tests. Imaging could have been discontinued at 6 or 9 hours because biliary obstruction had been excluded.

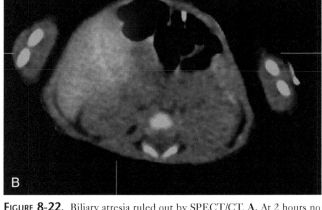

TABLE 8-8 Comparison of 3-, 15-, 30-, 60-Minute Sincalide Infusions (0.02 µg/kg) in Normal Subjects

Infusion length	Coefficient of variation (%)*	Range (%)	Abnormal (%)	Abdominal cramping (%)
3 minutes[†]	48	0-100	<0	50
15 minute[‡]	52	5-92	<17	5
30 minute[‡]	35	20-95	<19	0
60 minute[‡]	19[§]	50-96	<38	0

*Coefficient of variability (CV) as a measure of variability (SD/mean).
[†]Ziessman HA, Muenz LR, Agarwal AK, ZaZa A. Normal values for sincalide cholescintigraphy: comparison of two methods. *Radiology.* 2001;221(2):404-410; 2001 and Sostre S, Kaloo AN, Spiegler EJ, et al. A noninvasive test of sphincter of Oddi dysfunction in postcholecystectomy patients: the scintigraphic score. *J Nucl Med.* 1992;33(6):1216-1222.
[‡]Multicenter Investigation (Ziessman HA, Tulchinsky M, Lavely WC, et al. Sincalide-stimulated cholescintigraphy: a multicenter investigation to determine optimal methodology and gallbladder ejection fraction normal values. *J Nucl Med.* 2010;51[2]:229-236.)
[§]CV was statistically different (<0.0001) for 60 min vs. 30 min and 30 min vs. 15 min.

FIGURE 8-22. Biliary atresia ruled out by SPECT/CT. **A,** At 2 hours no definite biliary clearance is seen. Subtle increased uptake at the inferior border of the liver was noted. **B,** SPECT/CT acquired. The fused image demonstrates gallbladder filling, excluding biliary atresia.

Normal values depend on the amount of fat in the meal and the study length. Thus an established protocol and validated normal values should be used.

Many studies have shown that sincalide cholescintigraphy with calculation of GBEF can confirm the diagnosis of chronic acalculous gallbladder disease and predict response to cholecystectomy (Fig. 8-11). Scintigraphy should be performed on an outpatient basis when the patient is not having symptoms. Performing this test on an inpatient basis is fraught with potential for error, because the patient is likely to be on a variety of medications that may inhibit gallbladder contraction or may have illnesses that may adversely affect gallbladder function (Boxes 8-7 and 8-8).

Methodology for Sincalide Cholescintigraphy. When sincalide was used in conjunction with oral cholecystography

in the 1960s and 1970s, it was noted that bolus or rapid infusions can cause spasm of the gallbladder neck and ineffective gallbladder contraction. Thus it became common practice to infuse sincalide 0.02 µg/kg over 1 to 3 minutes. However, investigations have shown that 1- to 3-minute infusions of sincalide may result in poor contraction of the gallbladder in up to one third of normal subjects, whereas slower infusions of 30 to 60 minutes in the same subjects result in good contraction. The explanation is that 1-to 3-minute infusions are not physiological, producing similar effects to those of a bolus infusion. Another problem with short infusions is that approximately 50% of subjects who receive a 3-minute infusion have nausea or abdominal cramping. This does not occur with infusions of the same total dose for 30 to 60 minutes. Finally, normal values for 3-minute infusions cannot been established because of a very wide range of responses (0-100%) (Table 8-8)

A recent multicenter study of 60 normal subjects sought to determine the method with the least variability for sincalide infusion in normal subjects by comparing 15-, 30-, and 60-minute infusions in the same subjects (Table 8-8). Symptoms of nausea and cramping were sometimes seen with the 15-minute infusion, but never with the longer infusions. The 60-minute infusion had significantly less intersubject variability (coefficient of variation) and narrowest range of GBEF normal values (≥38%). A standardized method is described (Box 8-13).

Gallbladder emptying with sincalide may be inhibited if a patient has been on opiate drugs or recently received an opiate drug—for example, morphine. Other common therapeutic drugs can also inhibit gallbladder emptying and thus should not be taken before sincalide cholescintigraphy (Box 8-7).

Postoperative Biliary Tract
Postoperative Complications
Cholescintigraphy can provide valuable diagnostic information in patients with suspected complications presenting after laparoscopic or open cholecystectomy, biliary duct surgery, gallstone lithotripsy, and biliary enteric anastomoses.

Box 8-13. Consensus Methodology for Sincalide Cholescintigraphy: Gallbaldder Ejection Fraction Calculation

SINCALIDE ADMINISTRATION: STANDARDIZED PROTOCOL

1. Ensure that gallbladder has filled.
2. Position camera in left anterior oblique projection (35-40 degrees).
3. Draw 0.02 μg/kg sincalide into a 30- to 50-mL syringe and dilute with normal saline to the volume of the syringe.
4. Set up infusion pump so that the entire volume of the syringe will be infused over 60 minutes.
5. Set up computer acquisition for 60 one-minute frames (128 × 128).
6. Begin imaging at start of sincalide infusion and stop imaging at the end of 60-minute infusion.
7. Abnormal GBEF is less than 38%.*

COMPUTER PROCESSING GBEF

1. Select region of interest for the gallbladder and adjacent liver background.
2. Generate time–activity curve.
3. Calculate GBEF at 60 minutes = maximum counts – minimum counts divided by maximum counts, all corrected for background.

*From DiBaise JK, Richmond BK, Ziessman HA, et al. Cholecystokinin-cholescintigraphy in adults: consensus recommendations of an interdisciplinary panel. *Clin Nucl Med.* 2012;37(1):63-70.
GBEF, Gallbladder ejection fraction.

Biliary Leaks

Bile leaks occur most commonly after cholecystectomy or other biliary tract surgery. Obstruction can be a contributing cause. The laparoscopic method has become the procedure of choice for elective cholecystectomy; however, this approach is associated with a somewhat higher rate of bile duct injury than open cholecystectomy.

Although ultrasonography and CT can detect fluid collections, the type and origin of the fluid collection is sometimes unclear. Cholescintigraphy can determine whether the fluid collection is of biliary origin rather than a result of other causes, such as ascites or seroma. The rate of biliary leakage can be estimated visually, rapid versus slow. Slow bile leaks usually resolve spontaneously with conservative therapy; rapid leaks often require surgical correction.

Before percutaneous drainage of a biloma, cholescintigraphy can help ensure that central biliary obstruction is not present. With obstruction, it is unlikely that bile leakage can be effectively treated by percutaneous drainage without addressing the underlying cause of obstruction. Follow-up cholescintigraphy can confirm resolution or persistence of the leakage.

With cholescintigraphically, bile leakage is seen as a progressively increasing collection of radiotracer in the region of the gallbladder fossa or hepatic hilum. The activity may spread into the subdiaphragmatic space, over the dome of the liver, and into the colonic gutters or manifest as free bile in the abdomen (Fig. 8-23). Rapid leaks are detectable during the first 60 minutes of the study. Slower leaks may require delayed imaging. Positioning the patient on the right lateral decubitus for several minutes immediately before laying them flat under the camera positions camera closer for better image. Peritoneal tubing, drains, and collection bags may exhibit accumulation and should be imaged.

Biliary Diversion Surgery

Biliary enteric bypass procedures are performed in patients for benign and malignant diseases associated with biliary obstruction.

Ultrasonography has imaging limitations in the presence of gas in the anastomotic bowel segment or refluxed biliary air after surgery. Two thirds of attempts are reported as indeterminate. Biliary dilation may be present in more than 20% of patients even though obstruction has been adequately relieved by surgery. MRCP has become a standard diagnostic procedure because of its good accuracy in visualizing the postoperative stricture and detecting obstruction. Cholescintigraphy is well-suited to diagnose bile leakage, patency of the anastomosis, and recurrent obstruction in patients who have had biliary diversion surgery. It is important to know the postoperative anatomy of the patient being imaged. Although biliary scintigraphy is useful in a variety of anastomoses, it is particularly valuable in patients with intrahepatic cholangiojejunostomy or choledochojejunostomy. The latter is a direct anastomosis of the extrahepatic portion of the common bile duct or common hepatic duct to a Roux-en-Y jejunal loop. The intrahepatic cholangiojejunostomy requires direct anastomosis between the small bowel and intrahepatic ducts. Cholescintigraphy also can be helpful if ERCP cannot reach the biliary tract when a long Roux-en-Y loop has been created.

Cholescintigraphy is the only noninvasive method that can distinguish obstructed dilated ducts from those that are chronically dilated but not obstructed. With scintigraphy, intestinal excretion visualization by 1 hour with or without ductal dilation is consistent with functional patency. Intestinal excretion longer than 1 hour is suggestive of partial obstruction. However, retention of activity in biliary ducts is a more reliable indicator. Persistent or worsening biliary duct retention between 1 and 2 hours is very suspicious for obstruction. Stasis with minimal intestinal excretion and pooling in the region of the biliary enteric anastomosis normally may be seen at 1 hour. This may be positional and can be confirmed by imaging the patient upright. Persistent nonvisualization of the biliary system and intestine is seen with complete biliary duct obstruction.

Other Gastrointestinal Surgical Anastomoses

Cholescintigraphy can provide functional information about other surgical procedures involving the gastrointestinal tract—for example, Billroth I and II and Whipple resection. In Billroth II anastomoses, afferent loop patency can be determined. The afferent loop should fill readily in an antegrade direction from the common duct. Normally, there is progressive accumulation of activity within the loop. However, it should clear distally by 2 hours.

Liver Transplants

The major role for cholescintigraphy is to aid in detection of the postoperative complications of bile leaks and

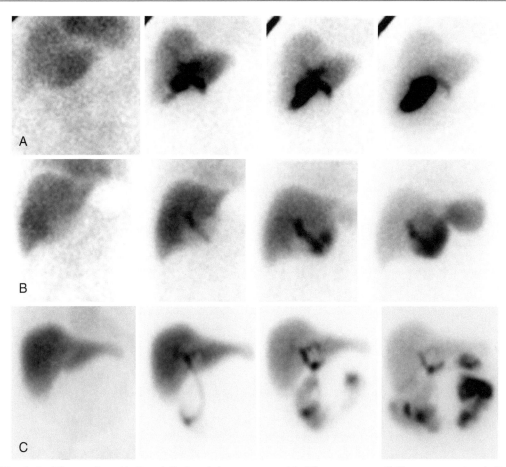

FIGURE 8-23. Biliary leaks. Three patients (**A**, **B**, and **C**) after cholecystectomy, with different patterns of biliary extravasation. **A**, Radiotracer extravasates along the inferior edge of the right lobe to the region of the gallbladder fossa. **B**, Leak transits inferior to the left lobe, extending to the left upper quadrant. **C**, Intraperitoneal extravasation.

obstruction. The findings of rejection on cholescintigraphy are nonspecific signs of liver dysfunction. Liver biopsy is necessary to make the diagnosis.

Trauma

Posttraumatic problems that must be clinically differentiated include hepatic laceration, hematoma, bile duct transection, extrahepatic biliary leakage, intrahepatic biloma formation, and perforation of the gallbladder. CT and ultrasonography can diagnose liver parenchymal injury. Only biliary scintigraphy can demonstrate communication between the biliary tree and space-occupying lesions that represent biloma formation.

Bile leakage is common after penetrating and blunt trauma. It may initially be occult and detected only after clinical deterioration or discharge of bilious material from surgical bed drains. Cholescintigraphy can differentiate between rapid and slow bile leakage, which can help the surgeon decide whether intervention or watchful waiting is indicated and assess resolution of leakage in patients treated conservatively.

Postcholecystectomy Pain Syndrome

Approximately 10% to 20% of patients who have had cholecystectomy for chronic cholecystitis develop recurrent abdominal pain. Sometimes the pain is not of biliary origin. Biliary causes include retained or recurrent biliary duct stones, inflammatory stricture, or sphincter of Oddi dysfunction (Box 8-14). Rarely, a cystic duct remnant acts like a small gallbladder and produces symptoms similar to those of acute or chronic cholecystitis. Cholescintigraphy can often confirm or exclude a biliary cause for the postcholecystectomy syndrome.

Retained or Recurrent Stones and Stricture

The most common biliary causes for this pain syndrome are retained or recurrent biliary duct stones, followed by inflammatory fibrotic stricture (Fig 8-24). On cholescintigraphy, they all show evidence of a partial biliary obstruction—delayed clearance from biliary ducts and often delayed biliary-to-bowel-transit. Delayed imaging at 2 hours shows no reduction activity in the common duct (Fig. 8-25).

Sphincter of Oddi Dysfunction

Sphincter of Oddi dysfunction occurs in approximately 10% of patients with the postcholecystectomy pain syndrome. It presents as intermittent abdominal pain and sometimes transient liver function abnormalities. It is a partial biliary obstruction at the level of the sphincter of Oddi, not caused by stones or stricture. It presents after cholecystectomy, possibly because the gallbladder had been acting as a pressure release valve, decompressing the biliary ducts with increases in pressure, preventing pain.

Patients have been classified clinically into 3 categories. In type I, enzyme elevations are seen, with pain episodes and dilated biliary ducts. In type II, either enzyme elevations or dilated biliary ducts occur. Type III presents with only pain. Patients with type I are the most easily diagnosed. Patients with types II and III are more diagnostically challenging; cholescintigraphy may have a role in these cases.

Therapy is usually sphincterotomy, particularly for a fixed obstruction (papillary stenosis), whereas a functional and

reversible obstruction (biliary dyskinesia) may temporarily respond to drugs (e.g., nifedipine) and toxins (e.g., Botox).

Sonography, CT, and MRCP often are not diagnostic. Sphincter of Oddi manometry has been regarded as the gold standard, with an elevated sphincter pressure (>40 mm Hg) being diagnostic. However, this technique is invasive, not widely available, technically difficult, prone to interpretative errors, and associated with a significant incidence of adverse effects, notably pancreatitis. ERCP is ultimately used to exclude cholelithiasis or stricture; however, it is invasive and associated with a high incidence of postprocedure complications, including pancreatitis.

The value of cholescintigraphy is controversial. Evidence-based data are lacking. However, multiple single-center studies have shown it to be useful and is routinely performed at some biliary referral centers. Early studies suggested that image analysis alone can be diagnostic with findings of a partial biliary obstruction—that is, delayed biliary duct clearance at 60 minutes with no further clearance between 1 and 2 hours (Fig. 8-25).

Box 8-14. Causes of Postcholecystectomy Pain Syndrome

Retained or recurrent choledocholithiasis
Inflammatory stricture
Sphincter of Oddi dysfunction
Cystic duct remnant (obstructed/inflamed)
Nonhepatobiliary origin

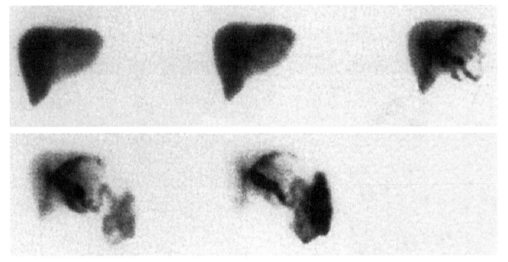

FIGURE 8-24. Postcholecystectomy biliary stricture causing moderate partial obstruction. Images at 5, 10, 20, 40, and 60 minutes. Common hepatic and bile ducts are dilated above an abrupt distal cutoff and tracer retention; however, biliary-to-bowel transit is present.

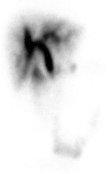 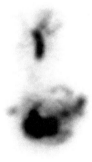

FIGURE 8-25. Partial biliary obstruction after cholecystectomy. HIDA images at 1 hour *(left)* and 2 hours *(right)*. At 1 hour considerable retained activity in the common duct and proximal ducts is seen. At 2 hours, the liver has cleared but, the common duct continues to retain activity. This patient had sphincter of Oddi obstruction that required subsequent sphincterotomy.

1 hour   2 hours

Various quantitative methods have been used to improve on image analysis—for example, bile duct half emptying time and percent emptying. One method uses sincalide as a pharmacological intervention before the study to improve diagnostic accuracy by increasing bile flow and stressing the capacity of the biliary ducts, thus bringing out more subtle abnormalities that might not otherwise be seen. The reported accuracy of the methodologies is varied, with no general consensus on the best method. One technique that incorporates image analysis and semiquantitative parameters is described (Fig. 8-26 and Box 8-15). It typically is used as a screening technique to determine if a patient needs more invasive diagnostic and therapeutic procedures.

TABLE 8-9 Differential Diagnosis of Primary Hepatic Tumors with Technetium-99m Hepatobiliary Iminodiacetic Acid

Lesion	Flow	Uptake	Clearance
Focal nodular hyperplasia	Increased	Immediate	Delayed
Hepatic adenoma	Normal	None	—
Hepatocellular carcinoma	Increased	Delayed	Delayed

Primary Benign and Malignant Tumors of the Liver

Liver tumors that contain hepatocytes take up Tc-99m HIDA. Thus cholescintigraphy can aid in the differential diagnosis of benign and malignant hepatic tumors—that is, focal nodular hyperplasia (FNH), hepatic adenoma, and hepatocellular carcinoma (Table 8-9).

Focal Nodular Hyperplasia and Hepatic Adenoma.

The presentation and therapy of these two benign tumors are quite different. FNH is usually asymptomatic, often discovered incidentally, and requires no specific therapy, whereas hepatic adenomas are often symptomatic and may cause serious hemorrhage that can be life threatening. Adenomas have a strong association with oral contraceptives; FNH has a weaker association.

FNH contains all hepatic cell types—that is, hepatocytes, Kupffer cells, and bile canaliculi. Characteristic findings seen with cholescintigraphy are increased blood flow, prompt hepatic uptake, and delayed clearance (Fig. 8-27). This characteristic pattern is seen in more than 90% of patients with FNH. Poor clearance may be due to abnormal biliary canaliculi. Evidence suggests that the overall accuracy is higher than the traditional Tc-99m sulfur colloid method used to diagnose FNH, which shows uptake in about two thirds of patients. Hepatic adenomas consist exclusively of hepatocytes; therefore it is surprising and not understood why it rarely exhibits uptake on cholescintigraphy. The benign tumors are cold.

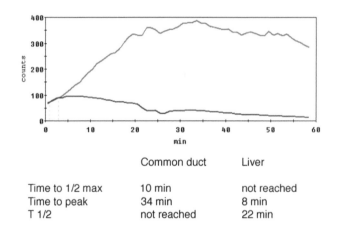

	Common duct	Liver
Time to 1/2 max	10 min	not reached
Time to peak	34 min	8 min
T 1/2	not reached	22 min

A

B

FIGURE 8-26. Sphincter of Oddi dysfunction. **A,** 2-minute sequential images demonstrate delayed clearance from the common duct. **B,** Regions of interest are drawn for the common duct and liver. *Below,* Time–activity curves of the common duct and liver. This patient had a scintigraphic score of 7, positive for sphincter of Oddi dysfunction. See Box 8-15 for the scoring method.

Box 8-15. Sphincter of Oddi Dysfunction: Sincalide and Semiquantification Protocol

PREPARATION
Fasting for 2 hours before study

COMPUTER SETUP
One-minute frames × 60

IMAGING PROTOCOL
1. Infuse sincalide 0.02 μg/kg × 10 minutes.
2. Fifteen minutes after sincalide infusion, inject 5 mCi Tc-99m HIDA intravenously.
3. Acquire 1-minute frames × 60 minutes (128 × 128).

COMPUTER PROCESSING ANALYSIS
1. Draw regions of interest around liver and common duct and derive time–activity curves.
2. Use image analysis for scoring. Time–activity curves provide ancillary information. Time–activity curves may sometimes help determine time to hepatic peak and percent of common bile duct emptying.

SCINTIGRAPHIC SCORING	SCORE
1. Peak liver uptake	
a. Less than 10 minutes	0
b. 10 minutes or greater	1
2. Time of biliary visualization	
a. Less than 15 minutes	0
b. Greater than 15 minutes	1
3. Prominence of biliary tract	
a. Not prominent	0
b. Prominence of major extrahepatic ducts	1
c. Prominence of major intrahepatic ducts	2
4. Bowel visualization	
a. Less than 15 minutes	0
b. 15 to 30 minutes	1
c. Greater than 30 minutes	2
5. CBD emptying	
a. More than 50%	0
b. Less than 50%	1
c. No change	2
d. Increasing activity	3
6. CBD-to-liver intensity ratio	
a. $CBD_{60\,min} \le liver_{60\,min}$	0
b. $CBD_{60\,min} > liver_{60\,min}$ but $< liver_{15\,min}$	1
c. $CBD_{60\,min} > liver_{60\,min}$ and $= liver_{15\,min}$	2
d. $CBD_{60\,min} >$ both $liver_{60\,min}$ and $liver_{15\,min}$	3

TOTAL SCORE ___

INTERPRETATION
Score of >5 is consistent with sphincter of Oddi dysfunction.*

*Sostre S, Kaloo AN, Spiegler EJ, et al. A noninvasive test of sphincter of Oddi dysfunction in postcholecystectomy patients: the scintigraphic score. *J Nucl Med*. 1992;33(6):1216–1222.
CBD, common bile duct.

Hepatocellular Carcinoma. Cholescintigraphy demonstrates characteristic findings with hepatocellular carcinoma (hepatoma). The malignant hepatocytes are hypofunctional compared to normal liver. Thus, during the first hour of imaging, no uptake is seen within the lesion (cold defect). Delayed imaging at 2 to 4 hours often shows filling in, or continuing uptake within the tumor, and concomitant clearing of adjacent normal liver (Fig. 8-28). This pattern is very specific for hepatoma. However, poorly differentiated hepatomas may not fill in on delayed imaging. Tc-99m IDA uptake may be seen at sites of hepatocellular metastases—for example, in the lung.

Enterogastric Bile Reflux

Cholescintigraphy can demonstrate bile reflux (Fig. 8-29). Some reflux may be seen in normal subjects on routine cholescintigraphy, particularly if morphine or sincalide has been administered. The more reflux and more persistent it is, the higher the likelihood that it is related to the patient's symptoms. Quantitative methods for estimating the amount of reflux have been described. Enterograstric reflux can produce an alkaline gastritis, seen most commonly after gastric resection surgery. Symptoms are often similar to those of acid-related disease.

■ TECHNETIUM-99M RED BLOOD CELL LIVER SCINTIGRAPHY

Cavernous hemangiomas are the most common benign tumor of the liver and the second most common hepatic tumor, behind liver metastases. They are usually asymptomatic and discovered incidentally on CT or ultrasonography during the workup or staging in a patient with a known primary malignancy or during evaluation of unrelated abdominal symptoms or disease. They require no specific therapy but must be differentiated from other more serious liver tumors.

Normal Hepatic Vascular Anatomy

The liver has a complex vascular system (Fig. 8-30). It receives two thirds to three fourths of its blood supply from the portal vein. The portal vein and hepatic artery flow into the liver sinusoids, which act as the capillary bed for the liver cells. Blood leaves the liver through the central veins and drain into the hepatic veins, emptying into the inferior vena cava.

Pathology

Cavernous hemangiomas of the liver consist of dilated, endothelium-lined vascular channels of varying sizes separated by fibrous septa. Histopathologically, they are not related to capillary hemangiomas, angiodysplasia, or infantile hemangioendotheliomas. Ten percent are multiple. Lesions larger than 4 cm are called giant cavernous hemangiomas.

Diagnostic Imaging

Noninvasive diagnosis of cavernous hemangioma of the liver can obviate the need for biopsy, which may result in hemorrhage and significant morbidity.

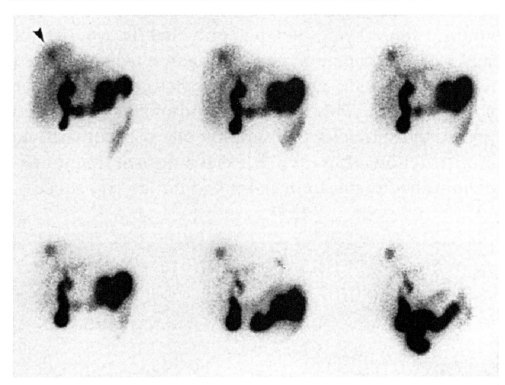

FIGURE 8-27. Focal nodular hyperplasia. Sequential 5-minute images show early uptake by the focal nodular hyperplasia tumor in the dome of the liver *(arrowhead)* that persists throughout the 60-minute study as the normal liver clears the tracer. Focal uptake persisted on delayed images at 3 hours.

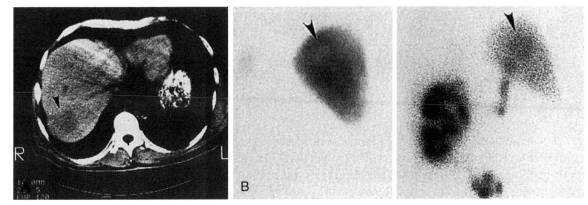

FIGURE 8-28. Hepatocellular carcinoma. **A,** CT shows a large mass in the posterior aspect of the right lobe *(arrowhead)*. **B,** *Left,* Tc-99m HIDA posterior view acquired at 5 minutes shows a cold defect in the same mass *(arrowhead)*. *Right,* Delayed images at 2 hours shows increased uptake within the lesion *(arrowhead)* compared to adjacent liver that is washing out. Surgery confirmed hepatocellular carcinoma.

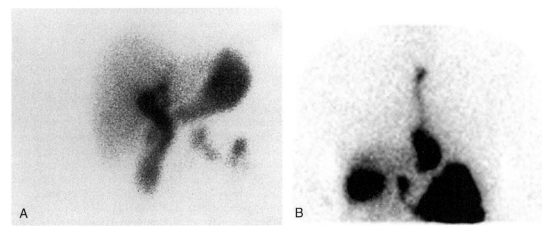

FIGURE 8-29. **A,** Enterogastric reflux. Sixty minutes after injection of Tc-99m IDA, reflux of labeled bile into the stomach. Bile gastritis was confirmed at endoscopy. **B,** Enterogastroesophageal reflux. The patient had a history of esophageal cancer and esophagectomy. Severe reflux into site of gastric pull-up occurred.

Ultrasonography

The typical sonographic pattern for hemangioma—a homogeneous, hyperechoic mass with well-defined margins and posterior acoustical enhancement—is neither sensitive nor specific for the diagnosis of cavernous hemangioma.

Computed Tomography

Strict CT criteria for hemangioma include hypoattenuation before intravenous contrast injection, early peripheral enhancement, progressive opacification toward the lesion center, and isodense fill-in usually by 30 minutes after contrast administration. Not all criteria are always satisfied. When these criteria are used to maximize specificity, the sensitivity of CT is 55%; less strict criteria result in a high false positive rate. Accuracy is poorer with multiple hemangiomas.

Magnetic Resonance Imaging

Cavernous hemangiomas have a characteristic appearance on magnetic resonance imaging (MRI) of high signal intensity on T2-weighted spin-echo images (light bulb sign). Gadolinium contrast shows findings similar to those seen with contrast CT. MRI is much more accurate than CT; however, various benign and malignant tumors can give false positive results. MRI is particularly useful for diagnosis of small lesions and those adjacent to major vessels or vascular organs.

Scintigraphy with Technetium-99m–Labeled Red Blood Cell

Scintigraphy has been used for decades to diagnose cavernous hemangiomas; it is less commonly used today because of the high accuracy of MRI. Dual-detector SPECT, Tc-99m red blood cell (RBC) imaging has good sensitivity and an extremely low false positive rate.

Radiopharmaceutical

Radiolabeling RBCs with Tc-99m pertechnetate is performed using methodology described in Chapter 13 in the discussion of gastrointestinal bleeding and labeling with Tc-99m RBCs.

Mechanism of Localization and Pharmacokinetics

After injection, Tc-99m RBCs take time to exchange and equilibrate within the large, relatively stagnant, nonlabeled blood pool of the hemangioma (Fig. 8-31). The equilibration time varies from 30 to 120 minutes. Early images typically show the cavernous hemangioma to be relatively cold, whereas delayed images will demonstrate increased uptake compared to that in liver.

Dosimetry

The total body radiation absorbed dose is approximately 0.4 rems (cGy). The target organ is the heart wall, which receives 1.2 rems (cGy), followed by the spleen and kidney (Table 8-4).

Methodology

With planar imaging, a three-phase study is performed with flow images, blood pool, and delayed multiple-view images (Box 8-16). Currently, SPECT during delayed imaging is mandatory for state-of-the-art Tc-99m RBC hepatic scintigraphy. Planar flow and early blood pool images are not necessary for diagnosis, although they illustrate characteristic pathophysiology.

Image Interpretation

Tc-99m RBC images should be correlated with anatomical imaging to ensure proper identification and interpretation of the abnormality.

Normal Distribution

With RBC blood pool imaging, organs with the highest activity are the heart, spleen, and kidney. The liver has less activity. The aorta, the inferior vena cava, and occasionally the portal vein can be seen with planar imaging. Portal branching vessels and hepatic veins can be seen with SPECT.

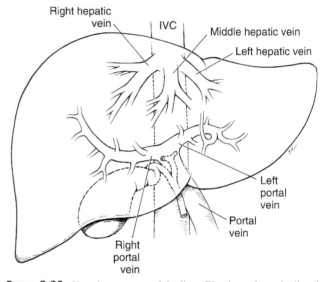

FIGURE 8-30. Vascular anatomy of the liver. Blood supply to the liver is largely from the portal vein (75%) and to a lesser extent from the hepatic artery (25%). Both enter the liver in the portal area. The hepatic artery and its branches are not shown. The portal vein divides into right and left branches and then subdivides. Smaller branches of portal vein with hepatic artery branches and canaliculi define the periphery of lobules (Fig. 8-1). Hepatic veins originate at the lobule center (central veins), feeding into right, middle, and left hepatic veins, which drain into the inferior vena cava *(IVC)*.

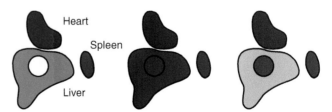

FIGURE 8-31. RBC schematic diagram of radiotracer pharmacokinetics that occur with liver hemangioma. *Left,* Immediately after injection the hemangioma is "cold." Time is required for the radiolabeled RBCs to equilibrate with the unlabeled RBCs in the blood pool volume of the hemangioma. *Middle,* As the Tc-99m–labeled RBCs increasingly enter the hemangioma and mix with the unlabeled cells, activity in the hemangioma becomes equal to normal liver. *Right,* When fully equilibrated (60-120 minutes), activity within the hemangioma exceeds that in the surrounding liver and is equal to activity in the heart and spleen.

Diagnostic Criteria

Radionuclide blood flow imaging typically shows normal arterial flow to a cavernous hemangioma. Immediate blood pool images show decreased activity within the hemangioma compared with adjacent liver. Early increased inhomogeneous uptake as a result of rapid

---

Box 8-16. Technetium-99m Red Blood Cell Liver Hemangioma Scintigraphy: Protocol Summary

PATIENT PREPARATION
None

RADIOPHARMACEUTICAL
Tc-99m RBCs (in vitro kit method), 25 mCi (925 MBq)
Inject Tc-99m–labeled RBCs intravenously; bolus injection for flow images

INSTRUMENTATION
Camera: large-field-of-view with SPECT capability
Energy window: 15% to 20% centered over 140-keV photopeak
Collimator: Low energy, high resolution, parallel hole

IMAGE ACQUISITION
Planar Imaging
1. Blood flow: 1-second frames for 60 seconds on computer and 2-second film images.
2. Immediate images: 750k to 1000k count planar image in same projection and other views as necessary to best visualize lesion(s).
3. Delayed images: 750k to 1000k count planar static images 1 to 2 hours after injection in multiple projections (anterior, posterior, lateral, and oblique views).
4. SPECT or SPECT/CT.

CT, Computed tomography; *SPECT,* single-photon emission computed tomography.

---

equilibrium is sometimes seen (Fig. 8-32). On 1- to 2-hour delayed imaging, hemangiomas show increased activity compared with that of adjacent liver. Activity is often equal to that of the blood pool of the heart and spleen. Giant cavernous hemangiomas may show heterogeneity of uptake on delayed images, with areas of both decreased and increased uptake. These cold regions, often located centrally, are caused by thrombosis, necrosis, and fibrosis. Benign and malignant liver tumors, abscesses, cirrhotic nodules, and cysts have decreased activity compared to that of normal liver (Fig. 8-33).

Accuracy

Tc-99m RBC scintigraphy has a positive predictive value approaching 100%—that is, a positive test is likely to be a true positive. Very few false positive study results have been reported.

Tc-99m RBC sensitivity for detection of cavernous hemangiomas depends primarily on lesion size and the imaging method used. SPECT is superior to planar imaging because of its improved contrast resolution (Fig. 8-34). It is especially useful for the detection of small hemangiomas, those located centrally in the liver, multiple hemangiomas, and those adjacent to the heart, kidney, and spleen. In seven comparison studies, the mean overall sensitivity for planar imaging was 55% and for SPECT, 88%.

Lesion size and location are critical determinants of detectibility (Table 8-10). Planar imaging can detect hemangiomas down to about 3 cm. Single-headed SPECT has good sensitivity for hemangiomas 2 cm and larger, whereas multidetector SPECT can visualize almost all hemangiomas larger than 1.4 cm and may be diagnostic for some as small as 0.5 cm, although sensitivity for detection is reduced (Table 8-10). SPECT/CT allows for better anatomical localization (Fig. 8-35).

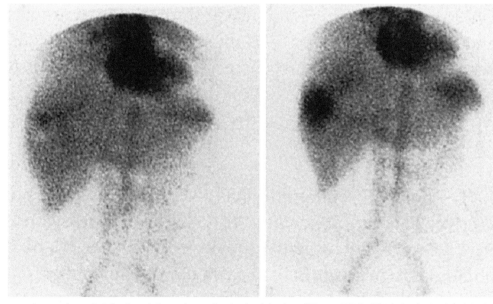

FIGURE 8-32. Cavernous hemangioma. *Left,* Static early image immediately after injection of Tc-99m RBCs. The lesion in the right lobe is partly cold and partly showing early filling. *Right,* Delayed image at 2 hours shows increased activity in the lesion compared to background liver, almost equal to heart blood pool.

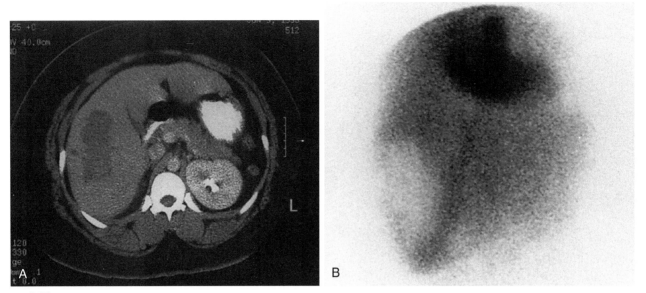

FIGURE 8-33. Negative Tc-99m RBC study for hemangioma. **A,** CT scan shows a large lesion in right lobe of the liver. **B,** Planar Tc-99m RBC scan is cold in the same region and negative for hemangioma. The diagnosis was metastatic colon cancer.

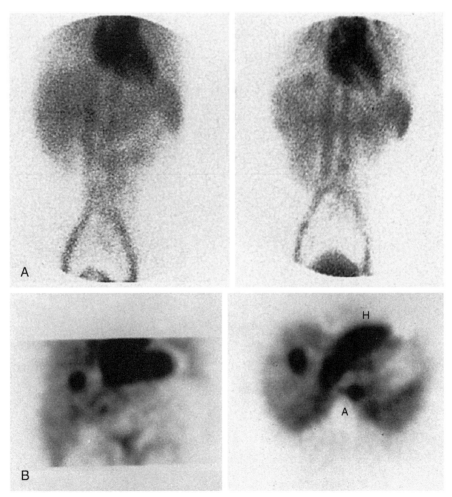

FIGURE 8-34. Improved visualization of hemangioma with SPECT. **A,** *Left,* Immediate postinjection planar image shows neither decreased nor increased uptake, probably because of small lesion size. *Right,* After 1.5-hour delay, planar study shows mildly increased focal uptake in the liver dome. **B,** SPECT coronal *(left)* and transverse *(right)* sections are strongly positive for hemangioma with high target-to-background ratio. *A,* Aorta; *H,* heart.

■ TECHNETIUM-99M SULFUR COLLOID LIVER AND SPLEEN IMAGING

Tc-99m sulfur colloid liver and spleen imaging was introduced in 1963 and became the standard clinical method for liver and spleen imaging until the advent of CT. Although not a frequently requested study today, it still has a few important clinical indications.

Mechanism of Localization and Pharmacokinetics

After intravenous injection, the Tc-99m–labeled sulfur colloid particles, 0.1 to 1.0 μm, are extracted from the blood by reticuloendothelial cells, the Kupfer cells of the liver (85%), and macrophages of the spleen (10%) and bone marrow (5%). Tc-99m sulfur colloid has a single-pass liver extraction efficiency of 95% and a blood clearance half-life of 2 to 3 minutes. Uptake is complete by 15 minutes. After phagocytosis, the Tc-99m sulfur colloid particles are fixed intracellularly.

Kupffer cells line the walls of the liver sinusoids (Fig. 8-1), make up less than 10% of liver cell mass, and are fixed phagocytic cells. However, most liver diseases affect hepatocytes and Kupffer cells similarly, causing local, diffuse, or heterogeneously decreased uptake as a result of destruction or displacement of normal liver. With severe diffuse liver disease, a generalized reduction in hepatic extraction and increased uptake by the spleen and bone marrow occur (*colloid shift*). Increased splenic uptake can be seen with immunologically active states.

Preparation

Tc-99m sulfur colloid is available in kit form and takes only 15 minutes to prepare. Acid is added to a mixture of Tc-99m pertechnetate and sodium thiosulfate, which is heated in a water bath (95°-100° F) for 5 to 10 minutes. Labeling efficiency is greater than 99%.

TABLE 8-10 Sensitivity for Hemangioma Detection by Lesion Size with Multiheaded Single-Proton Emission Computed Tomography

Lesion (cm)	Sensitivity (%)
>1.4	100
>1.3	91
1.0-2.0	65
0.9-1.3	33
0.5-0.9	20

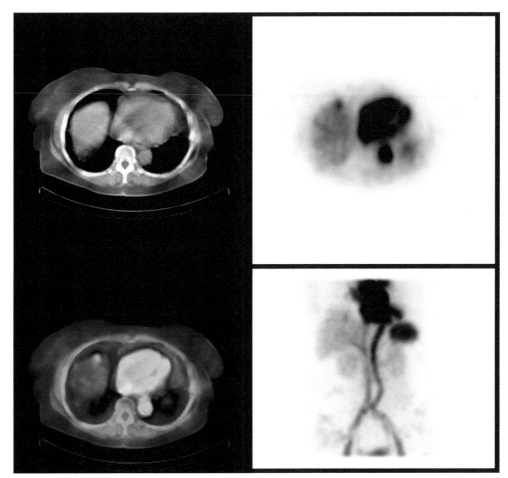

FIGURE 8-35. SPECT/CT cavernous hemangioma. Small focus of mildly increased Tc-99m RBCs on the MIP image *(bottom right)*. Small hypodense lesion seen on CT *(left upper)*. SPECT *(upper right)* shows increased focal uptake in anterior aspect of the dome of the liver. The fused SPECT/CT transverse image nicely confirms the cavernous hemangioma.

Dosimetry

Estimated radiation dose from Tc-99m sulfur colloid is 1.7 rem (cGy) to the liver and 1.1 rem (cGy) to the spleen (Table 9-3).

Clinical Applications

Currently, the clinical role for Tc-99m silver colloid liver and spleen imaging is in situations in which the functional study can add diagnostic information—for example, cirrhosis, focal nodular hyperplasia, and splenosis.

Methodology

No patient preparation is required. Imaging acquisition begins 15 to 20 minutes after Tc-99m sulfur colloid injection. Planar images are obtained in multiple views. SPECT is often performed. A standard protocol is described (Box 8-17).

Image Interpretation

Abnormal scintigraphic findings include hepatomegaly, heterogeneity of distribution, splenomegaly, colloid shift, focal defects, and focal increased uptake. Hepatomegaly is a nonspecific finding that suggests hepatic dysfunction or an infiltrating process.

Splenic uptake on the posterior view is normally equal to or less than that of the liver. Colloid shift (relatively increased splenic uptake compared to that in the liver) occurs in some hepatic diseases, such as cirrhosis (Fig. 8-36). A quantitative spleen-to-liver count ratio greater than 1.5 is abnormal. Bone marrow uptake is often not seen with optimal settings to view liver and spleen.

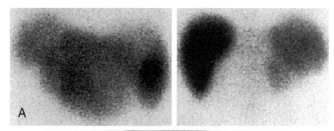

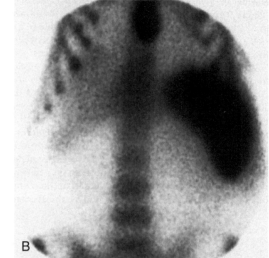

FIGURE 8-36. Hepatic parenchymal disease with Tc-99m sulfur colloid. **A**, 52-year-old man with hyperpigmentation and biopsy-proved hemochromatosis. Anterior *(left)* and posterior *(right)* views show small right lobe, hypertrophied left lobe, large spleen, and colloid shift. **B**, Severe cirrhotic liver disease. Anterior view shows very small liver with poor uptake, enlarged spleen, and prominent colloid shift to the marrow and spleen.

Liver
Decreased Uptake

Most benign and malignant lesions of the liver produce cold or "photopenic" defects on Tc-99m sulfur colloid liver imaging (Box 8-18 and Fig. 8-37). Radiation therapy results in characteristic rectangular port-shaped hepatic defect. Diffusely decreased uptake is usually caused by hepatocellular disease, although infiltrating tumor involvement appears similar.

Alcoholic liver disease involves the liver diffusedly, as will fatty infiltration, acute alcoholic hepatitis, and cirrhosis. Thus common findings are hepatomegaly, heterogeneous uptake, and colloid shift (Fig. 8-36). The scan pattern is related to the degree of pathological condition and the presence or absence of portal hypertension. With increasing severity, the liver, particularly the right lobe, shrinks; the left lobe compensates with hypertrophy, and colloid shift becomes marked.

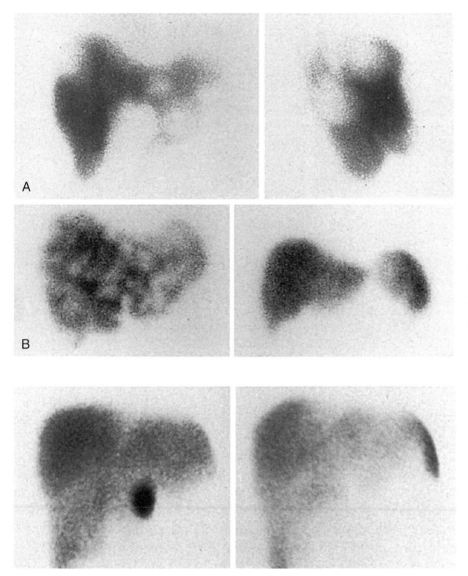

FIGURE 8-37. Colon cancer metastases on Tc-99m sulfur colloid scan. **A,** Anterior and right lateral views show large metastases in the right and left lobes. **B,** In another patient, extensive liver metastases are seen on initial Tc-99m sulfur colloid study *(left)*, and good response to therapy is seen on follow-up 4 months later *(right)*.

FIGURE 8-38. Liver hot spot in superior vena cava syndrome. *Left,* Tc-99m sulfur colloid liver spleen scan in a patient with lung cancer. Hot spot in the region of the quadrate lobe. Radiotracer was injected in the arm. *Right,* Repeat study with radiotracer injected in lower extremity shows that no hot spot is present.

Increased Uptake

Increased hepatic uptake on Tc-99m sulfur colloid imaging is uncommon but quite characteristic for specific pathological conditions (Box 8-18).

Superior Vena Cava Obstruction. Collateral thoracic and abdominal wall vessels communicate with the recanalized umbilical vein delivering Tc-99m sulfur colloid via the left portal vein to the region of the quadrate lobe. Thus relatively more concentrated Tc-99m sulfur colloid is delivered to that region compared to the remainder of the liver, producing a hot spot (Fig. 8-38). This same phenomenon is seen occasionally on fluorodeoxyglucose positron emission tomography (FDG-PET) and Tc-99m macroaggregated albumin (MAA) lung perfusion studies. Injection in the lower extremity rather than the upper extremity results in a normal scan.

Focal Nodular Hyperplasia. FNH typically has increased Tc-99m sulfur colloid uptake because of the vascular nature of the tumor and increased density of functioning Kupffer cells. This tumor has all three hepatic cell types. Tc-99m sulfur colloid uptake is seen in two thirds of patients (Fig. 8-39) with FNH (one third with increased

uptake and one third with normal uptake). Another third are cold, for unclear reasons. Hepatic adenoma is usually cold, comprising only hepatocytes.

Budd-Chiari Syndrome. Hepatic vein thrombosis is characterized by relatively more uptake in the caudate lobe than the remainder of the liver (Fig. 8-40). The impaired venous drainage of most of the liver results in poor hepatic function. The caudate lobe retains good function because of its direct venous drainage into the inferior vena cava.

▄ SPLEEN SCINTIGRAPHY

The spleen serves as a reservoir for formed blood elements, as a site for clearance of microorganisms and particle trapping, as a potential site of hematopoiesis during bone marrow failure, and as a source of humoral or cellular response to foreign antigens. It plays a role in leukocyte production, contributes to platelet processing, and has immunological functions.

Radionuclide imaging can confirm splenic remnants, accessory spleens, splenosis, splenules, polysplenia-asplenia

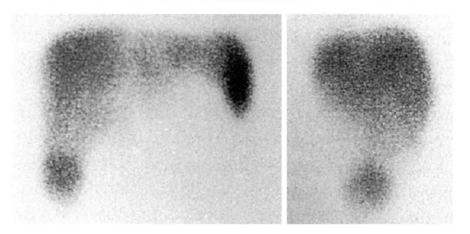

FIGURE 8-39. Focal nodular hyperplasia. Anterior *(left)* and right lateral *(right)* views show increased uptake in lesion at inferior tip of right lobe of liver. Angiography confirmed the diagnosis of focal nodular hyperplasia.

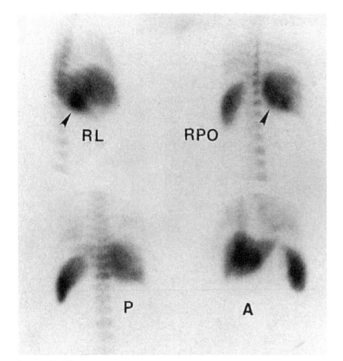

FIGURE 8-40. Budd-Chiari syndrome. Increased uptake of Tc-99m sulfur colloid in region of caudate lobe *(arrowheads)* in patient with hepatic vein thrombosis. Images acquired in the right lateral *(RL)*, right posterior oblique *(RPO)*, posterior *(P)*, and anterior *(A)* projections. Note increased marrow uptake (colloid shift).

syndromes, and splenic infarction. Tc-99m sulfur colloid is commonly used. Imaging with heat or chemically damaged Tc-99m is less frequently used, but can be useful to detect accessory spleens or splenosis immediately adjacent to the liver (Figs. 8-41 and 8-42).

Nonvisualization of the spleen may result from congenital absence or from acquired functional asplenia caused by interruption of the blood supply (splenic artery occlusion) or secondary to reticuloendothelial system (RES) dysfunction (sickle cell crisis). Asplenia may be irreversible (Thorotrast irradiation, chemotherapy, amyloid) or functionally reversible (sickle cell crisis). With sickle cell disease, discordance is seen between RES function and other splenic functions.

▬ TECHNETIUM-99M MACROAGGREGATED ALBUMIN HEPATIC ARTERIAL PERFUSION SCINTIGRAPHY

Oncologists have used regional intraarterial therapy to treat primary and metastatic cancer since the 1960s. The advantage of a selective intraarterial approach is based on the dual blood supply to the liver. As a tumor in the liver grows, it derives most of its blood supply from the hepatic artery, whereas normal liver cells are supplied predominantly by the portal circulation. Intraarterial chemotherapy, chemoembolization, and therapeutic radiolabeled microspheres deliver therapy directly to the tumor, thus minimizing exposure to normal liver and to drug-sensitive dose-limiting tissues (e.g., gastrointestinal epithelium and bone marrow), often the source of side effects from conventional intravenous chemotherapy.

Successful application of intraarterial therapy requires that it be reliably and safely delivered to the tumor. Contrast arteriography is used to position the therapeutic catheter; however, it is not a good indicator of blood flow at the capillary level. High flow rates required for angiography often do not reflect the actual physiological perfusion pattern of the tumor and liver. A high-pressure contrast bolus may result in streaming, reflux, or retrograde flow.

Incorrect positioning of the intraarterial catheter results in inadequate distribution to the tumor-involved liver and possible extrahepatic flow to the stomach, pancreas, spleen, and bowel. This may be due to problems of catheter placement or normal vascular anatomical variation. Tc-99m MAA infused into the hepatic artery catheter can estimate the adequacy of blood flow to the tumor and determine the presence or absence of extrahepatic perfusion, a frequent cause of gastrointestinal and systemic toxicity. Scintigraphy can also quantify arteriovenous shunting to the lung. This is most important before the infusion of therapeutic yttrium-90–radiolabeled therapeutic microspheres (Therasphere, SIR-Sphere) to minimize pulmonary irradiation.

Mechanism of Localization

Tc-99m MAA particles are larger than capillary size (range, 10-90 μm; mean, 30-50 μm). When infused into the hepatic artery, they distribute according to blood flow and are trapped

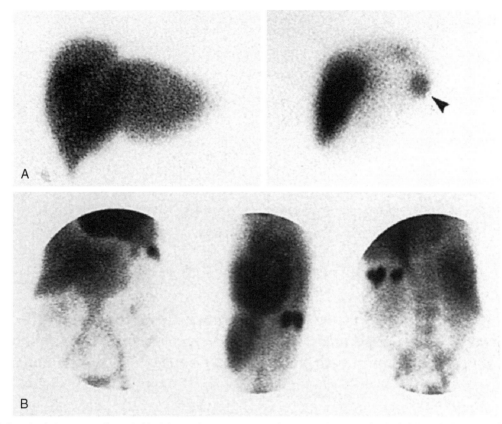

FIGURE 8-41. Splenosis. **A,** Tc-99m sulfur colloid with splenic remnant postsplenectomy best seen in the left lateral view *(arrowhead).* **B,** Autotransplantation of splenic tissue after trauma. Chemically damaged Tc-99m RBCs. Uptake in the left upper quadrant (anterior, left lateral, posterior views). Tc-99m–labeled RBCs and patient after splenectomy. Multiple foci of uptake in the left upper quadrant consistent with splenosis. Patient had prior posttrauma splenectomy.

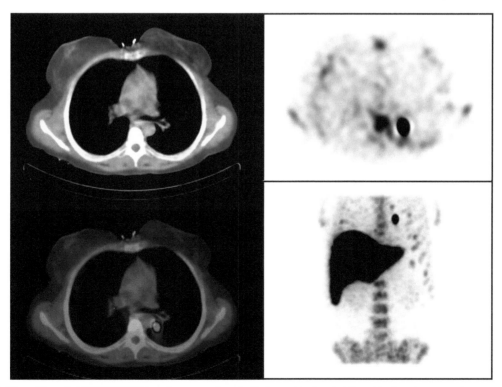

FIGURE 8-42. Tc-99m sulfur colloid SPECT/CT in pulmonary splenosis. Patient with chronic idiopathic thrombocytopenic purpura had persistently low platelet count in spite of splenectomy and predisone therapy. Several masses in her chest were confirmed to be splenic tissue.

on first pass in the arteriolar-capillary bed of the liver. The irregularly shaped and malleable particles partially occlude a small percentage of the liver capillary bed, break down into smaller particles (half-life of 4-6 hours), and eventually are taken up by macrophages or cleared through the kidney.

Methodology

After placement of the hepatic arterial catheter via contrast angiography, a small volume of Tc-99m MAA is slowly infused. The procedure is described in Box 8-19. Planar imaging is adequate to quantify right to left shunting. SPECT and SPECT/CT can sometimes aid in confirming or excluding extrahepatic perfusion—for example, to the stomach.

Study Interpretation

The typical pattern of intrahepatic tumor perfusion on Tc-99m MAA studies is greater uptake in the tumor than in normal liver (tumor-to-nontumor uptake ratio 3:1). Small tumor nodules show uniform uptake (Fig. 8-43, *A*), whereas larger tumors often have increased uptake at the periphery of the tumor and relatively decreased uptake centrally because of necrosis (Fig. 8-43, *B*). This hypervascular peripheral rim of tumor is where active growth occurs (neovascularity).

Symptoms of extrahepatic perfusion include pain, nausea, vomiting, or bleeding caused by gastritis, ulceration, and hemorrhage. Adverse symptoms are seen more commonly

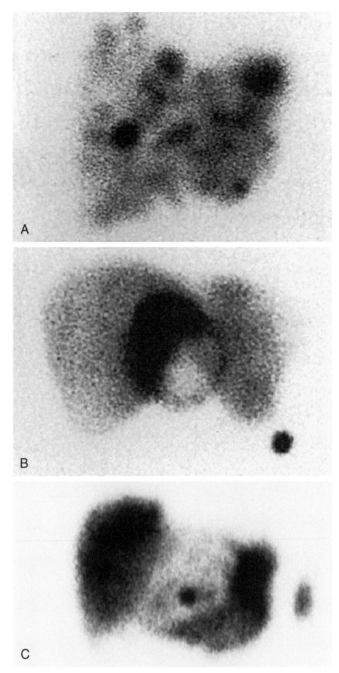

FIGURE 8-43. Tc-99m MAA hepatic arterial perfusion scintigraphy. **A,** Patient with colon cancer and liver metastases. Tc-99m MAA study shows solid tumor nodules involving both lobes of liver. **B,** Hyperperfusion of the periphery of the large tumor mass with a large, cold, necrotic center. **C,** Poor perfusion to the left lobe and extrahepatic perfusion to the stomach and small portion of spleen. The focal hot spot adjacent to the stomach is due to a small thrombus at the constant chemotherapy infusion catheter tip.

in patients with extrahepatic perfusion than those without it (70% vs. 20%). Extrahepatic perfusion on Tc-99m MAA perfusion imaging is seen as uptake in the stomach, spleen, or bowel (Fig. 8-43, *C*).

Although a small amount of atriventricular shunting to the lungs is common (1%-10%), abnormal shunting of 20% to 40% may occur (Fig. 8-44). For therapy with Y-90 microspheres, this can result in significant pulmonary irradiation and likely would require a reduction in administered dose.

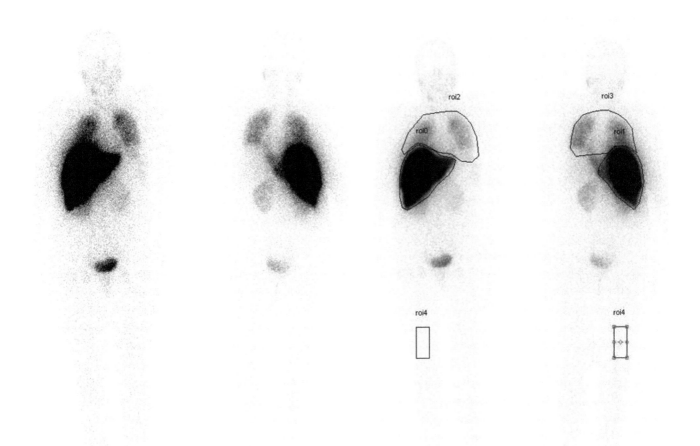

FIGURE 8-44. Hepatic shunting to the lung with calculation of percent lung shunt. Patient with colon cancer metastatic to the liver, unresponsive to chemotherapy, underwent this study before treatment with Theraspheres. Tc-99m MAA was injected via the hepatic artery catheter. Whole-body imaging was acquired. Regions of interest were selected for the lungs, liver, and background. The calculated shunting to the lung was 9%.

■ SUGGESTED READING

DiBaise JK, Richmond BK, Ziessman HA, et al. Cholecystokinin-cholescintigraphy in adults: consensus recommendations of an interdisciplinary panel. *Clin Nucl Med.* 2012;37(1):63-70.

Choy D, Shi EC, McLean RG, et al. Cholescintigraphy in acute cholecystitis: use of intravenous morphine. *Radiology.* 1984;151(1):203-207.

Fig LM, Stewart RE, Wahl RL. Morphine-augmented hepatobiliary scintigraphy in the severely ill: caution is in order. *Radiology.* 1990;175(2):473-476.

Sostre S, Kaloo AN, Spiegler EJ, et al. A noninvasive test of sphincter of Oddi dysfunction in postcholecystectomy patients: the scintigraphic score. *J Nucl Med.* 1992;33(6):1216-1222.

Yap L, Wycherley AG, Morphett AD, Toouli J. Acalculous biliary pain: cholecystectomy alleviates symptoms in patients with abnormal cholescintigraphy. *Gastroenterology.* 1991;101(3):786-793.

Ziessman HA. Acute cholecystitis, biliary obstruction, biliary leakage. *Sem Nucl Med.* 2003;33(4):279-296.

Ziessman HA. Functional hepatobiliary disease: chronic acalculous gallbladder disease and chronic acalculous biliary disease. *Sem Nucl Med.* 2006;36(2):119-132.

Ziessman HA, Muenz LR, Agarwal AK, ZaZa A. Normal values for sincalide cholescintigraphy: comparison of two methods. *Radiology.* 2001;221(2):404-410.

Ziessman HA, Tulchinsky M, Lavely WC, et al. Sincalide-stimulated cholescintigraphy: a multicenter investigation to determine optimal methodology and gallbladder ejection fraction normal values. *J Nucl Med.* 2010;51(2):229-236.

CHAPTER 9

Genitourinary System

Since the 1950s, it has been possible to measure renal function with radiopharmaceuticals. Techniques have evolved from urine counting and crude probe detectors to measurements of plasma clearance, dynamic functional imaging, and single-photon emission computed tomography (SPECT) cortical imaging. In recent years, some indications previously reserved for renal scintigraphy have been shifted to ultrasound, computed tomography (CT), or magnetic resonance imaging (MRI). However, the ability to image and quantify function can provide information not available by anatomical imaging methods. Nuclear medicine techniques still provide the best problem-solving tools in many clinical situations.

Indications for renal scintigraphy (Box 9-1) include differentiating obstructive from nonobstructive hydronephrosis, assessing the significance of renal artery stenosis, searching for postoperative leaks, and the evaluation of infection and scarring. Quantifying differential function and assessing viability is useful in the evaluation of complications that can occur after surgery or trauma. The ability to quantify function by effective renal plasma flow (ERPF) and glomerular filtration rate (GFR) can provide a better measurement of function than estimations based on serum creatinine.

Over the years, many radiopharmaceuticals have been developed to assess different aspects of renal function based on binding characteristics and clearance pathways. It is critical to have a solid understanding of renal anatomy and physiology to perform and interpret these examinations correctly.

RENAL ANATOMY AND FUNCTION

The kidneys are responsible for regulating water and electrolyte balance, excreting waste, secreting hormones (renin, erythropoietin), and activating vitamin D. They lie in the posterior abdomen at the level of L1-3, with the right kidney often slightly inferior to the left. The outer cortex contains the glomeruli and proximal convoluted tubules. The renal pyramids, consisting of the collecting tubules and the loops of Henle, make up the medulla. At the apex of the pyramids, papillae drain into the renal calyces. Cortical tissues between the pyramids are known as the columns of Bertin (Fig. 9-1, *A*).

The renal artery supplies blood flow to the kidney. End arterioles lead to tufts of capillaries forming glomeruli in the renal cortex (Fig. 9-1, *B*). The most proximal end of the renal tubule, Bowman capsule, surrounds the glomerulus. Each kidney contains more than 1 million of these basic functional units of the kidney—the nephron.

Normally, the kidneys receive 20% of cardiac output, with renal plasma flow (RPF) averaging 600 mL/min. The kidneys clear the plasma and body of waste products. The clearance, or rate of disappearance, of a substance can be measured as:

$$\text{Clearance (mL/min)} =$$
$$\frac{\text{Urine concentration (mg/mL)} \times \text{Urine flow (mL/min)}}{\text{Plasma concentration (mg/mL)}}$$

Box 9-1. **Clinical Indications for Genitourinary Scintigraphy**

Blood flow abnormalities
Function quantification
   Differential function
   Glomerular filtration rate, effective renal plasma flow
Mass vs. column of Bertin
Obstruction: Uteropelvic junction, ureteral
Pyelonephritis
Renal failure: Acute and chronic
Renovascular hypertension/renal artery stenosis
Renal vein thrombosis
Surgical complications
Transplant rejection
Transplant anastomosis assessment
Trauma
Vesicoureteral reflux
Volume quantification: Bladder residual volume

Plasma clearance occurs by glomerular filtration and tubular secretion (Fig. 9-2). If an agent undergoes 100% first-pass extraction, it can be used to measure RPF. However, because the actual extraction possible clinically is less than 100%, the term *effective renal plasma flow* (ERPF) is used to describe the measurement.

Approximately 20% of RPF (120 mL/min) is filtered through the semipermeable membrane of the glomerulus. A pressure gradient created by the RPF and resistance in the vessel drives filtration from the vascular space into the renal tubules. Larger material, such as protein-bound compounds, will not be filtered, whereas small molecules with a polar charge will be filtered. The resulting ultrafiltrate consists of water and crystalloids but no colloids or cells. The molecule inulin is the gold standard for glomerular filtration measurement.

The remaining plasma moves into the efferent arteriole, where active secretion occurs at the tubular epithelial cells. Molecules that could not be filtered may be cleared into the tubular lumen by active tubular secretion. Overall, tubular secretion accounts for 80% of renal plasma clearance. Paraaminohippurate (PAH) is the classic method for measuring ERPF because its high extraction mirrors the distribution of RPF—20% of PAH is cleared by glomerular filtration, and 80% is secreted into the renal tubules. PAH is actively secreted by anionic transporters on the proximal convoluted tubular cell membranes. It is not metabolized or retained in the kidney and is not highly protein-bound, so plasma extraction is high. However, PAH does have some plasma protein binding so clearance is 85% to 95%.

When urine passes along the tubule, essential substances such as glucose, amino acids, and sodium are conserved. The filtrate is concentrated because 65% of the water filtered at the glomerulus undergoes reabsorption in the proximal convoluted tubule. Active sodium pumping in the loop of Henle sets up an osmotic gradient allowing water to passively diffuse back into the interstitium. The remaining concentrated urine passes down the renal tubule, through the papillae of the medullary pyramids, and into the calyces. The calyces empty into the renal pelvis, and urine passes down the ureter into the bladder.

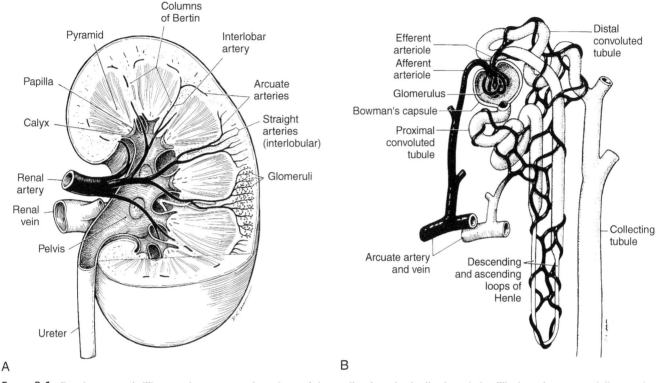

FIGURE 9-1. Renal anatomy. **A,** The outer layer or cortex is made up of glomeruli and proximal collecting tubules. The inner layer, or medulla, contains pyramids made up of distal tubules and loops of Henle. The tubules converge at the papillae, which empty into calyces. The columns of Bertin, between the pyramids, are also cortical tissue. The renal artery and vein enter and leave at the hilus. The interlobar branches of the renal artery divide and become the arcuate arteries, which give rise to the straight arteries, from which arise the afferent arterioles that feed the glomerular tuft. **B,** The nephron consists of afferent vessels leading to the tuft of capillaries in the glomerulus, the glomerulus itself, and efferent vessels. Bowman capsule surrounds the glomerulus and connects to the proximal and distal renal tubules and loops of Henle.

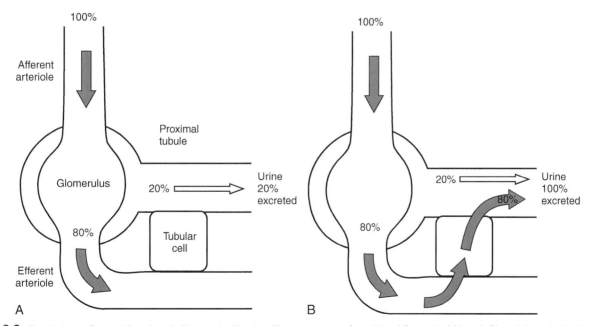

FIGURE 9-2. Renal plasma flow and function. **A,** Glomerular filtration. Twenty percent of renal blood flow to the kidney is filtered through the glomerulus. **B,** Tubular secretion. The remaining 80% of renal plasma flow is secreted into the proximal tubules from the peritubular space.

■ RENAL RADIOPHARMACEUTICALS

Numerous radiopharmaceuticals have been developed over the years that can assess renal function, some by measuring clearance in blood samples and others by imaging on a gamma camera (Box 9-2). Renal radiopharmaceuticals are classified by their uptake and clearance mechanisms as agents for glomerular filtration, tubular secretion, or cortical binding. A list of currently important renal imaging agents is found in Table 9-1. Because of their different clearance mechanisms (Fig 9-3), characteristic renal imaging patterns vary considerably (Fig. 9-4), as do clinical protocols used.

Technetium-99m Mercaptoacetyltriglycine

In the past, iodine-131 and subsequently I-123 hippuran were used to image and quantify renal function. Hippuran had a high first-pass extraction of 85%, but image quality was poor. Once Tc-99m mercaptoacetyltriglycine (MAG3) received approval from the U.S. Food and Drug Administration (FDA), it rapidly replaced hippuran.

Currently, Tc-99m MAG3 is the most commonly used renal radiopharmaceutical (Fig. 9-5). It is cleared almost entirely by tubular secretion and therefore does not measure

GFR. The extraction efficiency is considerably higher than that of filtration agents, which results in better performance and less radiation exposure when function is compromised. Tc-99m MAG3 images show significant anatomical detail while assessing function (Figs. 9-6 and 9-7).

Pharmacokinetics

Because Tc-99m MAG3 is protein-bound and not filtered, it is exclusively cleared from the kidney by tubular secretion. It has a much higher first-pass extraction than a glomerular filtration agent such as Tc-99m diethylenetriaminepentacetic acid (DTPA). Plasma protein binding is 97% for Tc-99m MAG3, keeping Tc-99m MAG3 in the vascular space and improving renal target-to-background ratios compared to those of Tc-99m DTPA. However, the clearance is only about 60% that of hippuran. The alternative path of Tc-99m MAG3 excretion is via the hepatobiliary route. Liver activity and biliary tract clearance are frequently noted. The normal time to peak activity is 3 to 5 minutes, with a time to half peak ($T_{1/2}$) of 6 to 10 minutes. Clearance is bi-exponential, and in patients with normal renal function, 90% of the dose is cleared in 3 hours.

Technetium-99m Diethylenetriaminepentaacetic Acid

The clinical applications of Tc-99m DTPA and Tc-99m MAG3 are often interchangeable, because they can both

---

Box 9-2. Agents Used to Quantify Renal Function

AGENTS FOR GLOMERULAR FILTRATION RATE
C-14 or H-3 inulin
I-125 diatrizoate
I-125 iothalamate
Co-57 vitamin B_{12}
Cr-51 EDTA
In-111 or Yb-169 DTPA
Tc-99m DTPA

AGENTS FOR EFFECTIVE RENAL PLASMA FLOW
H-3 or C-14 paraaminohippurate (PAH)
I-125 or I-131 iodopyracet
I-123, or I-131 orthoiodohippurate (hippuran)
Tc-99m mercaptoacetyltriglycine (MAG3)

TABLE 9-1 Mechanism of Uptake for Renal Scintigraphy Imaging Agents

Clearance	Agent	(%)
Glomerular filtration	Tc-99m DTPA	100
Tubular secretion	Tc-99m MAG3	100
Tubular secretion and glomerular filtration	I-131 hippuran	80 tubular
		20 filtered
Cortical binding	Tc-99m DMSA	40-50

DMSA, Dimercaptosuccinic acid; *DTPA*, diethylenetriaminepentacetic acid; *MAG3*, mercaptoacetyltriglycine.

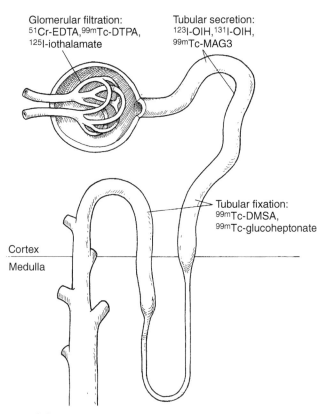

Glomerular filtration:
^{51}Cr-EDTA, ^{99m}Tc-DTPA, ^{125}I-iothalamate

Tubular secretion:
^{123}I-OIH, ^{131}I-OIH, ^{99m}Tc-MAG3

Tubular fixation:
^{99m}Tc-DMSA, ^{99m}Tc-glucoheptonate

Cortex
Medulla

FIGURE 9-3. Different mechanisms of renal radiopharmaceutical uptake and excretion include glomerular filtration, tubular secretion, and cortical tubular binding.

examine flow and renal function. However, only Tc-99m DTPA can be used to calculate GFR. Images also differ because the higher background activity and slower clearance lead to inferior images in comparison with Tc-99m MAG3. In cases in which renal function is impaired, the difference in quality is significant, and in such cases, target-to-background ratios may be so poor that no diagnostic information is gained. The lower extraction efficiency also results in higher patient radiation doses, which is particularly significant in cases of renal failure.

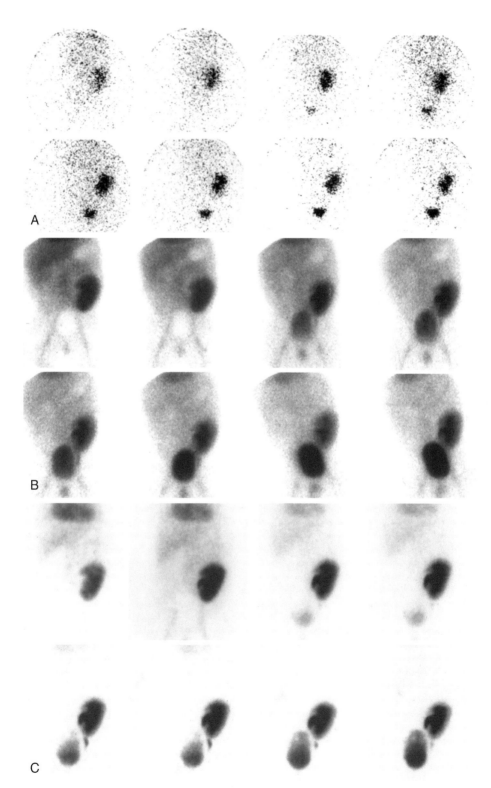

FIGURE **9-4.** Radiopharmaceutical comparison in a renal transplant patient. **A,** I-131 hippuran provides excellent functional information but has poor image quality compared to technetium agents. **B,** Tc-99m DTPA image from the same day shows higher resolution. **C,** Tc-99m MAG3 done 30 hours later reveals the highest level of detail as well as an improved target-to-background ratio compared to DTPA.

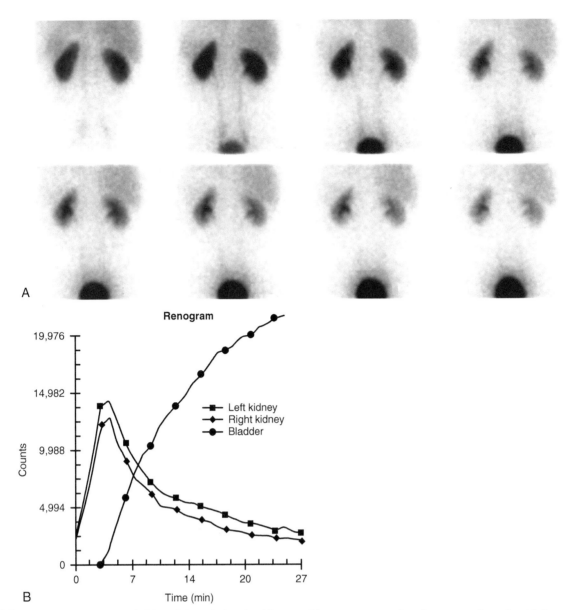

Figure 9-5. Normal Tc-99m MAG3. **A,** Normal dynamic functional images with prompt symmetric radiotracer uptake and rapid clearance over the study. **B,** Normal time-activity curves with a steep uptake slope, distinct peak, and rapid clearance confirming image analysis.

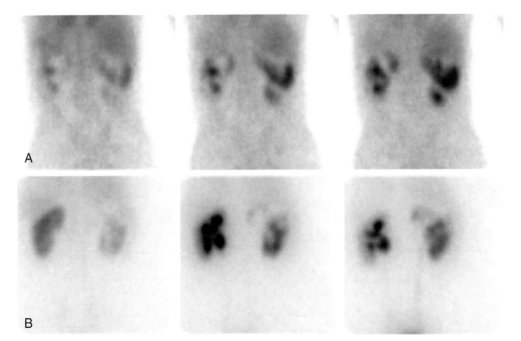

Figure 9-6. Abnormal Tc-99m MAG3 examples revealing cortical anatomic detail. **A,** Multiple cortical defects are seen throughout the examination from polycystic kidney disease in poorly functioning kidneys. **B,** Asymmetric cortical uptake, decreased on the right, with a right upper pole scar in a patient with a history of reflux and infection.

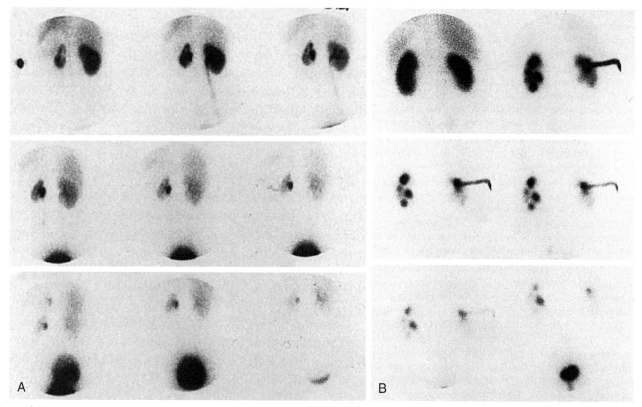

FIGURE 9-7. Abnormalities detected during the dynamic function portion of Tc-99m MAG3 imaging. **A,** Small scarred left kidney secondary to vesico-ureteral reflux contributes only 15% to overall function. **B,** Obstructed right kidney secondary to cervical carcinoma is draining well through a nephrostomy tube, and bilateral function is good. Prominent left pelvis and calyces mostly clear by the end of the study. The last image was taken with the bladder in view.

Chemistry and Radiolabeling
Technetiium-99m Diethylenetriaminepentaacetic Acid
DTPA is a heavy metal chelator used for treatment of poisoning. Like other chelators, it is cleared via glomerular filtration. A simple radiolabeling kit is available containing stannous tin as a reducing agent. The reduced Tc-99m forms a strong bond with DTPA. Contaminants such as hydrolyzed and oxidized Tc-99m (free pertechnetate) can be readily identified by chromatography.

Technetium-99m Mercaptoacetyltriglycine
A radiolabeling kit is used that entails adding sodium pertechnetate to a reaction vial. A small amount of air is added to the reaction vial to consume excess stannous ion for increased stability. Radiolabeling efficiency is 95%.

Pharmacokinetics
Following intravenous injection, normal peak cortical uptake occurs by 3 to 4 minutes. By 5 minutes, the collecting system is seen; the bladder is typically visualized by 10 to 15 minutes. The $T_{1/2}$ peak, or the time it takes for half of the maximal cortical activity to clear, is normally 15 to 20 minutes for Tc-99m DTPA.

Tc-99m DTPA is completely filtered at the glomerulus, with no tubular secretion or reabsorption. Because only 20% of renal function is the result of glomerular filtration, the first-pass extraction of a glomerular filtration agent is less than that of agents cleared by tubular secretion. In practice, normal first-pass Tc-99m DTPA extraction is less than the 20% of RPF because of factors such as the level of protein binding. The extraction fraction is only 40% to 50% that of Tc-99m MAG3.

The rate of Tc-99m DTPA clearance depends on the amount of impurities in the preparation, which bind to protein in the body. Protein binding leads to underestimation of GFR. Different preparations of Tc-99m DTPA may show highly variable protein binding that should be controlled. Although Tc-99m DTPA generally underestimates GFR, it is adequate for clinical use if properly prepared.

Technetium-99m Dimercaptosuccinic Acid

Renal cortical imaging with Tc-99m dimercaptosuccinic acid (DMSA) is most commonly used today to detect renal scarring or acute pyelonephritis and provide accurate differential renal function. Although other radiopharmaceuticals have been used for cortical imaging in the past, only Tc-99m DMSA is currently used clinically today.

The rapid transit of most renal radiopharmaceuticals such as Tc-99m DTPA and Tc-99m MAG3 does not allow high-resolution imaging of the cortex. On the other hand, the stable cortical uptake of Tc-99m DMSA produces high-quality images using either pinhole imaging (Fig. 9-8) or single-photon emission computed tomography (SPECT). Delayed imaging results in high target-to-background ratios and good resolution.

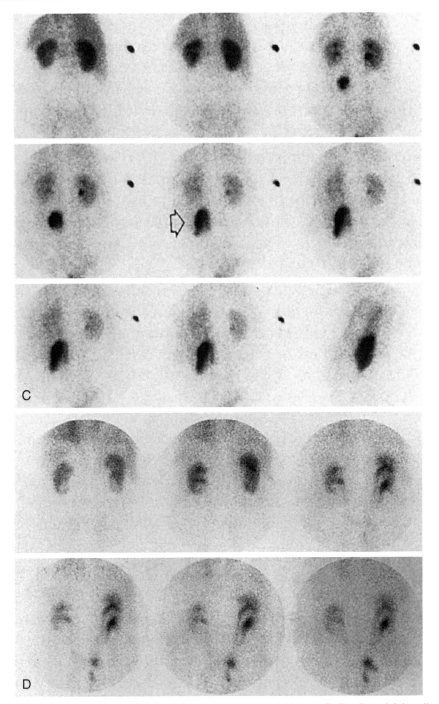

Figure 9-7, cont'd. C, Postoperative ureteral leak on left *(arrow)* detected on sequential images. **D,** Duplicated right collecting system, a congenital abnormality sometimes associated with lower pole reflux and upper pole obstruction.

Radiolabeling

A radiolabeling kit is available using stannous ion for Tc-99m pertechnetate reduction. The introduction of air can cause degradation of the label and increased background activity, including in the liver. Tc-99m DMSA radiolabeling produces multiple forms of the Tc-99m DMSA complex, which may vary slightly in their clearance.

Pharmacokinetics

Roughly 40% to 50% of the injected Tc-99m DMSA dose localizes in the cortex, predominantly in the proximal tubules. Imaging is generally done after a 2- to 3-hour delay to allow time for slow background clearance. In cases of decreased renal function, further delay may be needed. The low level of urinary excretion is not adequate for assessment of the collecting system and lower urinary tract.

Diseases affecting the proximal tubules, such as renal tubular acidosis and Fanconi syndrome, inhibit Tc-99m DMSA uptake. Nephrotoxic drugs, including gentamicin and cisplatinum, also may inhibit uptake. In patients with poor renal function, target-to-background ratios may be so poor that no useful diagnostic information can be gained.

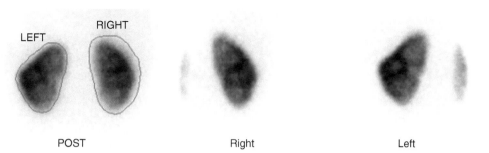

FIGURE 9-8. Normal appearance of the kidneys in a child using Tc-99m DMSA.

TABLE 9-2 Dosimetry for Renal Radionuclides

Organ	Tc-99m DTPA (mSv/MBq)		Tc-99m MAG3 (mSv/MBq)		Tc-99m DMSA (mSv/MBq)	
	Adult	5 yr	Adult	5 yr	Adult	5 yr
Kidney	0.0057	0.014	0.0041	0.0097	0.19	0.45
Bladder wall	0.077	0.86	0.14	0.0015	0.015	0.02
Marrow	0.0022	0.0050	0.0011	0.17	0.0041	0.0095
Effective dose	0.0082	0.012	0.012	0.015	0.016	0.039

Data from Radiation dose estimate to adults and children from common radiopharmaceuticals. Oak Ridge, TN: Radiation Internal Dose Information Center; 1996).
DMSA, Dimercaptosuccinic acid; *DTPA,* diethylenetriaminepentacetic acid; *MAG3,* mercaptoacetyltriglycine.

Dosimetry

Although the radiation dose to the patient from renal radiopharmaceuticals is low when renal function is normal, the absorbed dose rises significantly in the obstructed kidney or when renal function fails. Dosimetry of the important renal radiopharmaceuticals is listed in Table 9-2.

■ DYNAMIC RENAL IMAGING TECHNIQUES

Renal protocols must be tailored for specific clinical applications. This section provides a basic approach to these techniques and modifications.

Dynamic Renography

Dynamic functional studies are generally acquired in two parts. Renal blood flow is assessed in the first pass of the radiopharmaceutical bolus to the kidney. Then, over the next 25 to 30 minutes, uptake and clearance assess function. Similar protocols can be used for the dynamic functional agents Tc-99m DTPA and Tc-99m MAG3 (Box 9-3).

Method
Patient Preparation

Patients should be well hydrated before the study. While blood flow, radiopharmaceutical uptake, or functional calculations (ERPF or GFR) are not altered, excretion and washout can be delayed by dehydration, simulating obstruction or poor function.

It is important to document all medications the patient has taken that may affect the study, such as diuretics and

BOX 9-3. Protocol Summary for Dynamic Renal Scintigraphy

PATIENT PREPARATION
Hydration: Begin 1 hour before examination; give fluids over 30 minutes
Adults: Drink 300-500 mL water
Children: Intravenous hydration 10-15 mL/kg ⅓ normal saline (with 5% dextrose <1 years)
Void bladder before injection

RADIOPHARMACEUTICAL
Tc-99m MAG3
Children: 0.1 mCi/kg (3.7 MBq/kg), minimum dose 1 mCi (37 MBq)
Adult: 2.5-5 mCi (93-185 MBq)
Tc-99m DTPA
Children: 0.05 mCi/kg (1.9 MBq/kg), minimum dose 1 mCi (37 MBq)
Adults: 5-10 mCi (185-370 MBq)

INSTRUMENTATION
Gamma camera: Large field of view
Collimator: Low energy, high resolution, parallel hole
Photopeak: 15%-20% window centered over 140 keV

POSITIONING
Routine renal: Supine, camera posterior
Renal transplant: Camera anterior over allograft

COMPUTER ACQUISITION
Blood flow: 1- to 2-second frames for 60 seconds
Dynamic: 30-second frames for 25-30 minutes
Prevoid image: 500k count
Postvoid image

PROCESSING
Draw region of interest around kidneys.
Draw background area next to each kidney.
Generate time-activity curves for flow and dynamic phases.
Generate differential function calculation.

blood pressure medicines. Any known anatomic anomalies and prior interventions are important factors to consider in positioning and image interpretation.

In cases of neurogenic bladder or bladder outlet obstruction, bladder catheterization should be considered. This helps relieve retrograde pressure, which can cause delayed upper urinary tract washout. Catheterization is also often helpful infants and children who cannot void voluntarily.

Patient Positioning

A supine position is preferred because kidneys are frequently mobile (or "ptotic") and can move to the anterior pelvis when patients are upright. Patients are placed so that the kidneys are closest to the camera, with the camera posterior for normal native kidneys and anterior for transplants, pelvic kidneys, and horseshoe kidneys.

Dose

The administered dose of radiopharmaceutical varies with the agent. Doses of Tc-99m MAG3 range from 2 to 5 mCi (74-185 MBq). For Tc-99m DTPA, higher amounts are generally used, ranging from 10 to 20 mCi (370-740 MBq).

Image Acquisition

After a bolus injection of radiopharmaceutical, the image acquisition begins when activity is about to enter the abdominal aorta. Images are acquired at a rate of 1 to 3 seconds per frame for 60 seconds to assess renal perfusion. Then images are acquired at 60 seconds per frame for 25 to 30 minutes to evaluate parenchymal radiotracer uptake and clearance.

Computer Processing of Renal Studies

The uptake and clearance of radiopharmaceuticals is a dynamic process. Mentally integrating all the information in the many images of a renal scan is challenging, even for experienced clinicians. Computer-generated time-activity curves (TACs) provide a dynamic visual presentation of changes in activity over the course of the study. Usually, separate TACs are drawn for the blood flow and dynamic function portions of the study.

Perfusion Time-Activity Curve

The first-pass perfusion TAC shows the blood flow to each kidney compared with arterial flow. A region of interest is drawn around each kidney and the closest major artery (aorta for native kidneys, iliac artery for transplanted kidneys) on the initial 60-second portion of the study. Although absolute flow (milliliters per kilogram per minute) cannot be calculated with the radiotracers discussed, relative flow can be visualized or calculated using the upslope of the perfusion curve. A ratio of the activity compared to the aorta or kidney to arterial (K/A) ratio can help follow changes in perfusion.

Dynamic Renal Function Time-Activity Curve

A TAC is generated for the remaining portion of the examination by drawing on the computer a region of interest (ROI) around each kidney (Fig. 9-9). The selection of kidney ROI depends on the information needed. Whole-kidney regions can be used if the collecting system clears promptly. When a whole-kidney ROI is used in a patient with retained activity in the collecting system, clearance will appear delayed on the TAC. In cases of hydronephrosis and obstruction, a 2-pixel-wide peripheral cortical region of interest, excluding the collecting system, can be helpful, although some overlap with calyces is inevitable.

Various methods of background correction have been employed using a 2-pixel-wide region of interest. It may be placed beneath the kidneys, around the kidneys, or in a crescent configuration lateral to the region of interest. Background correction is less critical with delayed images, such as those obtained with Tc-99m DMSA, because of their high target-to-background ratio.

At any point in time, the renogram represents a summation of uptake and excretion. Three phases are normally seen in TACs. These include blood flow, cortical uptake, and clearance phases (Fig. 9-10). The TAC must be

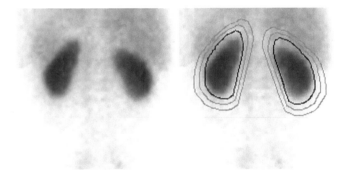

FIGURE 9-9. Regions of interest (ROI) for time-activity curves. *Left,* An image at 3 minutes with peak cortical activity is chosen for the ROIs. *Right,* Regions of interest are drawn for the kidney (*dark lines*) and for background correction (*gray lines*).

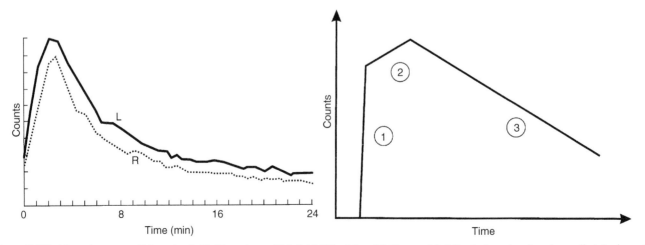

FIGURE 9-10. Normal renogram (*left*) can be divided into phases. *Right,* Initial blood flow (30-60 seconds). *2,* Cortical uptake phase (normally 1-3 minutes). *3,* Clearance phase representing cortical excretion and collecting system clearance.

interpreted in conjunction with the images because the curves may be affected by many factors, such as retained activity in hydronephrosis, which can alter the slope.

Numerous values can be derived from TACs and are used to help track functional changes. These include time to peak activity, uptake slope, rate of clearance, and percent clearance at 20 minutes. Ratios such as the cortical activity at 20 minutes divided by the peak activity (20/peak) and the amount of activity at 20 minutes by the activity at 3 minutes (20/3) are relative but can help follow function over time. For example, when a 20/3 gets very high (e.g., greater than 0.8), this suggests obstruction or marked cortical retention caused by a variety of disease conditions.

Differential Function

Differential or split function is a universally performed calculation. This calculation is particularly useful because estimated GFR and serum creatinine may not identify unilateral lesions (Fig 9-11). From the ROI drawn after the

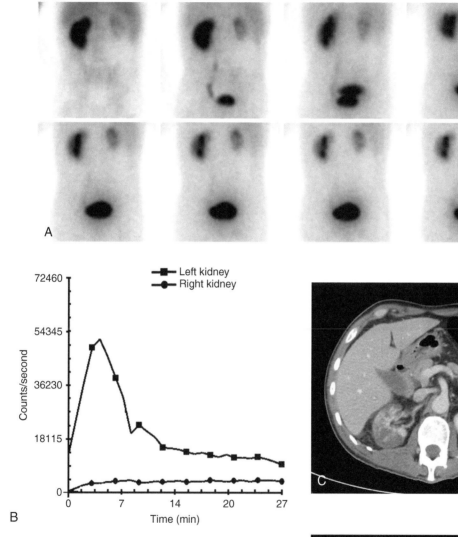

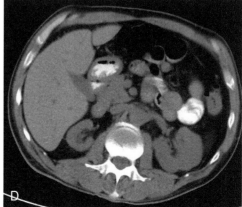

FIGURE 9-11. Differential function and viability. **A,** Tc-99m MAG3 images and time-activity curve **(B)** acquired shortly after injury from a car accident show little function in the right kidney (calculated at 6%). **C,** Postcontrast CT on admission revealed flow to the kidney but severe cortical injury. **D,** 3 months later, a non-contrast CT shows chronic effects with the right kidney, now small and scarred.

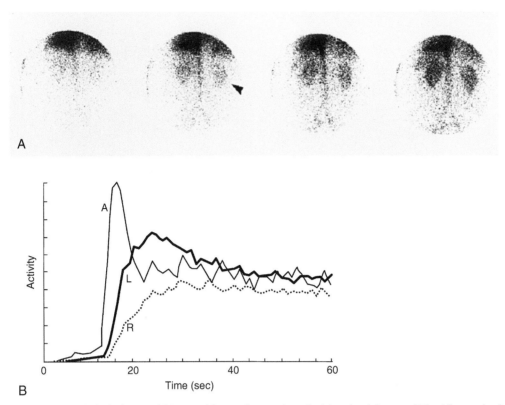

FIGURE 9-12. Renal blood flow analysis. **A,** Sequential 2-second frames show moderately delayed and decreased blood flow to the right kidney *(arrowhead).* **B,** Sixty-second time-activity curves confirm the imaging findings. Initial upslope of the right kidney *(R)* is delayed compared with the aorta *(A)* and left kidney *(L).*

blood flow phase and before excretion into collecting system (at the peak nephrogram activity 1 to 3 minutes after injection), the actual counts in each kidney are expressed as a fraction of 100% total function. Normally, the relative contribution for each kidney lies between 45% to 55%. This value does not indicate whether the overall or global renal function is normal or abnormal. A calculation of GFR or ERPF can be done as a separate study to quantify actual function.

Interpretation
Flow Phase
Blood flow to the kidneys is normally seen immediately after flow appears in the adjacent artery. In practice, arterial flow can be judged by the first few 2-sec flow frames. It is important to assess the quality of the injection bolus, because delayed renal visualization may be artifactual, as a result of suboptimal injection technique. If the slope of the arterial TAC is not steep or if activity visibly persists in the heart and lungs, the injection may have been given over too long a period. Any asymmetry in tracer activity suggests abnormal perfusion to the side of decreased or delayed activity. A smaller or scarred kidney will have less flow as a result of a decrease in parenchymal tissue volume (Fig. 9-12).

Cortical Function Phase
Normal kidneys accumulate radiopharmaceutical in the parenchymal tissues in the first 1 to 3 minutes. The cortex should appear homogeneous. The calyces and renal pelvis are either not seen in this initial phase or appear relatively photopenic. If decreased function is present on one side,

the rate of uptake and function are often delayed on that side relative to the better functioning kidney. This produces a "flip-flop" pattern; the poorly functioning side initially has lower uptake, but the cortical activity on later images is higher than on the better functioning side, which has already excreted the radiotracer. Cortical retention, or delayed cortical washout, is a nonspecific finding, occurring in acute and chronic renal failure (Fig. 9-13).

Clearance Phase
The calyces and pelvis usually begin filling by 3 minutes. Over the next 10 to 15 minutes, activity in the kidney and collecting system decreases. With good function, most of the radiotracer clears into the bladder by the end of the study. In some healthy subjects, pooling of activity in the dependent calyces can result in focal hot spots that usually clear at least partially over time. Lack of clearance or overlap of pelvocalyceal structures on the cortex suggests hydronephrosis. Because areas with increased activity appear larger, caution must be taken in diagnosing hydronephrosis on scintigraphic studies.

The normal ureter may or may not be seen. Prolonged, unchanging, or increasing activity suggests dilation. Because peristalsis and urine flow rates cause such variable visualization, care must be taken in diagnosing reflux into the ureters when activity remains in the kidney. On these studies, indirect determination of reflux can be done when ureteral activity persists after the kidneys have cleared. However, reflux is best detected on a direct vesicoureterogram (VCUG) with activity introduced directly into the bladder via a catheter.

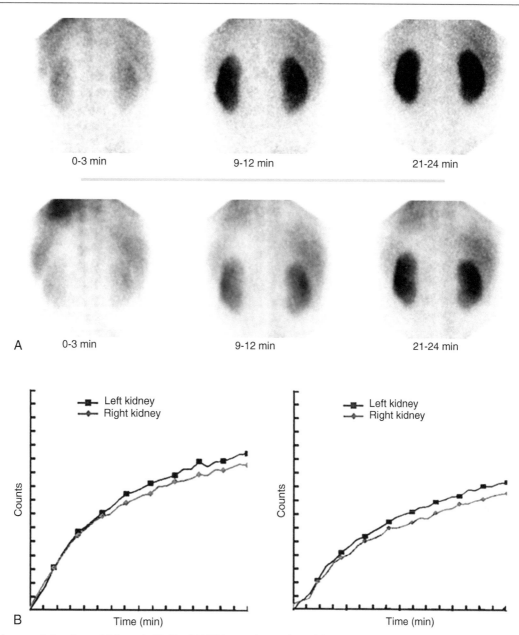

FIGURE 9-13. Acute and chronic renal failure. **A,** Tc-99m MAG3 images in a patient with newly elevated creatinine initially showed slow uptake and clearance with bilateral cortical retention *(top row)*. It is not possible to predict whether any improvement can be expected. No improvement occurred 6 months later, and uptake slightly diminished as function gradually worsened *(bottom row)*. **B,** The time-activity curves show poor uptake and clearance with a slight worsening between the two studies, with a more gradually rising slope on the right. In long-standing renal failure, uptake tends to diminish over time with kidneys appearing small, scarred, and less intense. *cts,* Counts.

The bladder must be monitored as well. Prevoid and postvoid bladder images evaluate emptying and postvoid residual. A distended bladder can cause an obstructed pattern. In a patient with neurogenic bladder or outlet obstruction, the renal scan is best performed with a urinary catheter in place. In infants and small children, the bladder may appear quite large and higher in position than might be expected when looking at the outline of the child's body

Clinical Applications of Renal Scintigraphy

Because the renal scan can monitor function over time and provides some quantitative information, it can provide data difficult to get by other means. Functional information

from the scan is often needed after trauma or vascular procedure. In many patients, the nuclear medicine scintigram compliments anatomical assessment done with CT, ultrasound, or angiography.

Urinary Tract Obstruction
Background
Obstruction can lead to recurrent infection, diminished function, progressive loss of nephrons, and parenchymal atrophy. Upper urinary tract obstruction results in backpressure from the pelvis onto the tubules and vessels. Within hours of onset, renal blood flow, glomerular filtration, and renal output are decreased. If a high-grade obstruction is corrected promptly, function can recover

fully; however, if it is left uncorrected for more than a week, only partial recovery is expected.

Ultrasound is a sensitive method of identifying hydronephrosis but cannot reliably indicate whether the dilation is due to mechanical obstruction or merely nonobstructive hydronephrosis (such as from reflux, primary megaureter, or a previous obstruction that has been relieved). Retrograde pyelography, endoscopy, and CT scans often can identify the cause of an obstructed system such as a ureteral calculus or tumor. However, assessment of the residual function and of the effects of treatment using radionuclide imaging is still often important. Contrast studies such as intravenous pyelogram and conventional radionuclide renography show findings that overlap between obstructed and nonobstructed systems: delayed filling, dilation, and decreased washout.

In a dilated system, prolonged retention of contrast or radiopharmaceutical is seen because of a reservoir effect. The addition of furosemide (Lasix) to the protocol allows accurate identification of patients affected by obstruction. Furosemide, a loop diuretic that inhibits sodium and chloride reabsorption, markedly increases urine flow and washout in normal patients. If mechanical obstruction is present, the narrowed lumen prevents augmented washout; prolonged retention of tracer proximal is seen and can be quantified on the time-activity curves. The ability to perform quantitation is an important advantage of functional radiotracer studies over those done with intravenous contrast dye. Box 9-4 lists conditions for which furosemide renography is indicated.

Methods

Numerous protocols for diuretic renography exist, and attempts to standardize methodology have been made by comparing data from multiple institutions, resulting in several consensus papers. Although some variability still exists among institutions, many general areas have been agreed on. An example protocol is listed in Box 9-5.

The furosemide injection is given slowly over 1 to 2 minutes, with an onset of action within 30 to 60 seconds, and a maximal effect is seen at 15 minutes. The time of diuretic administration varies at different centers—for example, 20 minutes after the radiopharmaceutical (F+20), at the same time as the radiopharmaceutical (F+0), and 15 minutes before the study (F-15). A commonly used method is the F+20 furosemide protocol, which allows an identifiable of washout of pooled activity. However, earlier administration may be useful in cases with diminished renal function, because this gives additional time for the diuretic effect to occur allowing radiotracer washout.

Interpretation

The interpretation of diuretic renography can be complex (Box 9-6). In a normal, nondilated kidney, the TAC rapidly reaches a sharp peak and spontaneously clears rapidly. Furosemide diuresis accelerates the rate of radiotracer washout in a normal kidney. If a region of interest is placed over the ureter, a transient spike after diuretic injection indicates passage of a bolus of accumulated activity from the renal pelvis.

A dilated but nonobstructed system may initially look like a normal kidney with a steep TAC uptake slope. However, a sharp peak is not seen and, as the dilated system fills, the TAC may show continued accumulation or a plateau 20 to 30 minutes after tracer injection. After furosemide infusion, a nonobstructed hydronephrotic kidney clears promptly as a result of increased urine flow (Fig. 9-14). An obstructed system, on the other hand,

---

Box 9-4. Urological Conditions Studied by Diuresis Renography

Ureteropelvic junction obstruction	Urethral valves
Megaureter: Obstructive, nonobstructive, refluxing	Postoperative states
	Pyeloplasty
	Ureteral reimplantation
	Urinary diversion
Horseshoe kidney	Renal transplant ureteral obstruction
Polycystic kidney	
Prune-belly syndrome	Obstructing pelvic mass
Ectopic ureterocele	Ileal loop diversion

Box 9-5. Diuretic Renography: Protocol Summary

PATIENT PREPARATION
Hydration should be as described in dynamic renography protocol.
Place Foley catheter in children; consider in adults.
If not catheterized, complete bladder emptying before diuretic injection.

FUROSEMIDE DOSE
Children: 1 mg/kg to maximum 40 mg (may require more in severe azotemia)
Adults: Base dose on creatinine level

Serum Creatinine (mg/dL)	Creatinine Clearance (mL)	Furosemide Dose (mg)
1.0	100	20
1.5	75	40
2.0	50	60
3.0	30	80

IMAGING PROCEDURE
Inject Tc-99m MAG 3-5 mCi (111-185 MBq).
Acquire study for 20 minutes.
Slowly infuse furosemide intravenously over 60 seconds.
Continue imaging 10 to 30 min.
Obtain prevoid and postvoid image in uncatheterized patients.

IMAGE PROCESSING
On computer, draw region of interest around entire kidney and pelvis.
Generate time-activity curves.
Calculate a half-emptying time or fitted half-time.

will not respond to the diuretic challenge; activity will continue to accumulate or sometimes stays at a plateau (Fig. 9-15). Different patterns can be seen in response to furosemide (Fig 9-16).

The distinction between obstruction and nonobstructed hydronephrosis decreases as the collecting system volume becomes larger. In very distended systems, delayed washout may be seen regardless of whether obstruction is present. An "indeterminate" clearance pattern is seen with little change on the images or TAC (Fig. 9-16, *D*).

Diuretic response may also be diminished in patients with azotemia. An increased furosemide dose or early diuretic infusion (F-15) may be used. However, even with additional modifications, it may not be possible to induce sufficient diuresis to exclude obstruction in a poorly functioning kidney (Figs. 9-17 and 9-18). Although elevated serum creatinine may indicate severe renal dysfunction, GFR or ERPF may be more accurate, especially is the lesion is unilateral. If the GFR on the affected side is less than 15 mL/min, diuretic renography is unreliable.

At times, it is useful to quantitate collecting system clearance half time or washout half time ($T_{1/2}$). Numerous

BOX 9-6. Diuretic Renography Pearls and Pitfalls

Diminished response to furosemide
  Dehydration
  Pressure from distended bladder
  Massive hydronephrosis
  Azotemia
  Infants
    Insufficient time for diuretic action
Diuretic given at T0 or before Tc-99m MAG3
  Acts steadily, does not give visible drop in curve
  $T_{1/2}$ values not applicable
  Useful with azotemia
Uteropelvic junction may present with partial obstruction, but often detected on serial examinations.
Use of diuretics in patients with spinal cord injury can result in dangerous hypotension.
Postoperative obstruction in renal transplants can be best assessed with diuretic scans.
  External fluid collections
  Anastamotic swelling or stricture

MAG3, Mercaptoacetyltriglycine.

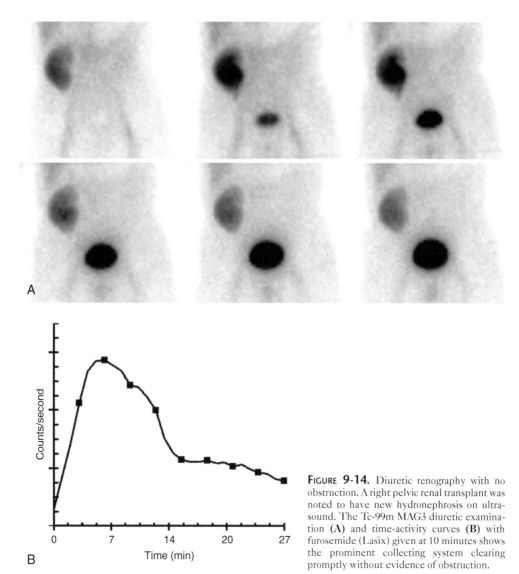

FIGURE 9-14. Diuretic renography with no obstruction. A right pelvic renal transplant was noted to have new hydronephrosis on ultrasound. The Tc-99m MAG3 diuretic examination (**A**) and time-activity curves (**B**) with furosemide (Lasix) given at 10 minutes shows the prominent collecting system clearing promptly without evidence of obstruction.

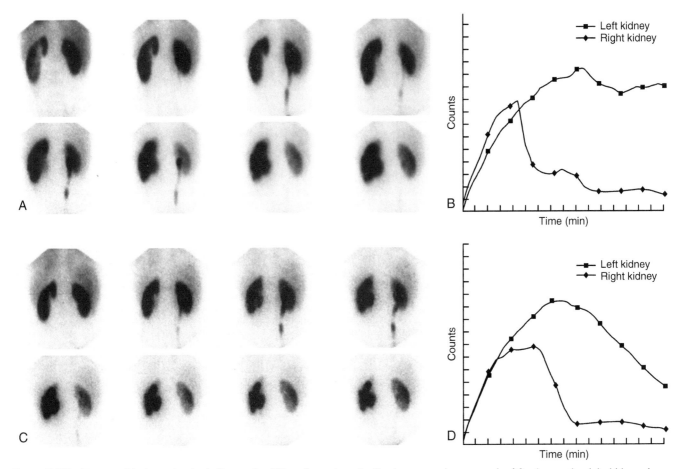

FIGURE 9-15. Obstructed hydronephrosis. **A,** Progressive filling of an enlarged collecting system is seen on the *left*, whereas the right kidney clears normally following furosemide (Lasix) administration at 10 minutes. **B,** Time-activity curves (TACs) show washout on the *right* but no overall clearance on the *left*, consistent with obstruction. **C,** Diuretic renography images following surgical correction of the left ureteropelvic junction obstruction in the same patient show hydronephrosis but improved uptake and clearance. **D,** Postoperative TACs are useful, confirming that no significant obstruction remains on the left.

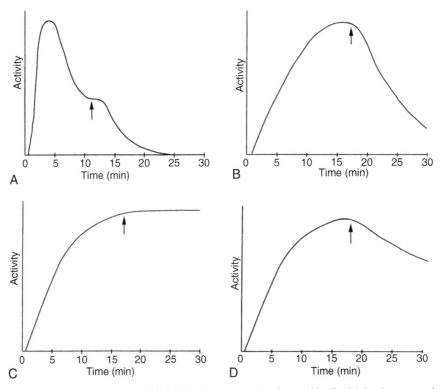

FIGURE 9-16. Diuresis renography time-activity curves (TACs). In these examples, furosemide (Lasix) is given at peak collecting system filling *(arrows)*. **A,** Normal kidney response to diuretic. The short plateau before further emptying represents diuretic-induced flow just before rapid clearance. **B,** Dilated nonobstructed kidney. The slowly rising curve represents progressive pelvocaliceal filling. With diuretic *(arrow)*, rapid clearance occurs. **C,** Obstructed kidney. The diuretic has no effect on the abnormal TAC. **D,** Indeterminate response. Following diuretic, very slow partial clearance is seen. This can be the result of an extremely distended system, but obstruction is not excluded.

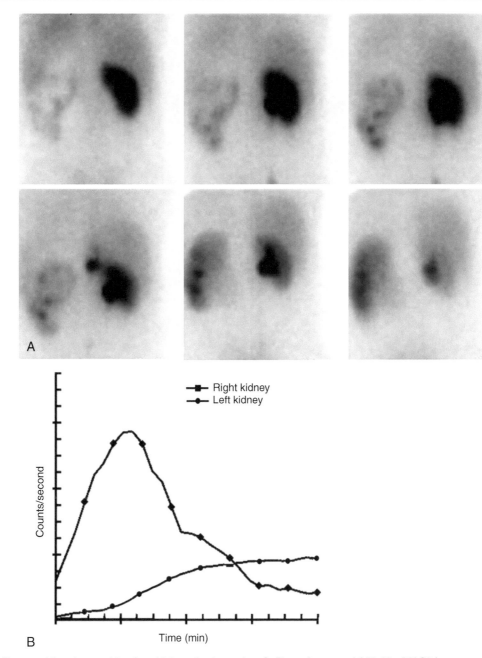

FIGURE 9-17. Decreased function resulting from high-grade obstruction. **A,** Dynamic sequential Tc-99m MAG3 images performed 15 minutes after giving furosemide (Lasix) reveal normal function on the right. The left kidney shows only a thin rim of cortex with delayed uptake, a photopenic hydronephrotic collecting system, and continual collecting system filling without washout consistent with obstruction. **B,** Findings are confirmed on the time-activity curve.

methods for calculating the $T_{1/2}$ have been described. The activity can be measured when the diuretic is given; then the length of time it takes to reach half that level can be used. However, this does not account for the delay in furosemide effect, a more precise method might be to fit a curve to the steepest portion of the washout time-activity curve. In general, a $T_{1/2}$ less than 10 minutes indicates that no clinically significant obstruction is present, whereas values greater than 20 minutes are considered obstructed. Values between 10 and 20 minutes fall in a gray zone or indeterminate range. Large capacitance collecting systems will clear slowly, even if not obstructed.

Serial studies may be used to monitor patients with partial obstruction, previously treated obstruction, or those at risk for worsening obstruction. Some situations in which this might be needed include cervical carcinoma and known partial ureteropelvic junction obstruction. Also, patients at high risk for functional deterioration from reflux, such as ileal loop diversions of the ureters, may be followed with interval studies. Periodic diuresis renography can help determine at what point aggressive intervention is needed. In neonates, congenital problems often result in irreparable damage. Surgeons generally prefer to wait until the child is larger for surgery when possible.

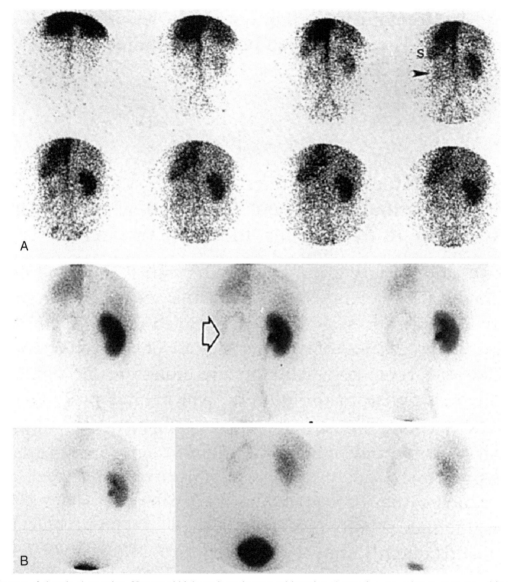

Figure 9-18. Impact of chronic obstruction. Untreated high-grade vesicoureteral junction obstruction secondary to tumor resulting in severely compromised renal function on the *left*. **A,** Flow study shows very decreased perfusion to the left kidney *(arrowhead)*. **B,** Dynamic sequential images show only a thin rim of cortex with poor uptake *(open arrowhead)* and a large photopenic collecting system consistent with hydronephrosis. Diuresis renography would not be useful as no tracer enters the collecting system.

Renovascular Hypertension
Physiology
When an arterial lesion causes significant vascular renal artery stenosis (RAS), glomerular perfusion pressure drops, causing the GFR to fall. The kidney responds by releasing the hormone renin from the juxtaglomerular apparatus. Renin converts angiotensinogen made in the liver to angiotensin I. In the lungs, angiotensin I is converted by angiotensin converting enzyme (ACE) to vasoactive angiotensin II, which acts as a powerful vasoconstrictor. This constriction raises blood pressure peripherally and acts on the efferent arterioles of the glomerulus to raise filtration pressure, thus maintaining GFR (Fig. 9-19). If renal blood flow remains low, the kidney will become scarred and contracted with time. If renovascular hypertension (RVH) is present, early intervention decreases arteriolar damage and glomerulosclerosis, increasing the chance for cure.

The development of ACE inhibition renography using captopril led to a sensitive, noninvasive functional method for diagnosing RVH. ACE inhibitors work by blocking the conversion of angiotensin I to angiotensin II (Fig. 9-20). This causes the GFR to fall in patients with RVH who rely on the compensatory mechanism to maintain perfusion pressure. Functional changes can be seen on the scintigram.

Indication
Although more than 90% of patients with hypertension have essential hypertension, RVH is common among patients who have a correctable cause. ACE inhibition renography should be considered for patients at moderate to high risk for RVH. This includes patients with severe hypertension, hypertension resistant to medical therapy, abrupt or recent onset, onset under the age of 30 years or over the age of 55 years, abdominal or flank

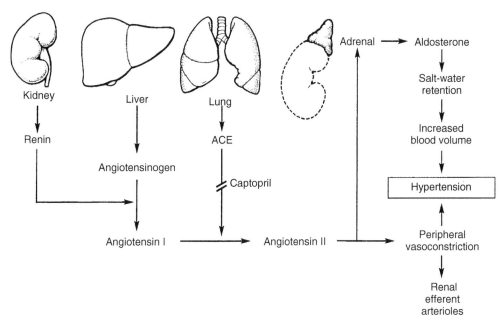

FIGURE 9-19. Renin-angiotensin-aldosterone physiology and site of angiotensin-converting enzyme (ACE) inhibitor (captopril). See text for details.

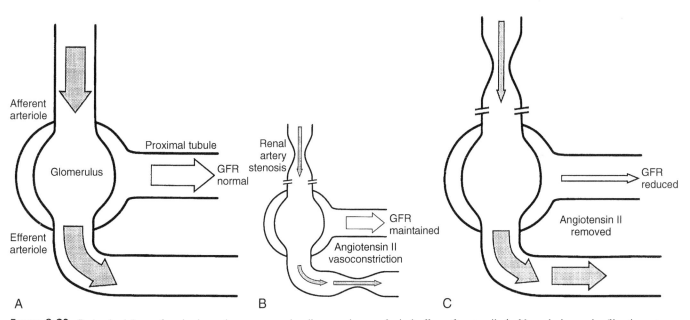

FIGURE 9-20. Pathophysiology of renin-dependent renovascular disease: pharmacological effect of captopril. **A,** Normal glomerular filtration rate (*GFR*). **B,** Renovascular hypertension. Because of reduced renal plasma flow, filtration pressure and GFR fall. Increased renin and resulting angiotensin II produces vasoconstriction of the efferent glomerular arterioles, raising glomerular pressure and maintaining GFR. **C,** Captopril blocks the normal compensatory mechanism and GFR falls.

bruits, unexplained azotemia, worsening renal function during ACE inhibitor therapy, and occlusive disease in other beds.

RAS often can be diagnosed with color Doppler ultrasound. It is sometimes also found incidentally during angiography or on diagnostic CT and MRI. Not all cases of RAS will cause RVH, and thus some patients will show no response to angioplasty or stenting. Therefore an ACE inhibition renography or a captopril scan is also indicated on patients with an anatomical lesion, to determine which cases will benefit from correction of a stenotic lesion.

Imaging Protocol
Patient preparation involves discontinuing all ACE inhibitors (2-3 days for captopril and 5-7 days for longer-acting agents such as enalapril and lisinopril) before the study. If ACE inhibitors are not discontinued, the sensitivity for diagnosis of RVH is reduced approximately 15%. Stopping angiotensin receptor blockers and halting calcium channel blockers also should be considered. False positive test results have been reported to result from calcium channel blockers. Diuretics should be stopped to prevent a dehydrated

condition. Otherwise, most antihypertensive agents have little or no effect on the results.

A decision must be made as to which imaging protocol to use. A 1-day protocol can be used by first doing a baseline examination using a low dose of 1 mCi (37 MBq) of Tc-99m MAG3 radiopharmaceutical followed by a post–ACE inhibitor study using 5 mCi (185 MBq) of Tc-99m MAG3 (185-370 MBq). Although this is convenient, interpretation is sometimes more difficult, and because most patients will have a negative post-captopril examination, they receive extra radiation from an unnecessary baseline examination. Alternatively, the two studies can be performed on separate days with 3 to 5 mCi (111-185 MBq) of Tc-99m MAG3 on the first day with the ACE inhibitor. A baseline study is done only in patients with an abnormal ACE inhibitor study. The radiotracer should be allowed to clear and decay, so at least 24 hours between the studies is needed.

In addition, a choice must be made as to which ACE inhibitor to use. Although oral captopril (25-50 mg) has been used traditionally, intravenous enalapril (Vasotec) examinations are faster and ensure reliable absorption of the drug. Intravenous access must be gained, which can be used for hydration and in hypotensive emergencies. After the ACE inhibitor is given, serial blood pressures measurements are taken, and the patient should be monitored until imaging is completed. An example ACE inhibitor renography protocol is listed in Box 9-7.

Image Interpretation

In patients with renin-dependent RVH, decreased blood flow to the affected kidney is most often *not* seen. In particular, on any noncaptopril renography, any decreased perfusion is usually related to a decrease in tissue volume being perfused. ACE inhibitors cause a drop in GFR, which leads to decreased urine flow that can be visualized during the functional portion of the study as a diminished function. However, because the kidney could have abnormal function from numerous causes, a baseline study is done. In patients with RVH, function generally improves in the absence of ACE inhibitors. In normal patients and those with renal disease from other causes (such as chronic scarring from pyelonephritis), function does not improve on a baseline study compared to the ACE inhibitor examination.

The diagnostic pattern seen depends on the type of radiopharmaceutical. If the glomerular agent Tc-99m DTPA is used, the ACE inhibitor–induced drop in GFR leads to a marked drop in radiotracer filtration and uptake. The most common pattern is an overall drop in function seen as slower uptake and a lower peak (Fig. 9-21). Looking at the degree of change from baseline is critical with Tc-99m DTPA, and the greater the change, the higher the probability that RAS is causing significant RVH. A 10% decrease in relative function (differential function or split renal function) or a decrease in absolute function (calculated GFR) greater than 10% is considered "high probability" or positive; a change of 5% to 9% is intermediate or borderline in significance.

Tc-99m MAG3 tubular uptake and secretion are not affected by GFR changes from the ACE inhibitor. The decreased urine flow causes delayed Tc-99m MAG3 washout and the primary finding will be cortical retention (cortical staining) (Fig. 9-22).

If bilateral cortical retention is seen, the finding is likely artifact and not bilateral renal artery stenosis. Among patients with bilateral cortical retention undergoing arteriogram, roughly two thirds had no significant stenosis. Usually, the causes are dehydration or hypotension (Fig. 9-23).

If the protocol has been properly followed, sensitivity and specificity of ACE inhibitor renography is reportedly 90% and 95%, respectively. However, the sensitivity and specificity are lower in patients with elevated creatinine. The kidney must function well enough to actually show a change in function when ACE inhibitors are given. Therefore a small shrunken kidney or one with poor baseline function can be difficult to interpret. In general, ACE inhibitor renography is accurate when the serum

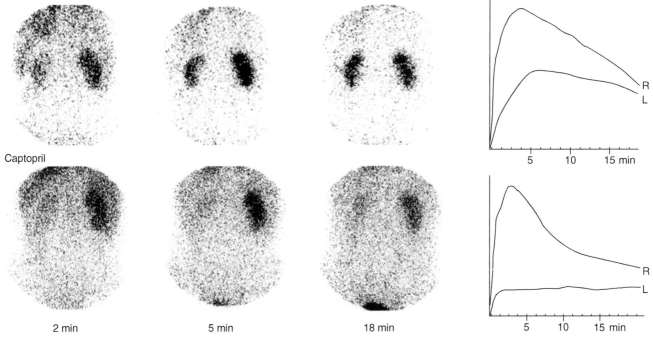

FIGURE 9-21. Effects of captopril on renovascular hypertension with Tc-99m DTPA. *Top,* The baseline study shows mildly decreased function on the left. *Bottom,* Examination after captopril reveals severe deterioration on the left kidney with diminished peak and overall function.

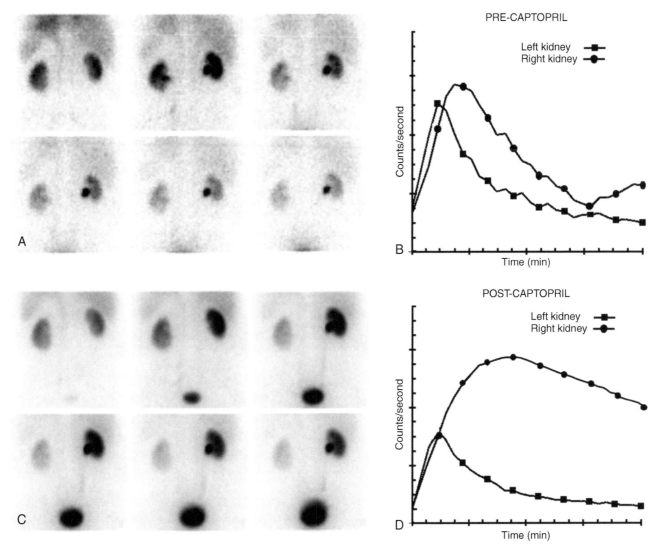

FIGURE 9-22. Positive Tc-99m MAG3 captopril study. **A** and **B,** The baseline study was performed first. Note prompt, fairly symmetric initial uptake and good washout over time. **C** and **D,** A follow-up examination performed later the same day with captopril shows marked cortical retention on the right considered "high probability" for renal artery stenosis as a cause for renovascular hypertension.

creatinine is normal or only mildly elevated (creatinine <1.7 mg/dL). False positive results are rare but have been reported in patients on calcium channel blockers.

Reporting

A normal ACE inhibitor study should be read as "low probability" of renin-dependent RVH. This means the posttest chance of RVH is less than 10%. In general, no additional workup is needed. If the 2-day protocol was used, the patient need not return for a baseline study. An "indeterminate" reading can be used for patients with very poor renal function or when an abnormal-appearing kidney does not change between baseline and ACE inhibitor examinations. When function markedly worsens on the ACE inhibitor challenge compared to the baseline study, the study is "high probability," with a greater than 90% chance of RVH. These patients are highly likely to improve with angioplasty or surgery.

Renal Transplant Evaluation

Renal transplantation is a well-established procedure (Fig. 9-24). When complications occur, transplanted kidneys are now usually evaluated by ultrasound and biopsy. However, radionuclide scintigraphy has been widely used to evaluate renal allograft function and remains an important screening tool.

Kidneys for transplantation come from one of three sources: a deceased donor (cadaveric kidney), a living related donor, or a living unrelated donor. All potential donors are carefully screened with immunological matching and undergo functional and anatomical evaluation. Although cadaveric kidneys are carefully screened and transported, allografts from living donors generally have the best prognosis. Allograft 1-year survival rates are 90% to 94% for living related donor kidneys and 88% to 90% for cadaveric transplants.

The development of improved immunosuppressive drug therapy over the years has resulted in a marked increase in allograft survival. These drugs act largely by suppressing the CD4 T-cell activity. Glucocorticoid steroids remain essential in the treatment and prevention of rejection. Additional agents used include calcineurin inhibitors (tacrolimus or cyclosporine), antiproliferative agents (such as azathioprine) that prevent mitosis and nonspecifically suppress lymphocyte proliferation, and

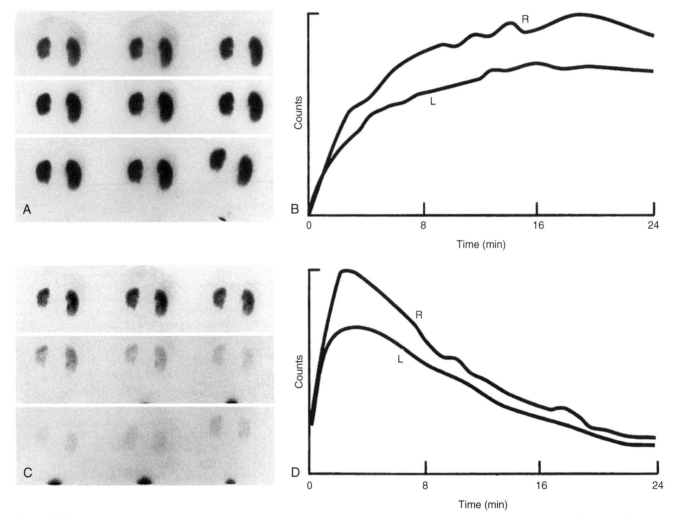

FIGURE 9-23. Bilateral cortical retention from dehydration. **A,** Captopril-stimulated study with Tc-99m MAG3 and the captopril time-activity curve (TAC) **(B)** show marked bilateral cortical retention and minimal urinary bladder clearance over 30 minutes. Further investigation revealed the patient had abstained from food and drink for nearly 12 hours before the examination. Repeat captopril images **(C)** and TAC **(D)** after the usual hydration protocol show normal cortical function and good clearance. The previous dehydration was presumed to cause the initial false-positive imaging pattern.

antiinterleukin (IL)-2 monoclonal antibodies and T-cell specific monoclonal antibody muromonab-CD3 (OKT3). However, it is critical to determine precisely when these agents are needed and how to monitor patients because of the potential serious acute and long-term side effects of these medications.

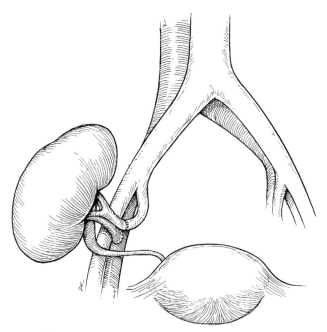

FIGURE 9-24. Renal transplant surgery. For technical reasons, the initial allograft is usually placed in the right iliac fossa. The vessels are attached end to end for the artery and side to side for the vein. The ureter is usually directly implanted into the recipient's bladder. After an initial failure, a second graft is usually placed in the left. If a pancreas is transplanted simultaneously, the pancreas is usually placed on the right.

Transplant Complications

A summary of transplant complications is provided in Table 9-3.

Vasomotor Nephropathy

A common early transplant complication is acute vasomotor nephropathy (also properly called ischemic nephropathy or delayed graft function). Although commonly referred to as acute tubular necrosis (ATN), ATN is just one possible component of the process. Ischemia before transplantation damages the kidney, worsening if the time between the donor's death and transplantation is prolonged. Vasomotor nephropathy is most common in cadaveric kidneys, occurring up to 50% of the time. However, it can be seen in grafts from living donors (5%), especially if the surgery was complicated. The functional impact ranges from a mild, rapidly resolving disorder to a slower recovery or total anuria. Although renal function will be impaired at the time of transplant in these cases, it should recover spontaneously during the first 2 weeks.

Hyperacute Rejection

Careful human leukocyte antigen (HLA) immunological matching has eliminated hyperacute rejection. Preformed antibodies in the recipient's circulation from a major histocompatibility or blood group mismatch cause renal vasculature thrombosis. The classic story is that of the surgeon witnessing the kidney turning blue in the operating room after performing the vascular anastomosis. The allograft cannot be salvaged, and the chance of patient survival is grim.

Accelerated Acute Rejection

Accelerated acute rejection is also uncommon but occurs in patients with antibodies already in their system, as in sensitization from pregnancy or multiple blood

TABLE 9-3 Complications After Renal Transplantation

Complication	Usual time of occurrence postoperatively	Comments
PRESURGICAL INSULT		
Vasomotor nephropathy (acute tubular necrosis)	Minutes to hours	Cadaveric transplants; may recover, days to weeks
AUTOIMMUNE: REJECTION		
Hyperacute rejection	Minutes to hours	Preformed antibodies; irreversible
Accelerated acute rejection	1-5 days	History of prior transplant or transfusion
Acute rejection	After 5 days, most common during first 3 months	Cell mediated, responsive to treatment
Chronic allograft nephropathy (chronic rejection)	Months to years	Humoral, irreversible, inevitable
Cyclosporine toxicity	Months	Reversible with drug withdrawal
SURGICAL		
Urine leak/urinoma	Days or weeks	
Hematoma	First few days	
Infection	First few days	
Lymphocele	2-4 months	
VASCULAR		
Renal artery stenosis	After first month	
Vascular occlusion	Days to weeks	
Infarcts		
Renal		
Obstruction (extrinsic mass, stricture or calculi)	Days, months, years	
Vesicoureteral reflux		

transfusions. The patient presents with clinical signs of acute rejection earlier than expected, in the first few days after transplantation. Unlike hyperacute rejection, accelerated rejection often responds to therapy.

Acute Rejection

Acute rejection is a relatively frequent transplant complication. Although it can occur at any time, acute rejection does not typically occur until 10 to 14 days (minimum of 5-7 days) after transplantation and is most common in the first 3 months. Two immunological pathways, T cells and humoral antibodies, can be involved causing arteritis, microinfarcts, hemorrhage, and lymphocytic infiltration. It is common for the patient to be febrile and the allograft to be swollen and painful. Typically, the patient becomes desensitized to the allograft over time, and acute rejection is rarely seen after 1 year in a patient taking appropriate immunosuppressive therapy.

Chronic Allograft Nephropathy

Commonly referred to as chronic rejection, chronic renal allograft nephropathy is a cumulative, delayed, and irreversible process. Vascular constriction, chronic fibrosis, tubular atrophy, and glomerulosclerosis from immunological and nonhumoral causes occur. Over months to years, this fibrosis causes cortical loss and decreased function. Dilation of the collecting system may occur as the cortex thins. Risk factors for early development (<1 year) include damage from early ischemic injury (severe ATN), prior severe acute rejection episodes, subclinical rejection, and long-term calcineurin-inhibitor therapy. No effective therapy exists for chronic renal allograft nephropathy, and it is now the leading cause of graft failure, given improved therapy and early transplant survival.

Immunosuppressive Drug Toxicity

Another important cause of allograft dysfunction is drug nephrotoxicity of therapeutic drugs. In the past, this was often due to high levels of cyclosporine. Cyclosporine toxicity is seldom seen because it has been largely replaced with other agents or is prescribed at lower, safer levels. Similar changes can be seen with other antirejection agents.

Surgical Complications

The rare arterial thrombosis demonstrates no flow or function. Renal vein thrombosis can occur as a postoperative complication or related to autoimmune problems. Unlike in renal vein thrombosis in native kidneys, there are no venous collaterals to drain the kidney and allow spontaneous recovery to occur. The thrombus leads to infarct and hemorrhage, and the effect is often severe, with loss of the allograft.

Postoperative RAS should be suspected in patients who develop hypertension after transplantation surgery and may occur in up to 10% of patients. Although the anastomosis is the most common site, stenosis in other locations (including the iliac artery) must be considered. The imaging protocol is similar to the renovascular hypertension workup for native kidneys described in Box 9-7, with anterior positioning of the camera over the allograft. Interpretation criteria are the same as for native kidneys.

Fluid collections associated with the transplant can be seen from necrosis of the ureteral anastomosis in the immediate postoperative period with urinary leakage. Although other imaging modalities, such as ultrasound, can identify fluid in the pelvis, nuclear medicine techniques are better able to specifically identify the source. Because the transplanted kidney has no lymphatic connections, lymphoceles can form in the transplant bed. This may occur in up to 10% of transplants and is seen typically 2 to 3 months after transplant. These are only clinically important if they impinge on the ureter or vasculature.

Although uncommon, ureteral obstruction may be caused by kinking of the ureter, extrinsic mass compression (e.g., hematoma, lymphocele), intraluminal obstruction (from blood clot or calculus), or periureteral fibrosis. Some degree of collecting system dilation without significant mechanical obstruction often is seen from postoperative hematomas and seromas. Hydronephrosis from obstruction can be differentiated from dilation caused by reflux or related to chronic rejection using diuretic renography. Ureteral obstruction often resolves spontaneously.

Methods

Renal allograft evaluation is performed using the dynamic scintigraphy protocol with Tc-99m MAG3 listed in Box 9-3, with the camera anterior, centered over the allograft in the lower pelvis. It is useful to include at least some of the native kidneys in the field of view because they may contribute to overall function. Some portion of the bladder should be seen, and the entire bladder is included on prevoid and postvoid images.

The protocol can be modified to answer any question that arises. If concern for RAS exists, the ACE inhibitor protocol is used. The diuretic renography protocol can be followed when hydronephrosis develops or obstruction is suspected. Delayed images over the course of 1 to 2 hours can help clarify the cause of fluid collections and assess possible urine leaks.

Interpretation

Because the medical and surgical complications described previously occur at certain times, renal transplant scintigrams must be interpreted with the age of the transplant as well as the clinical context (including physical symptoms, laboratory values, and current medications) in mind. The type of allograft (cadaveric or living related donor transplant) is especially important and needs to be considered when evaluating vasomotor nephropathy or the expected level of renal function. The expected level of perfusion and function will typically diminish over the years.

During the perfusion phase, the transplanted kidney normally becomes the "hottest" structure within 2 to 4 seconds of activity appearing in the adjacent iliac artery after a good bolus of radiopharmaceutical. However, achieving good perfusion images is extremely difficult, especially because most patients with renal transplants have limited vascular access as a result of prior dialysis. A living related donor allograft will usually function better and clear radiotracer more rapidly than a cadaveric allograft. However, both will normally clear slightly slower than a healthy native kidney.

The two most common issues to consider in the early posttransplant period are vasomotor nephropathy and acute rejection (Table 9-4). Both conditions manifest with

TABLE **9-4** Comparison of Acute Rejection and Vasomotor Nephropathy

Disease	Baseline scan	Follow-up scan	Perfusion	Renal transit time
Acute rejection	Normal	Worsens	↓	↑
Vasomotor nephropathy (acute tubular necrosis)	Abnormal	Improves	Normal	↑

decreased function and marked cortical retention: a diminished initial slope on the TAC, progressively increasing cortical activity over time, and a delay in appearance of collecting system and bladder activity from the expected 3- to 6-minute time frame. Unlike vasomotor nephropathy, acute rejection affects small renal parenchymal vessels, and the allograft should show diminished blood flow on the perfusion portion of the examination. The classic dynamic imaging pattern of acute rejection is decreased perfusion and then marked cortical retention with Tc-99m MAG3 (Fig 9-25). Vasomotor nephropathy, on the other hand, shows normal perfusion but poor function with delayed cortical clearance and decreased urine excretion immediately after surgery (Fig. 9-26).

Vasomotor nephropathy is the result of damage occurring before transplant insertion and so is present from the start. Usually, function improves in the first couple of weeks (Fig 9-27). However, dysfunction often persists, especially in severe cases, overlapping with the time frame expected of acute rejection. In these cases, worsening function suggests another process is developing. The degree of renal dysfunction can vary widely. Severe cortical retention or function that does not rapidly improve on serial studies has strong negative prognostic implications with increased transplant loss in the first 6 months.

When function is initially normal and then deteriorates, diagnosis of acute rejection is more certain, because it is not seen in the first several days (Fig 9-28). If the initial transplant function is not known or was poor from initial vasomotor nephropathy, it may be difficult to differentiate developing acute rejection from persisting vasomotor nephropathy or to identify acute rejection superimposed on persisting vasomotor nephropathy. For this reason and given the difficulty in ensuring a high-quality perfusion image, a 24- to 48-hour baseline study is extremely helpful, though seldom performed. While biopsy is quite sensitive, it is not without risk for complications.

Nephrotoxic effects of immunosuppressive therapy demonstrate a pattern of prompt uptake and delayed clearance similar to that of vasomotor nephropathy. The time frame of the examination usually allows these two processes to be differentiated. Vasomotor nephropathy is seen immediately, whereas time is required for nephrotoxicity or true ATN to occur.

In chronic renal allograft nephropathy, the blood flow and function images may initially appear normal, with change first revealed through quantitative means such as ERPF and GFR measurement (Fig. 9-29). As the chronic renal allograft nephropathy worsens on serial examinations, parenchymal retention is seen. Although mild to moderate cortical retention is often seen, more marked

retention is likely the result of another process. Over time, nephron loss and scar in chronic rejection causes the cortex to appear thinned and the central collecting system prominent. Uptake appears patchy or less intense than normal, the allograft appears small or scarred, and clearance is delayed (Fig. 9-30).

Although acute vascular complications are rare, they must be suspected in the patient with anuria. Renal artery occlusion leads to absent perfusion and a photopenic defect on the functional portion of scintigraphy. Although renal vein thrombosis in native kidneys has a variable appearance depending on severity and stage of resolution, the classic appearance is of an enlarged kidney with intense cortical retention initially. In a transplanted kidney, there are no venous collaterals to drain the kidney so the impact is more severe, causing the kidney to have an appearance similar to that of renal artery occlusion (Fig 9-31).

A postoperative leak may occur at the anastomotic site or result from rupture of an obstructed allograft. A progressive accumulation of activity occurs outside of the urinary tract on dynamic scintigraphic images. A slow leak may be seen as a photopenic defect from a nonradiolabeled urinoma (Fig. 9-32). If Tc-99m DTPA is being used or if function is poor, delayed imaging at 2 hours or later may be needed to detect increasing activity in this fluid collection. Delayed images with Tc-99m MAG3 may be misinterpreted as showing a leak because of the normal bowel activity appearance over time. Other fluid collections such as lymphoceles and hematomas may be noted as fixed pararenal, photon-deficient areas.

An obstructed allograft may present with hydronephrosis or diminished urine output. Diuretic renography can be useful in evaluating suspected obstruction in a manner similar to that in native kidneys (Fig. 9-33). It is important that acute rejection is not present and that function is adequate to respond to the diuretic.

▬ MEASURING RENAL FUNCTION: EFFECTIVE RENAL PLASMA FLOW AND GOMERULAR FILTRATION RATE

Normal GFR varies according to age, sex, and body size. Estimated GFR can be fairly reliably calculated using these factors and the serum creatinine (http://www.kidney.org/professionals/kdoqi/gfr_calculator.cfm). However, these estimations may not be reliable when function is very abnormal and changes from a unilateral abnormality may be difficult to detect.

Accurate quantification of GFR and ERPF with nonradioactive inulin and PAH is possible with continuous infusion to achieve a steady state and multiple blood and urine samples. Nuclear medicine techniques have evolved using

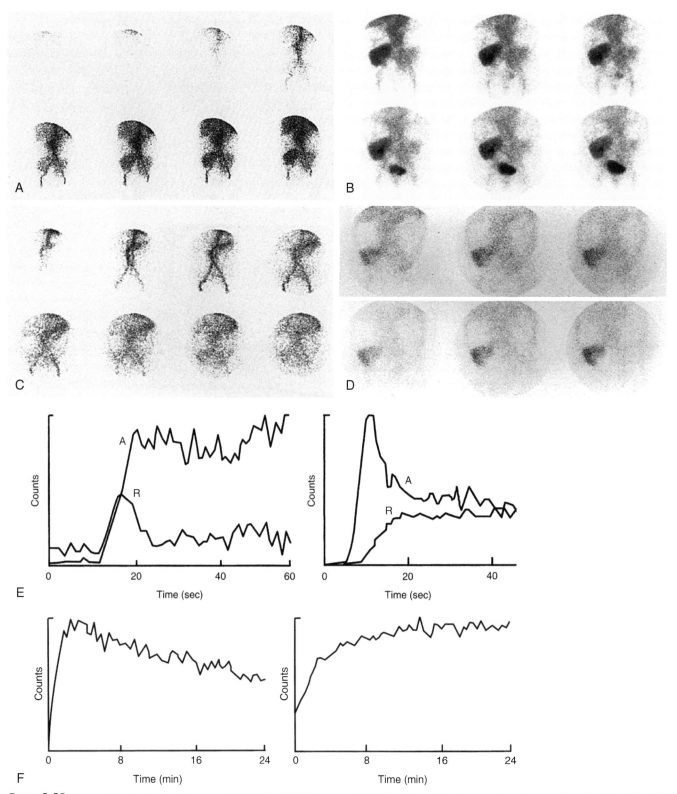

FIGURE 9-25. Acute allograft rejection. Postoperative Tc-99m MAG3 images of a right iliac fossa cadaveric transplant show good baseline blood flow (**A**) and reasonably good function (**B**). Six days later, the patient developed fever, allograft tenderness, and elevated serum creatinine. Repeat blood flow is diminished (**C**), and functional images show cortical retention (**D**). These findings are consistent with acute rejection. **E,** Perfusion time-activity curves show initial good blood flow *(left)* that falls on the follow-up study *(right)* as a result of acute rejection. **F,** The time-activity curves over the 25-minute study show adequate baseline function *(left)*, which deteriorates at the time of rejection *(right)*. *A*, Artery; *R*, right renal transplant.

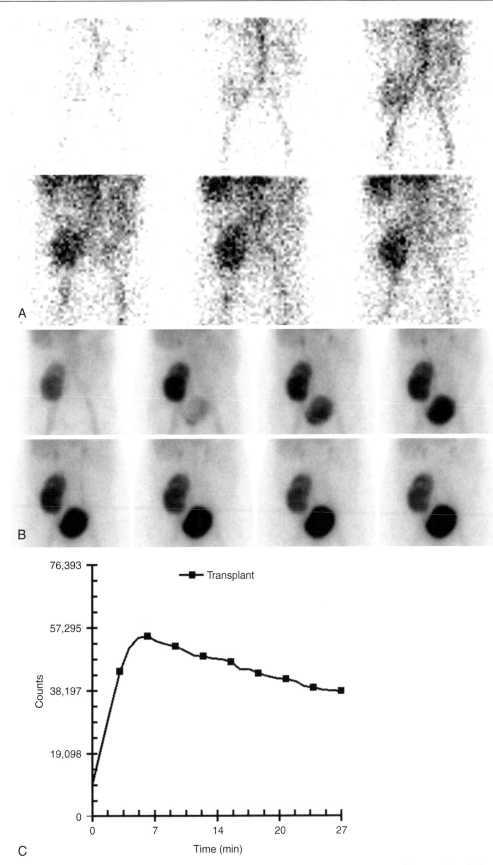

FIGURE 9-26. Postoperative function in a cadaveric transplant. Imaging 72 hours after transplantation reveal **(A)** normal perfusion but **(B)** slight cortical retention on functional images and on time-activity curves **(C)** typical of mild vasomotor nephropathy.

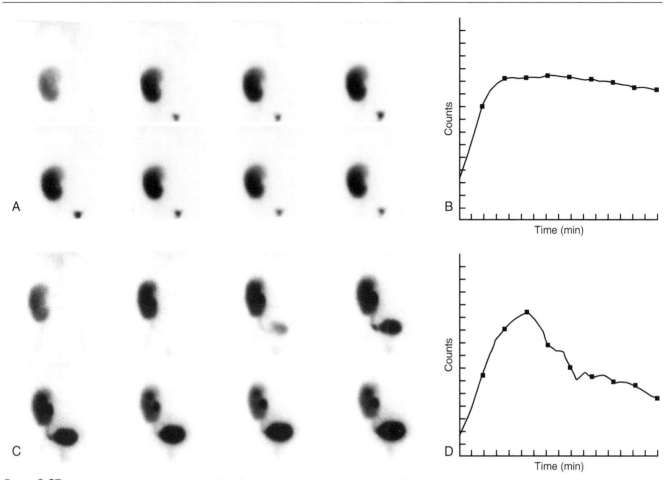

FIGURE 9-27. Acute vasomotor nephropathy. **A,** Baseline images and time-activity curve **(B)** obtained 24 hours after transplantation reveals significant cortical retention, confirming the diagnosis of vasomotor nephropathy, often called acute tubular necrosis. **C** and **D,** A follow-up examination shows improving function, with more rapid transit into bladder and decreased cortical retention. *Cts,* Counts.

analogs of inulin (Tc-99m DTPA) and PAH (I-131 OIH or Tc-99m MAG3). Different combinations of plasma sampling and imaging techniques are available. Most institutions do not have a wet laboratory setup for the more accurate blood sample methods; therefore camera-based techniques have become more popular. Camera-based methods require no blood sampling and only a few minutes of imaging time (Fig. 9-34). Precise adherence to protocol is necessary for these techniques, and they are more prone to error than the blood sampling methods.

To perform a camera-based GFR calculation, a small known dose of Tc-99m DTPA is counted at a set distance from the camera face to determine the count rate before injecting it into the patient. The actual administered dose is then corrected for the postinjection residual in the syringe and serves as a standard. If the dose is too large, it may overwhelm the counting capabilities of the system and lost counts would affect accuracy, causing overestimation of GFR.

After injection, images are acquired for 6 minutes. Regions of interest are drawn around the kidneys, and the counts are background subtracted. Attenuation of the photons caused by varying renal depth is corrected using formula based on patient weight and height. The fraction of the standard taken up by the kidneys in the 1- to 2.5-minute or 2- to 3-minute frames can be correlated with GFR measured by other methods (e.g., multiple blood sample, single blood sample, or less accurately by creatinine clearance). A similar camera-based approach can be used for ERPF calculation using Tc-99m MAG3.

These camera methods allow assessment when only one side is abnormal. The percent differential function can be applied to the GFR or ERPF data to calculate function contributed by each kidney. It should be noted that any method for measuring function may not be "accurate" measurements of function, but they are generally superior to estimates based on creatinine in difficult situations such as in the elderly or when function is poor. In addition, being highly reproducible in any one patient, patients can be followed over time using this method.

RENAL CORTICAL IMAGING

It is often difficult clinically to distinguish upper urinary tract infections from lower tract infections. However, the long-term complications and therapeutic implications of renal parenchymal infection are very different from those of lower urinary tract disease. Infection and reflux can lead to cortical scarring, renal failure, and hypertension.

Renal cortical lesions are usually evaluated with the structural imaging modalities ultrasound, CT, and sometimes MRI. However, in specific instances, nuclear medicine cortical imaging adds vital information by showing

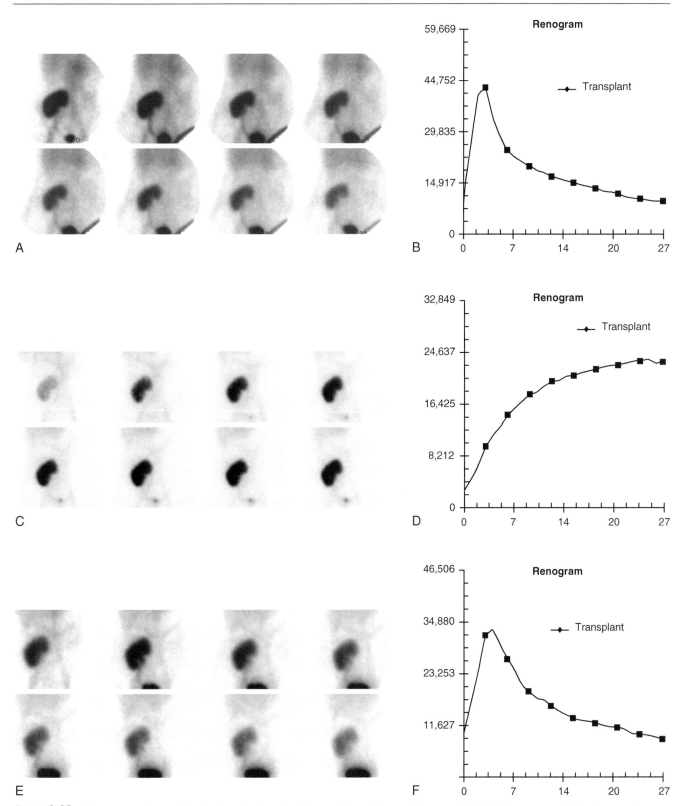

FIGURE 9-28. Time course of acute rejection. Baseline functional images **(A)** and time-activity curves (TACs) **(B)** are unremarkable. Two months later, images show delayed uptake and cortical retention **(C)**. This is confirmed on the TAC **(D)**. Function improves 1 week later with immunosuppressive therapy on the follow-up scan **(E)** and TAC **(F)**.

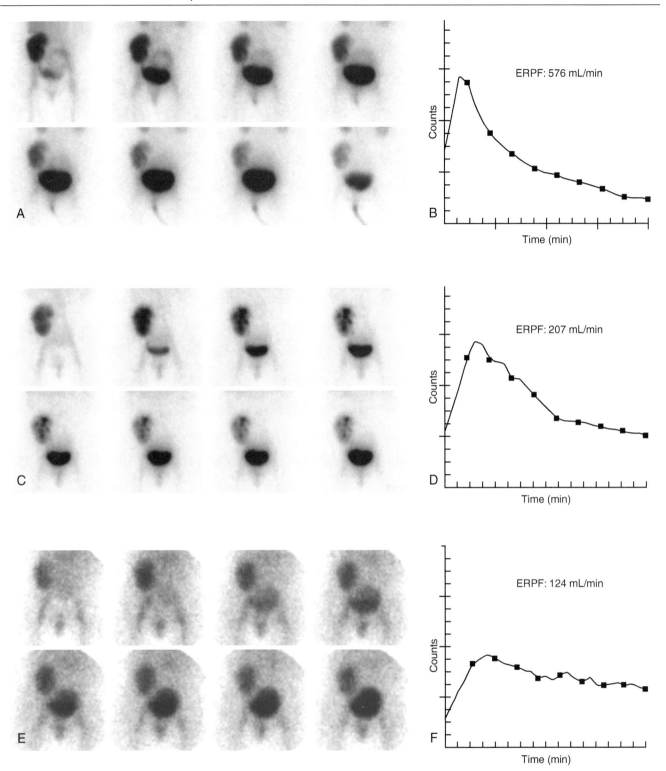

FIGURE 9-29. Chronic renal allograft nephropathy (chronic rejection). Baseline scan **(A)** and time-activity curve (TAC) **(B)** 24 hours after transplantation reveal good uptake and clearance. Note the presence of a Foley catheter draining the bladder and some native kidney function at the top edge of the image. Images over 1 year later are unremarkable **(C)**, although some decline is suggested on the TAC **(D)**. A steady decline in effective renal plasma flow *(ERPF)* is characteristic and often the only way to diagnose the early stages of disease. Four months later as creatinine continued to rise, a visible decline in function with diminished uptake and mild to moderate cortical retention is seen on the scan **(E)** and on the curve **(F)**. Cortical retention is usually less intense and transit to collecting system less delayed than in acute rejection.

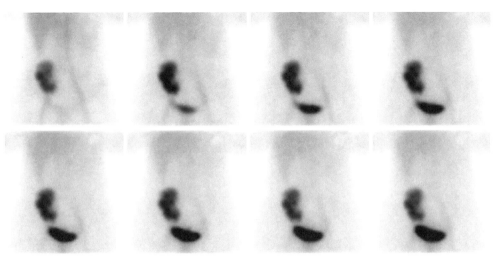

FIGURE 9-30. Chronic renal allograft nephropathy (chronic rejection) in a 3-year-old transplanted kidney showing cortical scarring and retention with diminished washout. The prominent collecting system often present at this stage is not well seen in this particular case.

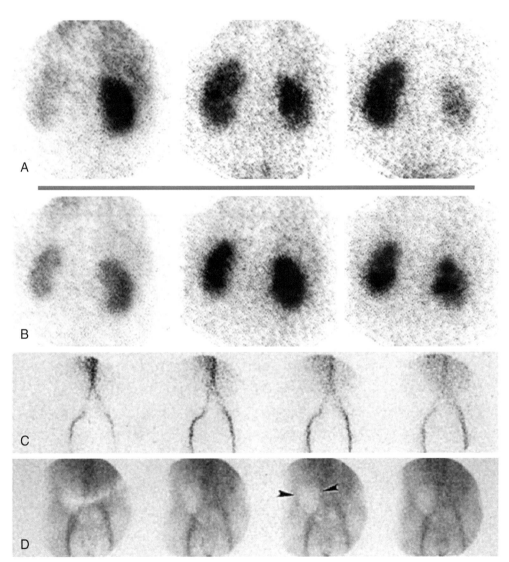

FIGURE 9-31. Renal vein thrombosis. **A,** Renal vein thrombosis in a native kidney. The Tc-99m DTPA scan reveals poor uptake and delayed clearance in the left native kidney. **B,** Function improves on a follow-up scan 4 months later. **C, D** Images from a renal allograft with renal vein thrombosis. The radionuclide angiogram **(C)** demonstrates no perfusion to the transplanted kidney. **D,** Dynamic images acquired immediately after the flow study and sequentially every 5 minutes show a photopenic defect *(arrowheads)* resulting from nonviable allograft causing attenuation but having no uptake. *LPO,* Left posterior oblique; *RPO,* right posterior oblique.

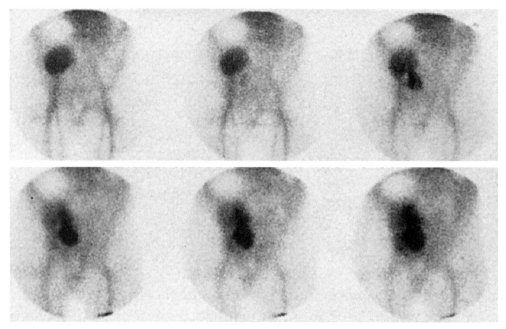

FIGURE 9-32. Postoperative urinary leak. Rapid leakage resulted from disrupted surgical anastomosis. Note accumulation of radiotracer just inferior to the transplant but superior and lateral to the bladder. No bladder filling is seen.

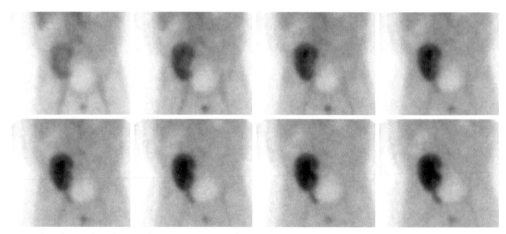

FIGURE 9-33. Postoperative obstruction. Images from a recent transplant reveal a photopenic area in the pelvis from a postoperative fluid collection pressing on the ureter and causing obstruction. Delayed images (not shown) failed to show active urine leak in the region.

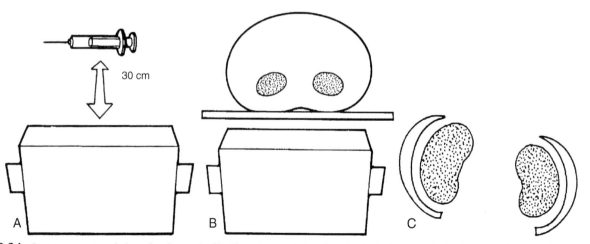

FIGURE 9-34. Gamma camera technique for glomerular filtration rate calculation. **A,** A 1-minute image of the Tc-99m DTPA syringe before and after injection are taken 30 cm distance from center of the collimator. **B,** After injection, 15 seconds per frame images are acquired for a total of 6 minutes. **C,** Kidney and background regions are selected on images to obtain counts. After correcting for background and attenuation, the net renal cortical uptake as a percentage of the total injected dose is calculated.

improvements and changes over time that are difficult to see with anatomical imaging modalities. Tc-99m DMSA offers superior cortical resolution over Tc-99m MAG3 because of its significant cortical binding. Commonly, Tc-99m DMSA is used to evaluate suspected pyelonephritis or to possibly detect renal scarring in a patient with reflux. Occasionally, cortical scintigraphy is used to differentiate a prominent column of Bertin seen on ultrasound from a true mass.

Acute Pyelonephritis

Acute pyelonephritis usually results from reflux of infected urine. The clinical diagnosis of acute pyelonephritis based on fever, flank pain, and positive urine cultures is unreliable and especially difficult in infants. Therefore recurrent infections often occur and lead to significant damage and scarring. This process is a significant cause of long-term morbidity, causing hypertension and chronic renal failure.

CT can often identify the inflammatory change in the kidney, as can radiolabeled white blood cells and gallium-67 citrate. However, these tests are not suitable for frequent use, especially in children. Ultrasound is widely used to assess the kidney and is generally considered an essential part of the pyelonephritis workup. However, sonography is relatively insensitive to the inflammatory changes of acute pyelonephritis and the residual cortical defects and scars. Reported ultrasound sensitivities range from 24% to 40% for pyelonephritis and are approximately 65% for the detection of scars.

Cortical scintigraphy with Tc-99m DMSA is significantly more sensitive than sonography. Sensitivities for acute pyelonephritis are difficult to determine because Tc-99m DMSA is considered the gold standard. Most frequently, cortical scanning is done in children with acute pyelonephritis, but it also may be performed as part of the workup in patients with vesicoureteral reflux who have no evidence of active pyelonephritis.

Method

With Tc-99m DMSA, dynamic imaging is not performed because background clearance is slow, and the kidney clears only a small percentage of the radiotracer. Delayed cortical planar or SPECT imaging is acquired. An example protocol is listed in Box 9-8.

Planar imaging usually requires at least both posterior and posterior oblique views. A pinhole collimator or converging collimator provides magnification and improved resolution. SPECT affords excellent image detail. However, children may require sedation for SPECT because they must be completely still for the entire acquisition.

Image Interpretation

The normal Tc-99m DMSA scan should show a homogeneous distribution throughout the renal cortex. The shape of the kidney is variable, as is the thickness of the cortex. The upper poles often may appear less intense because of splenic impression, fetal lobulation, and attenuation from liver and spleen. The central collecting system and medullary regions are photon deficient because Tc-99m DMSA tubular binding occurs in the cortex. The columns of Bertin will show radiopharmaceutical uptake and may appear quite prominent. In a study performed to differentiate the prominent column of Bertin from true mass, the

---

Box 9-8. Renal Cortical Imaging Protocol Summary

RADIOPHARMACEUTICAL
Tc-99m DMSA
  Child: 50 µCi/kg (minimum dose of 600 µCi)
  Adult: 5 mCi (185 MBq)

INSTRUMENTATION
Planar gamma camera: Large-field-of-view, parallel-hole collimator for differential calculation. Pinhole collimator for cortical images. Converging collimator may be used for adults.
SPECT: Dual- or triple-head preferred

IMAGING PROCEDURE
Patient should void before starting.
Inject radiopharmaceutical intravenously.
Image at 2 hours after injection.
Acquire parallel collimator images for 500k on anterior and posterior views for differential calculation.
Pinhole images acquire for 100k counts per view.
Position patient so each kidney is imaged separately, but camera is equidistant from patient.
Quantify function as geometric mean (square root of the product of anterior and posterior counts).

SPECT
Camera: Low-energy high-resolution collimator
Matrix: 128 × 128
Zoom: As needed
Orbit: Noncircular body contour, rotate 180 degrees, step and shoot 40 views/head, 3 degrees/stop, 40-second/stop
Reconstruction: 64 × 64 Hamming filter with high cutoff
Smoothing kernel
Attenuation correction

SPECT, Single-photon emission computed tomography.

Tc-99m DMSA scan will show radiotracer uptake in a column of Bertin but not in a mass caused by tumor.

Areas of cortical tubular dysfunction from infection or scar present as cortical defects (Figs. 9-35 and 9-36). This may be caused by localized mass effect and edema from the inflammatory process and by actual tubular dysfunction and ischemia. A tumor will present as a defect because cortical scanning is not specific. Therefore comparison with ultrasound is advisable.

Infection may present as a focal, ill-defined lesion or as a multifocal process. A diffuse decrease in activity also may be seen; if it occurs without volume loss, it would suggest a diffuse inflammatory process. Scars would be expected to have localized, sharp margins and may occur in a small kidney with associated cortical loss. However, it is extremely difficult to tell an area of acute inflammation from a scar without serial images, particularly in patients with clinically silent infections (Fig 9-37).

In the workup of acute abnormalities resulting from acute pyelonephritis, serial scans may also be useful to assess the extent of recovery. In general, it is advisable to wait 6 months from the acute infection to allow recovery. The acute inflammatory changes in pyelonephritis will usually resolve over time (nearly 40%) or significantly

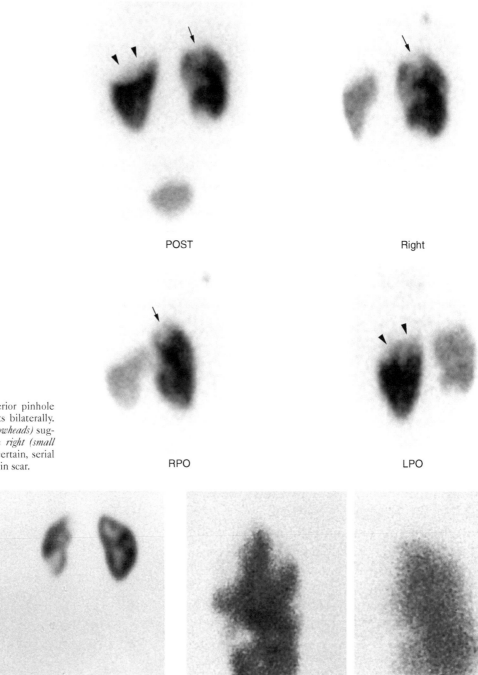

POST

Right

RPO

LPO

FIGURE 9-35. Cortical scar. Anterior pinhole DMSA images reveal focal defects bilaterally. The sharp margins on the *left (arrowheads)* suggest scar. Smaller defects on the *right (small arrow)* are also present. When uncertain, serial studies can confirm lack of change in scar.

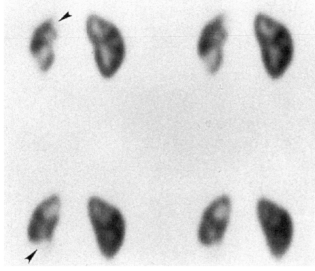

FIGURE 9-36. Tc-99m DMSA SPECT. Sequential 3.5-mm coronal sections show great detail such as cortical and medullary separation. Cortical defects in the upper pole and lower pole *(arrowheads)* are present in the slightly smaller right kidney from scar.

FIGURE 9-37. Acute pyelonephritis. Tc-99m DMSA pinhole images study in an 11-year-old child show **(A)** multiple cortical defects, particularly in the upper pole that nearly completely resolve on a follow-up study obtained 6 months later, after appropriate antibiotic therapy **(B).**

improve (*44%*). Any defect persisting after 6 months should be considered a chronic scar.

Multiheaded SPECT is more sensitive than planar techniques for detection of small defects because of its better contrast resolution. However, specificity may be somewhat lower because some apparent cortical defects actually may be caused by normal variations such as fetal lobulation and splenic impression. Pinhole collimator imaging gives high-resolution images of the renal cortex, superior to parallel-hole collimator imaging. Either method can give excellent clinical results, with experience often dictating preference.

▬ RADIONUCLIDE CYSTOGRAPHY

Vesicoureteral Reflux

Untreated reflux and infection are associated with subsequent renal damage, scarring, hypertension, and chronic renal failure. Vesicoureteral reflux (VUR) occurs in approximately 1% to 2% of the pediatric population. In patients with acute pyelonephritis, VUR is present in approximately 40% of patients. In untreated patients, VUR is responsible for 5% to 40% of end-stage renal disease in patients under 16 years of age and 5% to 20% of adults younger than 50 years of age.

VUR is caused by a failure of the ureterovesical valve. The normal ureter passes obliquely through the bladder wall and submucosa to its opening at the trigone. As urine fills the bladder, the valve passively closes, preventing reflux. If the intramural ureteral length is too short in relation to its diameter or if the course is too direct, the valve will not close completely and reflux results. As a child grows, the ureter usually grows in length more than in diameter, resulting in decreased reflux and eventual resolution in 80% of patients. Spontaneous resolution by 2 to 3 years of age is seen in 40% to 60% of VUR diagnosed prenatally. Even among patients with severe reflux, resolution occurs spontaneously in 20% within 5 years.

Renal damage is more likely in patients with severe rather than mild or moderate grades of reflux. Reflux by itself is not pathological; that is, sterile low-pressure reflux does not cause renal injury. The intrarenal reflux of infected urine is required for damage to develop. In patients without reflux, pyelonephritis has been presumed to be secondary to causes such as fimbriated bacteria, which can climb the ureter. Antibiotic therapy is the first line of defense. Renal scaring has been decreased from 35% to 60% in untreated patients down to 10% with therapy. The goal of therapy is to prevent infection of the kidney until reflux resolves spontaneously. However, antibiotics do not completely protect the kidney from infection and scar. Therefore patients must be carefully monitored, and serial Tc-99m DMSA scans may be helpful.

Radionuclide cystography was introduced in the late 1950s to diagnose VUR and is widely accepted as the technique of choice for evaluation and follow-up of children with UTIs and reflux. The radionuclide method is more sensitive than contrast-enhanced cystography for detecting reflux and results in considerably less radiation exposure to the patient. In many centers, contrast-voiding urethrocystography is reserved for the initial workup of male patients to exclude an anatomical cause for reflux, such as posterior urethral valves.

VCUG screening is recommended for siblings of patients with reflux. It must be remembered that reflux and pyelonephritis may be clinically silent. These siblings are at an increased risk of approximately 40% for VUR.

Methodology

Indirect radionuclide cystography can be performed as part of routine dynamic renal scintigraphy done with Tc-99m MAG3. The child is asked to not void until the bladder is maximally distended. When the bladder is as full as can be tolerated, a previoiding image is obtained. Then dynamic

---

---

images are acquired during voiding. A postvoid image is obtained once voiding is done. Although this test has an advantage because the bladder is not catheterized, upper-tract stasis often poses a problem for interpretation. In addition, the indirect method cannot detect the reflux that occurs during bladder filling (20%).

Direct radionuclide cystography is the most commonly used method for diagnosing reflux. It is done as a three-phase process with continuous imaging during bladder filling, during micturition, and after voiding. Besides diagnosing reflux, this procedure can quantitate postvoid bladder residuals.

The protocol for radionuclide retrograde cystography and residual bladder volume calculation is listed in Box 9-9. The high sensitivity depends on rapid and continuous imaging. Tc-99m sulfur colloid and Tc-99m DTPA are the radiopharmaceuticals most commonly used. Tc-99m pertechnetate may be absorbed through the bladder, particularly if the bladder is inflamed. A solution of 1 mCi of radiotracer in 500 mL normal saline provides sufficient concentration.

TABLE 9-5 Radiation Dosimetry for Technetium-99m Direct Cystography

Suggested dose MBq (mCi)	Organ receiving highest mGy/MBq (rad/mCi)	Effective dose mSv/MBq (rem/mCi)
	Bladder	
18.5-37 (0.5-1.0)	0.028 (0.10)	0.0024 (0.0089)

Data from the 2003 Society of Nuclear Medicine Procedure Guidelines. Available at: http://www.snm.org for children 5 years of age.

Dosimetry

The absorbed radiation dose is quite low. A list is provided in Table 9-5. From 50 to 200 times less radiation is delivered to the gonads from the radionuclide method than with contrast cystography.

Image Interpretation

In a normal study, no radiotracer is seen in the ureters or kidneys. Any reflux is abnormal and readily detected by the presence of activity above the bladder (Fig. 9-38).

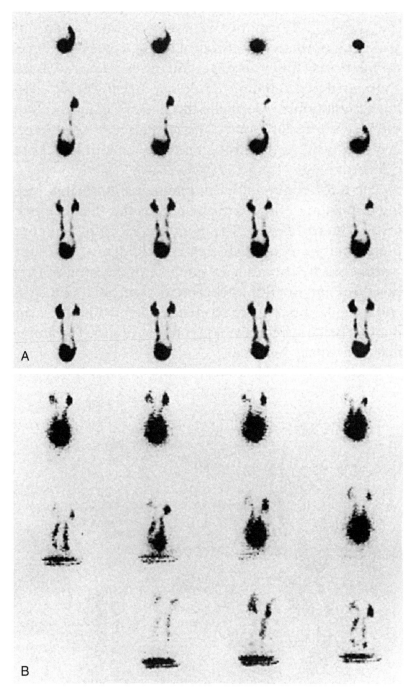

FIGURE 9-38. Vesicoureteral reflux. **A,** During the filling phase, reflux is seen first on the right, then bilaterally in **B.** On voiding, the left side clears better than the right. Reflux is seen in the renal pelvic region bilaterally from grade II to III reflux.

Reflux grades have been described for radiographic contrast studies (Fig. 9-39). In this system, criteria include the level the reflux reaches, the dilation of the renal pelvis, and ureteral dilation and tortuosity. However, anatomical resolution is much lower with scintigraphic methods and calyceal morphology is not well defined.

A radionuclide grading system would report activity confined to the ureter grade I reflux, similar to the radiographic grade I. A scintigraphic grade II would include reflux to the renal pelvis and corresponds to x-ray cystography grades II and III. If a diffusely dilated system is seen on the scintigrams, it corresponds to grades IV and V seen with contrast cystography.

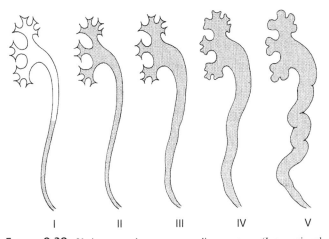

FIGURE 9-39. Vesicoureteral contrast grading system (International Reflux Study Committee). *I*, Ureteral reflux only. *II*, Reflux into ureter, pelvis, and calyces without dilation. *III*, Mild to moderate dilation/tortuosity of ureter and calyceal dilatation. *IV*, Moderate dilation and tortuosity of ureter and moderate dilation of the renal pelvis. The angles of the fornices obliterated, but the papillary impressions maintained. *V*, Gross dilation and tortuosity of the ureter and gross dilation of the renal pelvis and calyces. Papillary impressions no longer visible in most calyces.

Radionuclide cystography is more sensitive than the radiographic contrast technique. The radionuclide technique permits detection of reflux volumes on the order of 1 mL. In one study comparing the two techniques, 17% of reflux events were seen only on the radionuclide examination. Although radionuclide voiding cystography can miss low level I reflux because of the adjacent bladder activity, it is generally accepted that level I reflux is of little consequence. If a study is negative but clinical suspicion is high, refilling the bladder will improve sensitivity. This is not routinely done, however.

■ SUGGESTED READINGS

Blaufox MD, Aurell M, Bubeck B, et al. Report of the Radionuclides in Nephrology Committee on Renal Clearance. *J Nucl Med.* 1996;37(11):1883-1890.

Dubovsky EV, Russell CD, Bischof-Delaloye A, et al. Report of the radionuclides in nephrology committee for evaluation of transplanted kidney (review of techniques). *Semin Nucl Med.* 1999;29(2):175-188.

Fouzas S, Krikelli E, Vassilakos P, et al. DMSA scan for revealing vesicoureteral reflux in children with urinary tract infections. *Pediatrics.* 2010;126(3):e513-e519.

Gates GF. Glomerular filtration rate: estimation from fractional renal accumulation of Tc-99m DTPA (stannous). *AJR Am J Roentgenol.* 1982;138:565-570.

Liu Y, Blaufox MD. Use of radionuclides to study renal function. *Methods Mol Med.* 2003;86:79-117.

Maisey M. Radionuclide renography: a review. *Curr Opin Nephrol Hypertens.* 2003;12(6):649-652.

Perez-Brayfield MR, Kirsch AJ, Jones RA. A prospective study comparing ultrasound, nuclear scintigraphy and dynamic contrast enhanced magnetic resonance imaging in the evaluation of hydronephrosis. *J Urol.* 2003;170(4 Pt 1):1330-1334.

Prigent A, Cosgriff P, Gates GF, et al. Consensus report on quality control of quantitative measurements of renal function obtained from the renogram. International Committee from the Scientific Committee of Radionuclides in Nephrology. *Semin Nucl Med.* 1999;29(2):146-159.

Russell CD, Bischoff PG, Kontzen F, et al. Measurement of glomerular filtration rate using Tc-99m-DTPA and the gamma camera method. *Eur J Nucl Med.* 1985;10(11-12):519-521.

Sfakianakis GN, Sfakianakis E, Georgiou M, et al. A renal protocol for all ages and indications: mercapto-acetyl-triglycine (MAG3) with simultaneous injection of furosemide (MAG3-F0)—a 17 year experience. *Semin Nucl Med.* 2009;39(3):156-173.

Taylor A, Manatunga A, Morton K, et al. Multicenter trial of a camera-based method to measure Tc-99m mecaptoacetyltriglycine, or Tc-99m MAG3, clearance. *Radiology.* 1997;204(1):47-54.

Taylor A, Nally J, Aurell M, et al. Consensus report on ACE inhibitor renography for detecting renovascular hypertension. *J Nucl Med.* 1996;37(11):1876-1882.

Pulmonary System

PULMONARY EMBOLISM

It is estimated that more than 650,000 cases of pulmonary embolism (PE) are diagnosed each year, with more than 100,000 deaths annually. The mortality rate of approximately 30% can be reduced to 3% to 10%, with anticoagulation therapy or inferior vena cava filter placement. Predisposing factors include immobilization, recent surgery, underlying malignancy, and hypercoagulable states. In women, pregnancy and estrogen use are also risk factors.

The clinical diagnosis of PE is difficult. The classic triad of dyspnea, pleuritic chest pain, and hemoptysis is rarely encountered. Clinical signs span a spectrum from tachycardia and cough to cor pulmonale and circulatory collapse. Tests that might aid diagnosis are frequently nonspecific. Although a normal plasma D-dimer can exclude the diagnosis of PE in patients with low or intermediate clinical risk, the D-dimer can be elevated in many conditions apart from PE. Clinical grading systems such as the Modified Wells Criteria have been used to assess the clinical probability of PE (Box 10-1).

Pulmonary arteriography has been considered the gold standard for PE diagnosis, with a reported sensitivity of 98% and specificity of 97%. The arteriogram offers excellent imaging resolution and the opportunity to directly measure vascular pressures. However, interpretation can be difficult, and the invasive procedure carries a 0.5% risk for death and 2% risk for other major complications. Therefore less invasive imaging tests are more often used.

Chest radiographs are generally required when evaluating possible PE, often revealing other causes for the patient's clinical symptoms. Atelectasis, small effusions, or infiltrates may be seen, but normal radiographs are common. Changes from infarction after PE include an infiltrate from hemorrhage filling the alveolar spaces and the pleural-based *Hampton hump*.

Ready availability and lack of risk have contributed to the popularity of lower extremity ultrasound. Sonography with vein compression has a reported sensitivity of 94% and specificity of 99% for deep vein thrombosis (DVT) of the thigh veins but is less sensitive in the pelvic veins and below the knee. Although the presence or absence of DVT does not determine whether PE is present, a positive ultrasound would increase the likelihood of PE.

The nuclear medicine ventilation (V)/perfusion (Q), or V/Q, scan developed as an accurate method for PE diagnosis. In the rigorous multicenter Prospective Investigation of Pulmonary Embolism Diagnosis (PIOPED) trial, V/Q scans were performed and patients assessed for PE, with angiography required if the V/Q was abnormal. The PIOPED trial found the V/Q to be an accurate examination, but the interpretation criteria were complex. Since then, a number of modifications to the criteria have been suggested and attempts have been made to simplify reporting risk categories.

Computed tomography arteriography (CTA) has become widely used as the primary method for PE diagnosis. Emboli are seen as filling defects within the pulmonary arteries. Developments in multislice spiral CT technology and computer-guided administration of timed, powerful boluses of iodinated intravenous contrast with power injectors have contributed to high detection rates. Diagnostic accuracy with multidetector CT (MDCT) is high with the Prospective Investigation of Pulmonary Embolism Diagnosis (PIOPED) II study reporting a sensitivity, specificity, positive predictive value, and negative predictive value of 83%, 96%, 86%, and 95%, respectively. However, reports in the literature often exclude nondiagnostic or indeterminate scans from their sensitivity assessments. In the PIOPED II data, sensitivity for PE fell to 78% if indeterminate scans were included in the data. Reported rates of nondiagnostic CT scans average 6% but may be higher in some conditions, such as pregnancy, where it might reach as high as 25% due to difficulty timing the contrast bolus.

Other problems are associated with CTA. Many patients cannot have iodinated contrast because of allergy or renal failure. In the PIOPED II trial, 50% of eligible patients could not undergo MDCT. In addition, the conventional CT radiation effective dose of 3 to 5 mSv is associated with increased risk of cancer, especially of the breast in women, as well as other cancers for patients undergoing multiple scans.

Magnetic resonance angiography (MRA) offers the potential to diagnose vascular disease without ionizing radiation. However, attempts to replace CTA with MRA

Box 10-1. Modified Wells Criteria

Clinical symptoms of DVT: 3
Other diagnosis less likely than PE: 3
Heart rate >100 beats/min: 1.5
Immobilization or surgery <4 weeks: 1.5
Previous DVT or PE: 1.5
Hemoptysis: 1
Malignancy: 1

CLINICAL PROBABILITY ASSESSMENT
High: >6 (41%)
Moderate: 2-6 (16%)
Low: <2 (0.5-2.7%)

Data from Wells PS, Anderson DR, Rodger M, et al. Excluding pulmonary embolism at the bedside without diagnostic imaging: management of patients with suspected pulmonary embolism presenting to the emergency department by using a simple clinical model and d-dimer. *Ann Intern Med.* 2001;135(2):98-107.

have not yet been successful. The PIOPED III trial reported a sensitivity of only 63% for pulmonary emboli.

The V/Q scintigram remains an important tool for the diagnosis of PE. With an effective dose of approximately 2 mSv or less, the V/Q scan results in significantly lower radiation exposure to the chest than CT. In addition to patients who cannot have CTA, the V/Q scan is often recommended as a first-line test in patients with negative radiographs. These patients have a high likelihood of a diagnostic V/Q scan, and many sites utilize very low-dose techniques involving perfusion only techniques.

It should be noted that data from the PIOPED II trial failed to prove the superiority of CTA over VQ. The positive predictive value of CTA at 83% is similar to that of a high-probability V/Q lung scan at more than 85%. The negative predictive value of CTA at 95% is very close to the less than 10% chance of PE in a very-low-probability scan. Both CTA and V/Q lose value if the objective clinical evaluation is discordant or does not match the imaging results.

Experts also note that many of the prior V/Q trials, including PIOPED I, were performed on equipment that would not be considered acceptable by today's resolution

standards. Better ventilation delivery systems and agents have improved specificity and lowered nondiagnostic examination rates. Also, dual-headed single-photon emission computed tomography (SPECT) offers the possibility of improved sensitivity and specificity.

Yet a great deal of confusion remains over the interpretation of V/Q findings. Complex and periodically changing interpretation criteria have added to the difficulties the average physician faces when reviewing V/Q scan results. New, simplified interpretation criteria are being considered in the United States and are already recommended in Europe.

■ VENTILATION PERFUSION SCINTIGRAPHY

Ventilation and perfusion are normally coupled in the lungs. Gravity affects radiotracer distribution, with the lung apices receiving less perfusion and ventilation than the bases in a normal gradient. Areas of the lung that are well ventilated are also well perfused (Fig. 10-1), with the opposite being true as well.

Many diseases such as asthma, bronchitis, pneumonia, and emphysema affect aeration. The normal regional

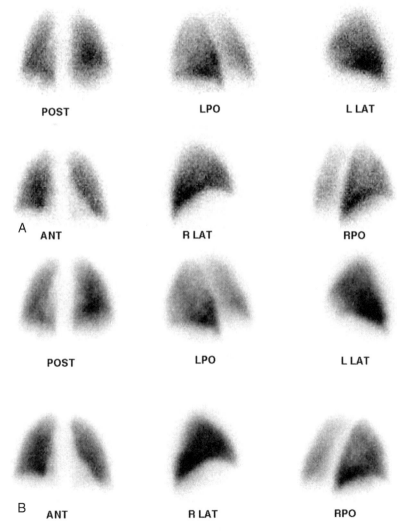

FIGURE 10-1. Normal V/Q scan. Ventilation (**A**) and perfusion (**B**) lung scans show homogeneous radiotracer distribution and the normal gradient of increasing activity in the bases relative to the apices. *ANT,* Anterior; *L LAT,* left lateral; *LPO,* left posterior oblique; *POST,* posterior; *R LAT,* right lateral; *RPO,* right posterior oblique.

response to acute hypoxia is vasoconstriction, which shunts blood flow away to other aerated areas of lung. This results in regions of reduced perfusion and reduced ventilation that are "matched." In a pulmonary embolus, pulmonary arterial perfusion is reduced. The ventilation is unaffected in such cases, so the alveolar spaces remain aerated. Ventilation and perfusion are uncoupled or "mismatched" in territories affected by the pulmonary embolus.

These physiological parameters form the foundation of interpretation of the V/Q scan. Intravenously injected radiolabeled microscopic particles large enough to be trapped on the first pass through the pulmonary capillary bed show the distribution of pulmonary blood flow. To determine whether a perfusion defect is secondary to a ventilation abnormality rather than primarily a vascular problem, inhaled radiopharmaceuticals can map ventilation. Because most mismatched perfusion abnormalities are the result of acute pulmonary emboli, the diagnosis can be made with a reasonably high degree of accuracy.

■ RADIOPHARMACEUTICALS

Perfusion Radiopharmaceuticals

Red blood cells have a diameter just under 8 μm, capillaries are just slightly larger at 7 to 10 μm, and precapillary arterioles are approximately 35 μm. For a perfusion agent to be trapped on the first pass, the particles must be larger than the size of the capillaries. However, if the particles are too large, becoming trapped in larger central arterioles, distribution may not fully reflect perfusion, potentially causing artifactual or exaggerated defects.

Several particulate agents have been used over the years, including iodine-131 macroaggregated albumin and technetium-99m (Tc-99m)–labeled human albumin microspheres. However, only Tc-99m macroaggregated albumin (Tc-99m MAA) is available for clinical use in the United States. Tc-99m MAA preparations contain particles ranging in size from 5 to 100 μm, generally with 60% to 80% between 10 and 30 μm. A kit containing MAA and stannous ion is available. Tc-99m pertechnetate is added to the reaction vial, resulting in rapid labeling of the MAA particles.

After peripheral intravenous injection, the Tc-99m MAA passes through the right atrium into the right ventricle, where mixing with blood occurs before particles are pumped into the pulmonary arteries. As the MAA move into smaller vessels, it is filtered out or trapped throughout the pulmonary bed. Where perfusion is decreased or absent, the lack of particles appears as a "cold" region on the scan.

The MAA particles have a biological half-life in the lungs of approximately 4 to 6 hours. Over time, the particles undergo degradation. They may lodge in smaller vessels or enter the circulation but eventually are phagocytized in the reticuloendothelial system.

The number of particles used for the scan is an important consideration. If the dose is too small, the distribution pattern will not be statistically valid. On the other hand, too many particles could theoretically obstruct a hemodynamically significant portion of the vessels. In practice, 200,000 to 500,000 particles are administered. Because there are an estimated 300 million precapillary arterioles and more than 280 billion pulmonary capillaries, this should result in no ill effects with obstruction of only 0.1% to 0.3% of vessels.

For children, the number of particles given is a reflection of age, decreased to 10,000 for neonates and 50,000 to 150,000 for children younger than 5 years of age. A reduction in the number of particles is also warranted in certain conditions in adults, such as in cases of pulmonary hypertension, right-to-left cardiac shunt, and pregnancy. Patients with pulmonary hypertension may have significantly fewer capillaries than normal. Theoretically, the condition could be worsened if too many more capillaries are blocked so the number is reduced to 100,000 to 250,000. In cases of right-to-left cardiac shunt in which particles enter the systemic circulation, the brain, kidneys, and other structures will be visualized. Although this seems alarming, investigators have long used Tc-99m MAA without ill effect to calculate the severity of cardiac shunts. Although it is prudent to decrease the number of particles to 100,000 to 150,000, right-to-left shunt is not a contraindication to V/Q.

In pregnant patients, a V/Q scan offers the ability to diagnose PE with low risk. Clearly, the minimum amount of radiation should be used, but simply requesting a lower dose of radioactivity is not sufficient. The request should indicate the reduced number of particles requested, maintaining the minimum of 100,000 particles. The amount of Tc-99m added to commercially available multidose vials changes after the first dose, so calculations change. In addition, fresh particles are desirable. Many patients can be diagnosed on the perfusion scan alone; therefore many sites advocate performing a reduced-dose perfusion-only scan with 1 to 2 mCi (37-74 MBq) of Tc-9m MAA in pregnant patients to reduce fetal exposure. If a ventilation scan is deemed necessary, it is performed the next day. Although the radiation dose to the fetus is low, it is higher than from CTA.

Ventilation Radiopharmaceuticals

An ideal ventilation radiopharmaceutical could be used after the perfusion examination was completed, once it was deemed a ventilation examination was necessary. It should have an optimal radiolabel for gamma camera imaging and closely model respiration, with activity rapidly moving to the lung periphery even in cases of turbulent flow or air trapping. Because of the need for imaging in multiple projections or possibly SPECT, it should not clear too rapidly from the lungs. Two classes of radiopharmaceuticals are available for ventilation imaging: radioactive gases and radioaerosols (Box 10-2).

Radioactive gases are generally preferred in cases of abnormal airflow, more often resulting in diagnostic images. Two of these are no longer in common use. The higher energy photopeaks of xenon-127 (172 keV and 375 keV) compared to Tc-99m MAA allows ventilation imaging after the perfusion scan. However, the long half-life (36.4 days) and the higher energies add to

Box 10-2. Ventilation and Perfusion Agents of Historical Interest

PERFUSION
Tc-99m human albumin microspheres
Tc-99m macroaggregated albumin (MAA)*

VENTILATION
Radioactive Gases
Xe-133*
Xe-127
Kr-81m

Radioaerosols
Tc-99m DTPA*
Tc-99m Technegas

*Currently available for clinical use in the United States.

TABLE 10-1 Comparison of Xenon-133 and Technetium-99m DTPA Ventilation Agents

Comparison factors	Xenon-133	Tc-99m DTPA
Mode of decay	Beta-minus	Isomeric
Physical half-life	53 days	6 hr
Biological half-life	30 sec	45 min
Photon energy	81 keV	140 keV
Multiple-view imaging	No	Yes
Useful for severe COPD	Yes	+/−
Used after perfusion scan	No	No

COPD, Chronic obstructive pulmonary disease; *DTPA*, diethylenetriaminepentaacetic acid.

patient exposure and special xenon traps and delivery systems are required. Krypton-81m (Kr-81m) has an ideal photopeak of 190 keV. It is continuously eluted from a rubidium-81/Kr-81m generator because of the short half-life of 13 seconds. It can reach true equilibrium in the lungs. However, the expensive generator has a half-life of only 4.6 hours. Neither of these agents ever achieved wide use.

Only one aerosol, Tc-99m diethylenetriamine pentaacetic acid (DTPA), and one gas, Xe-133, are commercially available in the United States. Comparative studies have not shown a significant difference in accuracy between the two agents. The choice depends largely on available equipment, room ventilation, and experience, as well as the prevalence of chronic obstructive pulmonary disease (COPD) in the referral population. Outside the United States, Tc-99m Technegas has been widely used for years and appears to provide superior images. A multicenter trial is ongoing in the United States.

Xenon-133

Xe-133 is the only gas currently commercially available in the United States. The physical characteristics of Xe-133 are listed in Table 10-1. The physical half-life of 5.3 days makes it easy for radiopharmacies to keep and supply. Xe-133 clears from the body rapidly, with a biological half-life of 30 seconds during washout. Xe-133 offers superior sensitivity to Tc-99m DTPA for detection of COPD, improving specificity. No central airway deposition occurs, and the photopeak is low at 81 keV; thus artifact from the ventilation agent does not interfere with perfusion image interpretation.

However, Xe-133 has several disadvantages. First of all, unlike a radioaerosol, the rapid washout limits the number of views and projections obtainable. The lower photopeak of 81-keV is not optimal for gamma camera imaging. Anterior images, in particular, may be limited by soft tissue attenuation. The photopeak is also less than that of Tc-99m MAA. Therefore the ventilation scan must be performed first, or the down scatter from the Tc-99m perfusion images would degrade the ventilation scan. Finally, special equipment (e.g., xenon traps [charcoal filters and tubing that retain xenon], negative pressure rooms, good airflow

mechanisms, and external exhaust ventilation or filters) is needed to maintain radiation safety.

Technetium-99m DTPA

The physical properties of Tc-99m DTPA are listed in Table 10-1. Liquid Tc-99m DTPA can be aerosolized using a commercially available nebulizer to produce nanoparticles capable of being readily inhaled. The ideal particle size is in the range of 0.1 to 0.5 μm. Particles larger than 1 to 2 μm tend to settle out in the large airways, including the trachea and bronchi, limiting the quality of the ventilation study and possibly "shining through" onto the subsequent perfusion examination. Particle clumping may still occur in patients unable to cooperate with deep breathing or who have asthma or COPD.

Tc-99m DTPA aerosol particles are cleared by crossing the airway membrane and entering the circulation, where they are cleared by the kidney. The biological half-life is approximately 80 ± 20 minutes in healthy people and 24 ± 9 minutes in healthy smokers.

Technetium-99m Technegas

The aerosol Technegas consists of Tc-99m–labeled solid graphite particles with a submicron diameter of approximately 100 nM (0.005-0.2 μm) in argon carrier gas. Once inhaled, the particles adhere to the walls of the alveoli. However, like a gas, the particles penetrate far into the lung periphery without the central clumping often seen in COPD with Tc-99m DTPA. In addition to having the advantages of a gas, multiple views or SPECT imaging is possible, adding appeal.

Exhaled Technegas is trapped by a filter in the mouthpiece and valve assembly. Because it must be used rapidly to prevent aggregation, Technegas is produced onsite by a generator. This generator requires regular maintenance. Tc-99m Technegas is widely used outside of the United States, and the images appear superior to those obtained with Tc-99m DTPA and Xe-133.

Dosimetry

Radiation dosimetry values are listed in Table 10-2. The V/Q lung scan results in low radiation exposure with any of the ventilation agents. The Tc-99m MAA dose to the lungs generally results in less than 1 cGy (1 rad).

TABLE 10-2 Dosimetry of Ventilation-Perfusion Scan Agents

Radiopharmaceutical	Administered activity mCi (MBq)	Organ receive largest dose rad/mCi (mGy/MBq)	Effective dose rem/mCi (mSv/MBq)
Tc-99m MAA	1-4 (40-150)	0.25 Lungs (0.067)	0.041 (0.011)
Tc-99m DTPA	0.5-1.0 (20-40)	0.17 Bladder (0.047)	0.023 (0.0061)
Xe-133	5-20 (200-750)	0.0041 Lungs (0.0011)	0.0026 (0.00071)
Kr-81m	1-10 (40-400)	0.00078 Lungs (0.00021)	0.0001 (0.000003)
Tc-99m Technegas[†]	0.5-0.8 (19-30)	0.41 Lungs (0.11)	0.555 (0.015)

*From The Society of Nuclear Medicine and Molecular Imaging Practice Guideline for Lung Scintigraphy, x4.0. http://interactive.snm.org/Lung_Scintigraphy_V4_Final. pdf; 2011.
[†]From EANM guidelines for ventilation perfusion scintigraphy. *Eur J Nucl Med Mol Imaging.* 2009.
DTPA, Diethylenetriaminepentaacetic acid; *MAA,* macroaggregated albumin.

Reports describe the effective whole-body dose for a V/Q scan to be 1.4 to 2 mSv compared to 2.2 to 6.0 mSv from CTA. In the breasts, the exposure from CT at 35 mGy for each breast may be particularly significant given that an increased risk for breast cancer is reported after 10 mGy in women younger than 35 years of age. In pregnant patients, fetal doses from V/Q are low, reportedly 350 to 570 μGy using a reduced 1 to 2 mCi (37-74 MBq)-MBq Tc-99m MAA dose. However, this is generally higher than with CT.

Technique

Xenon-133 Ventilation

The protocol for Xe-133 is outlined in Box 10-3. The examination is performed in three phases: the single breath or wash-in phase, the equilibrium phase, and the washout phase (Fig. 10-2, *A*). The patient is usually placed with the camera posteriorly because, while the location of perfusion defects is not known in advance, most PEs involve the lower lobes. Some laboratories perform the examination in the supine position, whereas others favor sitting because it allows better posterior oblique acquisitions. Positioning should be the same for both ventilation and perfusion imaging.

To begin with, a closed system is set up with a facemask or mouthpiece. This may be difficult for some patients to tolerate. The patient is asked to take a breath in and hold it. An initial image is obtained at maximal inspiration for 100,000 counts, if possible, or 10 to 15 seconds.

After the initial breath is completed, the next phase of the study is the equilibrium phase. The patient breathes a mixture of air and Xe-133 at tidal volume. Two images are usually obtained for 90 seconds each. Optional, posterior oblique images can be performed.

Then, the system is opened during the third phase. The patient breathes room air, and exhaled Xe-133 is delivered to a trapping system or evacuated to the exterior. Three or four sequential 45-second washout images are obtained as Xe-133 clears from the lungs.

Technetium-99m DTPA

Because the radiolabel is the same as the perfusion agent and the achievable count rates or the amount of aerosol that reaches the lungs from the nebulizer is significantly

---

Box 10-3. Xenon-133 Ventilation Scintigraphy: Protocol Summary

PATIENT PREPARATION
None

DOSAGE AND ADMINISTRATION
10-20 mCi (370-740 MBq) inhaled

INSTRUMENTATION
Collimator: Low-energy parallel hole
Photopeak: 20% window centered at 81 keV

POSITIONING
Supine; seated may be necessary.
Camera centered over chest posteriorly.
If dual-head camera, second head may be placed anteriorly.
Use tight-seal facemask or mouthpiece with attached spirometer and intake and exhaust tubing.

IMAGING PROTOCOL
First breath: Patient exhales fully and is asked to maximally inspire and hold it long enough (if possible) to obtain 100,000 counts or 10-15 seconds.
Equilibrium: Obtain two sequential 90-second images while the patient breathes normally.
Washout
  Turn system to exhaust.
  Obtain three sequential 45-second posterior images, then right and left posterior oblique images, and final posterior image.

---

less than the amount of injected Tc-99m MAA, the Tc-99m DTPA ventilation examination is performed first.

The lung ventilation protocol for Tc-99m DTPA is listed in Box 10-4. The radiopharmaceutical is placed within the nebulizer. Placing the patient in the supine position will minimize the gravity perfusion gradient in the lungs. However, an erect position may improve detection of lesions in the bases and allow the patient to be in better proximity to the camera heads during lateral and oblique images. The nose may be clamped, and the patient is asked to breathe through a mouthpiece in a closed system until sufficient radiotracer is delivered to the lungs, which may require

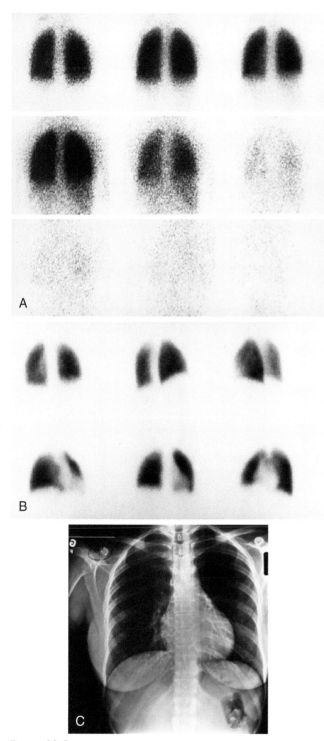

FIGURE 10-2. Normal VQ with xenon-133 ventilation. **A,** The initial breath and equilibrium images are in the *upper* row. The sequential washout images in the *middle* and *lower* rows show no evidence of air trapping. **B,** Corresponding Tc-99m MAA images show homogeneous distribution of tracer activity throughout the lungs. **C,** The chest radiograph was also normal.

several minutes. Although 30 mCi (1110 MBq) is placed in the nebulizer, only 0.5 to 1.0 mCi (18.5-37 MBq) is delivered to the patient. The goal is to deliver enough radioaerosol to the lungs to achieve 200,000 to 250,000 count images in 1 to 2 minutes. Usually, inhalation continues until (1 mCi [37 MBq]) is delivered to the lungs.

Box 10-4. Technetium-99m DTPA Ventilation Scintigraphy: Protocol Summary

PATIENT PREPARATION
None

DOSAGE AND ADMINISTRATION
30 mCi (1110 MBq) Tc-99m DTPA in nebulizer

INSTRUMENTATION
Collimator: Low energy, parallel hole.
Photopeak: 20% window centered at 140 keV.

POSITIONING
Place nose clamps on patient and connect mouthpiece with patient supine.

IMAGE PROTOCOL
Center camera over chest posteriorly.
Patient breathes continuously through mouthpiece for several minutes.
Acquire posterior image for 250,000 counts.
Obtain other views for same time as the posterior.
  Views: Posterior, anterior, right and left lateral, right and left posterior oblique, anterior oblique views recommended.

Technetium-99m MAA Perfusion

The perfusion protocol is described in Box 10-5. Immediately before injection, the dose syringe is inverted to mix the particles that have settled and to prevent clumping. A 23-gauge or larger needle should be used to prevent fragmentation of the dose during administration. The 2- to 5-mCi (74-185 MBq) dose containing 200,000 to 500,000 particles is injected slowly over the course of several respiratory cycles. Care must be taken not to draw blood back into the syringe, because this would cause clots in the syringe, resulting in hot emboli on the images (Fig. 10-3).

Once the injection is complete, imaging can begin immediately. Multiple projections are obtained in the same position as the ventilation if Tc-99m DTPA was used. Most nuclear medicine clinics obtain anterior, posterior, right and left lateral, right and left 45-degree anterior oblique, and both 45-degree posterior oblique images.

Single-Photon Emission Computed Tomography

With its increased sensitivity, SPECT V/Q imaging has gained popularity in many centers, especially outside of the United States. Generally, studies are done on a dual-head gamma camera using 0.6 to 0.8 mCi (25- to 30-MBq) Tc-99m Technegas immediately followed, without moving the patient, by the perfusion study using 100 to 120 MBq of Tc-99m MAA.

▬ IMAGE INTERPRETATION

A rigorous, systematic approach is needed to interpret V/Q scans. First, a chest radiograph less than 24-hours old must be reviewed. Any abnormality should be classified as acute or chronic if possible. Acute findings such as atelectasis,

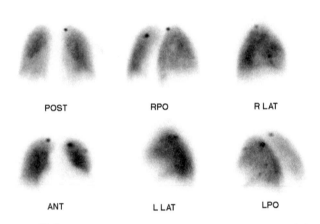

POST   RPO   R LAT

ANT   L LAT   LPO

Figure 10-3. Injected blood clot artifact with Tc-99m MAA. Blood clots formed from drawing blood back into the syringe appear as focal hot spots when they are reinjected into the patient. These have a variable appearance but can be quite large. *ANT,* Anterior; *L LAT,* left lateral; *LPO,* left posterior oblique; *POST,* posterior; *R LAT,* right lateral; *RPO,* right posterior oblique.

infiltrates, and effusions that might cause triple match defects are noted, as are potential causes of nonsegmental defects such as cardiomegaly, elevated diaphragm, and hilar enlargement.

Ventilation Scintigram

The normal distribution of Tc-99m DTPA should appear similar to that seen on the corresponding Tc-99m MAA perfusion image but with fewer counts on the image (Fig 10-1). The lung bases may appear more intense than the apices, and the heart causes a mild defect in the left anterior base.

The normal Xe-133 scintigram shows homogenous activity on all three phases, without defect, or significant retention during washout (Fig. 10-2, *A*). The initial single-breath image may appear slightly less intense than the subsequent equilibrium image because it has fewer counts. Washout should be rapid, with a clearance half-time of less than 2 minutes with good patient cooperation. The last image may have very faint or no discernable residual activity. Because of the low photopeak, attenuation occurring from anterior structures often degrades images. Even with dual-headed cameras, it may not be possible to image all regions of the lung in a single sitting as a result of the rapid washout and challenges of positioning the patient with the ventilator apparatus in place.

Differential Diagnosis of Ventilation Abnormalities

Destruction of the bronchial walls causes decreased ventilation in chronic bronchitis, bronchiectasis, and the bullae of COPD. Acute ventilation decreases can be seen from bronchospasm in COPD or asthma. Additionally, areas do not ventilate if the alveolar spaces are filled with fluid, such as in heart failure or pneumonia. Mucous plug impaction can affect large regions—from a lobe to a whole lung. The abnormal patterns seen in these processes vary in shape and size (Fig. 10-4). Often, the acute ventilation defects from mucous plugs are worse than the regional perfusion. Ventilation is not affected in PE, especially early on in the first 24 hours.

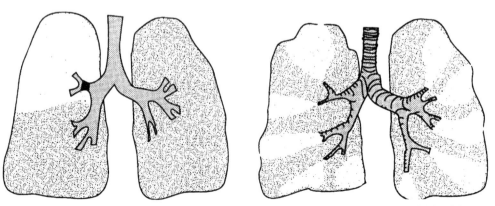

Figure 10-4. Effects of airway obstruction. Ventilation abnormalities may be due to obstructions in larger airways. This might present as a large defect *(left)* caused by bronchogenic carcinoma or mucous plugs. Constriction of smaller bronchi in asthma can also cause ventilation abnormalities *(right)*.

All airway processes may appear as a defect with either ventilation agent, but Xe-133 is more sensitive than Tc-99m DTPA. The Xe-133 washout phase is the most sensitive, detecting 90% of ventilation abnormalities compared with 70% on the initial single-breath image and 20% for equilibrium images. Although this improves specificity by proving perfusion defects to be matched, it can make the Xe-133 images more challenging because the abnormality can change over the course of the scan. An initial defect may fill in over time, and an area originally normal may fail to clear because air trapping. It is important to remember that a study is abnormal if there is an abnormality on any phase of the Xe-133 imaging.

Difficulties can occur when radiotracer is seen outside of the normal confines of the lungs. Swallowed Tc-99m DTPA in the mouth, esophagus, and stomach (Fig. 10-5) can shine through on the subsequent perfusion examination and mask perfusion defects. Central Tc-99m DTPA deposition in trachea and large bronchi also can limit the interpretation. Occasionally, Xe-133 retained activity is seen in the right upper quadrant, which is difficult to separate from lung base. This is the result of retention of the fat soluble Xe-133 in the liver in patients with fatty infiltration (Fig. 10-6) and should not be mistaken for air-way trapping in the right lower lobe.

Perfusion Scintigram

Normal perfusion images show homogenous, uniform distribution of radiotracer throughout the lungs (Figs. 10-1, B, and 10-2, B). The hilar structures are often seen as photopenic areas, and the heart causes decreased activity in the left base. The spine and sternum attenuate activity at midline. Differences in positioning during radiotracer administration cause variations in distribution from the effects of gravity, with activity greater in the lower lung fields.

Renal uptake can persist from the previous Tc-99m DTPA ventilation examination. Free pertechnetate from the Tc-99m MAA can be seen in the kidneys, stomach, and thyroid. However, contaminants and free pertechnetate cannot cross the blood–brain barrier. Tc-99m MAA uptake in the brain should be attributed to a right-to-left cardiac shunt (Fig. 10-7).

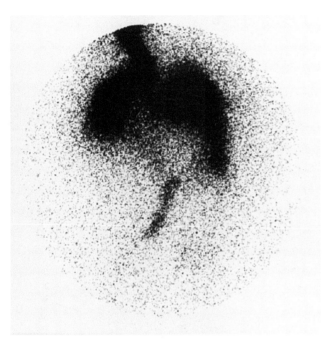

FIGURE 10-5. Swallowed Tc-99m DTPA. Intense uptake in the trachea and stomach may result from swallowed radiopharmaceutical.

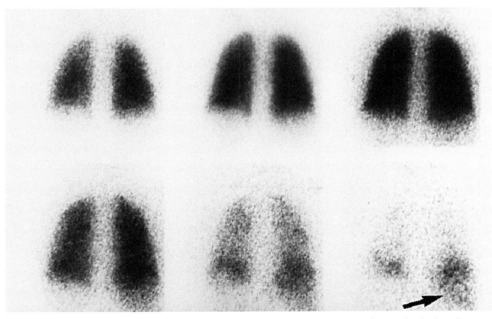

FIGURE 10-6. Xe-133 accumulation in the liver. Posterior ventilation images show delayed washout of xenon in the lung bases and significant xenon uptake in the region of the liver *(arrow)*.

Differential Diagnosis of Perfusion Abnormalities

Perfusion is considered abnormal not only when it is absent but also when it is diminished. Causes for perfusion defects are listed in Box 10-6, and many of the special terms used in the diagnostic schemes employed in V/Q interpretation are defined in Box 10-7. Pulmonary emboli typically cause multiple moderate to large defects, most common in the lower lungs (Fig. 10-8). In the acute stages after a pulmonary embolus occurs, ventilation is maintained in the corresponding region, resulting in V/Q mismatch (Fig. 10-9). Although patterns vary, the likelihood of PE increases as the number and size of mismatched perfusion defects increase. Knowledge of segmental anatomy is critical for correct interpretation and lesion description (Fig. 10-10).

While perfusion defects are unlikely to be from PE when matched by a ventilation defect, even when very numerous, sometimes small unmatched defects can occur without PE. This can occur in smokers or in the lung bases when restrictive air way disease is present.

Nonsegmental defects, those resulting from processes outside the pulmonary segments, must be recognized. The term *nonsegmental* should not be used to describe lesions that are within a segmental distribution but do not involve the entire segment. These are more correctly referred to as *small segmental* or *subsegmental*. Some causes of nonsegmental defects are listed in Box 10-8. Pleural effusions have a variable appearance. They may layer out in supine patients (Fig. 10-11). In other cases, effusions or fibrosis may cause a defect running along the fissures. Although this extends to the pleural surface, the characteristic "fissure" sign is clearly nonsegmental (Fig. 10-12). Breasts, arms, and soft tissues can all cause attenuation artifacts. Explanations for other perfusion defects, such as adenopathy, masses, and

---

Box 10-6. Causes of Perfusion Defects

PRIMARY VASCULAR LESION
Pulmonary thromboembolism
Septic, fat, and air emboli
Pulmonary artery hypoplasia or atresia
Vasculitis

PRIMARY VENTILATION ABNORMALITY
Pneumonia
Atelectasis
Pulmonary edema
Asthma
Chronic obstructive pulmonary disease, emphysema, chronic bronchitis, bullae
Mucous plug

MASS EFFECT
Tumor
Adenopathy
Pleural effusion

IATROGENIC
Surgery: Pneumonectomy lobectomy
Radiation fibrosis (also postinflammatory fibrosis)

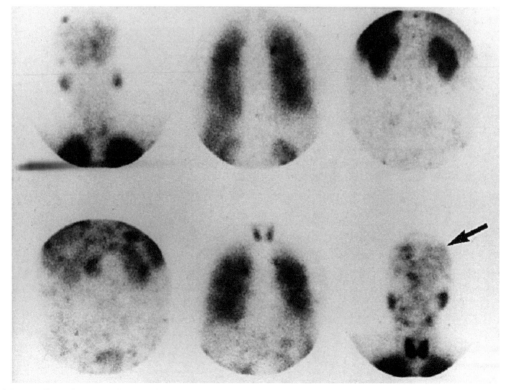

FIGURE 10-7. Right-to-left cardiac shunt. Tc-99m MAA images reveal abnormal uptake in the kidneys, liver, and brain *(arrow)* from a right-to-left shunt. Heterogeneous activity in the abdomen is also from shunting. Free pertechnetate activity is seen in the thyroid, salivary glands, and urine but does not explain the cerebral activity as free pertechnetate does not cross the blood brain barrier.

Box 10-7. Ventilation-Perfusion Terminology

V/Q matched defect: Both scans abnormal in same area and of equal size

V/Q mismatch: Abnormal perfusion in an area of normal ventilation or a much larger perfusion defect than ventilation abnormality

Triple-match: V/Q matching defects in a region of chest radiographic abnormality, in which the radiographic abnormality is of the same size or smaller than the perfusion defect

Segmental defect: Characteristically wedge shaped and pleural based; conforms to segmental anatomy of the lung; may be caused by occlusion of pulmonary artery branches

   Large: >75% of a lung segment

   Moderate: 25%-75% of a lung segment

   Small: <25% of a lung segment

Nonsegmental defect: Does not conform to segmental anatomy or does not appear wedge shaped

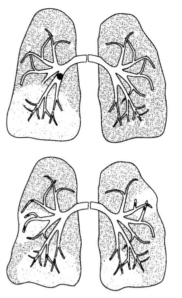

FIGURE 10-8. Effect of pulmonary artery branching pattern on the appearance of emboli. Emboli may be due to larger, more proximal clots *(top)* or showers of smaller clots lodging more distally *(bottom).* In either case, the resulting defects should be pleural-based and corresponding to the segments of the lung.

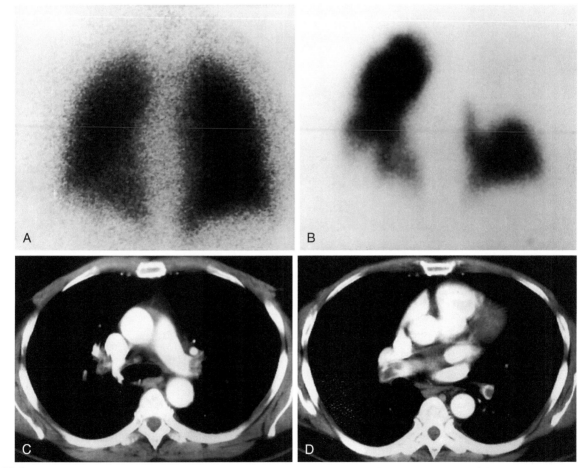

FIGURE 10-9. Effects from a pulmonary embolus. Posterior equilibrium ventilation image **(A)** and perfusion image **(B)** reveal an extensive mismatch in the left lung base and upper half of the right lung. **C,** Spiral CT shows contrast around a large partially obscuring clot in the left main pulmonary artery and right upper lobe pulmonary artery. **D,** Filling defects in the left descending pulmonary artery and right interlobar pulmonary artery are also present.

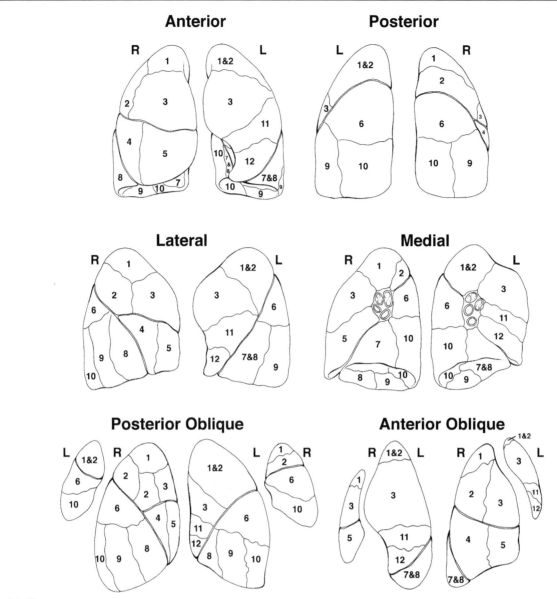

FIGURE 10-10. Segmental anatomy of the lungs. *Upper lobe: 1*, apical; *2*, posterior; *3*, anterior. *Right middle lobe: 4*, lateral; *5*, medial. *Lower lobe: 6*, superior; *7*, medial basal; *8*, anterior basal; *9*, lateral basal; *10*, posterior basal. *Lingula (left): 11*, superior lingual; *12*, inferior lingual.

BOX 10-8. Causes of Nonsegmental Defects

Pacemaker artifact	Cardiomegaly
Tumors	Hilar adenopathy
Pleural effusion	Atelectasis
Trauma	Pneumonia
Hemorrhage	Aortic ectasia or aneurysm
Bullae	

BOX 10-9. Causes of Severe Unilateral Lung Perfusion Abnormality

Pneumonectomy
Mediastinal fibrosis
Tumor
Pneumothorax
Mucous plug
Pulmonary embolus
Pulmonary artery stenosis or atresia
Swyer-James syndrome
Chylothorax
Massive pleural effusion

---

pacemakers, should be sought on the radiograph. This correlation should be made with a chest radiograph less than 24 hours old, given the rapid rate at which processes in the lungs can evolve.

Occasionally, perfusion defects predominantly involve one lung (Box 10-9). Such asymmetric abnormalities are often from surgery. However, a mucous plug can sometimes involve a whole lobe or lung, causing matched ventilation and perfusion defects. Although a large

saddle embolus could affect only one lung, this is extremely rare. If a perfusion defect without a corresponding ventilation abnormality only involves one lung, close scrutiny of the radiograph or CT is needed to exclude a centrally located bronchogenic carcinoma or

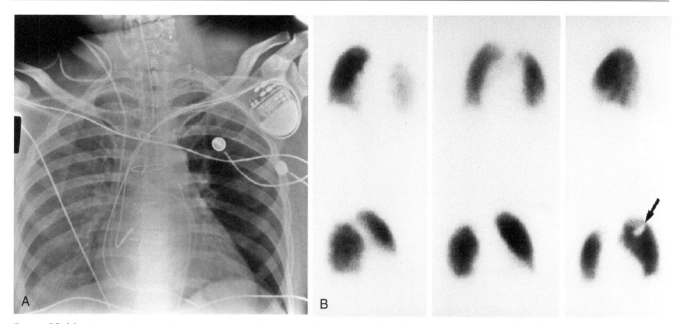

FIGURE 10-11. Pleural effusion effect. **A,** Anteroposterior chest radiograph reveals uniformly greater density in the right lung compared to the left caused by an effusion layering out posteriorly when the patient is supine. **B,** Corresponding Tc-99m MAA perfusion study shows decreased perfusion to the right lung on the posterior view *(upper left hand image)*, which is not seen on the other views, tipping off the observer to the explanation for the discrepancy. Blunting of the costophrenic angle is apparent. The pacemaker causes a well-defined defect *(arrow)*.

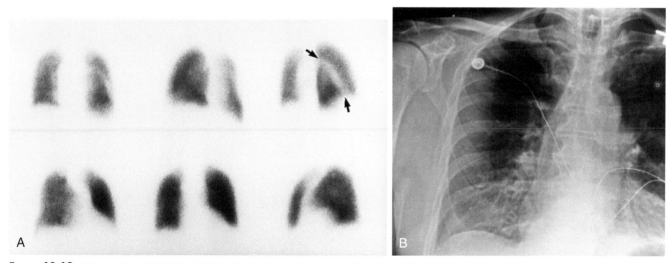

FIGURE 10-12. Fissure sign. **A,** Tc-99m MAA perfusion images show a curvilinear defect in the area of the major fissure of the right lung from the "fissure sign." **B,** Corresponding radiograph shows right costophrenic angle blunting but provides no indication of the extent of the fluid in the fissure.

hilar mass, which could impinge only on the vessel but spare the adjacent the airway.

If the patient's symptoms are less than 24 hours in duration, classic multiple, large mismatched perfusion defects on the V/Q scan can be expected. However, the appearance of PE varies over time. Because emboli may be intermittent or recurrent and are broken down with time, a mix of large and small defects is often present, possibly with some ventilation abnormalities at different stages of evolution. The speed at which clots resolve varies considerably, improving rapidly in some patients and never resolving in others, particularly the elderly. Defects should not resolve in less than 24 hours, whereas defects persisting for 3 to 6 months are unlikely to ever clear.

Perfusion defect size is an important consideration in the differential diagnosis. Because emboli usually cause larger defects, many assessment criteria include lesion size as an important parameter. By convention, a defect is considered large if it involves more than 75% of a lung segment, moderate if it is between 25% and 75%, and small if it is less than 25%. Size grading is made more difficult as the segments themselves vary considerably by size. Size estimates are subjective, although confidence increases with experience. Some authors suggest there is no difference between moderate and large defect significance, which simplifies interpretation.

Even if the embolus is more central, ensuing segmental defects should affect the entire lung beyond the occlusion in a wedgelike distribution. This is not the case in a process such as pneumonia, in which perfusion might persist

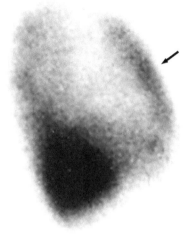

R LAT

Figure 10-13. Stripe sign. Perfusion on the right lateral view is seen anteriorly along the periphery of the lung *(arrow)*, beyond an extensive area of decreased perfusion posterior to it strongly suggesting that the decreased perfusion in the upper lobe is not caused by PE.

beyond a more central lesion. When preserved perfusion is seen at the periphery or pleural margin of a perfusion defect, it has been termed the "stripe sign" and used to help exclude the diagnosis of PE (Fig. 10-13). It may be difficult to determine whether a defect truly extends to the lung periphery given that a volume of tissue is being examined on the two-dimensional image. Defects overlapping with normal areas may be completely obscured. This is one reason why the increased sensitivity of SPECT has gained popularity at some institutions.

As has been stated, ventilation in the area of the PE should be normal, causing a V/Q mismatch. However, this may not remain true, and ventilation can decrease, especially as atelectasis develops. Correlation with the radiograph is helpful in identifying secondary atelectasis and infiltrates from hemorrhagic infarct that could cause a false negative V/Q result with a match on the ventilation. A *triple match* is the term used for matching abnormalities on ventilation, perfusion, and chest radiograph.

Triple matches must be considered differently when assessing the probability of a PE. If the perfusion defect is much smaller than a radiographic abnormality, it is unlikely to be from PE, which affects the vascular territory beyond the occlusion point. It is also important to try and discover whether the radiographic abnormality is acute or chronic. Acute findings that can be seen with PE include atelectasis, infiltrate, and effusion, whereas chronic scar, long-standing effusion, and masses are obviously not consistent with acute PE. In addition, studies have shown that triple matches in lower lobes are more likely caused by PE than those in upper lung zones.

▬ VENTILATION-PERFUSION INTERPRETATION CRITERIA

The PIOPED trial resulted in widely accepted criteria for assigning a risk for PE based on the V/Q scan and chest x-ray findings (Box 10-10). The categories of risk

---

Box 10-10. PIOPED Criteria for Pulmonary Embolus Diagnosis

HIGH-PROBABILITY SCAN
Two or more large mismatched segmental defects (or equivalent in moderate or large defects) with normal radiograph
Any perfusion defect substantially larger than radiographic abnormality

INTERMEDIATE PROBABILITY SCAN
Multiple perfusion defects with associated radiographic opacities
More than 25% of a segment and fewer than two mismatched segmental perfusion defects with normal radiograph:
  One moderate segmental defect
  One large or two moderate segmental defects
  One large and one moderate segmental defect
  Three moderate segmental defects
Solitary moderate to large matching segmental defect with matching radiograph (triple match)
  Later analysis suggested
    Upper and mid-lung zone triple match = low probability
    Lower lung zone triple match = intermediate probability
Difficult to characterize as high probability or low probability

LOW PROBABILITY SCAN
Nonsegmental defects: tiny effusion blunting costophrenic angle, cardiomegaly elevated diaphragm, ectatic aorta
Any perfusion defect with substantially larger radiographic abnormality
Matched ventilation and perfusion defects with normal chest radiograph
Small subsegmental perfusion defects with normal radiograph

NORMAL SCAN
No perfusion defects

PIOPED, Prospective Investigation of Pulmonary Embolism Diagnosis.

---

for PE were high probability (>80% risk for PE), intermediate probability (20%-80% risk), low probability (<20% risk), and normal. Scans also could be indeterminate if technically inadequate.

A subsequent retrospective analysis of the PIOPED data led to some additional suggested changes. These modified PIOPED criteria were found to be more accurate, although based on limited data. For example, it was recognized that the 20% cited risk of the low probability category was too high to base clinical decisions on, and an additional category—very low probability (<10% risk)—was proposed. Use of the very low probability category has varied widely in clinical practice.

Revised PIOPED criteria have been used in the PIOPED II trial to assess the accuracy of CTA. The modified PIOPED II criteria are widely used in the United States. The latest

TABLE **10-3** Comparison of 2011 PIOPED and Modified Criteria for Ventilation and Perfusion Scan Interpretation Risk or Probability Criteria

PIOPED criteria	Modified PIOPED II criteria
HIGH LR	**HIGH LR**
More than two large mismatched segmental defects	Two or more large mismatched segmental defects
BORDERLINE HIGH	
Two large mismatched segmental defects	
INTERMEDIATE LR	**NONDIAGNOSTIC**
One large or two moderate mismatched defects Difficult to categorize as high or low	All other findings not listed in High, Very low, or Normal categories
BORDERLINE LOW LR	
One matched defect, normal radiograph	
LOW LR	
Matched V/Q defects, clear chest radiograph Single moderate to large matched perfusion defect Perfusion defect much less than radiographic abnormality Any number of small perfusion defects Nonsegmental perfusion defects*	Moderate effusion (more than one third of a hemithorax)
	VERY LOW LR
	Nonsegmental defects* 1-3 small segmental defects Single triple matched defect upper zone ≥2 Matched defects normal radiograph Stripe sign
NORMAL	**NORMAL**
No perfusion defects	No perfusion defects

From Society of Nuclear Medicine and Molecular Imaging Practice Guideline for Lung Scintigraphy v4.0. http//interactive.snm.org/Lung_Scintigraphy_v4_Final.pdf
*Nonsegmental defects = enlarged heart, tortuous vessels, hilar mass.
PIOPED, Prospective Investigation of Pulmonary Embolism Diagnosis; *V/P*, ventilation-perfusion. *LR*, Likelihood ratio

V/Q scan Procedure Guidelines by the Society of Nuclear Medicine and Molecular Imaging propose some additional changes in the Modified PIOPED II criteria listed in Table 10-3. One significant difference in the Modified PIOPED II criteria is the nondiagnostic category. This reflects a move to read V/Q scans as being positive (PE highly likely to present: high probability) or negative (PE very unlikely to be present: normal or very low probability) whenever possible. Because it is difficult to base treatment decisions on the V/Q scan findings alone for the other categories of low and intermediate probability, the study could be considered nondiagnostic. Caution should be used, however, as many such "nondiagnostic" cases are actually very suspicious (e.g., a single segment mismatched defect in a patient with a clear radiograph) or are unlikely to be from PE (e.g., matched perfusion and ventilation defects with a clear radiograph). The patient would be better served with a description of risk that incorporates an explanation of findings and includes clinical factors rather than a simple "nondiagnostic" reading.

Over the years, proposed changes to the PIOPED criteria have often added to the confusion experienced by those learning to read V/Q scans. Even among expert readers, use of the various interpretation criteria has long differed. At our institutions, we prefer to follow the revised PIOPED criteria listed in Box 10-10, with attempts to use very low probability generally limited to nonsegmental defects (e.g., enlarged hearts, tortuous vessels, hilar masses) rather than the Modified PIOPED II criteria. Other centers that utilize SPECT or perfusion-only techniques (discussed later) may favor other criteria.

High Probability

Examples of high-probability scans are shown in Figures 10-9, 10-14, and 10-15. Interpretation of high probability requires two or more large, segmental mismatched perfusion defects with a clear radiograph. This category also includes cases in which a combination of large and moderate defects adds up to two large defects (e.g., one large and two moderate or four moderate areas). The chance of PE increases as the number and size of mismatched defects increase. However, other processes can result in mismatched perfusion defects; differential diagnoses are listed in Box 10-11. One of the most common causes for mismatched defects is a previous PE that did not resolve fully. Therefore establishing a new baseline after the PE resolves and reviewing old lung scans along with the current examination is wise (Fig. 10-16).

This category was originally set to carry at least an 80% risk of PE. In practice, however, the risk is much higher. The high probability category is generally associated with an 85% to 90% risk of PE. However, as with any test, the pretest probability significantly affects results. When the clinical suspicion for PE is very high, there is an approximately 96% risk of PE given a high probability V/Q reading. In the PIOPED trial, the specificity for PE was 97% and the positive predictive value was 88%. Although the sensitivity is low, with only 41% of PEs falling into the high probability category, a high probability reading is not only very specific, but there is also little discrepancy across experienced readers in how it is used. Therefore treatment can be based on these results with confidence.

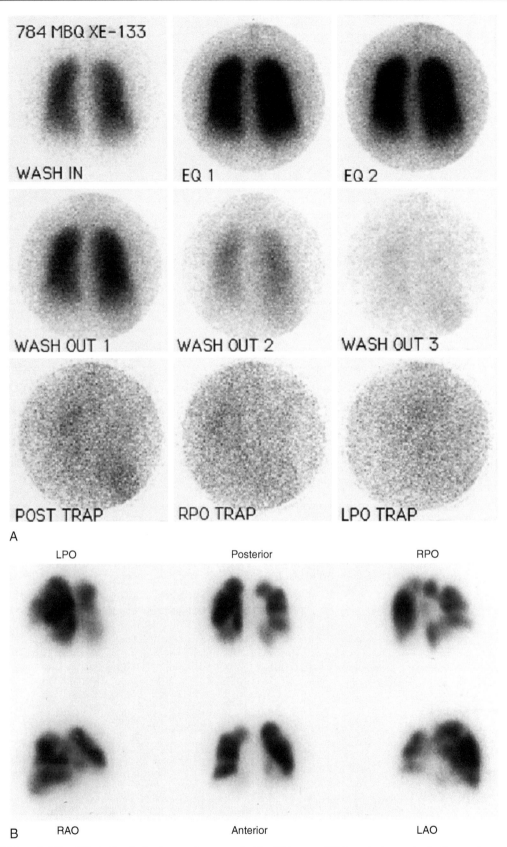

FIGURE 10-14. High probability V/Q. **A,** Ventilation is normal on posterior Xe-133 images. Mild uptake is seen in the liver at the very end of washout. **B,** Corresponding Tc-99m MAA perfusion study reveals multiple bilateral large pleural-based mismatched defects. This pattern fits the high-probability diagnosis category. *EQ,* Equilibrium; *LAO,* left anterior oblique; *LPO,* left posterior oblique; *POST,* posterior; *RAO,* right anterior oblique; *RPO,* right posterior oblique; *TRAP,* delayed trapping.

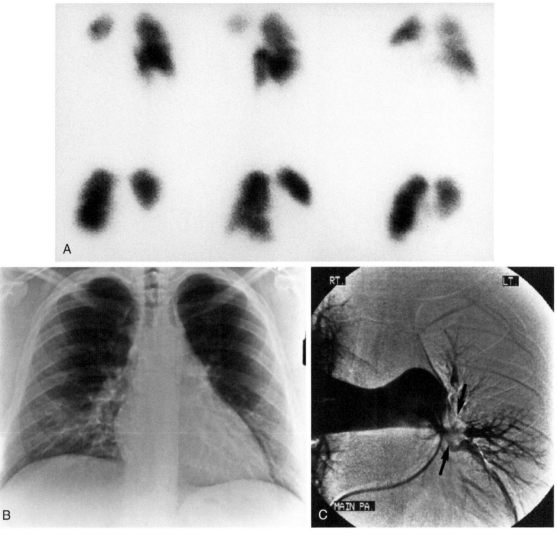

FIGURE 10-15. High-probability V/Q image. **A,** Tc-99m MAA perfusion studies reveals absent perfusion to the left lower lobe and lingula as well as a moderate-size segmental defect in the right base and a small one in the right middle lobe. **B,** Corresponding chest radiograph was normal. **C,** Pulmonary arteriogram with injection of the main pulmonary artery shows the large left-sided clot *(arrows)*. Some contrast is seen distal to the clot, which does not completely occlude the involved arteries in this case.

Box 10-11. Conditions Associated with Ventilation-Perfusion Mismatch

Acute pulmonary embolus	Mediastinal or hilar adenopathy (with obstruction of
Chronic pulmonary embolus	pulmonary artery or veins)
Other causes of embolism (septic, drug abuse, iatro-	Swyer-James syndrome (occasional)
genic, fat)	Postradiation therapy
Bronchogenic carcinoma (and other tumors)	Vasculitis
Hypoplasia or aplasia of pulmonary artery	

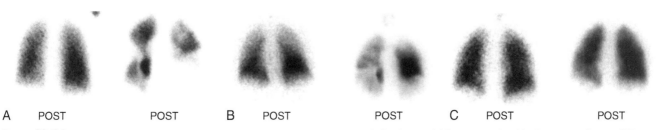

FIGURE 10-16. Resolution of PE. Normal ventilation images *(left)* and abnormal perfusion images *(right)* were obtained in the same patient at different times. **A,** The symptomatic patient had a high-probability V/Q scan. **B,** Ten years later, recurrent symptoms led to another V/Q scan, with marked mismatches. It is difficult to tell how many of these are new because no follow-up baseline study was performed after the original episode. **C,** Near complete resolution of these defects 7 days later confirms the mismatches were new and the result of recurrent PE. *POST,* Posterior.

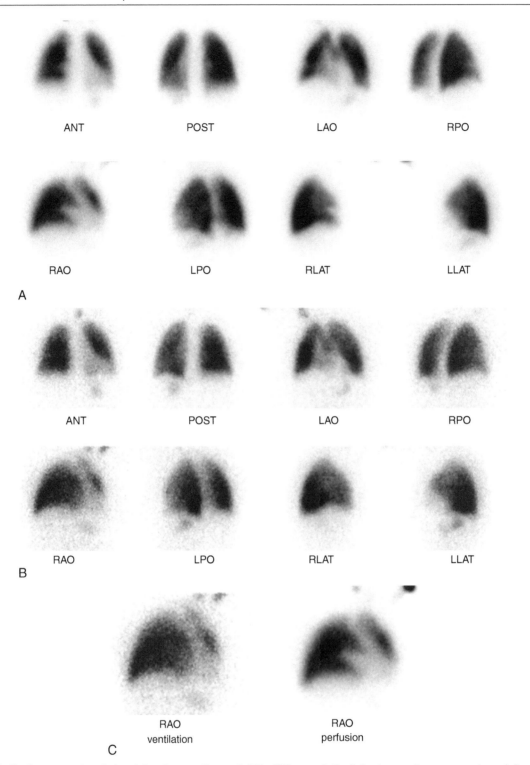

FIGURE 10-17. Single segmental perfusion defect. Intermediate-probability V/Q scan. **A,** Perfusion images demonstrate a large defect in the medial segment of the right middle lobe. **B,** Ventilation was unremarkable. **C,** Close-up views show the utility of the anterior oblique view for visualizing anterior medial defects. *ANT,* Anterior; *LAO,* left anterior oblique; *LLAT,* left lateral; *LPO,* left posterior oblique; *POST,* posterior; *RAO,* right anterior oblique; *RLAT,* right lateral; *RPO,* right posterior oblique

Intermediate Probability

A technically adequate abnormal study by PIOPED criteria is placed in the intermediate probability category when it does not fit in high probability, low, very low, or normal groups. This includes single large segmental defects (Fig. 10-17) and mismatched defects that do not add up to two segments. When a triple-matched defect is present with radiographic, ventilation, and perfusion defects, retrospective analysis of the PIOPED data suggests that it should be placed in the intermediate probability category when occurring in the lower lung fields

TABLE 10-4 Positive Predictive Value of Triple-Matched Perfusion Defects Based on Location

Lung zone	Defects from PE (%)	95% Confidence interval (%)
Upper	11	3-26
Middle	12	4-23
Lower	33	27-41

PE, Pulmonary embolism.

(Table 10-4). In addition, unless it is known to be chronic, a small but significant pleural effusion (less than one third of the lung) should technically be in this category. While the Modified PIOPED II criteria now place large effusions, greater than one third of the hemithorax, into the very low probability category, data is limited. Many readers still place larger, acute effusions into the intermediate or low probability categories. A tiny effusion is put in the very low probability category by many expert readers.

The intermediate probability category carries a reported risk for PE of 20% to 80%. Although this is a very wide range, the risk actual incidence has been found to be 30% to 35% but varies depending on pretest clinical suspicion. When the pretest probability is high, the likelihood of PE has been reported to be 66% while it may be as low as 16% when suspicion is low.

Low Probability

The risk of PE in the low probability category was designed to be less than 20%. This group includes most perfusion defects matched by ventilation abnormalities and cases with small perfusion defects. Examples of low probability scans are shown in Figures 10-18 and 10-19. As long as some perfusion to a lung occurs, even very extensive matched V/Q abnormalities can be considered low probability when the chest radiograph is clear. If all defects are small, the study is at least low probability, without regard to the ventilation examination or radiograph. For example, multiple small mismatched defects unrelated to emboli can be seen in restrictive airway disease.

When the radiograph is abnormal, the situation is more difficult. If the radiograph abnormality is much larger than the perfusion defect, the examination result is in the low probability category. If a triple match is present, defects in the lower lung fields are properly classified as intermediate probability. Those triple matches in the upper lung zones carry a lesser risk and can be placed in the low probability category (Fig. 10-20).

As mentioned previously, pretest clinical suspicion should be considered when evaluating V/Q findings. In cases in which the pretest clinical probability of PE is high, the incidence of PE has been found to be much higher than the 20% expected in a low-probability read. In fact, the probability of PE has been reported to be as high as 40% in such cases. In the opposite case, if objective clinical suspicion is low, the incidence of PE is only 2%.

Very Low Probability

It has long been recognized that a 20% chance of PE is too significant not to treat or pursue further. In an effort to

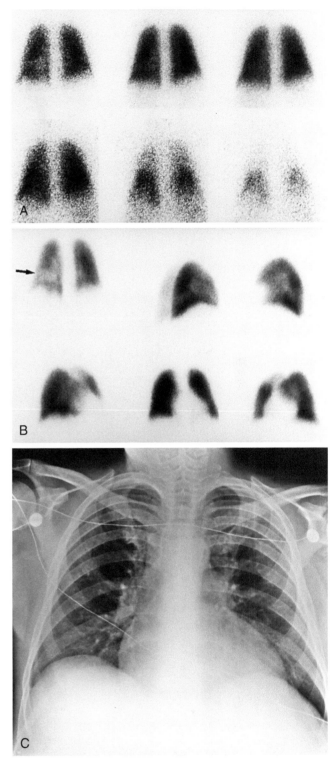

FIGURE 10-18. Low-probability V/Q image. **A,** Xe-133 ventilation images are normal on initial single-breath and equilibrium images *(top row)* but bibasilar air trapping is seen on washout *(bottom row).* **B,** Tc-99m MAA shows a large area of relatively decreased perfusion in the left lower lobe *(arrow)* and a smaller area in the right base in the general area of ventilation abnormalities. **C,** The radiograph showed no abnormalities in these matched ventilation-perfusion abnormalities.

improve patient management, the very low probability category carrying a less than 10% chance of PE was proposed after retrospective review of the PIOPED data. This category includes cases with nonsegmental defects, such as those related to the heart, vessels, costophrenic blunting

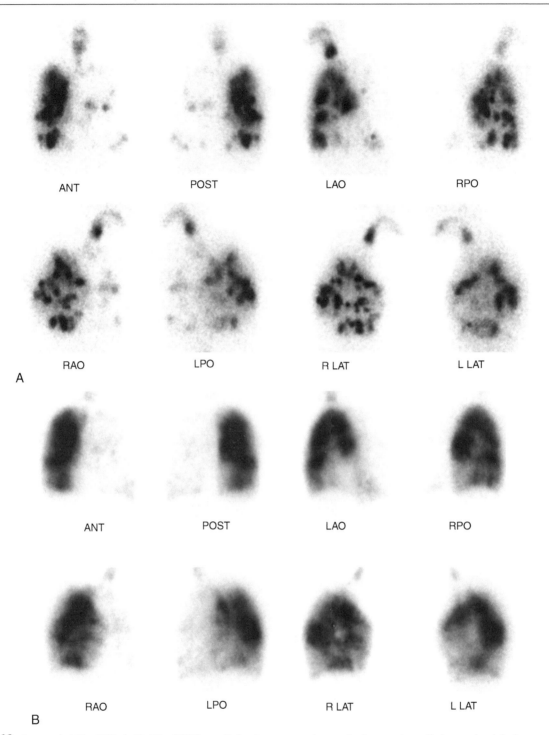

Figure 10-19. Low-probability V/Q. **A,** Tc-99m DTPA ventilation images reveal severely decreased ventilation to the right lung and essentially absent ventilation to the left lung. Significant clumping is present. **B,** Perfusion images show matching defects, although the abnormalities are less severe than the ventilation defects on the right. The clumping of the ventilation agent is seen faintly persisting. *ANT,* Anterior; *LAO,* left anterior oblique; *L LAT,* left lateral; *LPO,* left posterior; *POST,* posterior; *RAO,* right anterior oblique; *R LAT,* right lateral; *RPO,* right posterior oblique.

from a small effusion, and elevated diaphragm. Matched V/Q abnormalities in two or three zones of a single lung and cases with 1 to 3 small segmental (<25% of a segment) defects can be placed in this category. Data supporting the elements of this category are limited. The Modified PIOPED II data places large pleural effusions into the very low probability category. However, this is based on limited retrospective data and other studies have called these low or intermediate probability. Because PE cannot be excluded

with an effusion of any size, a pleural effusion can be placed in the intermediate probability or nondiagnostic category. A known chronic effusion is unlikely to represent PE and may be placed in low or very low categories.

In clinical use, what constitutes very low, low, and even sometimes normal can vary widely among readers. However, the clinical outcome is not likely to significantly vary because a near-normal V/Q scan essentially excludes clinically significant emboli.

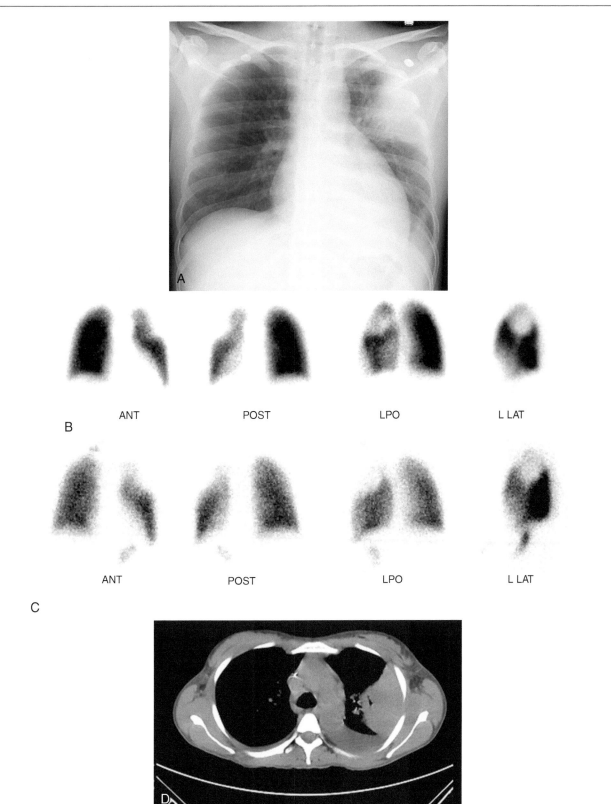

ANT POST LPO L LAT

ANT POST LPO L LAT

FIGURE 10-20. Triple-match V/Q in the upper lobes. **A,** An anteroposterior radiograph raised suspicion for infarct with a large pleural-based, upper-lobe wedge-shaped opacity and a left hazy density from an effusion layering. **B,** Perfusion shows a large wedge-shaped perfusion defect in the left upper lobe and a mild overall decrease on the left corresponding to radiographic abnormalities. **C,** The ventilation images show complete matching of the abnormalities on the left. **D,** A noncontrast CT the next day also has the same left upper lobe consolidation and effusion. The clinical suspicion was low in this febrile, immunocompromised patient. The study was interpreted as low probability, although the Modified PIOPED II criteria suggests this could even be called very low probability. The patient was later found to have aspergillosis not PE. *ANT,* Anterior; *L LAT,* left lateral; *LPO,* left posterior oblique; *POST,* posterior.

TABLE **10-5** Ventilation-Perfusion Scan Sensitivity and Specificity

Probability category	Sensitivity (%)	Specificity (%)
High	41	97
High + intermediate	82	52
High + intermediate + low	98	10

TABLE **10-6** 2009 European Association of Nuclear Medicine Guidelines for Ventilation-Perfusion Interpretation

No PE	Normal perfusion conforming to anatomical lung boundaries
	Matched or reverse mismatch V/Q defects of any size in absence of mismatched defects
	Mismatch without lobar, segmental, or subsegmental pattern
PE present	V/Q mismatch at least one segment or two subsegments conforming to pulmonary vascular anatomy
Nondiagnostic for PE	Multiple V/Q abnormalities not typical of specific diseases

From Bajc M, Neilly JB, Miniati M, Schuemichen C. EANM guidelines for ventilation/perfusion scintigraphy. I. *Eur J Nucl Med Mol Imaging*. 2009;36(8):1356-1370. *PE,* Pulmonary embolism; *V/Q,* ventilation-perfusion.

Normal

When a perfusion study is completely normal (Figs. 10-1 and 10-2), the diagnosis of PE is essentially excluded with an incidence of 2% to 4%. In addition, the chance of significant morbidity or mortality from PE is less than 1%.

Nondiagnostic Category

Many readers advocate having fewer categories in the interpretive criteria. This trend is reflected in the Modified PIOPED II criteria. It leads to readings of "PE present" (high probability) or "PE absent" (near normal/ very low probability or normal) while placing scans from the low and intermediate probability groups in a "nondiagnostic" category. Because a significant number of emboli occur in low and intermediate probability categories (Table 10-5), further workup is warranted. Since even expert readers frequently disagree whether to place a scan in the low probability or intermediate probability category, this overlap may make sense. However, clinicians will still want guidance on the chance a PE is present based on clinical factors and findings. For example, in a young patient with no cardiovascular disease, a single segment of mismatch must be considered highly suspicious.

■ OTHER ADDITIONAL V/Q INTERPRETATION CRITERIA

Several studies have shown that if a perfusion defect conforms to a vascular segment distribution, then only one segment of mismatched perfusion deficit is sufficient to diagnose a PE, rather than the two segments of the Modified PIOPED II criteria in patients without evidence of

TABLE **10-7** Proposed Trinary Interpretation of Ventilation-Perfusion Scans in Patients with No Radiographic Findings

Previous interpretation	New interpretation
Normal, very low, and low probability	No evidence of PE
High probability	PE present
Intermediate and indeterminate probability	Nondiagnostic study

From Glaser JE, Chamarthy M, Haramati LB, Esses D, Freeman LM. Successful and safe implementation of a trinary interpretation and reporting strategy for V/Q lung scintigraphy. *J Nucl Med*. 2011;52(10):1508-1512. *PE,* Pulmonary embolism.

cardiovascular disease. The 2009 European Association of Nuclear Medicine Guidelines (Table 10-6) have a reported sensitivity of 96% to 99%, specificity of 97% to 99%, and negative predictive value of 97% to 99%. Rates of nondiagnostic examinations were low, at 1% to 3%.

In cases in which no cardiopulmonary disease is present otherwise, as evidenced by a clear chest radiograph, a new "trinary" approach has been used at one site (Glaser et al, 2011), with the group reporting examinations as "no evidence of PE" (rather than normal, very low probability, or low probability), "PE present" (instead of high probability), or "nondiagnostic" (in place of intermediate probability and indeterminate) (Table 10-7). In this protocol, a single moderate to large mismatched defect is considered sufficient evidence that a PE is present. This seems reasonable given the chance of another explanation was low in the presence of a normal x-ray. Clinicians were told in advance that "no evidence of PE" was associated with a 90% negative predictive value (or <10% chance of PE), and when discordance occurred between the V/Q scan report and pretest probability, additional workup was required. On follow-up, this trinary approach in patients with normal radiographs had a reported 1.2% false negative rate. Further studies are needed to confirm whether this approach can be used more widely.

Despite these additional criteria recommendations, the Modified PIOPED criteria remain the most widely used standards for V/Q reporting. Additional prospective trials are needed to determine what changes will be made to V/Q scan interpretation criteria.

■ OTHER APPLICATIONS OF VENTILATION-PERFUSION SCINTIGRAPHY

Quantitative Lung Scan

Quantification of lung perfusion and ventilation can be valuable in the preoperative assessment of high-risk patients before planned lung resection for malignancy, dead-space lung volume reduction in severe COPD, and lung transplantation. This information is used in conjunction with respiratory spirometry to determine how much function each lung or lung region contributes. Quantitation also can be useful in assessing relative pulmonary perfusion before and after operations for congenital heart disease (e.g., correction of pulmonary stenosis).

Right to left lung differential function is commonly performed by acquiring anterior and posterior views, drawing

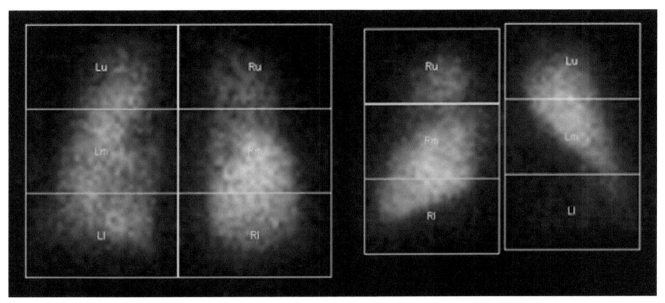

FIGURE **10-21.** Preoperative quantitative lung scan. Anterior and posterior projections. Geometric mean quantification is performed for left to right lung differential function and upper, mid, and lower lung regions.

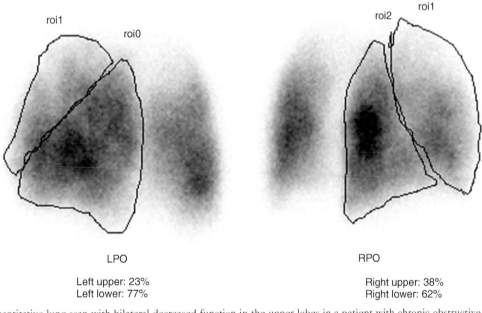

LPO

Left upper: 23%
Left lower: 77%

RPO

Right upper: 38%
Right lower: 62%

FIGURE **10-22.** Quantitative lung scan with bilateral decreased function in the upper lobes in a patient with chronic obstructive pulmonary disease. *LPO,* Left posterior oblique; *roi,* region of interest; *RPO,* right pulmonary oblique.

regions of interest around the right and left lungs, and calculating the geometric mean to correct for attenuation (Fig. 10-21).

$$\text{Geometric mean} = \sqrt{\text{Counts}_{\text{anterior}} \times \text{Counts}_{\text{posterior}}}$$

However, the anterior and posterior views do not allow for good separation of the upper and lower lobes. Posterior oblique views allow better separation of the upper and lower lobes (Fig. 10-22).

Adult Respiratory Distress Syndrome

The clearance of Tc-99m DTPA is significantly affected by the presence of pulmonary disease. The clearance half-time is approximately 45 minutes in healthy adults. Patients with adult respiratory distress syndrome have more rapid clearance, probably because of the rapid diffusion of Tc-99m DTPA across the airspace epithelium to the pulmonary circulation. Other conditions associated with increased Tc-99m DTPA clearance are cigarette smoking, alveolitis, and hyaline membrane disease in infants. This technique has not found a clear-cut clinical use.

Detection of Deep Venous Thrombosis

Although this chapter mainly concerns the diagnosis of PE, diagnosis of DVT is a related topic. In the past, traditional contrast venography and radionuclide venography were used for diagnosis. Radionuclide venography involves

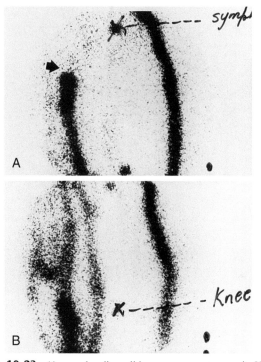

FIGURE 10-23. Abnormal radionuclide venogram patterns. **A,** Venous obstruction *(arrow)* on the right caused by thrombus. **B,** Extensive collateralization on the right indicates obstruction of the deep venous system.

placing a tourniquet above the ankle and injecting radiopharmaceutical, Tc-99m MAA, into a small vein in the foot; this procedure has shown high sensitivities above the knee (Fig. 10-23). Doppler sonography imaging in combination with various compression techniques is useful in the veins above the knee in the lower extremity. Contrast CT can be used to assess pelvic veins. Images of the pelvis can be obtained after pulmonary arterial imaging is completed. It may be technically difficult to time the study to achieve adequate venous opacification for diagnosis. PIOPED II also examined utility of CT venography (CTV) for the pelvic and thigh veins. Preliminary reports found CTV to be 95% sensitive, with a positive predictive value of 86% overall. However, the majority of lesions were found in the thighs. These would be potentially visualized by ultrasound without the exposure to ionizing radiation.

Various radiolabeled agents have been developed that bind to components of an active clot. These have included radiolabeled platelets, fibrin, and various peptides. Tc-99m apcitide (AcuTect) was approved by the U.S. Food and Drug Administration for diagnosis of DVT. Although advocated for use in equivocal ultrasound findings or for detection of thrombus in the calf, it did not achieve widespread use.

▬ SUGGESTED READING

Bajc M, Neilly JB, Miniati M, Schuemichen C. EANM guidelines for ventilation perfusion scintigraphy. *Eur J Nucl Med Mol Imaging.* 2009;36(8):1356-1370.

Freeman LM. Don't bury the VQ scan: it's as good as multidetector CT angiography with a lot less radiation exposure. *J Nucl Med.* 2008;49(1):5-8.

Freeman LM, Krynyckyi B, Zuckier LS. Enhanced lung scan diagnosis of pulmonary embolism with the use of ancillary scintigraphic findings and clinical correlation. *Semin Nucl Med.* 2001;31:143-157.

Glaser JE, Chamarthy M, Haramati LB, Esses D, Freeman LM. Successful and safe implementation of a trinary interpretation and reporting strategy for V/Q lung scintigraphy. *J Nucl Med.* 2011;52(10):1508-1512.

Gottschalk A, Sostman HD, Coleman RE, et al. Ventilation-perfusion scintigraphy in the PIOPED study. II. Evaluation of the scintigraphic criteria and interpretations. *J Nucl Med.* 1993;34(7):1119-1126.

Gottschalk A, Steine PD, Sostman HD, et al. Very low probability interpretation of VQ lung scans in contribution with low probability objective clinical assessment reliably excludes pulmonary embolism: data from PIOPED II. *J Nucl Med.* 2007;48(9):1411-1415.

Gray HW. The natural history of venous thromboembolism: impact on ventilation/perfusion scan reporting. *Semin Nucl Med.* 2002;32(3):159-172.

Groves AM, Yates SJ, Win T, et al. CT pulmonary angiography versus ventilation-perfusion scintigraphy in pregnancy: implications from a survey of doctors' knowledge of radiation exposure. *Radiology.* 2006;240(3):765-770.

Howarth DM, Lan L, Thomas PA, Allen LW. ^{99m}Tc Technegas ventilation and perfusion lung scintigraphy for the diagnosis of pulmonary embolus. *J Nucl Med.* 1999;40(4):579-584.

Miniati M, Pistolesi M, Marini C, et al. Value of perfusion lung scan in the diagnosis of pulmonary embolism: result of the prospective investigation of acute pulmonary embolism diagnosis (PISA-PED). *Am J Respir Crit Care Med.* 1996;154(11):1387-1393.

Mores LK, King CS, Holley AB. Current approach to the diagnosis of acute nonmassive pulmonary embolism. *Chest.* 2011;140(2):509-518.

Perrier A, Bounameaux H. Accuracy or outcome in suspected pulmonary embolism. *N Engl J Med.* 2006;354:2383-2385.

The PIOPED Investigators. Value of the ventilation/perfusion scan in acute pulmonary embolism: results of the prospective investigation of pulmonary embolism diagnosis (PIOPED). *JAMA.* 1990;263(20):2753-2759.

Stein PD, Chenevert TL, Fowler SE, et al. Gadolinium-enhanced magnetic resonance angiography for pulmonary embolism: a multicenter prospective study (PIOPED III). *Ann Intern Med.* 2010;152(7):434-443.

Stein PD, Fowler SE, Goodman LR, et al. Multidetector computed tomography for acute pulmonary embolism. *N Engl J Med.* 2006;354(22):2317-2327.

Wells PS, Anderson DR, Rodger M, et al. Excluding pulmonary embolism at the bedside without diagnostic imaging: management of patients with suspected pulmonary embolism presenting to the emergency department by using a simple clinical model and d-dimer. *Ann Intern Med.* 2001;135(2):98-107.

Worsley DF, Alavi A. Comprehensive analysis of the results of the PIOPED study: prospective investigation of pulmonary embolism diagnosis study. *J Nucl Med.* 1995;36(12):2380-2387.

Worsley DF, Kim CK, Alavia A, Palevsky HI. Detailed analysis of patients with matched ventilation-perfusion defects and chest radiographic opacities. *J Nucl Med.* 1993;34(11):1851-1853.

CHAPTER 11

Oncology: Positron Emission Tomography

■ BACKGROUND

For decades, positron emission tomography (PET) was used for many research applications. In recent years, changes in reimbursement and availability have led to the rapid expansion of PET for clinical patient care. The majority of these PET scans are performed to evaluate cancer using the glucose analog fluorine-18 fluorodeoxyglucose (F-18 FDG). In most cases, cancer cells are more metabolically active and divide more rapidly than normal tissues. By using radiopharmaceuticals that target physiological parameters such as glucose metabolism, PET enables imaging and quantification of cellular function and tumor detection. This approach has several potential advantages over anatomical modalities such as computed tomography (CT).

CT imaging relies on size and architectural changes to diagnose malignancy, which limits sensitivity and specificity. For example, when lymph nodes are identified in patients with cancer, enlarged nodes are assumed to harbor malignancy and normal-size nodes are characterized as benign. Therefore nodes seen on CT are often inaccurately characterized as benign because they are not pathologically enlarged. In addition, it is often difficult to determine whether a residual mass seen on CT after therapy contains tumor as a change in the size of a mass does not accurately predict tumor response to therapy. Evaluation after therapy may also be difficult because scarring from surgery and radiation can obscure malignant disease. PET, on the other hand, permits monitoring of activity levels on serial studies. Changes in metabolic activity better characterize a mass and better predict therapy outcome than anatomical measurements of size.

However, PET is limited by a lack of anatomical detail. Normal uptake in structures such as bowel, muscles, and ureters can be mistaken for tumor. Therefore correlation with CT or magnetic resonance imaging (MRI) is critical for image interpretation. Although PET images can be fused to the CT when performed separately, most PET scans are currently acquired sequentially with the CT on a dedicated PET/CT scanner. This allows the most precise image fusion because differences in position are minimal. The combination of anatomical information with metabolic data is the most accurate method for evaluating malignancy.

Although F-18 FDG is highly sensitive for many tumors, reimbursement policy development for PET in the United States has been complicated (Table 11-1). In response to government requirements for evidence development before authorizing PET reimbursement, medical imaging societies formed the National Oncologic PET Registry (NOPR), which allowed payments for PET scans for patients on Medicare participating in the project and gathered data on the clinical impact of PET. When looking at large numbers of patients with many different tumors, initial results from the NOPR showed that PET changed patient management 36.5% of the time. The impact included avoiding biopsy, a major change in therapy, and a change in overall treatment goal. Based on the overall success of the NOPR trial, most solid tumors are eligible for at least one initial assessment and many others may qualify for subsequent evaluations.

Radiopharmaceuticals

Many commonly used positron-emitting radioisotopes are based on atoms found in organic substances: oxygen-15, nitrogen-13, carbon-11, and the hydroxyl analog, F-18 (Table 11-2). Short half-lives limit the clinical usefulness of many positron emitters, requiring a cyclotron to be in close proximity. However, F-18 has a 110-minute half-life and can be delivered from regional, commercial cyclotrons.

The various positron emitters can be attached to biological carrier molecules. Carrier molecules such as nucleosides, amino acids, fatty acid components, and glucose analogs are chosen to form radiopharmaceuticals that target components of cellular metabolism and division. Targets include DNA synthesis, membrane synthesis, and glucose metabolism (Table 11-3). The chemistry of labeling carrier molecules with positron emitters is usually much simpler than labeling with gamma emitters such as technetium-99m. Although F-18 sodium fluoride (F-18 NaF) was also approved by the U.S. Food and Drug Administration, F-18 FDG is the only PET radiopharmaceutical in wide clinical use for oncological imaging.

Fluorine-18 Fluorodeoxyglucose

Cancer cells generally have a higher level of metabolic activity than normal tissues and use more glucose. In malignant cells, higher levels of glucose membrane transporters increase intracellular glucose uptake. Within the cancer cell, hexokinase (hexokinase II) activity levels are increased, and the phosphorylated glucose then moves through the glycolysis pathway.

F-18 FDG is a glucose analog that is taken into the cell and phosphorylated by the same mechanism as glucose. Increased F-18 FDG activity is seen in tumors for several reasons. First of all, increased glucose transporter activity is present. In addition, glucose-6-phosphatase levels are low in cancer cells, and the phosphorylated

TABLE 11-1 History of Positron Emission Tomography Coverage by Centers for Medicare and Medicaid (CMS) in the United States

Date	Clinical indication	Coverage
March 1995	Myocardial perfusion	Coronary artery disease (Rubidium-82)
January 1998	Solitary pulmonary nodule	Characterization
	Non–small cell lung cancer	Initial staging
July 1999	Colorectal cancer and melanoma	Suggested recurrence
	Lymphoma	Staging/restaging as alternative to gallium scan
July 2001	Non–small cell lung cancer, esophageal cancer, colorectal cancer, lymphoma, melanoma, and head and neck cancer (excluding CNS and thyroid)	Diagnosis, staging, restaging
July 2001	Refractory seizures	Presurgical
July 2001	Myocardial viability	Following inconclusive SPECT
October 2002	Myocardial viability	Initial diagnosis
	Breast cancer	Staging, restaging, response to therapy
October 2003	Thyroid cancer	Restaging (negative I-131 scan, rising thyroglobulin)
September 2004	Alzheimer disease and dementia	In CMS approved clinical trial
September 2005	Brain, cervical, ovarian, pancreatic, small cell lung, testicular, and all other cancers and indications not previously specified	Coverage with evidence development (NOPR)
November 2009	Cancers of the following: Brain, breast, colorectal, esophageal, head and neck, lymphoma, melanoma, myeloma, non–small lung, ovary, and thyroid (follicular with negative I-131 and rising thyroglobulin)	Initial treatment strategy and subsequent treatment strategy
November 2009	Cancers of the following: Anus, bladder, bile duct, bone/cartilage, brain/CNS, cervix, connective/soft tissue, eye, gallbladder, genitalia (male/female), Kaposi's sarcoma, kidney, liver, neuroendocrine tumor, pancreas, pleura, retroperitoneum and peritoneum, skin (non-melanoma), small cell lung, small intestine, stomach, testis, thymus, heart, unknown primary, ureter, uterus, adnexa; all other solid tumors	Initial treatment strategy covered and subsequent treatment strategy NOPR
	Prostate	Initial treatment strategy not covered; subsequent treatment strategy NOPR
	Leukemia and all other cancers not listed	NOPR
February 2010	Bone metastases	F-18 sodium fluoride (NaF)

CEA, carcinogen embryonic antigen; *CNS,* central nervous system; *NOPR,* National Oncologic PET Registry; *SPECT,* single-photon emission tomography.

TABLE 11-2 Physical Characteristics of Positron-Emitting Isotopes Important in Oncology

Radioisotope	Half-life (min)	Decay mode (%)	γ (keV)	β^+ E max (MeV)	Range (mm)
O-15	2.07	β^+ (99.9) EC (0.1)	511	1.72	8.0
N-13	9.96	β^+ (100)	511	1.19	5-4
C-11	20.4	β^+ (99.8) EC (0.2)	511	0.96	4.1
F-18	109.7	β^+ (97) EC (3)	511	0.635	2.4

β^+, Positron emission; *EC,* electron capture.

TABLE 11-3 Carrier Molecules for Positron Emission Tomography Imaging in Oncology

Agent	Target	Label
Deoxyglucose	Glucose metabolism	F-18
Thymidine	DNA synthesis	F-18, C-11
Acetate	Lipid synthesis	F-18, C-11
Choline	Lipid synthesis, membrane synthesis	C-11
Tyrosine	Protein synthesis	F-18, C-11
Methionine	Protein synthesis	C-11

FDG cannot diffuse out of the cell. Unlike glucose, F-18 FDG is not metabolized further and remains trapped (Fig. 11-1).

After intravenous injection, F-18 FDG rapidly distributes throughout the body. Cellular uptake and phosphorylation occur as background activity clears. The primary route of radiotracer excretion occurs by the kidneys, although F-18 FDG excretion also takes place through the bowel. Optimal imaging time is usually 40 to 60 minutes, based on maximum uptake, background clearance, and physical half-life. Some studies have suggested additional delayed images at 90 to 120 minutes may identify

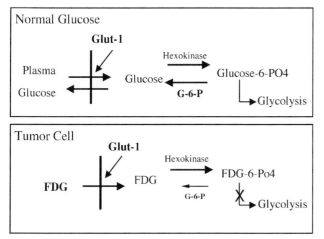

*G-6-P: Glucose-6-Phosphatase

FIGURE 11-1. Glucose and F-18 FDG intracellular kinetics. F-18 FDG uses the same uptake and phosphorylation pathways as glucose, although it cannot be metabolized through glycolysis. In cancer cells, greater accumulation is seen due to different levels of enzymatic activity. *G-6-P,* Glucose-6-phosphatase.

additional tumors because they continue to accumulate F-18 FDG, while activity clears from tissues and benign processes.

Many factors affect F-18 FDG uptake, distribution, and clearance. Serum glucose actively competes with F-18 FDG uptake. Insulin occurring endogenously after eating or administration to diabetics will increase uptake to the liver and muscles, thereby decreasing uptake in tumors. Also, inflammation and infection may result in uptake that rivals or exceeds that of a malignancy.

Investigational Positron Emission Tomography Imaging Agents

F-18 FDG uptake in tumor is not specific for malignancy. Clinically, it is often critical to differentiate cancer from inflammation. Many radiotracers that are more specific for malignancy by imaging the increased cellular division seen with cancer are under investigation. Other agents are being examined that may be superior to F-18 FDG because of more specific tumor uptake or reduced background activity. Additionally, PET radiopharmaceuticals are being developed that bind to receptors or reveal areas of tumor hypoxia. Some of these experimental agents are available for purchase through commercial radiopharmacies, and several more are expected to become available in the next few years. However, much work will be needed before these agents are approved or widely reimbursed for clinical use, as is discussed in Chapter 2.

In addition to these newer agents, F-18 NaF is gaining renewed interest (see Chapter 7). F-18 NaF was originally used as a bone scan agent, but it fell out of favor with the introduction of Tc-99m methylene diphosphate (MDP). However, with the rapid spread of dedicated PET/CT cameras, F-18 NaF may be more sensitive than Tc-99m MDP or F-18 FDG in evaluation of several skeletal tumors, including highly lytic tumors such as multiple myeloma. Work is being done to assess its actual utility.

TABLE 11-4 Fluorine-18 Fluorodeoxyglucose Dosimetry

Organ receive highest dose	Exposure	Effective dose
Bladder	0.17 mGy (0.63 rad)	0.027 mSv (0.10 rem)

Fluorine-18 Fluorodeoxyglucose Positron Emission Tomography Dosimetry

Radiation dosimetry values for F-18 FDG are listed in Table 11-4. The whole-body effective dose from a standard 400-MBq scan is 1.6 mSv (160 mrem). CT scans, used for anatomical localization, are generally performed using a low-dose technique. The effective radiation dose of a low-dose whole-body CT performed for PET/CT varies, but may be 2 mSv (200 mrem). This compares to typical diagnostic or optimized chest CT, in which the effective dose frequently reaches 8 mSv because increased radiation used to visualize structures optimally.

Protocol

An example of a protocol for F-18 FDG PET in patients with cancer is included in Box 11-1. Patient preparation generally includes fasting overnight or for at least 4 to 6 hours before injection and avoiding carbohydrates in the meal before injection. Because glucose competes with F-18 FDG, protocols include measures to limit the impact of serum glucose of the scan. The glucose level of patients should be checked before injection. The upper-limit cutoff varies among institutions, but a value under 200 mg/dL is generally considered acceptable. Patients with diabetes must be carefully scheduled, usually early in the morning after fasting and before taking insulin. Short-acting insulin should not be given within 2 hours of radiotracer injection and long-acting insulin should be held overnight. Patients with non–insulin-dependent diabetes are treated in a similar fashion. However, if the oral hypoglycemic medication metformin could be withheld for 2 days, this will decrease bowel background activity related to the drug.

Claustrophobic patients may require sedation, particularly when a PET/CT is performed, because the machine has a deep bore. Sedatives and beta-adrenergic blockers are sometimes used to decrease uptake in the supraclavicular fat (brown fat), although this is often with limited effectiveness. Patients should be kept warm, quiet, and relaxed for 30 to 60 minutes before injection and uptake phases to decrease muscle and brown-fat uptake. Patients should be instructed to avoid strenuous exercise for a couple of days before the study.

The standard F-18 FDG dose is 10 to 15 mCi (370-555 MBq) intravenously. A weight-based approach has been instituted to decrease pediatric exposure using 0.14 to 0.20 mCi/kg (5.18-7.4 MBq/kg). An absorption and clearance period necessitates a delay of 40 to 60 minutes before scanning. Patients must void immediately before being placed on the scanner.

Patients are usually imaged in the supine position. Because attenuation correction with CT causes beam-hardening artifact when the arms are in the field of view, arm position always must be taken into consideration. Arms are placed above the head when the pathology is in the chest, abdomen, and pelvis. When the tumor is in the

Box 11-1. Protocol for Fluorine-18
Fluorodeoxyglucose Imaging in Oncology

PATIENT PREPARATION
Avoid strenuous exercise for several days
Diabetics well controlled, stop long-acting insulin 8
  to 12 hours before scan, and no short-acting insulin
  within 2 hours of FDG injection
NPO except for water 4 to 6 hours or overnight, avoid
  carbohydrates
Check serum glucose (<200 mg/dL)
Patient kept warm, quiet, and relaxed
Consider sedation for claustrophobia, anxiety or tense
  muscles, cancer in head and neck, prior brown fat
  uptake

RADIOPHARMACEUTICAL
Children: 150 µCi/kg (5.3 MBq/kg)
Adults: 10-15 mCi [0.14-0.21 mCi/kg (5.18-7.77 MBq/
  kg)] intravenously
Wait 45 to 60 minutes, patient to avoid movement
  and speech
Void

IMAGE ACQUISITION AND PROCESSING
Field of View
Varies by patient size (50 cm)

Transmission Scan
Dedicated PET Only Scanner
External rod source 3 to 5 minutes per bed position

PET/CT
Low-dose CT (70-80 mA, 140 kvP)

Emission Scan
5 to 10 minutes per bed position
Repeat imaging each section or bed position until
  area covered

Processing
Filtered backprojection or iterative reconstruction

FDG, Fluorodeoxyglucose; *NPO,* nil per os.

head and neck, patients are imaged with arms at their sides. Scanning usually begins at the head but will begin at the thighs when tumor is in the pelvis, to minimize the impact of urine activity accumulating in the bladder.

The imaging is done in two stages. First, a transmission scan using an external positron or x-ray source (e.g., CT) is performed for attenuation correction. The positron emission scan is then acquired, which detects the photons from the F-18 FDG. As the administered dose is known and can be time-decay corrected, the number of photons striking the detector will reflect the metabolic activity of a lesion once a correction for differences in tissue attenuation is applied. Therefore attenuation correction allows the levels of activity in the patient to be accurately quantified. An attenuation correction factor is calculated by comparing the counts striking the detector from the transmission scan through the patient to a blank scan where no patient is present: attenuation correction factor = (counts blank scan)/(counts transmission scan).

External rods (germanium-68 or cesium-137) rotating around the patient have been used for this attenuation correction transmission scan. The process requires 4 to 6 minutes per image level (or bed position), with a typical whole-body scan requiring 5 to 7 bed positions. A PET/CT scanner uses the CT transmission data for attenuation correction and for image fusion for anatomical localization. The CT takes only seconds to complete.

The emission scan data are then acquired from the F-18 FDG patient activity. Depending on patient size, camera technology, and radiopharmaceutical dose, the emission scan takes 5 to 10 minutes per bed position on traditional PET/CT scanners. A whole-body scan has traditionally been considered a scan from skull base to midthigh, requiring approximately 15 to 40 minutes, depending on the type of scanner. If the entire brain or the lower extremities are included, more bed positions are added. This acquisition can be done more quickly with new time-of-flight cameras.

Currently, most PET/CT scans are performed without intravenous contrast. Contrast administration requires additional time, support personnel, equipment, and patient supervision. Also, CT contrast agents cause increased attenuation on the transmission scan, which can lead to areas of artifactually increased activity on attenuation-corrected PET images when the contrast is dense or concentrated. However, use of intravenous contrast has been increasing because it helps identify normal structures and make pathological conditions more conspicuous. Water can be used to distend the stomach and proximal bowel. Otherwise, dilute oral contrast or water-equivalent negative oral contrast agents are acceptable. Performing the attenuation-correction CT scan after the arterial phase of the intravenous contrast bolus will reduce the artifact from intravenous contrast material. In practice, examining the non–attenuation contrast images should allow an experienced reader to avoid confusion caused by contrast artifact.

Data are displayed as a maximal intensity projection (MIP) rotating image or as transaxial, coronal, and sagittal slices. Both attenuation-corrected images and non–attenuation-correction images should be reviewed because artifacts and lesions may be more obvious on one or the other. PET/CT scanners will automatically provide images fused to the CT in each orthogonal plane. If the CT is done in a separate imaging session, postimage fusion software may require manual or may semiautomatic alignment. A current correlative CT is helpful for optimal interpretation.

◼ IMAGE INTERPRETATION

Normal Distribution and Variants of F-18 Fluorodeoxyglucose

The normal distribution of F-18 FDG reflects glucose metabolism (Fig. 11-2). The brain is an obligate glucose user, so uptake is high. The kidneys, ureters, and bladder also show intense activity from urinary clearance of F-18 FDG. Moderate and sometimes heterogeneous activity is seen in the liver. Variable activity occurs in the heart, gastrointestinal tract, salivary glands, and testes. The uterus may show endometrial uptake depending on the menstrual cycle stage. Low-level activity is normal in the bone marrow.

The urinary activity can lead to interpretation difficulties. Although the ureters usually appear as long tubular structures, they may be seen as very focal areas of activity that may be confused with a pathological condition. CT correlation or PET/CT can help localize the activity to a visible ureter or show that no mass or lymph node is present. F-18 FDG in the bladder and kidneys can prevent visualization of tumors in those structures. The bladder may also limit evaluation of other tumors in the pelvis.

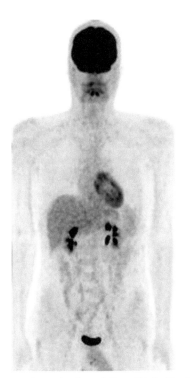

FIGURE 11-2. Normal distribution of F-18 FDG. Uptake is normally intense in the brain and urinary tract, moderately intense in the liver, and variable in muscles (especially of the oropharynx), heart, and bowel.

When imaging tumors located near the heart, minimizing cardiac activity is desirable. The myocardium uses glucose as an optional fuel. In a fasting state, fatty acid metabolism dominates over glucose use, leading to decreased FDG uptake. However, fasting yields inconsistent results. In fact, significant cardiac uptake is seen in up to 50% of fasting patients. Myocardial uptake is usually not seen in the right ventricle and may be heterogeneous in the left ventricle.

Normal excretion of F-18 FDG is highly variable throughout the gastrointestinal tract. Low-level activity can be seen focally or diffusely in the esophagus. In general, this normal uptake is less than that seen with esophagitis or cancer. Significant activity in the stomach sometimes limits the use of F-18 FDG PET in the evaluation of gastric adenocarcinoma and gastric lymphoma. Activity in both large and small bowel is especially problematic because it may obscure tumor in the bowel and mesentery (Fig. 11-3, *A*). Patients on the oral diabetic medication metformin frequently show intense activity in the small bowel. Focal accumulation of F-18 FDG may be caused by malignant and villous adenomas, but it is frequently an unexplained, transient finding.

Activity in the oropharyngeal cavity is highly variable. Low-level activity is normally seen in the salivary glands. Nonspecific diffuse uptake is occasionally seen in the parotid glands bilaterally in patients undergoing therapy. Marked uptake is often seen in oropharyngeal lymphoid tissue, including palatine and lingual tonsils (Fig. 11-3, *B*). Although uptake is most often symmetric, asymmetry can occur normally or as a result of therapy and inflammation. This may make it difficult to evaluate a tumor.

Benign Variants

Many processes alter F-18 FDG distribution (Box 11-2) and may affect the scheduling of a PET scan (Table 11-5).

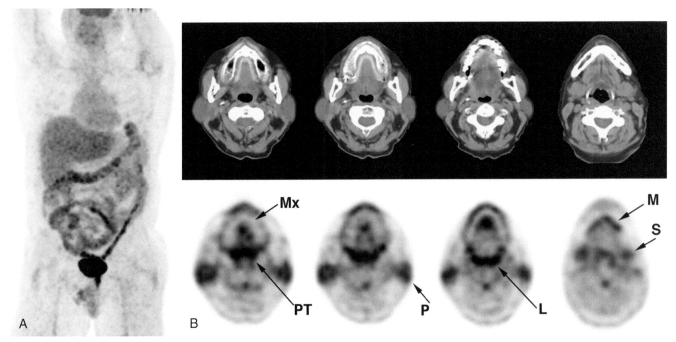

FIGURE 11-3. Normal variants. **A,** Normal intense uptake can be seen in small and large bowel. Bowel uptake is increased with metformin use. **B,** Axial PET and corresponding CT images show normal uptake in the oropharynx. Normal uptake is often symmetric and may be very intense when patients swallow excessively or talk. *L,* Lingual tonsils; *M,* mandible; *Mx,* maxilla; *P,* parotid gland; *PT,* palatine tonsils; *S,* submandibular gland.

Box 11-2. Factors Affecting Fluorine-18 Fluorodeoxyglucose Uptake

INCREASED UPTAKE	DECREASED UPTAKE
Higher tumor grade	Benign lesion/scar
Large number of viable cells	Necrosis
Increased tumor blood flow	Low-cellularity or low-grade tumor, mucinous tumors, bronchoalveolar carcinoma
Inflammation	Hyperglycemia
Tumor hypoxia	High insulin
Radiation (acute)	Chronic radiation
Recent chemotherapy	Prior chemotherapy
Recent surgery	Scar
	Decreased dose availability: Infiltrated injection, muscle uptake

TABLE 11-5 Clinical Factors Altering Patient Scheduling

History	Course of action
Prior surgery	Delay scan 4-6 weeks
Chemotherapy	Delay scan several weeks or schedule scan just before next cycle
Radiation therapy	Delay scan at least 3 months
Colony-stimulating factor	Delay scan 1 week for short-acting agents or several weeks for long-acting
Serum glucose >200	Reschedule scan to control glucose
Insulin administration	Wait at least 2 hours
Breastfeeding	Discontinue feeding at least 6 hours

In addition, radiotracer distribution may be altered for various reasons in clinical use. Activity is frequently seen in muscles that can sometimes pose interpretative problems. The muscles of the oropharynx show variable activity, and patients should avoid speaking after injection to decrease artifact. The skeletal muscles may show prominent uptake resulting from recent exertion and tension. Insulin administered to patients with diabetes or increased endogenous insulin occurring after eating also may cause intense levels of muscle activity, necessitating a repeat examination (Fig. 11-4). In vocal cord paralysis, unilateral uptake may occur in the normal vocal cord in a patient with contralateral vocal cord paralysis (Fig. 11-5).

One interesting and common variant is supraclavicular F-18 FDG accumulation in brown fat (Fig. 11-6). This activity was originally thought to occur in the muscles of the neck, but fused PET/CT images showed the uptake actually localized to areas of fat on the CT scan. This variant occurs more commonly in cold weather and in young, thin patients, relating to adrenergic stimulation of the

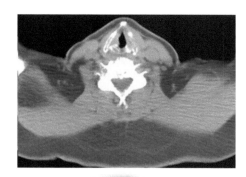

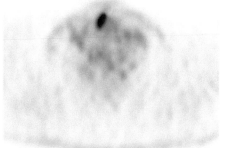

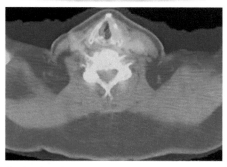

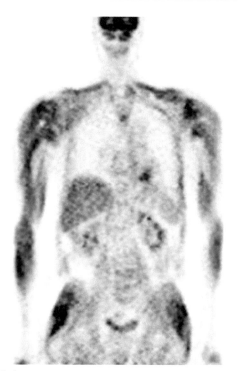

FIGURE 11-4. Muscle activity from increased insulin levels. Intense, diffuse uptake in the muscles caused by eating before radiotracer injection might obscure malignancy and require a repeat examination.

FIGURE 11-5. Paralyzed vocal cord artifact on PET. Axial CT, PET, and fused PET/CT images reveal unilateral uptake localizing to the right vocal cord. On physical examination, the left vocal cord was found to be paralyzed from left recurrent laryngeal nerve damage in this patient with left lung cancer and prior radiation therapy. This uptake could be confused with a lymph node metastasis or a laryngeal head and neck carcinoma on PET if CT correlation is not used.

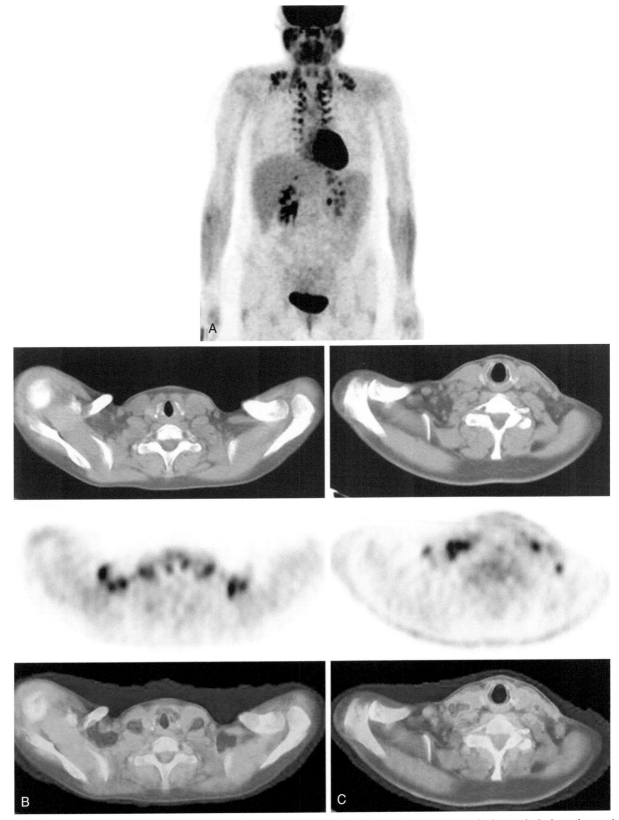

FIGURE 11-6. Brown fat uptake versus adenopathy. **A,** Maximum intensity projection image demonstrates marked supraclavicular and costophrenic region activity and more mild activity in the suprarenal fat, as can be seen in severe cases of brown fat uptake. On axial images **(B),** activity clearly localizes to fat, unlike in lymphoma **(C),** in which activity in the same region is within abnormal lymph nodes.

cells that may have originated as a primitive, nonshivering warming mechanism. Brown fat contains adrenergic receptors that contribute to uptake in anxious patients. Although the pattern is simple to recognize, it may decrease sensitivity for tumor detection in the region. Variable degrees of improvement have been obtained with sedation such as valium and with adrenergic blocking agents in anxious patients or those with a previously abnormal scan. Warming patients for 30 to 60 minutes before injection and keeping them warm is often effective in diminishing this uptake.

Focal F-18 FDG accumulation may localize to vessels, particularly in the aortic arch. This may be associated with calcifications from atherosclerotic disease. In general, this activity is nonspecific, although intense uptake could indicate arteritis.

A lack of significant thyroid activity is normal; however, the thyroid gland may show multiple uptake patterns (Fig. 11-7).

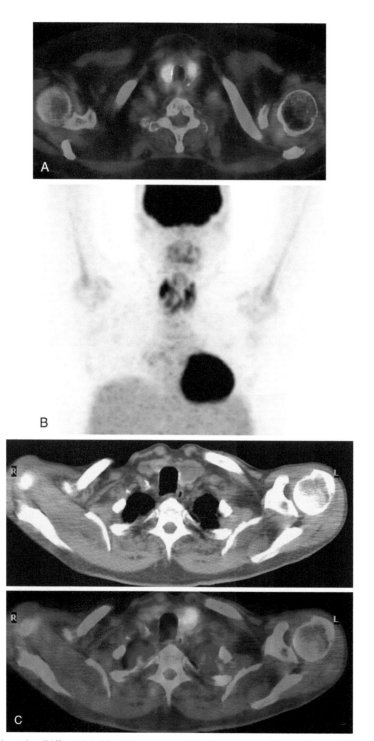

Figure 11-7. Patterns of thyroid uptake. Diffuse thyroid uptake suggests a benign process, as in a patient with Hashimoto thyroiditis **(A)** or multinodular goiter **(B)**. However, focal uptake requires follow-up with ultrasound and probable biopsy because of a significant risk for a thyroid malignancy, as in the thyroid nodule in **C.** A benign adenoma in this patient could have a PET appearance similar to that of a malignant nodule.

Diffusely increased uptake may be seen in thyroiditis, goiter, and Graves disease. The significance of low-level diffuse activity in patients without identifiable thyroid disease is uncertain; it may be normal or the result of subclinical thyroiditis. Focal uptake can be seen in benign nodules. However, focal activity can be the result of malignancy in up to 50% of cases and evaluation is warranted.

Benign adenomas and tumors outside the thyroid gland may also accumulate F-18 FDG. This includes adenomas in the colon, the parotid gland, and benign ovarian tumors.

Effects of Inflammation and Therapy

F-18 FDG uptake is not specific for tumor. Increased activity can be seen in inflammation and infection, with the cause attributed to glycolytic activity in leukocytes. Infections such as pneumonia will have intense radiotracer accumulation. Inflammatory uptake in a lymph node or mass cannot be differentiated from malignancy. Such uptake may be problematic in sarcoidosis and granulomatous disease in the chest (e.g., histoplasmosis and tuberculosis). Other inflammatory processes in the lungs, such as occupational lung diseases and active interstitial fibrosis and pneumonitis, may also cause markedly abnormal uptake (Fig. 11-8).

Increased activity around a joint in the soft tissues or joint capsule may be confused with a metastatic lesion. This pattern is most common in the hip and shoulder. Fused PET/CT images can help localize the uptake. Activity involving the joint surface or both sides of the joint may be present with degenerative disease. Acute and healing fractures normally accumulate F-18 FDG (Fig. 11-9). Correlation with the CT can usually help differentiate this from a metastatic lesion, because the fracture will be seen radiographically.

Therapy often causes an inflammatory response with resulting increased activity (Figs. 11-10 and 11-11). No definitive rules indicate how long to wait after therapy to perform a PET scan. At times, repeat or even serial imaging may be needed to confirm that increased activity is iatrogenic. Radiation therapy causes intense F-18 FDG uptake acutely. Because this uptake may vary as the inflammatory response evolves, delaying the PET scan for

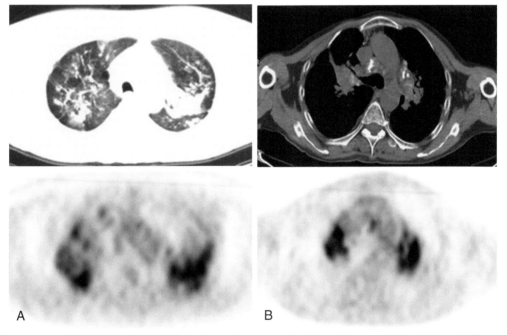

FIGURE 11-8. Inflammation on F-18 FDG PET. **A,** Marked changes from occupational lung disease on CT *(top)* show significant radiotracer uptake *(bottom)*. **B,** A different patient with bulky adenopathy from sarcoid *(top)* has high levels of uptake *(bottom)*, similar to lymphoma.

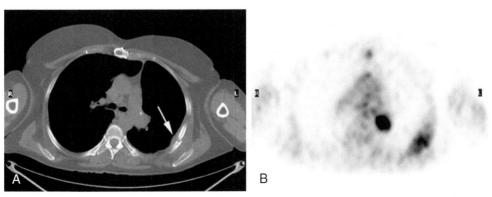

FIGURE 11-9. F-18 FDG uptake in fracture. **A,** CT shows a left rib fracture *(arrow)* after biopsy of lung cancer. **B,** PET shows uptake in the fracture and the left suprahilar mass, which is not well seen on the single noncontrast CT slice.

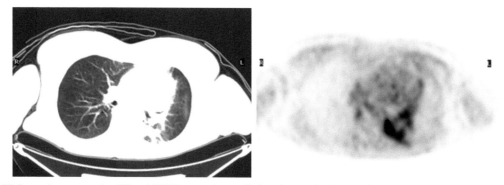

FIGURE 11-10. FDG posttherapy uptake. CT and PET images show radiation changes in the posterior medial left lung 3 months after external beam radiation therapy. The uptake may decrease slightly on follow-up scans, but marked uptake typically persists in the lungs.

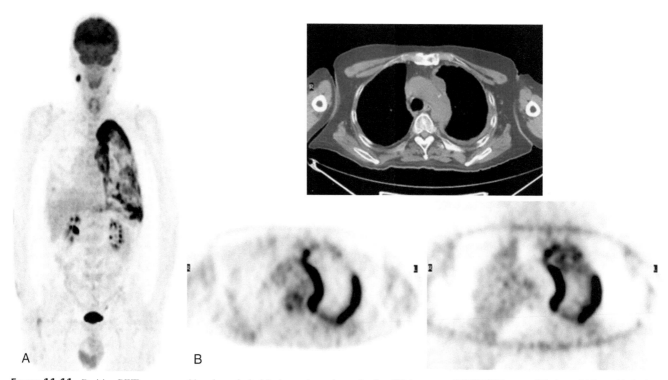

FIGURE 11-11. Positive PET scan caused by pleurodesis. Maximum intensity projection **(A)** images and PET/CT images **(B)** show thickened left pleura on the CT *(top)* and intense FDG uptake on attenuation corrected images *(bottom left)*. This uptake may be difficult to differentiate from tumor and can persist indefinitely. Note the typical differences on the non–attenuation-corrected image *(bottom right)* where the lungs *appear* "hotter," as does the skin.

2 to 3 months is recommended. However, radiation effects may persist indefinitely in the lungs. Chemotherapy may cause a lesion to show a transient apparent worsening. A delay in scanning of at least 2 weeks is recommended, but in some cases several weeks or until just before beginning the next chemotherapy cycle is optimal. However, increasing data indicate that imaging early after therapy can better predict therapeutic response in some tumors, such as lymphoma. The postoperative inflammatory response in the wound healing process results in F-18 FDG uptake that is usually mild to moderate (Fig. 11-12), and a delay of at least 2 to 4 weeks to minimize the effects of inflammation on uptake is recommended.

Bone marrow evaluation may be limited by the effects of therapy. When marrow-stimulating drugs (filgrastim [Neupogen] or epoetin alfa [Procrit]) are used in patients with anemia or undergoing chemotherapy, a diffuse increase in radiotracer uptake may result. Usually this pattern is easily differentiated from that of metastatic disease (Fig. 11-13). However, increased marrow background can mask actual lesions from tumor involvement. If possible, scans should be delayed until the effects of marrow-stimulating therapy has resolved. In short-acting agents, this typically takes 5 to 7 days but it is prolonged with newer, long-acting drugs.

Low-level activity with a characteristic shield shape in the anterior mediastinum may be seen in the thymus in young patients (Fig. 11-14). In cases in which activity appears after therapy, careful correlation with the CT can help determine whether normal-appearing thymic tissue is present in the anterior mediastinum. Increased uptake after therapy is known as *thymic rebound* and can be seen as an increase in size on CT as well. It may be difficult to differentiate from tumor involvement even on follow-up examinations.

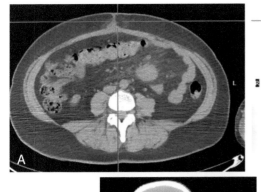

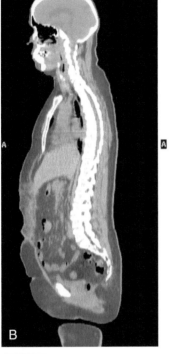

Figure 11-12. Postoperative change. **A,** Two months after laparotomy, the CT shows secondary changes in the midline anterior abdominal wall and stranding of the left lower quadrant peritoneal fat. The corresponding PET image has mild anterior soft tissue uptake and normal uptake in bowel and marrow. **B,** More intense uptake can be seen in the sagittal image done 6 days after surgery.

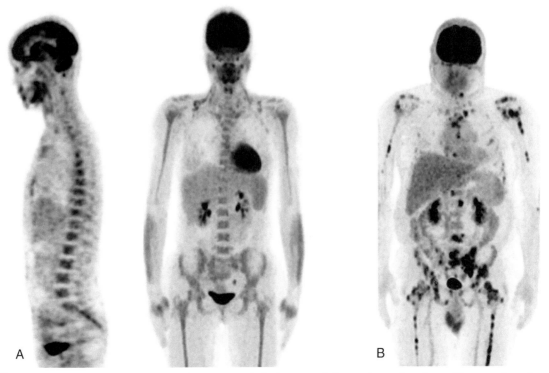

Figure 11-13. Patterns of bone marrow FDG uptake. **A,** Diffuse uptake in the marrow is frequently seen in patients with cancer after colony-stimulating factor therapy. **B,** Osseous metastases usually present with heterogeneous focal lesions.

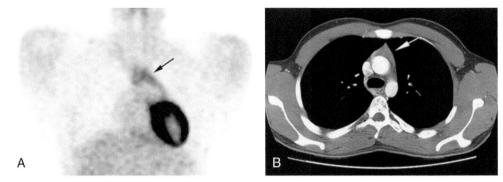

FIGURE 11-14. Benign FDG uptake in the thymus. Area of uptake above the heart *(arrow)* in the typical configuration of the thymus **(A)** corresponds to a normal thymus **(B)** on CT. After chemotherapy, this uptake may be even more intense, the so-called thymic rebound.

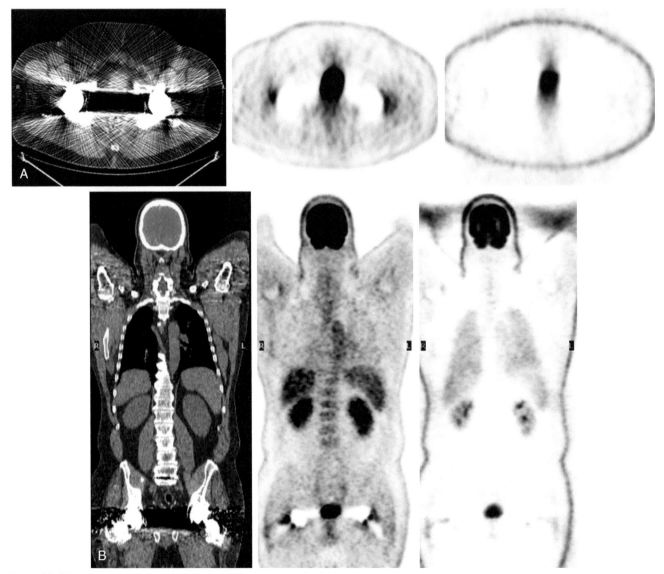

FIGURE 11-15. Metal artifact. Axial **(A)** and coronal **(B)** CT and PET images show beam hardening artifact on the CT *(left)* from bilateral hip prostheses. The attenuation corrected PET images *(middle)* show artifactually increased uptake along the lateral margins of the prostheses, which is significantly decreased on non–attenuation-corrected images *(right)*.

Artifacts

When metal or dense-iodinated contrast is present, the attenuation-correction images may mistakenly show increased radiotracer activity around the area (Fig. 11-15). Examining the non–attenuation-corrected images, which

will show no increased activity, can lead to the correct interpretation. Correlation with a current CT will help identify sources of such artifact.

Areas of intense F-18 FDG activity, such as in the bladder and infiltration at the injection site, can cause a

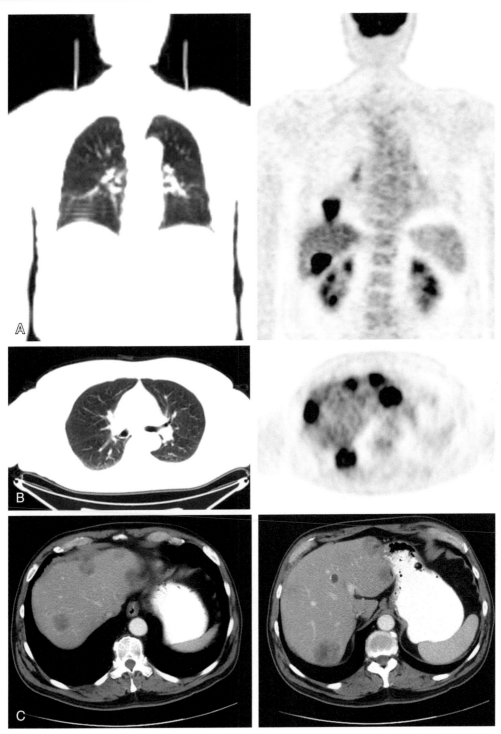

FIGURE 11-16. Respiratory motion artifact. Coronal **(A)** and axial **(B)** CT scans in lung windows and corresponding PET scans show intense FDG activity in liver metastases and the right lung base. However, no lung mass is seen on CT. **C,** Two axial enhanced CT images show liver metastases. Differences in respiration have caused misregistration and a posterior liver lesion projects over the lung on PET.

reconstruction artifact manifested by a band of artifactually decreased activity across the patient. This was more common with older systems that relied on filtered back-projection and is less of a problem with iterative reconstruction. The non–attenuation-corrected images show less effect.

Hybrid PET/CT systems can generate certain artifacts. A common artifact is caused by misregistration of PET and CT caused by respiration. A CT acquired with breath holding will greatly alter the position of organs compared with the PET scan, which must be done in quiet respiration. If the CT is done in quiet respiration, structures more closely match the PET images, but motion and low lung volumes may obscure lesions. Respiratory motion artifact also can cause abnormal uptake from a lesion to appear in an incorrect location on the CT, particularly for pathology near the diaphragm. This most frequent involves a liver lesion projecting over the lung or rib on the CT (Fig. 11-16). If the patient is large or imaged with arms at the sides, truncation artifact may lead to thin linear bands of activity running the length of the patient on the MIP image. CT beam-hardening artifact is a common problem that affects the quality of CT and fused PET/CT images (Fig. 11-17). This can be minimized by moving the arms out of the field of view. Another common, subtle artifact is a thin horizontal band or seam perpendicular to the patient's axis from motion at adjoining bed positions.

Patterns of Malignancy

Aggressive tumors usually have greater uptake because of higher levels of metabolic activity. This pattern must be differentiated from the intense activity often seen in

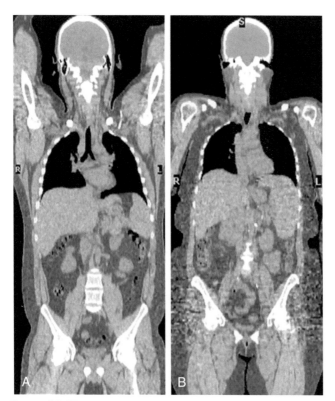

FIGURE 11-17. Effects of arm position and beam hardening on CT images. Soft tissue window CT image with the patient's arms up (**A**) compared with arms down (**B**) demonstrates the effect of beam hardening with artifact throughout the abdomen on **B**.

infection or after radiation therapy. Low-level activity may be seen in low-grade tumors and tumors with a lower relative numbers of cells such as bronchoalveolar carcinoma and mucinous adenocarcinoma. Malignant pleural effusions most often have low-level F-18 FDG activity, and some are even negative, which may be due to the dispersion of tumor cells in the fluid so uptake is not detected.

Areas of tumor necrosis will have diminished F-18 FDG accumulation. This is often seen as absent activity centrally in very large masses. By determining areas of necrosis and intense activity, PET scans can help direct biopsy for more sensitive accurate sampling. It may not be possible to differentiate a cavitary infectious process from a necrotic tumor on PET, because both will have a cold center and a peripheral rim of increased activity (Fig. 11-18).

Levels of background activity play a role in the detection of malignant lesions. For example, the high background activity of the brain limits sensitivity for metastatic disease, with perhaps only a third of lesions being visualized. Also, if background uptake is heterogeneous, as may happen in the liver, it can make lesion detection more difficult. It is helpful to describe or grade the severity of abnormal activity in terms of lesion-to-background differential. For example, lymph node activity in the hila and mediastinum are compared to the background mediastinal activity. The uptake can be graded as mild, moderate, or severe, depending on the level above normal adjacent tissue.

Lesion activity can be quantified with a lesion-to-background ratio, lesion-to-liver ratio, or standard uptake value (SUV). Quantification can help confirm the visual impression and help follow abnormalities.

Quantitation with the Standard Uptake Value

The SUV is a measure of the relative uptake in a region of interest. This calculation depends on a precise knowledge of the injected dose quantity and time. Therefore the dose calibrator quality control must be maintained and dose infiltration must be avoided during injection. Software will automatically time-decay the amount of dose given minus the postinjection residual in the syringe.

$$SUV = \frac{\text{Tissue activity (millicurie/milliliter)}}{\text{Injected dose (millicurie)/weight (grams)}}$$

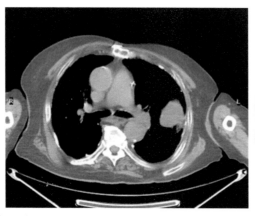
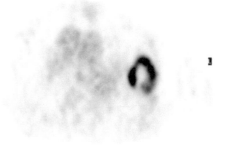

FIGURE 11-18. Central tumor necrosis on PET. A left upper lung carcinoma seen as a solid mass on CT actually contains significant central necrosis that is revealed as absent uptake on PET. Visualization of regional differences in tumor metabolic activity with PET can help direct a biopsy.

F-18 FDG distribution is very low in fat, which leads to higher values in tumor and normal tissues in heavier patients than in thin patients. Correction applied for body mass or body surface area can eliminate this problem (SUV_{lean} or SUV_{bsa}).

In general, an SUV greater than 2.5 is considered suspicious for malignancy. Most tumors have an even higher SUV. However, considerable overlap occurs with inflammatory processes. Numerous factors affect SUV levels (Table 11-6). For example, when comparing serial examinations, image acquisition at different times after injection may alter SUV values. Thus, to minimize variability in SUV, imaging should be done after the same time delay in patients undergoing serial examinations. Generally, this delay is 50 to 65 minutes after injection for patients with cancer. Some studies have shown improved detection of malignancy by dual-point acquisition with further delayed imaging at 90 to 120 minutes after injection. Lesion size is also an important consideration. Volume averaging can artifactually lower SUV values because regions of interest may include pixels from normal surrounding tissue in small tumors or from motion. In the past, SUVs were measured with a two-dimensional area, but software on current workstations allows assessment of three-dimensional regions, which is often superior. However, the region of interest must be selected with care to include only structures of interest.

Activity in a lesion often is reported in terms of the SUV_{max}, or the value of the most intense pixel in the region of interest. This allows exclusion of low counts from areas of necrosis or adjacent normal structures. An SUV_{mean} is an average of all counts in the region of interest, which may be more representative because a spurious single hot area will not cause incorrect data to be recorded. Many experts advocate using an SUV_{peak}, which is calculated as an average of the counts from a circular volume (often 1 cm) surrounding the hottest pixel. The SUV_{peak} may more accurately represent maximal tumor metabolism with a higher degree of statistical significance than the SUV_{max}.

When evaluating a response to therapy on serial scans or when comparing data from multiple sites participating in a trial, SUV accuracy is critical. All parameters that could alter the SUV must be controlled. However, variability still occurs and most consider that the SUV must change at least 20% to be significant. Reports describe greater difficulties when considering a multicenter trial. Because of difficulties maintaining protocol compliance and other issues, a 34% change was required before it could be considered significant.

CLINICAL USES OF POSITRON EMISSION TOMOGRAPHY IN ONCOLOGY

The use of PET scanning in primary tumors of the brain is discussed in Chapter 15. Evaluation of lung cancer in solitary pulmonary nodules was the first clinical indication for F-18 FDG PET scanning in the United States approved by the Centers for Medicare and Medicaid (CMS). Since that time, the number of approved applications for PET has increased. Although the list continually changes, indications for F-18 FDG PET approved by the CMS are listed in Table 11-1. Private insurers may cover other indications. Box 11-3 lists tumors that show a low degree of F-18 FDG uptake, causing a lower sensitivity.

Lymphoma

Malignant lymphoma is classified as either Hodgkin disease (15%) or the more common non-Hodgkin lymphoma (85%). For Hodgkin disease, 10-year survival rates are 80% to 85% for the early stages and approximately 40% for very advanced (stage IV) disease. Survival rates are much lower for non-Hodgkin lymphoma, with a 60% 5-year survival for the potentially curable tumors, which are the high-grade, more aggressive forms of the disease.

Hodgkin disease tends to spread in an orderly fashion in contiguous lymph node chains. Staging of Hodgkin disease is important in treatment planning and assessing prognosis, but surgical staging has largely been replaced by imaging (Box 11-4). Prognosis is good for stage I and stage II disease, which can be treated with local radiation therapy. More advanced disease requires the addition of chemotherapy.

Non-Hodgkin lymphoma is often widespread at the time of diagnosis and is more frequently fatal. Prognosis is closely related to histopathological classification and tumor grade. High-grade and intermediate-grade tumors are treated with chemotherapy and radiation therapy with the goal of a cure. Patients with low-grade tumors typically

TABLE 11-6 Factors Affecting Standard Uptake Value Levels

Factor	Change in SUV
↑ Serum glucose	↓
↑ Body mass	↑
↓ Dose delivery: Extravasated dose	↓
↑ Uptake period	↑
↓ Region-of-interest size	↑
↓ Pixel size	↑

SUV, Standard uptake value.

Box 11-3. Tumors with Frequently Lower Fluorine-18 Fluorodeoxyglucose Uptake

Prostate cancer
Renal cell carcinoma
Bronchoalveolar cell lung cancer
Mucinous adenocarcinomas
Carcinoid
Low-grade sarcomas
Low-grade lymphoma
  Mucosa-associated lymphoma (MALT)
  Small cell lymphocytic non-Hodgkin lymphoma
Differentiated thyroid cancer (iodine-avid)
Hepatocellular carcinoma
Metastasis to brain

have an indolent course initially. Although therapy may prolong survival, low-grade tumors relapse and eventually transform to aggressive and fatal tumors.

Imaging

Developments in imaging and therapy have led to significant improvements in the treatment of lymphoma. Gallium-67 was once widely used in the evaluation of lymphoma but was essentially replaced by CT in the 1990s and cannot compete with F-18 FDG PET/CT (Fig. 11-19). Although CT is often still a critical component of diagnosis and staging, F-18 FDG PET/CT alone is increasingly used to monitor lymphoma.

Detection

F-18 FDG PET is highly sensitive in the detection of Hodgkin disease and high-grade non-Hodgkin lymphoma and usually shows high levels of uptake. Some low-grade follicular non-Hodgkin lymphoma cases are also accurately evaluated. Other low-grade non-Hodgkin lymphoma tumors such as small cell lymphocytic lymphoma and mucosa-associated lymphoma tissue (MALT) have much less uptake and are not visualized reliably with F-18 FDG PET. Diagnosis of lymphoma generally relies on histopathological characterization of tissue samples, and PET has not played a significant role in lymphoma diagnosis. PET might be useful in directing biopsy to the most accessible site.

Staging, Monitoring Therapy, and Restaging

PET consistently has been found superior to CT in assessment of lymphoma. The accuracy of PET is 96% compared to 56% with CT, with a sensitivity greater than 91%, or 10% more sensitive than CT. The disease stage may be altered based on PET in 10% to 40% of cases. F-18 FDG PET is more accurate in assessing extranodal disease, including soft tissue lesions, bone marrow, and spleen (Fig. 11-20). Focal lesions are generally caused by tumor, whereas diffuse uptake may be the result of therapy. Although bone marrow biopsy is the gold standard, it can miss disease. A combination of PET and biopsy may provide the most accurate evaluation of marrow.

FDG PET can accurately evaluate the effectiveness of therapy. Decreased uptake is seen in patients responding to therapy (Fig. 11-21). This can be evaluated after as little as one cycle of chemotherapy or less. Responders identified

by PET have longer disease-free remission periods or are cured, whereas nonresponders and patients with residual disease relapse or progress. Clinicians may want to alter therapy early on based on a lack of response seen on F-18 FDG PET.

PET can assess for tumor viability in a residual mass found on CT after therapy. PET is much more specific than CT (86% vs. 31%) in these cases (Fig. 11-22). PET is often used in the restaging of disease as information complements that were gained by CT scanning.

Multiple Myeloma

Several diseases are included in the spectrum of plasma cell neoplasms, ranging from benign to highly aggressive tumors. These diseases originate from a single B cell and secrete monoclonal proteins. Multiple myeloma accounts for 24,000 deaths per year worldwide, with an incidence of 4 per 100,000. It may be detected during routine blood testing or may present with a variety of musculoskeletal, hematological, immunological, or neurological complaints. Patient workup consists of evaluation of immunoglobulin levels, 24-hour urine protein evaluation, serum and urine electrophoresis, whole-body skeletal survey, and bone marrow aspiration. Radiographic findings may begin with osteoporosis, but eventually numerous lytic lesions are seen. Bone scans are relatively insensitive.

Limited data suggest that F-18 FDG PET/CT may add information to that seen on MRI, CT, or radiographs. It detects bone involvement in 25% of newly diagnosed patients with negative skeletal surveys and extramedullary involvement in up to 25%. PET/CT scans are often negative in patients in remission or in patients with monoclonal gammopathy not related to malignant myeloma. PET/CT is also superior to skeletal surveys in the detection of active disseminated bone disease.

Box 11-4. **Ann Arbor Classification of Lymphoma**

I	Single lymph node or lymphoid structure
IE	I+: Growth into adjacent tissue or extralymphatic involvement (not liver)
II	Involving ≥2 regions on the same side of the diaphragm
IIE	II+: Extralymphatic involvement
III	Disease on both sides of the diaphragm (IIIS: Splenic involvement)
IIIE	III+: Involvement extranodal tissue localized
IV	Nonlocalized or disseminated disease

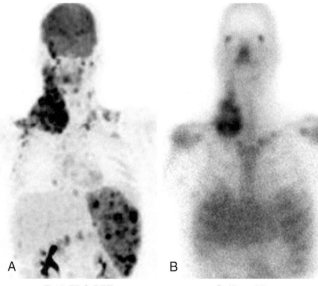

F-18 FDG PET   Gallium-67

FIGURE 11-19. Improved sensitivity of FDG PET over Ga-67. PET shows a large right neck mass and involvement in the left neck, spleen, and abdomen from lymphoma (**A**) whereas a 10-mCi Ga-67 scan at 96 hours has inferior image quality and fails to detect lesion outside of the right neck (**B**).

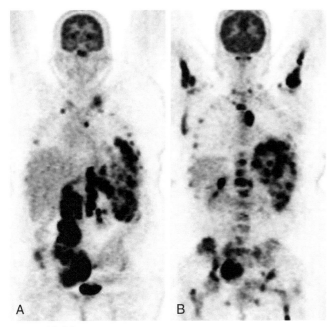

FIGURE 11-20. Restaging lymphoma. **A,** The initial PET image in a patient with non-Hodgkin lymphoma shows extensive abdominal adenopathy and involvement of the spleen, chest, and supraclavicular nodes. **B,** After two cycles of chemotherapy, much of the adenopathy has resolved in the abdomen, but worsening disease is seen in spleen, bone marrow, and mediastinum, requiring a change in therapy protocol.

Melanoma

The incidence of malignant melanoma is increasing dramatically. Survival depends on the stage at the time of diagnosis. The thickness of the primary lesion is the most important prognostic factor, and this is graded according to the Breslow classification. Prognosis is extremely poor, with nodal or distant metastases. Even after potentially curative surgery is performed, patients frequently present with metastatic disease because of early hematogenous spread. Some patients would benefit from further surgery or directed therapy if their disease were accurately restaged. Diagnosis of these metastases is difficult by conventional modalities alone, such as CT. Metastatic disease may occur in unusual locations, such as other cutaneous and subcutaneous sites, spleen, distant nodes, liver, and gallbladder. Metastases are frequently found in high-risk patients (i.e., >4-mm Breslow depth) on PET, sometimes widespread or distant from the primary tumor location (Fig. 11-23). Thus many sites perform head-to-toe imaging on patients with melanoma. Lesions that are not detected are likely microscopic. Although PET is generally more sensitive than conventional imaging methods, CT is more sensitive than PET in detecting small parenchymal lung lesions and MRI best identifies brain metastases. The sensitivity of PET is reported to be greater than 90%, with a specificity of 87%. PET alters therapy in approximately 25% of patients and is useful in staging disease in patients at high risk for metastases or who relapse.

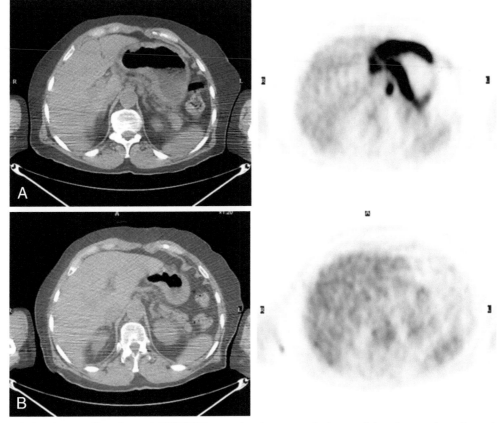

FIGURE 11-21. Monitoring therapy of lymphoma. **A,** PET/CT images show intense uptake in a gastric lymphoma and an adjacent lymph node. Gastric involvement may not be detected, but, when present, PET may be useful for follow-up. **B,** After one cycle of chemotherapy, no tumor could be identified. This suggests a better prognosis than for a late responder or nonresponder.

PET does not replace sentinel lymph node scintigraphy in intermediate-risk (>1.4-mm Breslow depth) or high-risk patients diagnosed with melanoma. Lymphoscintigraphy involves Tc-99m sulfur colloid injection around the primary lesion to identify the first draining sentinel lymph node. Evaluating the resected sentinel lymph node with histochemical staining is the most sensitive method to determine patients at risk for metastatic disease. This allows detection of microscopic disease not detected with PET.

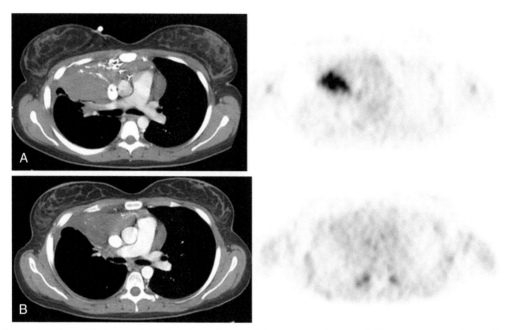

FIGURE 11-22. Evaluation of a residual mass. **A,** During chemotherapy for lymphoma, a large partially enhancing anterior mediastinal mass on CT showed persistently abnormal FDG accumulation in one region of the mass. **B,** When the follow-up CT showed residual mass, a repeat PET was done. No FDG uptake was seen consistent with fibrosis and scar.

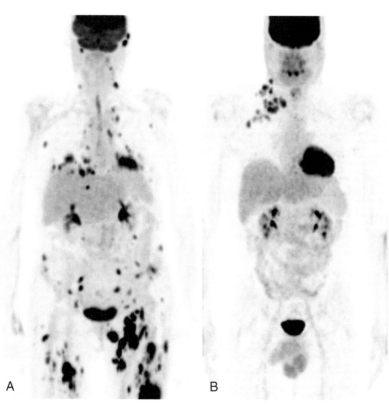

FIGURE 11-23. FDG PET in melanoma. **A,** Diffuse tumor involvement including uptake near the primary tumor in the left thigh, multiple lymph nodes, organs, and soft tissue metastases from melanoma. This result led to changing planned radiation therapy to systemic chemotherapy. PET can also identify subtle disease not found on CT. **B,** Regional metastases are seen in numerous right cervical lymph nodes in a patient with a recently resected melanoma of the right ear.

Head and Neck Carcinoma

The prognosis of head and neck cancer depends on the disease stage. As distant metastases at initial diagnosis occur only 5% of the time, assessing local cervical lymph node status is most critical in determining whether a patient is a candidate for surgical resection. At diagnosis, roughly 40% of patients have localized disease and 60% have advanced cases (Figs. 11-24 and 11-25). F-18 FDG PET has been found useful in staging, monitoring therapy response, and detecting recurrence of head and neck cancers (Table 11-7). PET reportedly changes patient management in 20% to 30% of patients with head and neck cancer.

Although FDG PET is sensitive, it plays a limited role in the diagnosis of head and neck cancer. Conventional modalities adequately visualize most tumors and are generally better able to assess tumor size. However, head and neck cancer often presents with palpable adenopathy.

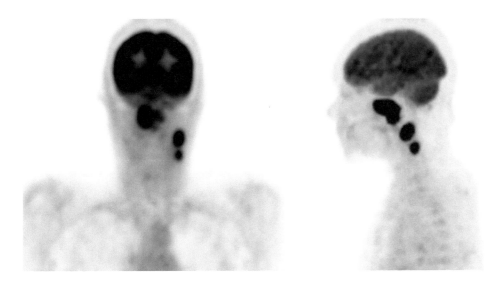

FIGURE 11-24. Recurrent squamous cell carcinoma of the head and neck. Coronal and sagittal PET images demonstrate tumor activity in enlarged palpable left cervical lymph nodes and in the primary tumor posteriorly along the oropharynx extending up to the skull base.

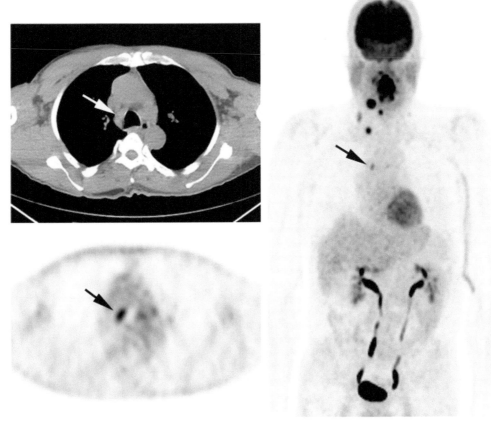

FIGURE 11-25. Head and neck carcinoma staging. PET images reveal several abnormal lymph nodes in the right cervical and supraclavicular region and an unexpected mediastinal metastasis to a normal-size lower paratracheal node *(arrows)*.

These lymph node metastases may be much larger than the primary tumor in head and neck cancer. In 5% to 10% of cases, the primary cannot be identified by endoscopy, CT, or MRI, which means that a patient might have to undergo large-field radiation therapy. Although small primary tumors may not be detected, PET can identify the unknown primary tumor in 20% to 50% of patients.

In staging of head and neck cancer, F-18 FDG PET/CT appears superior to CT and MRI. When lymph nodes are normal in size, this is particularly helpful. For restaging, PET consistently has been found superior to conventional imaging modalities. When the anatomy is distorted from surgery and radiation, restaging and detection of recurrent tumor by PET is better than by CT. The reported sensitivity of F-18 FDG for recurrence ranges from 79% to 96%, with a negative predictive value greater than 90%. CT, on the other hand, has a sensitivity of 54% to 61%.

PET/CT is particularly useful in evaluating the postoperative neck (Fig. 11-26). With a loss of symmetry, evaluation for recurrence is difficult; fusion images allow better identification of increased uptake in normal structures, such as discriminating muscles, from sites of tumor

recurrence or metastases. Recent studies suggest that additional imaging after a further delay of an hour or so may increase specificity. Use of F-18 FDG PET for monitoring therapy provides superior results over CT or MRI, but can be complicated by normal tissue response to therapy. The ability of PET to predict survival is promising, but additional work is needed.

Consistent terms must be used to describe the location of head and neck cancer. Different methods of describing the location of cervical lymph nodes have been used over the years. Currently, an imaging-based method of lymph node classification proposed by Som and colleagues optimizes recent updates by the American Joint Committee on Cancer (Table 11-8; Figs. 11-27 and 11-28).

Thyroid Carcinoma

Thyroid cancer must be considered separately from other cancers occurring in the head and neck. In most cases, thyroid cancer derives from the follicular cells of the gland, giving rise to papillary, follicular, or mixed cellularity variants. These differentiated tumors accumulate iodine-131 (I-131) and are best evaluated and treated with radioactive iodine. The sensitivity of F-18 FDG in these patients is low.

The clinical utility of F-18 FDG PET scanning is limited to thyroid malignancies that do not accumulate I-131—that is, poorly differentiated, aggressive tumors. This may occur in metastatic and recurrent tumors that transform from a previously well-differentiated, iodine-avid tumor. In cases in which the I-131 scan is negative but serum thyroglobulin levels remain elevated, the sensitivity of PET is greater than 90%. PET may help direct surgical resection or external beam radiation therapy. Unlike I-131 scanning, patients do not need to undergo thyroid hormone replacement therapy withdrawal or stimulation with recombinant thyroid-stimulating hormone. PET also may be of some benefit in the more aggressive Hürthle cell variant of follicular carcinoma and in some anaplastic tumors.

F-18 FDG PET scanning may be useful in medullary thyroid carcinoma. This tumor arises from the parafollicular cells of the thyroid and does not accumulate I-131. The

TABLE 11-7 Fluorine-18 Fluorodeoxyglucose Imaging in Head and Neck Carcinoma

Indication	Utility of FDG PET
Surveillance	Very useful
Restaging recurrence	Very useful, especially postoperative neck, but limited by radiation change
Response to therapy	May be useful
Diagnosis in unknown primary	Useful; positive only 20%-50%
Staging	
Clinical N1-N3 neck	Useful, detect distant metastasis
Clinical N0 neck	Low yield

FDG, Fluorodeoxyglucose; *PET,* positron emission tomography.

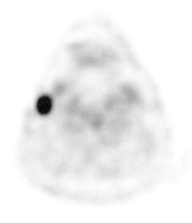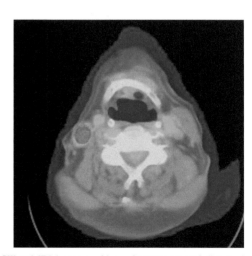

Figure 11-26. Recurrent or residual head and neck cancer is often difficult to diagnose by CT or MRI because of loss of symmetry and distorted anatomy from surgery and radiation. PET/CT makes detection easier as in the right-sided lymph node in this patient with prior radical neck dissection.

TABLE 11-8 Comparison of Nodal Classification Systems for Head and Neck Cancer

Rouviere system	AJCC system	Imaging-based system	
Submental	**I**	**IA:** Medial to medial edge anterior belly digastrics	Below mylohyoid muscle, above hyoid bone
Submandibular	**I**	**IB:** Lateral to IA and anterior to back of submandibular gland	
Internal jugular	**II:** Skull base to hyoid, anterior to back edge sternocleidomastoid	**II:** Skull base to bottom of hyoid, anterior to back edge sternocleidomastoid	**IIA:** Anterior, lateral, or inseparable from internal jugular vein
			IIB: Posterior to internal jugular vein with fat plane between
Retropharyngeal	**III:** Hyoid to cricothyroid membrane, anterior to back edge sternocleidomastoid	**III:** Bottom of hyoid to bottom of cricoid arch, anterior to back edge sternocleidomastoid	Lateral to carotid, level VI nodes medial to carotids
Midjugular	**IV:** Cricothyroid membrane to clavicle, anterior to back edge of sternocleidomastoid	**IV:** Bottom of cricoid arch to top of manubrium, anterior to back edge sternocleidomastoid	Lateral to carotids, level VI nodes medial to carotids
Spinal accessory	**V:** Posterior to sternocleidomastoid, anterior to trapezius, above clavicle	**V:** Posterior to sternocleidomastoid, anterior to trapezius, above clavicle	**VA:** Skull base to bottom of cricoid arch
			VB: Bottom cricoid arch to level clavicle
Anterior compartment	**VI:** Below hyoid, above suprasternal notch, between carotid sheaths	**VI:** Below bottom of hyoid, above top of manubrium, medial to carotid arteries	Visceral nodes
Upper mediastinal	**VII:** Below suprasternal notch	**VII:** Below top manubrium and above innominate	Overlaps highest mediastinal nodes of chest classification between carotids
Supraclavicular		Clavicles in field of view, above and medial to ribs	

All systems use facial, parotid, retropharyngeal, and occipital groups.
AJCC, American Joint Committee on Cancer.

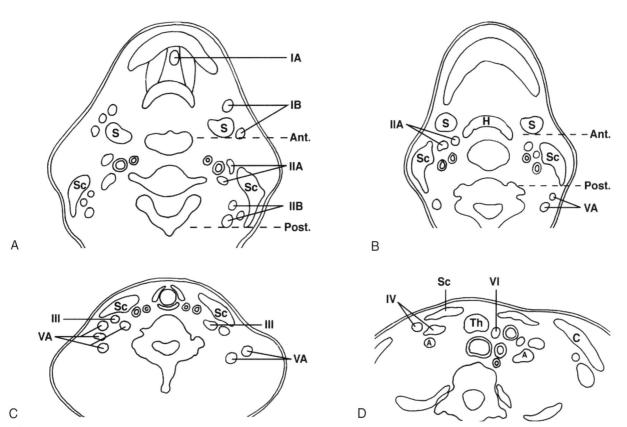

FIGURE 11-27. Transaxial diagram of cervical lymph node stations at **(A)** the level of the floor of the mouth and submandibular gland *(S),* **(B)** the hyoid bone *(H),* **(C)** the thyroid cartilage and cricoid cartilage, and **(D)** just above the clavicles *(C)* with a portion of the thyroid gland *(Th)* in view. Note the appearance of the sternocleidomastoid muscle *(SC),* which is a key landmark. *A,* arteries; *Ant,* anterior.

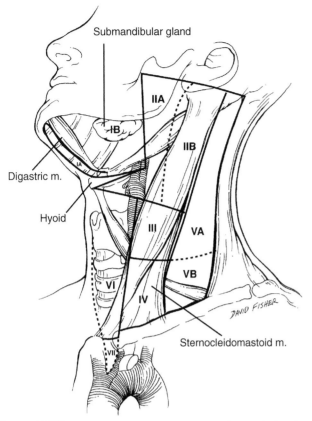

FIGURE 11-28. Cervical lymph node levels according to the imaging-based classification system described in Table 11-8. *m*, Muscle.

BOX *11-5.* **World Health Organization Histological Classification of Lung Carcinoma**

SMALL CELL
Pure small cell (oat cell)
Mixed (small cell and large cell)
Combined (small cell and squamous cell or adenocarcinoma)

NON–SMALL CELL
Large Cell
Undifferentiated large cell
Giant cell
Clear cell

Squamous Cell Carcinoma
Epidermoid
Spindle cell

Adenocarcinoma
Acinar
Papillary
Bronchoalveolar
Solid carcinoma with mucus production

Adenosquamous Carcinoma
Bronchial gland carcinoma
Adenoid cystic carcinoma
Mucoepidermoid tumor

Carcinoid

sensitivity of PET has been reported to be 78%, with a specificity of 79%.

F-18 FDG may accumulate with equal intensity in benign adenomas, thyroiditis, and malignant lesions. Although an incidentally detected F-18 FDG–avid nodule should be pursued to exclude malignancy, PET has no role in the diagnosis of thyroid cancer.

Lung Carcinoma

Lung carcinoma is the most common malignancy and has the highest cancer-related death rate. The histological classification of lung cancer is outlined in Box 11-5. Non–small cell lung carcinoma (NSCLC) accounts for roughly 80% of cases and small cell lung carcinoma (SCLC) accounts for the remaining 20%. Approximately 75% of SCLC cases are initially diagnosed with disseminated disease. Therefore surgery is rarely indicated and chemotherapy and radiation therapy are used. NSCLC, on the other hand, is often resectable. Early diagnosis and proper staging are critical to therapeutic planning in NSCLC.

Presenting clinical and radiographic findings are variable in lung cancer. Patients may be asymptomatic or experience hemoptysis, cough, weight loss, and symptoms of metastatic disease. Radiographic findings are also nonspecific. A mass with an irregular, spiculated border is malignant in up to 85% of cases, but lesions with smooth margins may be cancerous over a third of the time.

Workup for patients with these abnormal radiographs might include sputum cytology, bronchoscopy, transthoracic needle biopsy, and mediastinoscopy. Each of these procedures has limitations. For example, although bronchoscopy has a sensitivity of 85% for central tumors, it is much lower for small and peripheral lesions. The false negative rate for transthoracic needle biopsy is approximately 25%. Transthoracic needle biopsy also carries a 10% to 25% risk for pneumothorax requiring a chest tube. Patients may require thoracotomy and surgical biopsy for definitive diagnosis.

Diagnosis of Solitary Pulmonary Nodule
A pulmonary nodule is defined as a well-circumscribed lesion measuring less than 4 cm. With the increased use of CT, the incidental detection of these nodules has risen tremendously; about half will prove to be malignant. The presence of central calcifications in some nodules indicates they are benign granulomas. However, most pulmonary nodules are indeterminate based on radiographic appearance. The conventional workup of an indeterminate nodule is biopsy or serial radiographic follow-up for 2 years. If the size of a nodule is stable over a 2-year period, the nodule is presumed benign. Suspicious-appearing nodules and those that seem to increase in size are sent for biopsy. This method results in biopsy of many benign lesions and delayed diagnosis of some malignant cases. F-18 FDG PET has proved to be an accurate method to differentiate benign from malignant nodules and decrease biopsy of benign lesions (Fig. 11-29, *A*).

Malignant nodules generally have increased F-18 FDG uptake with an SUV greater than 2.5, although in most

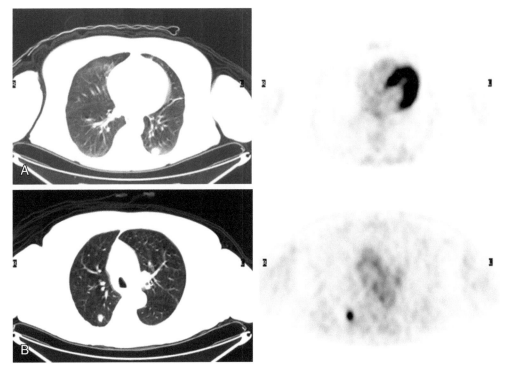

FIGURE 11-29. Characterization of solitary pulmonary nodules. **A,** A left lung nodule on CT had no FDG uptake on PET, consistent with a benign process. This lesion remained stable on CT follow-up, confirming this impression. **B,** A small, well-circumscribed right lower-lobe nodule with increased FDG accumulation on PET was later found to be an adenocarcinoma.

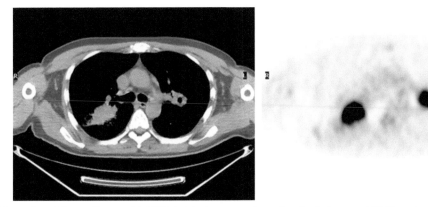

FIGURE 11-30. Detection of distant disease with PET. A right-lung mass showed markedly increased FDG uptake consistent with tumor. Contralateral hilar lymph nodes were also abnormal, which meant this patient was not a candidate for surgical resection.

cancers the SUV is considerably higher (Fig. 11-29, *B*). The sensitivity of PET alone is reported to be 95% to 96% and the specificity 77% to 81%. PET/CT compares favorably with multidetector CT (MDCT) when categorizing a nodule as benign or malignant with a 96% versus 81% sensitivity and a comparable specificity (88% PET/CT vs. 93% CT). PET has a high negative predictive value in evaluating a solitary pulmonary node (SPN), reported to be greater than 97%. This high value means that biopsy usually can be avoided when the PET scan is normal. The incidence of malignancy in patients with a negative PET scan depends on the prevalence of disease; it may be as low as 1% for patients at low risk for cancer, but can be 10% in high-risk cases. Because a chance remains that malignancy is present, these patients are often followed with CT.

F-18 FDG PET scans can change the surgical approach for nodules demonstrating increased uptake. This includes identification of mediastinal lymph nodes with abnormal uptake and distant metastases (Figs. 11-30 and 11-31). In these patients, plans for thoracotomy and surgical biopsy may be changed to mediastinoscopy.

However, F-18 FDG PET has some limitations. False negative results can be seen in lesions smaller than 1 cm. The resolution of PET is on the order of 7 to 8 mm, and volume averaging of small tumors with surrounding normal tissue may result in low or normal-appearing uptake. Motion occurring with tachypnea or in the more mobile lung bases may accentuate volume averaging. New respiratory gating techniques may improve the accuracy of SUV measurements in lung nodules. False negative PET results can occur in certain tumors. In the lungs, the most common of these are bronchoalveolar cell carcinoma and carcinoid.

The positive predictive value of PET is not as high as the negative predictive value, and a positive result cannot be assumed to represent malignancy. An inflammatory process such as granuloma commonly causes false positive findings. In some areas of the country where granulomatous disease is highly prevalent, this is a very significant problem.

A malignant solitary nodule is most commonly caused by primary bronchogenic carcinoma, although a single metastatic lesion is also a possibility. In some cases, a patient with known cancer develops new lung nodules. Even if the nodules are large enough to be characterized by PET, negative F-18 FDG uptake alone cannot rule out

metastases and follow-up is needed. Close examination of the PET scan and correlative CT are essential to detect any unexpected primary tumor outside of the lungs.

Staging Non–Small Cell Lung Cancer

Staging of NSCLC is critical in assessing prognoses and deciding the appropriate course of therapy. Lung cancer staging is based on the tumor-node-metastasis (TNM) classification (Box 11-6 and Table 11-9). Generally, in patients with stage I or II disease the tumors are

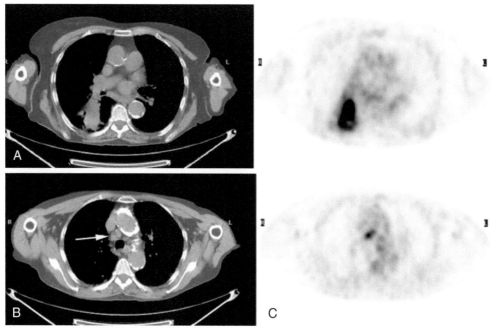

FIGURE 11-31. PET improves lung cancer staging. **A,** The right upper lobe bilobed pulmonary nodule appears malignant on PET. **B,** Small lymph nodes *(arrow)* on CT would not be read as positive based on size criteria alone. **C,** However, PET revealed these small lower paratracheal lymph nodes to be abnormal. Biopsy confirmed malignancy in both regions.

Box 11-6. **Tumor-Node-Metastasis Staging of Lung Carcinoma**

PRIMARY TUMOR (T)
Tx: Malignant cells; primary not seen
T0: No evidence of primary tumor
T1: ≤3 cm; surrounded lung or visceral pleura; not in mainstem bronchus
    T1a: ≤2 cm
    T1b: >2 cm but ≤3 cm
T2: >3 cm but <7 cm
    T2a: >3 cm but ≤5 cm
    T2b: >5 cm but ≤7 cm
    Other descriptors: Involves mainstem bronchus >2 cm from carina, invades visceral pleura
    Associated atelectasis or obstructive pneumonia extends to hilar region but does not involve whole lung
T3: >7 cm
    or <7 cm but with additional nodule same lobe or tumor invading chest wall, pericardium, mediastinal pleura, diaphragm
    <2 cm from carina
    Atelectasis entire lung

T4: Tumor any size with a nodule in a different ipsilateral lobe or invading mediastinum, heart, trachea, major vessels, esophagus

REGIONAL LYMPH NODES (N)
N0: No involvement
N1: Nodes within lung, ipsilateral bronchopulmonary or hilar
N2: Ipsilateral mediastinal, prevascular, retrotracheal, paratracheal and/or subcarinal
N3: Contralateral mediastinal, contralateral hilar, contralateral scalene, supraclavicular

METASTASIS (M)
M0: No distant metastasis
M1: Distant metastasis
    M1a: Nodule contralateral lung, pleural nodules, malignant effusion
    M1b: Distant metastasis such as brain or bone

Data from Edge S, et al, eds. *AJCC Cancer Staging Manual.* 7th ed. New York: Springer; 2010.

considered resectable, although a subset of patients with stage III disease might benefit from surgery. Only approximately 25% of patients have stage I or II disease at the time of diagnosis. Improved methods of staging are needed because up to 50% of patients with NSCLC who undergo surgery expected to be curative will suffer a recurrence.

CT and F-18 FDG PET often have complementary roles in the staging, restaging, and surveillance of NSCLC. CT better assesses tumor size, invasion of the pleura and mediastinum, and distance of the tumor from the carina. Also, abnormalities such as atelectasis and aspiration pneumonia can cause abnormal F-18 FDG uptake that may be confused with that of the primary tumor are often clear on CT.

However, radiographic staging has limitations. For example, CT examination of the lymph nodes depends on size criteria to determine if tumor involvement is present. Any lymph node larger than 1 cm is considered abnormal and suspicious for tumor involvement. Patients with normal-size lymph nodes are frequently understaged by CT. PET often detect abnormal uptake from tumor in normal-size lymph nodes. The sensitivity of PET for tumor involvement in any one lymph node is 75%, but it averages 91% for overall mediastinal involvement. This compares well to reported sensitivities of CT at 63% to 76%. PET/CT can help direct biopsy away from locations typically sampled to focus on areas with the highest likelihood of yielding disease.

The results of PET can help direct the method of biopsy and aid in surgical planning. Patients with no mediastinal involvement or distant metastases can go to thoracotomy for curative resection at the time of biopsy. Whereas N1 disease may be curable, resection in N2 disease results in cure much less frequently. In some cases, biopsy access can be achieved through endobronchial ultrasound to differentiate N1 from N2 disease. Although more invasive, mediastinoscopy is still considered the gold standard and may be needed to further evaluate the mediastinum when PET is positive. It is important to describe lymph node involvement in uniform terms. The commonly used classification system is outlined in Table 11-10 and Figures 11-32 and 11-33.

Biopsy is required when PET is positive, because specificity is lowered by uptake in inflammatory processes. However, it should be noted that both CT and PET can have false positive results for the lymph nodes. Inflammatory conditions can cause enlarged lymph nodes on CT, with false positive interpretations occurring in up to 40% of patients.

Inflammatory processes and the effects of therapy also cause increased uptake of radiotracer. However, lymph nodes may remain enlarged after disease has resolved and PET has normalized. After therapy, PET provides information on response that CT often cannot. Patients who respond to therapy will show PET changes more quickly than on CT.

FDG PET is superior to conventional imaging modalities for the detection of distant metastases (Fig. 11-34). A whole-body PET scan may detect distant lesions not seen on a chest and abdomen CT examination. Unexpected metastases outside of the thorax have been reported in 6% to 20% of cases in the literature. This includes retroperitoneal and pelvic lymph nodes, soft tissue lesions, and small adrenal metastases. Assessment of the adrenal glands is important, because they are a frequent site of lung cancer metastasis. CT reveals adrenal lesions in approximately 20% of cases, but the majority are later proved to be benign adenomas. PET can help differentiate benign and malignant adrenal gland lesions with a high degree of accuracy based on the level of uptake. Bone involvement is detected

TABLE 11-9 Staging of Lung Carcinoma Based on Tumor-Node-Metastasis Classification Scheme

Stage	TNM
Ia	T1 N0 M0
Ib	T2 N0 M0
IIa	T1a N1 M0, T1bN0M0, T2aN1M0
IIb	T2bN0-1 M0
IIIa	T3 N1 M0, T1-3 N2 M0, T4N0-1M0
IIIb	T1-4 N3 M0, T4 N2 M0
IV	Any T, any N, M1a or M1b

Based on the American Joint Committee on Cancer staging system, 1997.
TNM, Tumor-node-metastasis.

TABLE 11-10 Classification of Lymph Node Stations in the Chest

Station	Designation
SUPERIOR MEDIASTINAL NODES	
1 Highest mediastinal	Above top of left brachiocephalic vein crossing trachea
2 Upper paratracheal	Below station 1 to top of aortic arch
3 Prevascular	Anterior to great vessels, cranial to superior aortic arch
Retrotracheal	Behind trachea, thoracic inlet to bottom of azygous vein
4 Lower paratracheal	Below top of aortic arch to superior right upper lobe bronchus
	Azygous arch divides superior from inferior
AORTIC NODES	
5 Subaortic or AP window	Medial to first branch pulmonary artery, lateral ligamentum arteriosum
6 Paraaortic	Anterior and lateral to aortic arch
INFERIOR MEDIASTINAL NODES	
7 Subcarinal	Below carina, adjacent to lower paraesophageal nodes
8 Paraesophageal	Lateral to esophagus or anterior if below subcarinal nodes
9 Pulmonary ligament	In pulmonary ligament posteriorly
N1 NODES: DISTAL TO MEDIASTINAL PLEURAL REFLECTION	
10 Hilar	Along mainstem bronchus/bronchus intermedius
11* Interlobar	Between lobar bronchi and adjacent to lobar bronchi
12* Lobar	Adjacent proximal lobar bronchi
13* Segmental	Adjacent to lobar bronchi distally
14* Subsegmental	Adjacent subsegmental bronchi

*Intrapulmonary
AP, Aortopulmonary

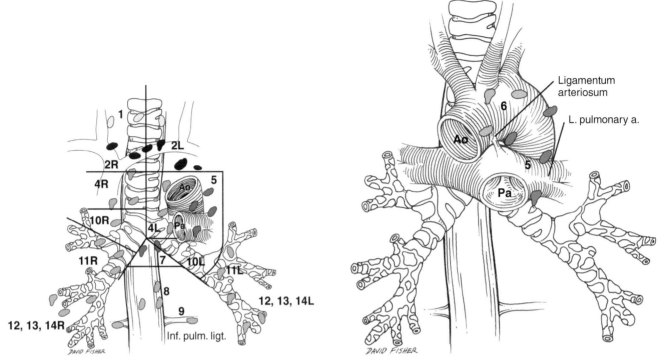

FIGURE 11-32. Lymph node classification of the chest. Anterior images of the chest outline the location of lymph node stations described in Table 11-10. *Ao*, Aorta; *a*, artery; *Inf. pulm. Ligt.*, inferior pulmonary ligament; *Pa*, pulmonary artery.

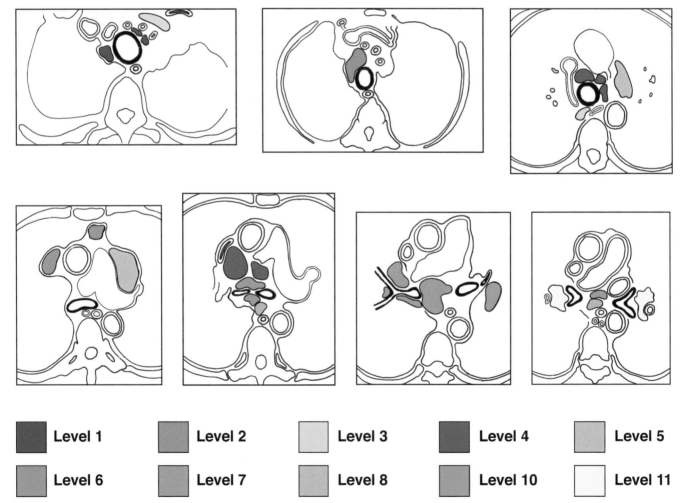

FIGURE 11-33. Transaxial diagram of chest lymph node station positions as outlined in Table 11-10 (pulmonary ligament [level 9] not included) and Figure 11-32.

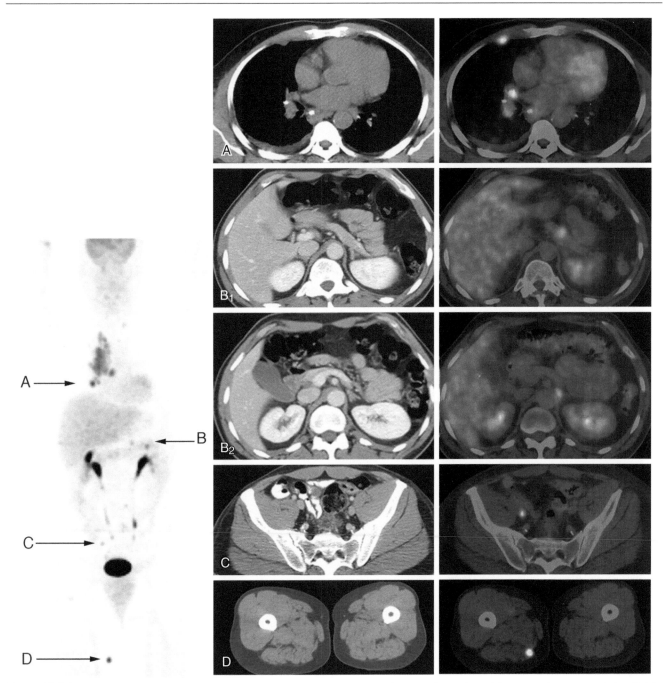

FIGURE 11-34. FDG PET/CT can be used to detect subtle and unexpected lesions such as these in a patient with recurrent lung cancer. **A,** Small right anterior pleural implant (note low-level activity in malignant right effusion). **B₁,** Peripancreatic metastasis. **B₂** Left adrenal gland (unremarkable on CT), **C,** Normal-size pelvic node lateral to the ureter and **(D)** right thigh. Soft tissue metastases are often overlooked on contrast-enhanced CT. *Note:* Some images shown are from the enhanced CT performed 2 weeks earlier.

with a somewhat higher sensitivity than the bone scan and a considerably higher specificity. Overall, F-18 FDG PET has a significant effect on staging and management. Unsuspected metastases are detected 10% to 14% of the time. A significant change in management has been reported in 19% to 50% of cases based on PET findings, including a decrease in futile thoracotomies.

Restaging Non–Small Cell Lung Cancer and Assessing Response to Therapy
When surgery and therapy distort anatomy, PET can detect residual and recurrent tumor not found on CT. Caution

must be used because increased F-18 FDG accumulation may occur after therapy, most significantly after radiation. Immediately after radiation, patchy areas of uptake can be seen corresponding to ground-glass appearing infiltrates. With time, these coalesce and contract with a final appearance on CT of a sharply marginated infiltrate containing air-bronchograms. The PET findings also change over time, but intense activity often does not resolve. It is generally advised to delay F-18 FDG PET until at least 3 months after therapy, although imaging can be done sooner if needed. The background uptake from radiation decreases sensitivity for residual and recurrent tumors and can persist

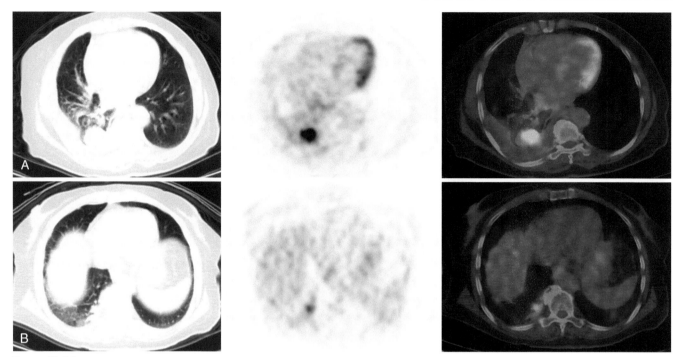

FIGURE 11-35. PET/CT images before **(A)** and during **(B)** chemoradiation therapy for a non–small cell lung cancer with mediastinal involvement (not shown) reveal the value of PET for monitoring therapy, with some residual active disease seen on PET even though a residual mass was not well seen on CT.

long term. Even given these limitations, PET can provide valuable information by identifying residual disease or relapse. For example, distant recurrence after complete resection of tumor occurs more than 20% of the time. PET restaging frequently leads to changes in management.

Data on the use of PET to measure a response to treatment are more limited. Although a decrease in the size of a mass on CT has been used to assess response, this does not always provide the best indicator of the efficacy of therapy (Fig. 11-35). A partial response to therapy has been defined as a decrease in F-18 FDG uptake of at least 20% to 40%. Data suggest a decrease in F-18 FDG activity may provide a better measure of response and normalization of uptake may be associated with a favorable prognosis. Nonresponders can rapidly be shifted to an alternative therapy.

Small Cell Lung Carcinoma

SCLC staging usually involves categorizing the disease as limited or extensive. If disease is confined to one hemithorax, it can be treated more successfully by adding radiation to the chemotherapy. Small cell lung carcinoma shows intense F-18 FDG accumulation. In general, data on the use of F-18 FDG PET in SCLC are more limited than for NSCLC. PET may help detect additional metastasis and lead to upstaging of disease in some patients originally thought to be surgical candidates with localized disease.

Breast Carcinoma

The general types of breast cancer are listed in Box 11-7. Breast cancer is classified as being a noninvasive or invasive tumor of ductal or lobular type. Of invasive carcinomas, ductal carcinoma accounts for 80%, lobular 10%, and medullary 5%. Noninvasive carcinoma, or carcinoma in situ, may be detected by mammography when microcalcifications are

---

Box 11-7. Types of Breast Cancer

Ductal carcinoma in situ
Infiltrating ductal carcinoma
Medullary carcinoma
Infiltrating lobular carcinoma
Tubular carcinoma
Mucinous carcinoma
Inflammatory breast cancer
Paget disease of the nipple

TABLE 11-11 Molecular Subtypes of Breast Cancer

Luminal A	ER+ and/or PR+, HER2–	Most common Less aggressive, good prognosis Hormone responsive
Luminal B	ER+ and/or PR+, HER2+	More frequent ER+/PR– than luminal A Worse prognosis than luminal A
HER2+ (ER–)		Highly aggressive, less common Often <40 years old African American possible risk factor HER2 improves outcome
Basal-like	Triple negative, cytokeratin 5/6+ and/or EGFR+	Aggressive Often <40 years old, African American

EGFR, Epidermal growth factor receptor; *ER*, estrogen receptor; *HER2*, human epidermal growth factor receptor 2; *PR*, progesterone receptor; *triple negative*, ER–, PR–, HER2–.

present (i.e., ductal carcinoma in situ [DCIS]), but may be difficult to detect when it presents as architectural distortion found in lobular carcinoma in situ (LCIS). Prognosis is related to many staging factors, as well as the genomic breakdown of the tumor (Table 11-11). Hormone receptor expression, such as estrogen receptor, and overexpression of tumor markers has been found highly predictive of outcome. Understanding these factors also helps guide therapy.

Diagnosis

Mammography is a sensitive screening tool for detecting breast carcinoma (81%-90%). However, the specificity of mammography is low and biopsy performed after an abnormal mammogram results in a histopathological diagnosis of malignancy only 10% to 50% of the time. MRI continues to be investigated because of its high sensitivity (up to 90%-95%) for the detection of breast cancer, although its specificity is low. MRI is recommended for patients with dense breasts, in which the diagnostic ability of mammography is limited. It also can better visualize multifocal disease, recurrence, and disease in patients with implants. Ultrasound has added considerably to the evaluation of the breast in cases of palpable masses and discrete masses found on the mammogram. F-18 FDG PET imaging has proved useful in breast carcinoma staging and restaging.

Primary Breast Cancer

The ability of F-18 FDG PET to detect primary breast cancer is related to tumor size. One metaanalysis of the literature suggests the sensitivity of PET is 88% and the specificity 79% for detecting primary tumors. Reported sensitivity of PET is 92% for tumors measuring 2 to 5 cm but is only 68% for tumors smaller than 2 cm. The false negative rate of F-18 FDG PET is not sufficient for a screening test. The histological type of the tumor also affects the sensitivity of F-18 FDG PET, with detection of lobular carcinoma and ductal carcinoma in situ being much more limited than in invasive ductal carcinoma. For example, in lobular cancers a sensitivity of approximately 40% has been reported.

Dedicated PET breast imaging systems are being developed, which may significantly improve detection rates compared to whole-body scanners. Positron emission mammography (PEM) performed with these dedicated PET breast cameras has reported resolution of 1 to 2 mm. The higher sensitivity over whole-body scanners aids in following patients during therapy. Promising reports suggest these devices can accurately identify multifocal disease or provide more specificity than breast MRI. However, commercial scanners do not have CT for attenuation correction, so quantitation is done with ratios of activity compared to normal background rather than SUV. In addition, the scans are not clinically approved for reimbursement in tumor diagnosis.

Lymph Node Evaluation

Lymph node involvement has important prognostic and therapeutic implications in breast carcinoma. Axillary lymph node dissection fully evaluates the draining lymph nodes. However, this is a highly invasive procedure with serious side effects (e.g., lymphedema). In patients with nonpalpable lymph nodes, sentinel lymph node localization with Tc-99m sulfur colloid, with or without blue dye, is still the best method to select which lymph nodes to selectively biopsy. A negative PET scan does not exclude the need for further workup.

F-18 FDG PET imaging is able to visualize lymph node metastases by detecting changes in metabolism, often before any anatomical change occurs on CT. Not all lymph

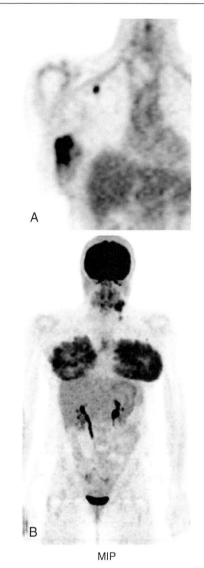

MIP

FIGURE 11-36. Breast cancer staging. **A,** F-18 FDG PET often identifies malignant adenopathy in advanced and recurrent breast cancer. In this case, the large right breast tumor shows markedly increased uptake, as does an axillary lymph node. **B,** This postpartum patient presented with lymphoma in the left cervical region. Intense breast uptake was seen resulting from hormonal stimulation rather than tumor.

nodes will be visualized, because microscopic metastases will not be seen, and the resolution of PET prevents evaluating the number of nodes involved. If scans are interpreted in a highly sensitive mode, specificity is lowered because inflammatory conditions frequently affect the axillary lymph nodes and cause increased FDG accumulation.

Clinical Use of Fluorine-18 Fluorodeoxyglucose Positron Emission Tomography

Because of the limitations of F-18 FDG PET, it is not generally recommended in the initial diagnosis or screening of most patients. However, it was proved useful for staging in patients with advanced disease, monitoring response to therapy, restaging, and detecting recurrent disease. Although PET cannot detect every metastatic deposit, it frequently adds significant information to that obtained with conventional imaging such as CT, MRI, and bone scan. One study reported that PET added information in 29% of cases (Fig. 11-36).

PET detects distant metastases better than conventional modalities in chest, liver, and bone. In bone, PET is best able to identify more aggressive or lytic lesions and the technetium bone scan visualizes sclerotic disease. Therefore PET compliments rather than replaces bone scan in patients at highest risk for metastases. When abnormalities are detected by CT, PET is often able to differentiate benign from malignant processes.

More accurate assessment of tumor response to therapy is possible with PET. Although CT can be used to monitor therapy, it can only examine changes in size. PET reveals changes in metabolic activity, which is a more accurate indication of response. Several studies have shown that PET can differentiate responders from nonresponders early in the course of therapy. This allows rapid protocol modifications to optimize therapy.

The detection of local recurrence is often difficult because of distortion of the anatomy from surgery and radiation. Yet, detection is critical, with recurrence seen in up to 30% of patients. PET has a sensitivity over 90% for the detection of recurrence (Fig. 11-37). Caution must be exercised, because false positive results can occur from therapy.

Gastrointestinal Tumors

Esophageal Carcinoma

Esophageal carcinoma is most commonly due to squamous cell cancer in the upper two thirds of the esophagus, whereas adenocarcinoma typically occurs in the lower third. It frequently presents as dysphagia or is detected by endoscopic biopsy in patients with Barrett esophagus, a known precursor of many cases of esophageal cancer. Because whole-body scanners have limited sensitivity and specificity for detecting tumor in patients with Barrett esophagus, PET has not proved useful in screening these patients. However, F-18 FDG PET has been used in cases of equivocal biopsy or to assess patients with biopsy-confirmed tumor.

Diagnosis

Overall, the sensitivity of PET is greater than 90% in esophageal cancer. The diagnosis of the primary esophageal tumors by PET may be limited by a small tumor volume. In adenocarcinoma, 10% to 15% of patients may have false negative PET results because of the low uptake in mucinous and signet cell varieties. PET is not able to determine the extent of the primary tumor and may not offer any substantial advantage over the standard diagnostic modalities such as endoscopic ultrasonography.

Staging

Esophageal cancer most commonly spreads to regional lymph nodes. The location of these nodes depends to a certain extent on the level of the primary tumor. For example, cervical metastases are more common in proximal tumors and abdominal lymph node involvement may be more frequent in distal masses. However, disease spread may occur in unexpected locations.

The accuracy of detecting lymph node involvement with F-18 FDG PET, particularly with PET/CT, has been consistently shown to be higher than that of CT and MRI. Nodes may be inseparable from the primary mass, and small lesions may be below the resolution of the PET detection systems (Fig. 11-38). However, the detection of distant metastases with PET has been reported to be 83%, compared to 68% with CT. PET may result in a change in patient management in approximately 20% of cases.

Restaging and Monitoring Response to Therapy

PET has proven value in assessing patients during therapy and after therapy for recurrence. A scan following neoadjuvant chemotherapy may better predict patient survival than standard imaging methods (Fig. 11-39). The ability to detect residual and recurrent disease is also significant. Although microscopic residual tumor may be present with a negative scan, a positive scan is a sign of macroscopic residual disease. However, caution must be taken when evaluating patients immediately after therapy because an artifactual increase in activity may be seen (Fig. 11-40).

Normal physiological activity or uptake related to inflammation in the esophagus may confound interpretation. Similarly, moderate F-18 FDG uptake in a normal stomach limits the usefulness of PET in evaluating tumors of the stomach and gastroesophageal junction. Some gastric adenocarcinomas may show only low-level activity on PET/CT. However, when a gastric tumor is F-18 FDG avid, PET scanning may be used in monitoring therapy.

Colorectal Carcinoma

Colon cancer develops in colon polyps, with dysplastic elements found in approximately one third of adenomatous polyps. A progression to invasive cancer occurs slowly. The diagnosis of colorectal carcinoma depends on direct visualization by colonoscopy as well as imaging with CT and barium enema. Staging with CT often identifies regional adenopathy and distant metastases. The staging of

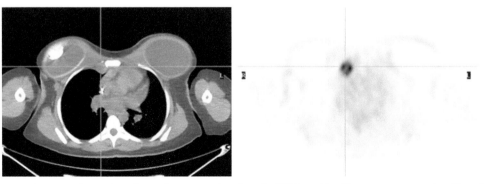

FIGURE 11-37. Recurrent breast carcinoma in an internal mammary lymph node. PET can identify metastases to regional lymph nodes and distant disease. Internal mammary node involvement is frequent in cancers of the inner or medial breast.

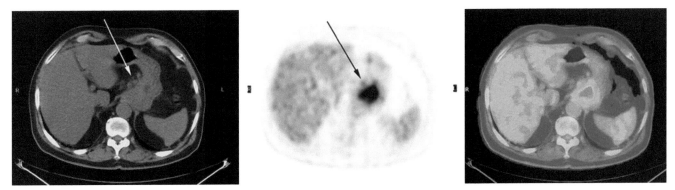

FIGURE 11-38. Identification of regional lymph nodes in esophageal cancer. *Left,* Small but suspicious nodes along the lesser curvature of the stomach *(arrow)* are seen on CT. *Middle,* Marked F-18 FDG uptake is present in the primary tumor at the gastroesophageal junction *(arrow).* However, as best seen on fused images *(right),* only low-level FDG activity was present despite the presence of metastases on endoscopic biopsy. The difficulty in identifying regional nodes may relate to activity in adjacent tumor or microscopic amounts of tumor present.

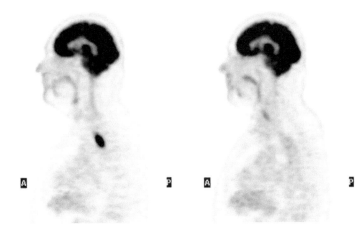

FIGURE 11-39. Monitoring esophageal tumor response to therapy. Sagittal F-18 FDG PET scans *(left)* before and *(right)* after chemotherapy show rapid resolution of the abnormal activity within an esophageal tumor. This type of response has been linked to a better prognosis.

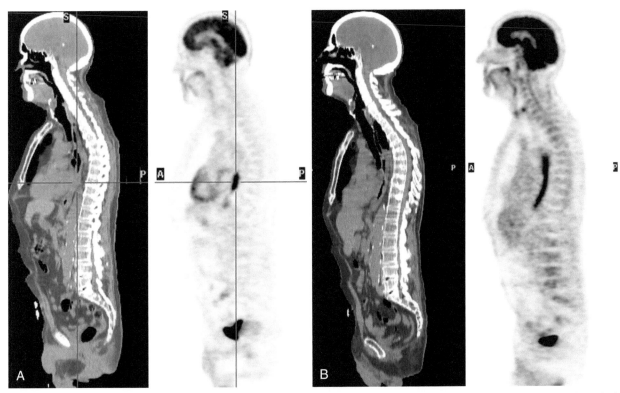

FIGURE 11-40. Effects of radiation therapy on PET interpretation. **A,** Initial sagittal CT and F-18 FDG PET images reveal abnormal uptake in the esophagus from tumor. **B,** Two months after radiation therapy, diffusely increased activity is seen in an extensive region of thickened esophagus. Although this was presumed secondary to therapy, underlying tumor could go undetected and further follow-up was suggested.

colorectal carcinoma is important in determining therapy and prognosis (Table 11-12 and Box 11-8).

The ability of PET to diagnose primary colorectal tumors may be limited because small tumors (especially <1 cm) and cancerous polyps are frequently not detected as high levels of normally occuring F-18 FDG activity in the bowel results in decreased sensitivity. Although not recommended for colorectal carcinoma diagnosis or screening, PET-CT is more accurate than CT. Incidentally detected areas of focal uptake in the colon often require follow-up to exclude the presence of cancer. False positive uptake can be seen in areas of inflammation, such as diverticulosis, and in benign polyps.

Although contrast-enhanced CT is the primary modality for the staging of colorectal carcinoma, it often fails to identify nodal disease. F-18 FDG PET is superior to CT for initial staging and the detection of recurrent colon cancer. Local recurrence can be difficult to detect on CT because of scarring after therapy, but may be easily visible on PET images. The obturator and iliac nodal regions of the pelvis are often particularly difficult to evaluate on CT, whereas PET is very helpful in evaluating these regions. F-18 FDG PET is also superior to CT in the retroperitoneal nodes. The detection of hepatic metastases is excellent with CT, but PET often complements this information or detects new lesions (Fig. 11-41). Sensitivity of PET has been reported at 85% to 99%, with specificity of 71% to 87%. PET may directly alter patient management in 29% to 36% of staging and restaging cases. Caution must be taken because recurrent tumor can occur at the anastomosis, where it can be mistaken for bowel. In some cases, residual tumor could be mistaken for infection or posttreatment inflammation. Data are limited concerning the use of PET in monitoring therapy effects.

TABLE **11-12** Tumor-Node-Metastasis Classification of Colon and Rectal Carcinoma

Primary tumor	Regional lymph nodes	Distant metastases
Tx: Cannot be assessed	Nx: Cannot be assessed	Mx: Cannot be assessed
T0: No evidence of tumor	N0: None	M0: None
TIS: Carcinoma in situ	Nl: 1-3 positive nodes	Ml: Distant metastases
Tl: Submucosal invasion	N2: ≥4	
T2: Invades muscularis propria	N3: Central nodes	
T3: Through propria		
T4: Invades other organs		

Box **11-8.** Dukes' Staging of Colorectal Carcinoma

A	T1, T2; N0; M0
B	T3, T4; N0; M0
C	T1-4; N1; M0
D	Any T; any N; M1

Other Tumors of the Gastrointestinal Tract

The use of F-18 FDG PET in other tumors of the gastrointestinal tract is more limited, and CT remains critical in the analysis of these tumors. However, PET may be helpful in tumors of pancreatic, biliary, and hepatic origin. PET is often used in patients with CT scans that are difficult to evaluate or in patients with elevated serum tumor markers, including alpha-fetoprotein in hepatocellular carcinoma and Ca 19-9 in pancreatic cancer.

Pancreatic Cancer

PET is highly sensitive for the detection of adenocarcinoma of the pancreas (Fig. 11-42). However, CT is essential in defining tumor extent and vascular involvement, as well as in determining resectability. Detection of hepatic and lymph node metastasis is usually done with CT or MRI. However, PET may identify lymph nodes difficult to visualize on CT, such as in the upper portal regions, and can identify undiagnosed distant metastases in 14% of cases. These factors can lead to alterations in surgical management in a significant number of cases. PET is often limited by poor sensitivity in small tumors and in acute pancreatitis. The uptake in acute pancreatitis can be as intense as in malignancy and can mask underlying tumor. Acute pancreatitis often accompanies therapy or obstruction by tumor, and PET in these cases is often nondiagnostic.

Some pancreatic masses seen on CT are benign, and PET can often differentiate benign and malignant processes (with accuracies of 85%-93%). This can support a negative fine-needle biopsy finding. PET may also detect occult cancers not seen on CT in symptomatic patients.

Primary tumors of the liver are much less common than involvement by metastases and are most often evaluated by CT. The two most common primary liver tumors are hepatocellular carcinoma and cholangiocarcinoma. F-18 FDG PET is highly accurate for detecting metastases to the liver but has low sensitivity for the detection of primary hepatic tumors. PET may detect 50% to 70% of hepatocellular carcinomas.

Cholangiocarcinoma is a rare cancer of the bile ducts that may not be detected on CT. It may occur in extrahepatic or intrahepatic locations. Tumors arising peripherally have a better prognosis because they may be resected, whereas those near the hilum are infrequently resectable. Tumors can be infiltrating, exophytic, or a polypoid intraluminal mass. The sensitivity of PET is lower for the infiltrating type in particular. Gallbladder cancer is a rare tumor that is generally diagnosed late in the course of disease and may present with distant metastases. PET usually shows intense uptake and may identify nodal metastases difficult to detect with CT, including distant nodes and those high along the common biliary duct.

One tumor in which PET has proved quite useful is the gastrointestinal stromal tumor (GIST). These tumors usually show high levels of F-18 FDG accumulation. In cases in which tumors respond to imatinib (Gleevec) therapy, markedly decreased F-18 FDG accumulation is seen with PET in a matter of days. PET more accurately assesses early response than CT and predicts improved patient survival (Fig. 11-43).

Genitourinary Tumors

Ovarian Carcinoma

Tumors may arise from any of the cellular elements of the ovary (Box 11-9). Ovarian carcinoma diagnosis is challenging because physical examination may not reveal disease and symptoms do not present until late in the course of disease. Tumor staging is outlined in Box 11-10.

Hematogenous spread is rare, but direct spread and seeding of the omentum and organ surfaces is common (Fig. 11-44). Lymphatic spread can lead to malignant pleural effusions. Although patients with localized disease have a more than 90% survival chance, most patients present with stage III or IV disease. The prognosis of ovarian carcinoma is poor, with overall survival of only 46% at 5 years.

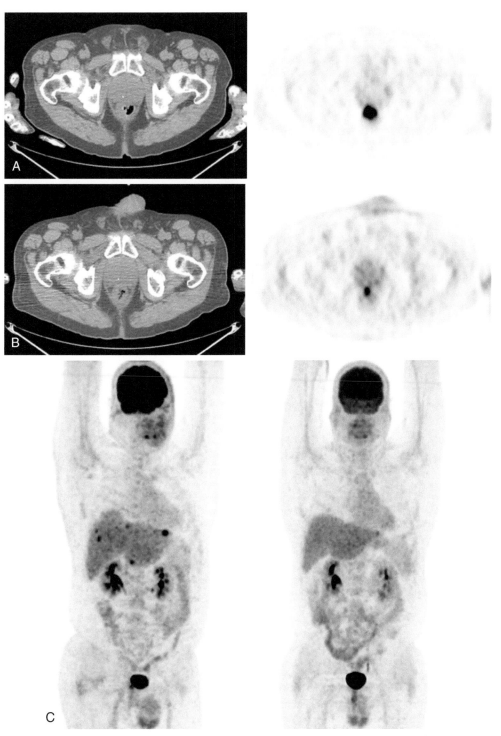

FIGURE 11-41. Evaluation of metastatic rectal carcinoma. Axial-enhanced CT and PET images before **(A)** and after **(B)** chemotherapy show a decrease in activity in a malignant rectal mass. **C,** Coronal images before *(left)* and after therapy *(right)* in this patient show a decrease in hepatic lesions, only one of which was ever detected by CT.

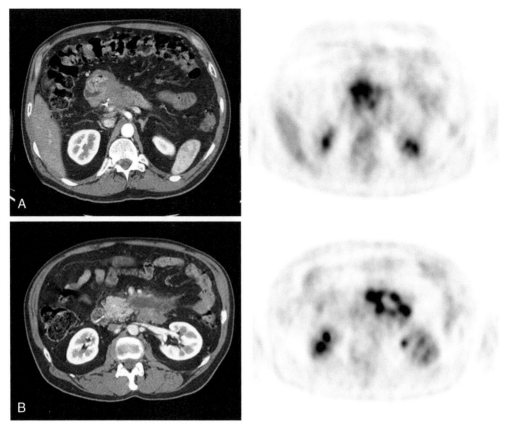

Figure 11-42. PET imaging of the pancreas. **A,** A malignant pancreatic head mass seen on contrast-enhanced CT had a high level of F-18 FDG uptake consistent with malignancy. However, the inflammation that accompanies pancreatitis also can cause intense uptake. **B,** CT following biopsy of a pancreatic mass showed inflammatory changes around the pancreatic tail positive on PET. Note the central "cold" area corresponding to a pancreatic duct dilated as a result of proximal obstruction from the mass.

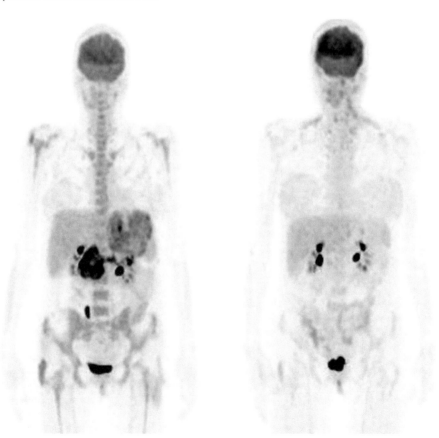

Figure 11-43. FDG PET in gastrointestinal stromal tumor (GIST). PET has proved useful in monitoring the remarkable effects of imitinib (Gleevec) therapy on GIST tumors. A baseline study *(left)* is needed to confirm the tumor is FDG avid. Unlike with CT, rapid improvement is often seen within days of therapy. In this case *(right)*, uptake has resolved even though the mass has decreased on CT only after 4 weeks of therapy.

Preoperative evaluation of patients often includes imaging with sonography, CT, and MRI. Staging with CT has 70% to 90% accuracy. However, small peritoneal lesions found with surgical exploration are frequently overlooked or undetectable by CT. PET/CT often highlights abnormal activity in lesions that were overlooked on CT.

F-18 FDG PET has been used for staging and restaging but is most widely used to detect recurrent disease. Often, this involves patients with elevated serum markers (Ca-125, Ca 19-9, alpha fetoprotein, and human chorionic gonadotropin) and negative or inconclusive CT findings. The reported sensitivity of PET varies from 50% to 90% and the specificity from 60% to 80%. The accuracy of PET depends on tumor size and cell type. As with CT, small peritoneal nodules seen during laparoscopy and small primary tumors confined to the ovary may be missed. Well-differentiated and mucinous tumors may not be seen, causing false negative results (Box 11-11). Also, PET scanning may not be useful for initial tumor diagnosis because several benign conditions may accumulate F-18 FDG (Table 11-13). Despite these limitations, PET is especially helpful in cases in which CT is negative but suspicion for

---

Box 11-9. Histopathological Classification of Ovarian Carcinoma

EPITHELIAL TUMORS
Serous
Mucinous
Endometrioid
Brenner
Transitional cell
Mixed epithelial
Small cell
Clear cell

SEX CORD–STROMAL TUMORS
Granulosa cell
Serotoli-Leydig cell

GERM CELL
Dysgerminoma
Yolk sac
Embryonal
Teratomas

Box 11-10. Ovarian Carcinoma Staging

Stage I: Growth limited to ovaries with an intact capsule
Stage II: Extension onto pelvic organs or into ascites
Stage III: Peritoneal implants outside of the pelvis; retroperitoneal or inguinal lymph node involvement
Stage IV: Distant metastasis

Box 11-11. Processes Causing False Negative Results in Ovarian Cancer

Well-differentiated serous cystadenocarcinoma
Mucinous cystadenocarcinoma
Disseminated peritoneal carcinomatosis
Borderline tumors
Stage I tumors confined to the ovary

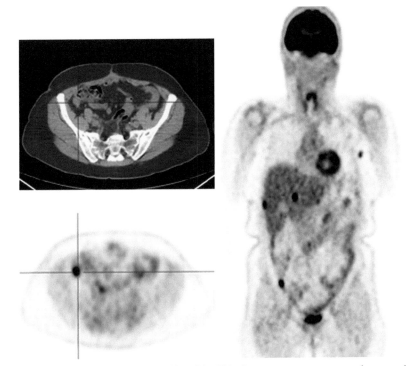

FIGURE 11-44. Recurrent ovarian carcinoma. A patient with a rising CA-125 had numerous metastases on the coronal PET, including a left axillary lymph node, metastases studding the surface of the liver, and a right lower quadrant peritoneal lesion studding the right colon on axial images.

TABLE 11-13 Fluorine-18 Fluorodeoxyglucose Positive Processes Mimicking Ovarian Carcinoma

Gastrointestinal activity
Infection/inflammation
Benign tumors

Germ cell: Benign teratomas

Epithelial tumors: Mucinous cystadenoma, serous cystadenoma
Dermoid cysts, hemorrhagic follicle cyst, corpus luteum cyst

Endometrioma
Fibroma
Benign thecoma
Schwannoma

recurrence is high. Overall, PET alters management in approximately 15% of cases.

Cervical Carcinoma

Cervical carcinoma is the most common gynecological cancer. It may be treated effectively by surgery when localized, but radiation and chemoradiation may be required for locally advanced disease. The spread of cervical carcinoma usually occurs by local extension or lymphatic spread to pelvic, paraaortic, and retroperitoneal lymph nodes. However, distant metastases occur, such as to the supraclavicular lymph nodes. Detection of nodal involvement is important in planning therapy but may be difficult by CT.

F-18 FDG PET has shown greater than 90% sensitivity for detection of cervical cancer, with marked uptake in primary tumors and lymph node metastasis. In patients whose disease appears to be confined to the pelvis on CT and MRI, PET has been shown to be useful in more accurate disease staging (Fig. 11-45) and can identify disease that might otherwise be outside of the field of treatment for radiation therapy. In patients who have had prior resection, scar may make detection of recurrent disease by CT difficult. Evaluation may be complicated by normal uptake in the bowel and urinary tract. Although increased uptake can occur in tissues affected by radiation therapy, usually tumor response is evident (Fig. 11-45, *B* and *C*).

Testicular Carcinoma

Testicular cancer can be divided into seminoma and non-seminoma germ-cell tumors. The spread of testicular tumor is most commonly to retroperitoneal lymph nodes. Although the overall prognosis for these tumors is good, accurate staging and surveillance are necessary. Disease is frequently incorrectly staged by CT. Disease initially classified as stage I is commonly then found to have nodal involvement at surgery. Other patients placed incorrectly in high-risk groups may undergo unnecessary therapy. For example, it has been common practice to treat all patients with seminoma with radiation.

Standard imaging of testicular carcinoma consists of ultrasound for diagnosis and CT for staging. However, F-18 FDG PET is accurate for tumor staging and detecting recurrence in seminomas. In comparison with CT, PET has shown superior sensitivity (80% vs. 70%), specificity (100% vs. 74%), positive predictive value (100% vs. 37%), and negative predictive value (96% vs. 92%) in the

multicenter SEMPET trial. The high negative predictive value of PET is useful for evaluation of residual masses, which are frequently seen on CT after therapy. F-18 FDG uptake is lower in nonseminomatous germ cell tumors, with a sensitivity of perhaps 59%. Detection of small tumors and well-differentiated teratomas is especially limited with PET. Relapse of testicular carcinoma is a frequent occurrence, and PET is useful for surveillance.

Prostate Carcinoma

F-18 FDG PET has very limited sensitivity for prostate carcinoma. Uptake in primary tumor is often low and similar to that in benign prostatic hypertrophy. In terms of staging, F-18 FDG PET detected fewer than two thirds of osseous metastases found on bone scintigraphy and approximately half of nodal metastases found on CT. CT is superior to F-18 FDG for the detection of pulmonary metastases.

However, F-18 FDG PET is often abnormal in advanced prostate carcinoma that has escaped hormonal control. In such cases, abnormal lesions may be identified in many areas, including bone and lymph nodes.

Renal and Bladder Carcinomas

CT is the most common imaging modality for the diagnosis and staging of renal cell carcinoma and bladder carcinoma. F-18 FDG PET is not useful in the diagnosis of primary tumors. Although some have suggested that the urinary excretion of F-18 FDG might obscure adjacent tumors, these masses often show no radiotracer uptake (Fig. 11-46). The cause for this finding, such as variations in glucose transporter expression, is being investigated. However, PET may play a role in diagnosing distant metastases and detecting recurrent disease.

Data are limited concerning the use of F-18 FDG PET in bladder and renal tumors. While transitional cell tumors reportedly should have increased F-18 FDG accumulation, detection of primary tumors is limited by excreted activity in urine; PET shows a high sensitivity for distant metastases. In renal cell carcinoma, only about 60% of primary tumors are identified by PET, although 65% to 80% of recurrent or metastatic lesions may be detected, many of which are not seen on CT. Cell type may affect sensitivity.

Musculoskeletal Tumors

Malignant primary bone tumors are usually F-18 FDG avid, as are many benign conditions. Benign tumors such as giant cell tumor, fibrous dysplasia, and eosinophilic granulomas have been shown to accumulate F-18 FDG. PET may be useful in both evaluating patients who cannot undergo MRI imaging and monitoring the effects of therapy. If a nonresponder is identified early by showing little change in SUV values on PET, the course of therapy can be altered. F-18 FDG may influence therapy by identifying other sites of disease, such as in patients with plasmacytoma.

For the evaluation of soft tissue sarcomas, the accuracy of F-18 FDG PET appears related to tumor grade. The increased uptake in high-grade tumors such as malignant

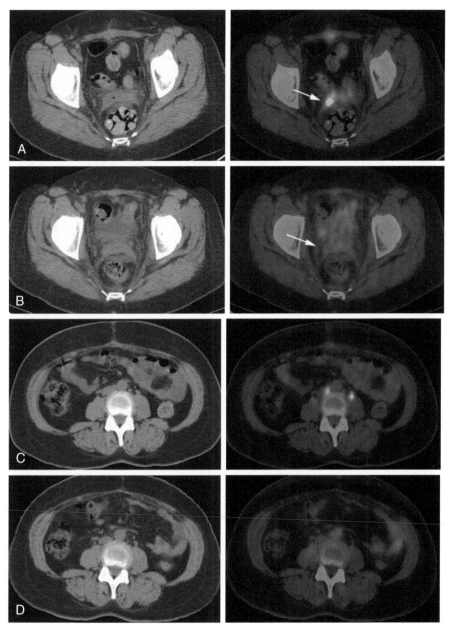

FIGURE 11-45. A, PET images of vaginal cuff show tumor *(arrow)* responding to radiation therapy **(B)** in a patient with cervical cancer. In the same patient, the detection of F-18 FDG uptake in a normal-size right paraaortic lymph node **(C)** lead to the disease being upstaged, requiring chemotherapy in addition to radiotherapy of the pelvis. **D,** Follow-up showed resolution of the active tumor.

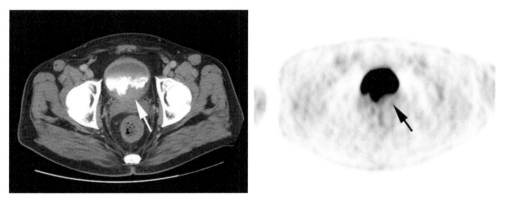

FIGURE 11-46. Bladder carcinoma. Renal cell carcinoma and bladder tumors are often negative on FDG PET. A mass along the posterior bladder *(arrow)* on CT *(left)* shows no FDG uptake on the PET portion of the examination *(right)*.

fibrous histiocytoma allows detection with a high degree of sensitivity. Low-grade tumors, on the other hand, show minimal or nonexistent uptake, leading to poor sensitivity. Although MRI remains the main imaging modality of the primary tumor, the ability of MRI to detect recurrence is limited in the postoperative patient. PET may help detect recurrent tumors, although the effects of surgery and radiation therapy lower sensitivity.

▰ SUGGESTED READING

Alessio AM, Kinahan PE, Manchanda V, et al. Weight-based, low dose pediatric whole body PET/CT protocols. *J Nucl Med.* 2009;50(10):1570-1577.

Coleman RE, Hillner BE, Shields AF, et al. PET and PET/CT reports: observations from the National Oncologic PET Registry. *J Nucl Med.* 2010;51(1):158-163.

Delbeke D, Martin WH. PET and PET-CT for the evaluation of colorectal carcinoma. *Semin Nucl Med.* 2004;34:209-223.

Delbeke D, Coleman RF, Guiberteau MJ, et al. Procedure guideline for tumor imaging with ^{18}F-FDG PET/CT 1.0. *J Nucl Med.* 2006;47(5):885-895.

Eary JF, Conrad EU. Imaging in sarcoma. *J Nucl Med.* 2011;52(12):1903-1913.

Eubank WB, Mankoff DA. Evolving role of positron emission tomography in breast cancer imaging. *Semin Nucl Med.* 2005;35:84-95.

Gupta NC, Maloof J, Gunel E. Probability of malignancy in solitary pulmonary nodules using fluorine-18-FDG and PET. *J Nucl Med.* 1996;37:943-947.

Hillner BE, Siegel BA, Liu D, et al. Impact of positron emission tomography/computed tomography and positron emission tomography (PET) alone on expected management of patients with cancer: initial results from the National Oncologic PET Registry. *J Clin Oncol.* 2008;26(13):2155-2161.

Ko JP, Drucker EA, Shepard JO, et al. CT depiction of regional node stations for lung cancer staging. *AJR Am J Roentgenol.* 2000;174(3):775-782.

Kresnik E, Mikosch P, Gallowitsch HJ, et al. Evaluation of head and neck cancer with F-18 FDG PET: a comparison with conventional methods. *Eur J Nucl Med.* 2001;28(7):816-821.

Kumar R, Kubota K, Yokoyama J, Yamaguchi K, et al. FDG-PET delayed imaging for the detection of head and neck cancer recurrence after radio-chemotherapy: comparison with MRI/CT. *Eur J Nucl Med.* 2004;31(4):590-595.

Alavi A. PET imaging in gynecologic malignancies. *Radiol Clin North Am.* 2004;42(6):1155-1167.

Macapinlac HA. FDG PET and PET/CT imaging in lymphoma and melanoma. *Cancer J.* 2004;10(4):262-270.

Pantvaidya GH, Agarwal JP, Deshpande MS, et al. PET-CT in recurrent head and neck cancers: a study to evaluate impact on patient management. *J Surg Oncol.* 2009;100(5):401–401.

Shankar LK, Hoffman JM, Bacharach S, et al. Consensus recommendations for the use of ^{18}F-FDG PET as an indicator of therapeutic response in patients in National Cancer Institute trials. *J Nucl Med.* 2006;47(6):1059-1066.

Som PM, Curtin HD, Mancuso AA. Imaging-based nodal classification for evaluation of neck metastatic adenopathy. *AJR Am J Roentgenol.* 2000;174(3):837-844.

Velasquez LM, Boellaard R, Kollia G, et al. Repeatability of ^{18}F-FDG PET in a multicenter phase I study of patients with advanced gastrointestinal malignancies. *J Nucl Med.* 2009;50(10):1646-1654.

Vesselle H, Pugsley JM, Vallieres E, et al. The impact of fluorodeoxyglucose F-18 positron-emission tomography on the surgical staging of non-small cell lung cancer. *J Thorac Cardiovasc Surg.* 2002;124:511-519.

Wahl RL. *Principles and Practice of Positron Emission Tomography.* 2nd ed Baltimore: Lippincott Williams & Wilkins; 2009.

Wong RJ, Lin DT, Schüder H, et al. Diagnostic and prognostic value of F-18 fluorodeoxyglucose positron emission tomography for recurrent head and neck squamous cell carcinoma. *J Clin Oncol.* 2002;20(20):4199-4208.

CHAPTER 12

Oncology: Non–Positron Emission Tomography

Many tumor imaging topics are described elsewhere, including thyroid cancer in Chapter 6, "Endocrinology"; bone tumors in Chapter 7, "Skeletal Scintigraphy"; brain neoplasms in Chapter 15, "Central Nervous System"; and a variety of uses of whole-body and brain fluorine-18 fluorodeoxyglucose (F-18 FDG) in Chapter 11, "Oncology: Positron Emission Tomography." This chapter covers a range of additional topics, including agents that accumulate in tumors without specific binding and molecules designed to target a characteristic attribute of the tumor cell for imaging or therapy. An overview of some imaging and therapeutic radiopharmaceuticals used in oncology is provided in Box 12-1. Although F-18 FDG positron emission tomography (PET) has replaced many agents clinically, the use of non-PET radioisotopes for oncology applications is also showing a surge in clinical growth.

PEPTIDE RECEPTOR IMAGING

Numerous endogenous peptides that modulate tumor cell growth and metabolism have been identified, including several hormones and growth factors that interact with receptors on the tumor cell membrane. Among these are somatostatin, vasoactive intestinal peptide (VIP), tumor necrosis factor, and angiogenesis factor. This section discusses somatostatin derivatives that are available for neuroendocrine tumor imaging and therapy.

Neuroendocrine Tumors

Neuroendocrine tumors can arise in most organs. Although the histologic grade is important, they are most often classified by their site of origin, as unique pathologic and clinical features of the tumors are often dependent on where the tumors arise. However, other shared characteristics are seen, including the presence of membrane-bound secretory granules and an ability to produce specific peptides and hormones. Examples of these neoplasms include carcinoid, several gastropancreatic tumors (e.g., gastrinoma, insulinoma), and small and large cell neuroendocrine cancers. Tumors arising from the neural crest, including those deriving from chromaffin cells such as pheochromocytoma and paraganglioma and those of neuroectodermal origin such as neuroblastoma and ganglioneuroblastoma, are often included in these discussions. Neuroendocrine tumors have long been associated with the inheritable multiple endocrine neoplasia (MEN) syndromes and other tumors (Table 12-1).

Somatostatin receptors are found on many different cells and tumors of neuroendocrine origin (Fig. 12-1). Somatostatin, a peptide 14 amino acids in length, is produced in the hypothalamus, pituitary gland, brainstem, gastrointestinal tract, and pancreas. In the central nervous system, it acts as a neurotransmitter. Outside of the brain, it functions as a hormone inhibiting release of growth hormone, insulin, glucagon, gastrin, serotonin, and calcitonin. It appears to play a role in angiogenesis inhibition, is involved in the immune function of white blood cells, and has an antiproliferative effect on tumors.

Box 12-1. Radiopharmaceuticals for Oncology Applications

ORGAN-SPECIFIC
Cold Spot Imaging
Thyroid: I-123, Tc-99m pertechnetate
Liver: Tc-99m sulfur colloid

Hot Spot Imaging
Bone: Tc-99m MDP, Tc-99m HDP

NONSPECIFIC
Ga-67: Lymphoma, others
Tl-201 chloride: Bone sarcomas, brain tumors
Tc-99m sestamibi: Breast cancer, parathyroid adenomas, and Tl-201 applications
Tc-99m tetrofosmin: Similar to sestamibi
F-18 fluorodeoxyglucose: Multiple tumors, especially aggressive disease

TUMOR-TYPE SPECIFIC
I-131: Papillary and follicular thyroid cancer
I-131 MIBG: Neural crest tumors (adrenal medulla imaging)
I-131 iodomethylnorcholesterol (NP-59)*: Adrenal cortical tumor imaging
Tc-99m HIDA: tumors of hepatocyte origin

Radiolabeled monoclonal antibodies: Tumor antigens

In-111 satumomab*: Ovarian and colorectal cancer
Tc-99m arcitumomab (CEA-Scan)*: Colorectal cancer
In-111 capromab pendetide (ProstaScint): Prostate cancer
Tc-99m Veraluma*: Small cell lung cancer
In-111 ibritumomab tiuxetan (Zevalin): Lymphoma
I-131 tositumomab (Bexxar): Lymphoma

Radiolabeled peptides: Somatostatin receptors

In-111 pentreotide (OctreoScan): Neuroendocrine tumors
Tc-99m depreotide*: Lung cancer

---

*No longer clinically available in the United States.
CEA, Carcinoembryonic antigen; *HDP*, hydroxyphosphonate; *HIDA*, hepatobiliary iminodiacetic acid; *MDP*, methylene diphosphonate.

Several agents have been developed that readily bind to somatostatin receptors (Fig. 12-2). Octreotide is an 8-amino-acid peptide that maintains the ability to bind to native hormone receptors but is resistant to enzymatic

degradation with a 1.5- to 2-hour half-life, as opposed to the 2- to 3-minute half-life of endogenous somatostatin. Nonradiolabeled octreotide (Sandostatin) has been approved by the U.S. Food and Drug Administration (FDA) as a therapeutic agent, suppressing growth in acromegaly and controlling symptoms in carcinoid syndrome.

TABLE 12-1 Multiple Endocrine Neoplasia (MEN) Syndromes

Lesion	MEN-I	MEN-IIA	MEN-IIB
Pituitary adenoma	+		
Pancreatic islet cell tumor	+		
Parathyroid adenoma	+	+	
Pheochromocytoma		+	+
Medullary thyroid cancer		+	+
Ganglioneuroma			+

Indium-111 Pentetreotide (Indium-111 OctreoScan)

Pharmacokinetics and Dosimetry

Radiolabeling indium-111 pentetreotide In-111-DTPA-pentetreotide (In-111 pentetreotide [OctreoScan; Mallinckrodt, Hazelwood, MO]) involves complexing octreotide with diethylenetriaminepentaacetic acid (DTPA) to bind In-111. In-111 pentetreotide is rapidly cleared by the kidneys, with 50% of the dose excreted by 6 hours and 85% by

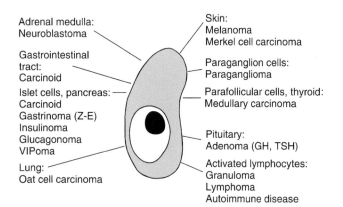

FIGURE 12-1. Somatostatin receptors are found on many tumors, including those derived from neuroendocrine cells. *GH*, Growth hormone; *TSH*, thyroid-stimulating; *VIPoma*, vasoactive intestinal polypeptide-secreting tumors; *Z-E*, Zollinger Ellison.

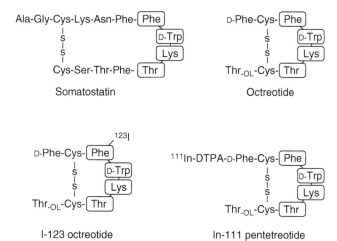

FIGURE 12-2. Comparison of somatostatin analogs octreotide, I-123 pentetreotide, and In-111 pentetreotide.

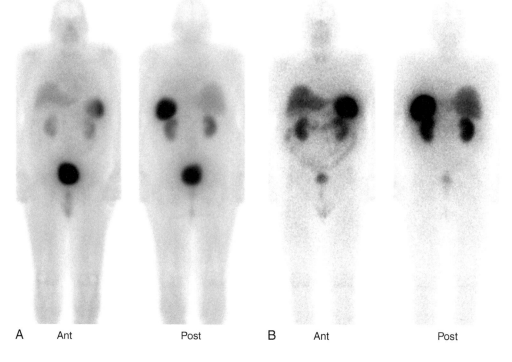

FIGURE 12-3. Normal In-111 pentetreotide whole-body scans at **(A)** 4 hours and at **(B)** 24 hours. Note increasing bowel activity over time. Significant renal uptake is classic but may be less intense in some patients. Activity in the spleen is more intense than in the liver in this case, although this varies. *Ant*, Anterior; *Post*, posterior.

24 hours after injection. A low level (2%) of hepatobiliary excretion also occurs. At 4 hours after injection, 10% of the dose remains in circulation; at 20 hours, less than 1% is in circulation. Whereas rapid clearance enhances the target-to-background ratio, bowel activity increases over time and can cause problems detecting abdominal lesions (Fig. 12-3). Estimates of radiation dosimetry are provided in Table 12-2.

At least five different subtypes of human somatostatin receptors (SSTR) have been identified (SSTR1 to SSTR5). These receptors are expressed to varying degrees on different tumors. The commercially available radiopharmaceutical In-111 pentetreotide binds with high affinity to the SSTR2 and SSTR5 subtypes, to a lesser extent with SSTR3, and not at all with SSTR1 or SSTR4. Identifying

TABLE 12-2 Indium-111 Pentetreotide (Indium-111 Octreotide) Radiation Dosimetry

Administered dose mCi (MBq)	Organ receiving highest dose rad/mCi (mGy/MBq)	Effective dose rem/mCi (mSv/MBq)
6 (222)	Spleen 2.1 (0.57)	0.20 (0.054)

Data from SNM Procedure Guideline version 2.0. 2011. Modified from ICRP 106(37).

Box 12-2. Indium-111 Pentetreotide (Octreotide): Protocol Summary

PATIENT PREPARATION
Hydrate patient before injection and at least 1 day after
Consider:
    Oral laxative (e.g., bisacodyl) for abdominal lesions (when no active diarrhea present)
    Discontinuing octreotide therapy 24 hours before injection

RADIOPHARMACEUTICAL
Children: 0.14 mCi/kg (5 MBq/kg)
Adults: 6 mCi (222 MBq) In-111 octreotide, intravenously

INSTRUMENTATION
Gamma camera: Large field of view,
Collimator: Medium energy
Windows: 20% centered at 173 keV and 247 keV

ACQUISITION
Imaging at 24 hours preferable but 4-hour images may be helpful; 48-hour images may be used if gut activity is initially limiting.

Planar Spot Views
10 to 15 minutes per view
512 × 512 or 256 × 256 word matrix

Whole-Body Images
Dual-head camera 3 cm/min (approximately 30 minutes head to below hips)
1024 × 512 or 1024 × 256 word matrix

SPECT Critical Areas
128 × 128 matrix, 3-degree angular sampling, 360-degree rotation, 20 to 30 sec/stop
Fusion to CT or SPECT/CT preferable

the specific receptor subtypes on tumors is also important as future targeted therapeutic agents.

Methodology
A sample protocol for imaging In-111 pentetreotide is provided in Box 12-2. Although early imaging allows visualization of the abdomen in the absence of significant bowel activity, 24-hour images are generally most sensitive. Additional images at 48 hours can be done with further bowel cleansing if needed. The addition of single-photon emission computed tomography (SPECT) adds considerably to specificity and may improve sensitivity, as well. Fusing SPECT images to a CT or, ideally, acquisition with SPECT/CT allows the best localization and identification of lesions.

Image Interpretation and Applications
Normal activity can be seen not only in the kidneys, bladder, liver, spleen, and colon but also occasionally in the thyroid and gallbladder. False positive uptake can occur in benign inflammatory conditions such as granulomatous disease, inflammatory bowel disease, chest radiation, bleomycin therapy, and sites of recent surgery. Close correlation with history is needed to avoid confusion.

Approximately 80% to 90% of tumors are visible by 4 hours. Because of decreasing background, more lesions are seen by 24 hours. Many tumors can be diagnosed with planar imaging (Figs. 12-4 and 12-5). However, SPECT is essential in the abdomen and can help identify disease in normal-size nodes in any area (Fig. 12-6). Lesions around the kidneys can be difficult to visualize because of the high renal uptake.

Overall, the sensitivity of In-111 pentetreotide is highest for carcinoid at 85% to 95%. This is particularly the case for extrahepatic sites of disease because liver lesions may show only background levels of activity. Neuroendocrine tumors of the pancreas such as gastrinomas, glucaganomas, vasoactive intestinal polypeptide-secreting tumors (VIPomas), and nonfunctioning islet cell tumors are also detected approximately 85% of the time (75%-100%). Pheochromocytomas, neuroblastomas, and paragangliomas can be evaluated with iodine-123 meta-iodo-benzyl-guanidine (MIBG), but In-111 pentetreotide may be preferable for the detection of extraadrenal lesions. The use of In-111 pentetreotide is more limited in insulinomas, with low sensitivity. In addition, sensitivity for medullary thyroid cancer is only moderate (Box 12-3).

False negative examination results are seen in tumors that do not express sufficient receptor quantities or the appropriate receptor subtype (e.g., SSTR2). Tumors that do demonstrate In-111 pentetreotide uptake are good candidates for octreotide drug therapy. Sensitivity appears to be lower in patients on octreotide therapy during imaging; however, many clinicians do not want to stop treatment for imaging examinations.

Experimental protocols with beta-emitters such as iodine-131, yttrium-90, and lutetium-177 labeled to octreotide have been used to treat poorly controlled neuroendocrine tumors. Some sites have used even higher doses of In-111 with its Auger electron emissions for therapy.

Although the use of F-18 FDG PET has grown in most areas of tumor imaging, the sensitivity is low for many neuroendocrine tumors. F-18 FDG PETCT may be useful in

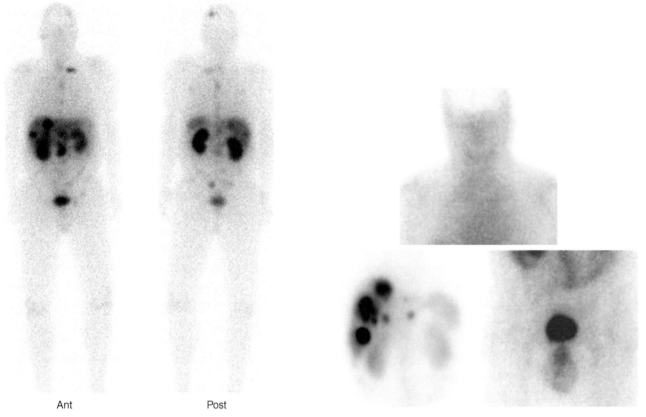

Ant   Post

FIGURE 12-4. Whole-body In-111 pentetreotide images reveal numerous metastases from carcinoid. The primary tumor was not seen with lesions in the abdomen corresponding to adenopathy. *Ant*, Anterior; *Post*, posterior.

FIGURE 12-5. Metastatic gastrinoma with diffuse hepatic lesions on In-111 pentetreotide. *Note:* Normal renal activity is variable and less intense in this example.

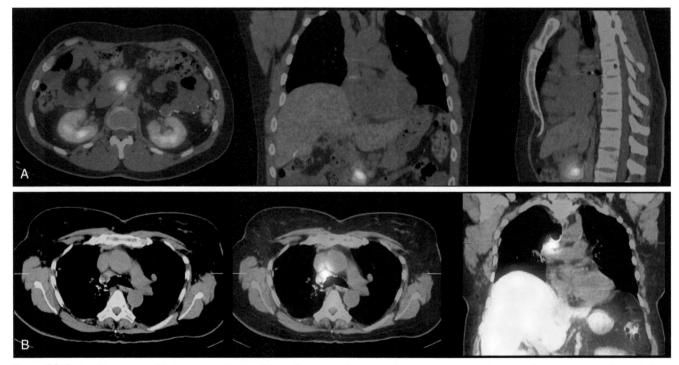

FIGURE 12-6. In-111 pentetreotide SPECT/CT images **(A)** localize a small focus of activity to a peripancreatic retroperitoneal lymph node, difficult to see on planar images and **(B)** show marked uptake in a precarinal nodal metastasis, which would be falsely called normal by CT size criteria.

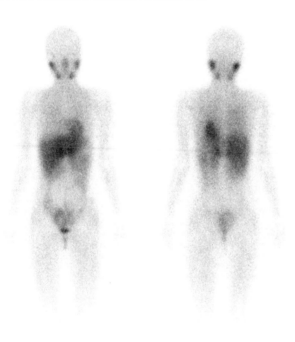

FIGURE 12-7. Normal I-123 MIBG study. Prominent uptake in salivary glands, heart, liver, both adrenals (faint in posterior view, on *right*), and colon and bladder clearance.

more aggressive, poorly differentiated cases. In addition, new gallium-68 labeled DOTA-TOC agents show superior sensitivity to In-111 pentetreotide.

ADRENAL SCINTIGRAPHY

In the previous edition of this text, adrenocortical imaging with I-131-6β-iodomethyl-19-norcholesterol (NP-59) was described. NP-59, most commonly used to localize tumors causing Cushing disease or hyperaldosteronism, is presently no longer available for clinical use in the United States and thus is not discussed here. However, I-123 MIBG is now FDA approved and widely available.

I-123 and I-131 Meta-iodo-benzyl-guanidine

Use of adrenal medullary scintigraphy has been increasing at many centers, because it has proved valuable for the diagnosis, staging, and management of adrenergic neuroectodermal tumors, particularly pheochromocytomas, extraadrenal paragangliomas, and neuroblastomas. MIBG is a norepinephrine analog that accumulates in adrenergic and neuroblastic tumors. Although it has been labeled for clinical use with both I-131 and I-123, the I-123 radiolabel is generally preferred. The major advantage is improved image quality, but dosimetry is a consideration as well, especially in children.

Radiopharmaceutical Localization and Dosimetry
Adrenal uptake occurs via a type I, energy-dependent, active amine transport mechanism. MIBG localizes in cytoplasmic storage vesicles in presynaptic adrenergic nerves. In addition to normal uptake in the adrenal medulla, the tracer localizes avidly in organs with rich adrenergic innervation, including the heart, salivary glands, and spleen (Fig. 12-7). Unlike I-131 MIBG, the normal adrenal medulla is frequently visualized with I-123 MIBG, particularly with SPECT. Normal uptake is seen in the liver, spleen, kidneys, heart, and salivary glands. Genitourinary and colon clearance is often seen. Variable activity has been reported in lungs, gallbladder, salivary glands, and nasal mucosa. The bones are not normally seen. Dosimetry for I-123 and I-131 MIBG is outlined in Table 12-3.

Methodology
Numerous drugs interfere with MIBG uptake, and a careful drug history should be obtained before imaging. Interfering drugs include tricyclic antidepressants, reserpine, guanethidine, certain antipsychotics, cocaine, and the alpha- and beta-blocker labetalol (Table 12-4).

A sample imaging protocol is supplied in Box 12-4. The patient is required to take potassium iodide (SSKI) or other thyroid-blocking medications starting at least 1 day

TABLE 12-3 Radiation Dosimetry of Iodine-123 and Iodine-131 Meta-iodo-benzyl-guanidine

	Organ with highest absorbed dose: bladder (mGy/MBq)			Effective dose(mSv/MBq)		
Agent	5 yr old	15 yr old	Adult	5 yr old	15 yr old	Adult
I-123	0.084	0.061	0.048	0.037	0.017	0.013
I-131	1.70	0.73	0.59	0.43	0.19	0.14

Data from the Society of Nuclear Medicine Procedure Guidelines.

TABLE **12-4** Medications Discontinue Before MIBG Imaging

Drug	Related drugs	Mechanism	No. days to stop
Antihypertensive/cardiac agents	Bretylium, guanethidine, reserpine Calcium channel blockers (amlodipine, nifedipine, nicardipine) Labetalol	Deplete granules Deplete granules Deplete granlues and inhibit uptake	7-14
Antipsychotics	Butyrophenones (droperidol, haloperidol) Loxapine Phenothiazines (chlorpromazine, fluphenazine, promethazine, others)	Inhibit uptake Inhibit uptake Inhibit uptake	21-28 7-21 21-28
Cocaine/opioids		Inhibit uptake	7-14
Sympathicomimetics	Amphetamine, dopamine, ephedrine, isoproterenol, phenoterol, phenylephrine, phenylpropanolamine, pseudoephedrine, salbutamol, terbutaline, xylometazoline	Deplete granules	7-14
Tramadol		Inhibit uptake	7-14
Tricyclic antidepressants	Amitriptyline (and derivatives), amoxapine, doxepine, others	Inhibit uptake	7-21

MIBG, Meta-iodobenzylguanidine.

Box 12-4. Iodine-123 and Iodine-131 MIBG: Summary Protocol

PATIENT PREPARATION
Hydration
Thyroid blockade (Table 12-5) with Lugol solution or potassium iodide. Begin day before injection and continue 1 to 2 days for I-123 and 3 to 6 days for I-131 MIBG
Discontinue interfering medications (Table 12-4)

RADIOPHARMACEUTICAL
IV dose injections must be done slowly, over at least 5 minutes
I-123 MIBG
  Children: 0.14 mCi/kg (5.2 MBq/kg); minimum 1.0 mCi (20 MBq) and maximum 10.8 mCi (400 MBq)*
  Adults: 10.8 mCi (400 MBq)
I-131 MIBG: Adults 1.2-2.2 mCi (40-80 MBq)

INSTRUMENTATION
Gamma camera: Large field of view for planar images
Modern SPECT/CT hybrid systems recommended for SPECT
Collimator:
  I-123: Medium energy, parallel hole
  I-131: High energy, parallel hole

ACQUISITION
I-123: Image at 20 to 24 hours. Delayed images less than 2 days for equivocal cases.
I-131: Image 1 to 2 days after injection. Repeat images at day 3 if needed.
Spot views: 75,000 to 100,000 counts for I-123 preferred, 256 × 256 matrix or 128 × 128 with zoom.
Whole body planar images (5 cm/sec) and limited spot views (500,000 counts or 10 minutes) can be done in adults.
SPECT: 3-degree steps, 25 to 35 sec/step, 120 projections, 128 × 128 matrix.
Uncooperative patients: consider 6-degree steps, or 64 × 64 matrix with shorter time per frame.

*Data from Gelfand MJ, Parisi MT, Treves ST. North American consensus guidelines for administered radiopharmaceutical activities in children and adolescents. *J Nucl Med.* 2011;52(2):318-322.
MIBG, Meta-iodo-benzyl-guanidine.

TABLE **12-5** Daily Doses of Thyroid Blockade Compounds

Drug	Adults	Child (15-50 kg)	Child (5-15 kg)	Child (<5 kg)
CAPSULES*				
Potassium iodate	170	80	40	20
Potassium iodide	130	65	32	16
Potassium perchlorate	400	300	200	100
SOLUTION				
Lugol solution 1%	1 drop/kg to max 40 (20 drops twice daily)			

*Dose in milligram per day. Data from Giammarile F, Chiti A, Lassmann M, et al. EANM procedure guidelines for I-131 MIBG therapy. *Eur J Nucl Med Mol Imaging.* 2008;35(5):1039-1047.

---

before injection to prevent uptake of free radioiodine by the thyroid and continuing for 3 to 6 days to prevent free radioiodine uptake in thyroid (Table 12-5). Although I-123 can be imaged with a low-energy collimator, a small fraction of the photons (<3%) may be high energy (440-625 keV [2.4%] and 625-784 keV [0.15%]), reducing image quality. Therefore a medium-energy collimator may be preferable. Images are acquired 24 hours after injection. For pheochromocytoma, posterior and anterior views of the abdomen are most important. Additional images from the pelvis to the base of the skull are indicated to detect extraadrenal pheochromocytoma and neuroblastomas. Whole-body imaging is indicated for patients with neuroblastoma. SPECT and or SPECT/CT are routine at many centers, improving sensitivity and accuracy.

Clinical Applications
Pheochromocytoma
Pheochromocytoma is an uncommon catecholamine-secreting tumor derived from chromaffin cells. When these tumors arise outside of the adrenal gland, they are termed *extraadrenal* pheochromocytomas, or paragangliomas. Because of excessive catecholamine secretion, they can precipitate life-threatening hypertension or cardiac arrhythmias. Ten percent of pheochromocytomas are bilateral, 10% are extraadrenal (paragangliomas), and 10% are malignant. Paragangliomas may be found from the bladder up to the base of the skull.

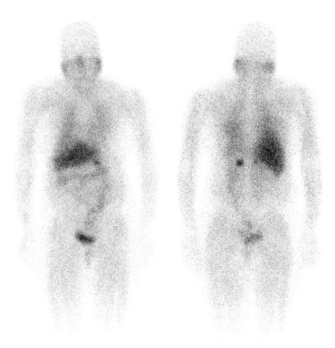

FIGURE 12-8. Pheochromocytoma on I-123 MIBG scan. Patient with poorly controlled hypertension and very elevated serum and urinary catecholamines. Focal increased uptake is noted in the region of the left adrenal consistent with a pheochromocytoma.

Paragangliomas are often associated with multiple endocrine neoplasia (MEN) types IIA and IIB, von Hippel-Lindau disease, neurofibromatosis, tuberous sclerosis, and Carney syndrome. Adrenomedullary hyperplasia develops in patients with MEN type IIA and can be difficult to diagnose with CT or magnetic resonance imaging (MRI). MIBG scintigraphy is uniquely suited to detect medullary hyperplasia and has been used to assist decision making for timing of surgery.

The diagnosis of pheochromocytoma is suggested by detection of elevated blood or urinary catecholamines, although there are many other causes for these laboratory findings. CT or MRI is often the first imaging modality used. If an adrenal mass is demonstrated in this setting, the diagnosis is inferred and further workup before surgery is often unnecessary. I-131 or I-123 MIBG can sometimes be helpful to confirm the cause of a detected mass on anatomical imaging and detect extraadrenal tumors and less commonly, metastatic disease.

The characteristic scintigraphic appearance of a pheochromocytoma or extraadrenal paraganglioma is focal intense MIBG uptake (Figs. 12-8 and 12-9). The tumor-to-background ratio is quite high. The sensitivity for detection is approximately 90% and specificity greater than 95%.

Neuroblastoma

Neuroblastoma is an embryonal malignancy of the sympathetic nervous system, typically occurring in children younger than 4 years of age. Seventy percent of tumors originate in the retroperitoneal region, from the adrenal or the abdominal sympathetic chain, and 20% occur in the chest, derived from the thoracic sympathetic chain (Fig. 12-10). Patients with localized tumors have good prognosis and outcome; however, those with metastatic disease fare

poorly. At the time of diagnosis, more than 50% of patients present with metastatic disease, 25% have localized disease, and 15% have regional extension. Metastatic disease typically involves lymph nodes, liver, bone, and bone marrow. Most patients present with signs and symptoms related to tumor growth.

Bone scans are used to detect osseous metastases. However, a common location for metastases is in the metaphyseal areas of long bones, which can be hard to detect due to high normal uptake in growth plates. MIBG has superior sensitivity for detection of metastases compared to the bone scan, partly because these tumors initially involve the bone marrow. The combination of the two studies results in the highest sensitivity for metastatic detection.

MIBG sensitivity for detection of neuroblastoma is greater than 90%, with specificity of 95%. The study is used for staging, detecting metastatic disease, restaging, and determining patient response to therapy. Whole-body scanning is routine for imaging patients with this disease (Fig. 12-11). SPECT and SPECT/CT for specific areas can be quite useful (Fig. 12-12).

Other tumors that take up MIBG include carcinoid and medullary carcinoma of the thyroid. However, the sensitivity for tumor detection is considerably lower than for neuroblastoma or pheochromocytoma.

The high uptake of MIBG in neuroectodermal tumors has led to investigations of the use of high-dose I-131 MIBG therapy to treat metastatic neuroblastoma in patients who have failed prior conventional therapies. Investigations are ongoing.

▬ MONOCLONAL ANTIBODY IMAGING AND THERAPY

In recent years, important radiolabeled antibodies have been developed and approved by the FDA for tumor imaging and therapy. Although some are no longer clinically available, agents for treating lymphoma and imaging prostate cancer remain valuable problem-solving tools.

Background

Antibodies are proteins produced by lymphocyte plasma cells in response to exposure to foreign antigens. An IgG antibody consists of two identical heavy (H) and two light (L) chains linked by a disulfide bridge (Fig. 12-13). Each chain is made up of two regions. The *variable* region (Fab') is responsible for specifically binding to a cell surface antigen. The *constant* region (Fc) is involved with cell destruction through complement fixation and antibody-dependent cell cytotoxicity.

A desired monoclonal antibody can be produced by fusing myeloma cancer cells with lymphocytes from the spleen of a mouse immunized with a particular antigen. These "hybridoma" cells retain both the specific antibody production capacity of the lymphocytes and the immortality of cancer cells. Immunoassay screening identifies the murine (or mouse) monoclonal antibody clone desired. A monoclonal antibody with high affinity and specificity for the antigen of interest is then harvested.

However, the human immune system recognizes these murine monoclonal antibodies as foreign and mounts an

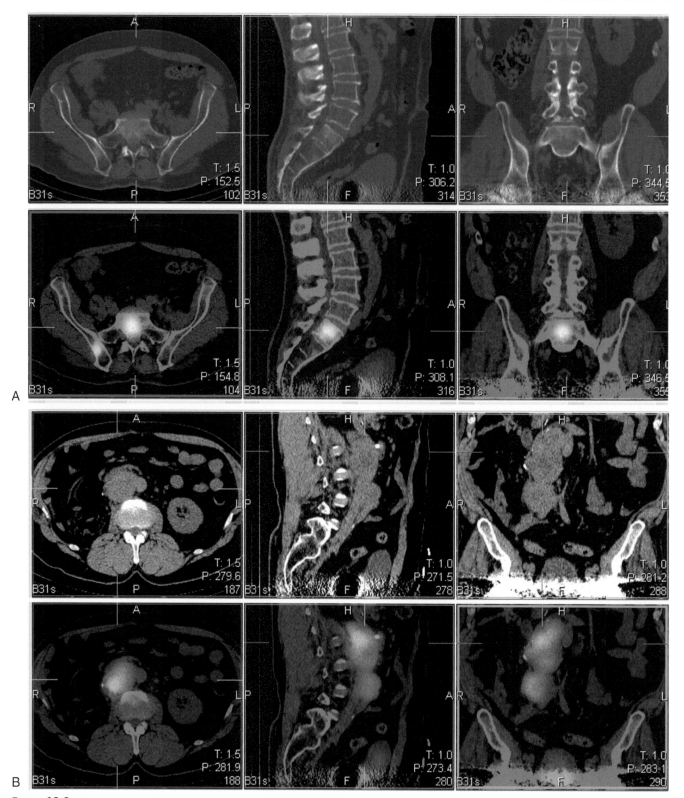

FIGURE 12-9. Metastatic pheochromocytoma on I-123 MIBG SPECT/CT scan. A 70-year-old man with extensive metastases. CT *above* and fused images *below*, transverse *(left)*, sagittal *(middle)*, and coronal *(right)* selected slices. **A,** Metastases noted in the ischium, sacrum, and lumbar spine. **B,** Conglomeration of retroperitoneal nodes with metastases.

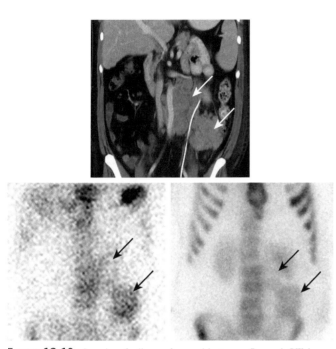

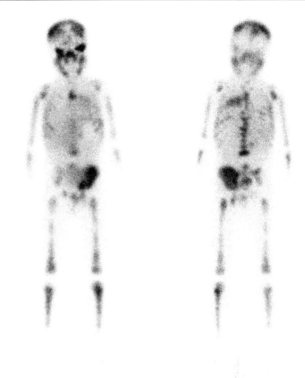

FIGURE 12-10. Imaging findings of neuroblastoma. Coronal CT image *(top)* reveal a large left abdominal mass *(arrows)* that had arisen from the retroperitoneum in an adult. I-131 MIBG images *(bottom left)* show increased uptake in the mass as well as throughout the bones from diffuse metastases. Tc-99m MDP bone scan *(bottom right)* shows abnormal soft tissue uptake in the mass, which is not uncommon. The bone lesions are seen but were harder to detect in some areas.

FIGURE 12-11. Metastatic neuroblastoma on I-123 MIGB whole-body scan. A 7-year-old boy with stage IV tumor after two bone marrow transplants. Extensive metastases are seen throughout the bones.

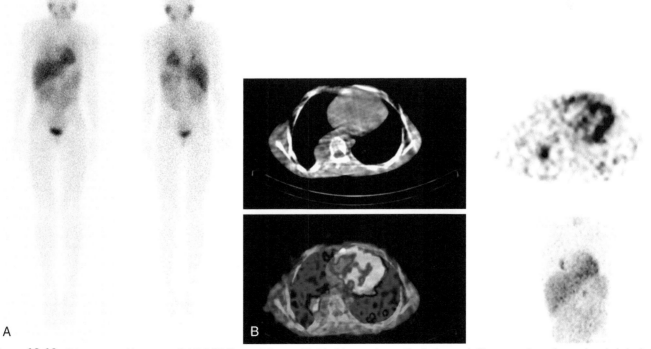

FIGURE 12-12. Primary neuroblastoma on I-123 MIBG scan. A 9-year-old girl with posterior mediastinal mass. **A,** Planar anterior and posterior whole body images. The posterior planar image shows uptake in the chest just above the liver. **B,** Low-resolution SPECT/CT clearly localizes the paraspinal mass.

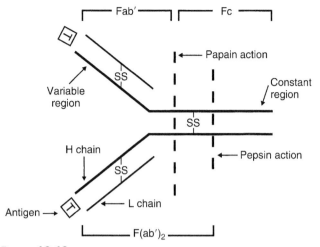

FIGURE 12-13. IgG antibody. The molecule can be digested enzymatically by papain, resulting in three parts, two Fab′ fragments and one Fc fragment, or by pepsin to produce one F(ab′)₂ and one Fc subfragment. Fab′ may be produced by splitting the disulfide bond of F(ab′)₂. *SS,* disulfide bond.

TABLE 12-6 Comparison of Monoclonal Antibody Lymphoma Therapy Agents

Factors compared	Y-90 rituximab (Zevalin)	I-131 tositumomab (Bexxar)
Radionuclide half-life	64 hr	8 days
Beta particle	2.293 MeV 5-mm path	0.606 MeV 8-mm path
Gamma emission	No	Yes, 364 keV
Pretreatment dosimetry	No	Yes
Pretreatment unlabeled antibody	Rituximab chimeric	Tositumomab murine
HAMA	1%-2%	60%
Outpatient therapy	+	+/−

HAMA, Human antimouse antibody.

immunological response known as a human antimouse antibody (HAMA) response. This can range from mild, with fever and hives, to severe, with shortness of breath and hypotension, or even fatal anaphylaxis. The HAMA response is related to the amount of antibody and the antibody size. Antibody fragments formed from the smaller active regions contribute less to the HAMA response. However, the potential for serious reactions remains a concern even with fragments. Chimera monoclonal antibodies replacing the murine Fc portion of the antibody with a human component and fully human monoclonal antibodies created through phage display recombinant DNA technology are being explored.

Fragment antibodies not only have fewer immunogenic side effects but are also better suited for imaging, clearing more rapidly from the background. Because of this rapid clearance, same-day imaging can be performed, and these agents can be labeled with technetium-99m. Several Tc-99m–labeled antibody fragments have been used clinically in the past, such as Tc-99m carcinoembryonic antigen (CEA) scan for colon cancer, but are no longer available.

The monoclonal antibody imaging agents currently in clinical use are derived from whole murine antibodies. Because these whole antibodies clear more slowly, they are labeled with radioisotopes with longer half-lives, such as In-111. Normal distribution on images also differs. Whereas antibody fragments demonstrate significant renal activity because of their clearance, whole antibodies tend to be seen in the liver.

Whatever the antibody type, it is designed for specific targets associated with the tumor. Examples include the surface antigens, such as CEA on colon cancer cells. Other tumors express increased numbers of normal antigens or receptors on their surfaces, such as the CD20 receptor on certain lymphomas.

Lymphoma

Non-Hodgkin lymphoma is the most common hematological cancer and the sixth most common cause of death. Whereas high-grade non-Hodgkin lymphoma can be cured, the low-grade form is generally considered incurable. Patients ultimately relapse after initial positive responses, tumors become refractory, and transformations to high-grade tumors are common. The mean survival is 8 to 10 years with conventional chemotherapy and radiation therapy.

Of the several immunological targets available, the CD20 antigen is present on 90% of the B-cell lymphomas but is not highly expressed on the membranes of normal hematopoietic cells, antibody-producing mature plasma cells, early B-cell precursors, or other lymphoid tissues. The nonradiolabeled antibody agent rituximab (Rituxan) has been successful in treating patients by recruiting the immune system to aid in killing the cell. Similar antibodies labeled with beta-emitters such as Y-90 and I-131 can directly kill the tumor cell (Table 12-6). Because beta radiation travels only a short distance, only nearby cells are irradiated. This limits damage to normal cells but causes a "cross-fire" effect, killing adjacent tumor cells not bound by the antibody. Therefore radiolabeled monoclonal antibody therapies show better tumor response than treatment with a nonradiolabeled monoclonal antibody.

Yttrium-90 Ibritumomab Tiuxetan (Zevalin)
Ibritumomab tiuxetan (Zevalin) was the first FDA-approved radiolabeled antibody therapy agent (Fig. 12-14). The murine immunoglobulin IgG1 kappa monoclonal CD20 antibody uses the chelator molecule tiuxetan to form a stable link to either In-111 or Y-90. The In-111 label (In-111 ibritumomab tiuxetan or In-111 Zevalin) can be used for an initial biodistribution scan. However, no imaging can be done with Y-90 because it is a pure beta-emitter. It has a high-energy (2.29 MeV) beta-particle that travels only 5 mm, depositing an effective dose of radiation very close to the binding site.

Indications and Contraindications
Y-90 ibritumomab tiuxetan was originally indicated for the treatment of relapsed, refractory, or transformed CD20+ non-Hodgkin lymphoma. However, it is now approved as a first-line therapy. It is absolutely contraindicated in patients with a known hypersensitivity reaction to murine

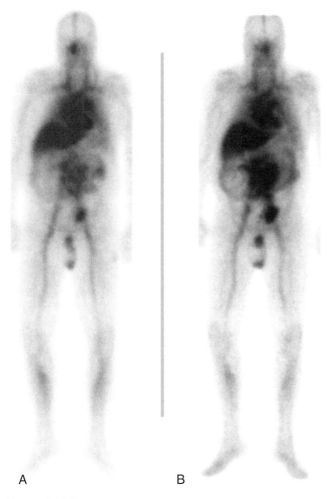

A   B

FIGURE 12-14. Before therapeutic infusion of the pure beta-emitter, Y-90 ibritumomab tiuxetan, an initial biodistribution scan with In-111 ibritumomab tiuxetan was required in the past. Images at 24 hours (**A**) and 48 hours (**B**) show normal activity in the kidneys, liver, and blood pool. Expected uptake is present in the lymph nodes involved with tumor in the midabdomen, left groin, and left pelvis

TABLE 12-7 Radiation Dosimetry of Indium-111 Ibritumomab Tiuxetan (In-111 Zevalin)

Administered dose	Organ receiving highest dose rad/mCi (mGy/MBq)	Effective dose rem/mCi (mSv/MBq)
	Spleen	
5 mCi (185 MBq)	2.11 (0.57)	0.19 (0.05)

proteins (HAMA), greater than 25% tumor involvement of marrow, and impaired marrow reserves. Patients should not have had myelotoxic therapies with autologous bone marrow transplant or stem cell rescue. External beam radiation should not have involved more than 25% of the marrow. The neutrophil count must be over 1500 cells/mm³, and the platelet count must be over 100,000.

TABLE 12-8 Yttrium-90 Ibritumomab Tiuxetan: Summary Protocol

I Day 1	II Biodistribution scans*	III Therapy (day 7-9)
Pretreatment: Acetaminophen 650 mg Diphenhydramine 50 mg	1. First scan 2-24 hr 2. Second scan 48-72 hr 3. Optional third scan 48-72 hr	Pretreatment: Unlabeled rituximab 250 mg/m²
Unlabeled rituximab (Rituxan) 250 mg/m² At initial test rate 50 mg/hr	Expect: • Blood pool activity first scan to decrease • Moderate liver or spleen uptake • Low uptake in kidneys	After 4 hr: Y-90 Zevalin 0.4 mCi/kg platelets >150k 0.3 mCi/kg platelet 100-150k
After 4 hr: In-111 Zevalin 5 mCi (185 MBq)	Unacceptable lung uptake	

*No longer mandatory in the United States.

Dosimetry and Radiation Safety

Y-90 ibritumomab tiuxetan has an average half-life in the blood of 27 hours (14-44 hours) and a biological half-life of 46 to 48 hours, resulting in a typical dose to the tumor of 15 to 17 Gy. Elimination is primarily through the urine (7%), although most of the agent remains in the body. The radiation dosimetry is listed in Table 12-7.

No special shielding is needed with this pure beta-emitter, and treatment can be done as an outpatient. In fact, few special radiation safety precautions are needed. This situation contrasts with I-131 tositumomab (Bexxar) therapy, which is stored and administered through heavily shielded equipment.

Patients should remain well hydrated and void frequently. Even though radiation exposure is limited, patients should limit prolonged close contact, sleep apart from others, and restrict time in public places for the first 4 to 7 days. They should be encouraged to prevent exchange of bodily fluids in the first week and use careful hygiene in the bathroom because of the urinary clearance.

Methodology

The full protocol originally consisted of three parts (Table 12-8), although biodistribution scans with In-111 are no longer mandatory in the United States. Many times the tumor was difficult to see on these images, but therapy was still indicated and effective. Unlabeled rituximab (Rituxan) is given to block CD20 antigens on cells circulating in the blood and spleen before therapy and before any biodistribution scan. The patient must be closely monitored during this infusion because serious, potentially fatal reactions can occur.

If biodistribution scans are to be done, 5 mCi (185 MBq) of In-111–labeled ibritumomab tiuxetan is administered over 10 minutes within 4 hours of the rituximab. Whole-body planar images are done within 2 to 24 hours and between 48 and 72 hours later to assess distribution of the radiopharmaceutical. An optional third image can be obtained over the next 90 to 120 hours. Normally, urinary tract and bowel activity are low, but fairly high liver and spleen uptake are present. The blood pool activity should markedly decrease over the studies. Altered blood pool

TABLE 12-9 Therapy Protocol for I-131 Tositumomab

Day 0	Day 1	Day 2, 3, or 4	Day 6 or 7	Day 7 up to 14
Thyroid blockade (continue 2 wk)	1. Premedicate acetaminophen 650 mg, tositumomab 450 mg over 60 min 2. I-131 tositumomab 5 mCi over 20 min 3. Prevoid whole-body dosimetry scan	Dosimetry scan	Dosimetry scan Calculate drug dose: >150k, 75 cGy 100-150k, 65 cGy	Therapy administration: 1. Pretreat with tositumomab 450 mg over 60 min 2. Therapy dose I-131 tositumomab over 20 min

distribution would include activity increasing rather than decreasing over time in lung, liver, heart, urinary tract, or bowel uptake. Any of these changes could lead to unacceptable radiation to the organ in question, such as the kidneys.

Toxicity

Significant side effects may occur from this therapy. Usually within 7 to 9 weeks, blood counts reach a nadir with a 30% to 70% reduction in platelets and neutrophils (median neutrophil count 800, platelet count 40,000, hemoglobin 10.3). The cytopenia may last from 7 to 35 days. Roughly 7% of neutropenic patients are prone to febrile neutropenia and infections. Thrombocytopenia may result in hemorrhage. Up to one third of patients will subsequently experience disease transformation to a more aggressive lymphoma. It is unclear whether this is a side effect of therapy or the natural course of the disease. A small number (1.4%) of patients will develop myelodysplasia or acute myelogenous leukemia.

Patients treated with Y-90 ibritumomab tiuxetan experience a HAMA response only 1% to 2% of the time. This low level could be due to the protective effects of the predosing administration of rituximab or the immunocompromised status of the patient.

Results

This is a very effective therapy. Overall, 75% (67%-83%) of patients experience some response, with 15% to 37% of patients showing complete remission. These values are significantly better than the results of nonlabeled rituxan monoclonal antibody therapy alone. The duration of response ranges from 0.5 to 24.9 months.

Iodine-131 Tositumomab (Iodine-131 Bexxar)

I-131 tositumomab (I-131 Bexxar) is a murine IgG2a monoclonal antibody developed to target CD20, which is the same target for Y-90 ibritumomab tiuxetan. Y-90 ibritumomab tiuxetan and I-131 tositumomab have several similarities and differences. I-131 tositumomab is recommended for CD20+ follicular non-Hodgkin lymphoma (with or without transformation) refractory to rituximab but is not considered a first-line therapy.

Method

A protocol outline is provided in Table 12-9. Unlike Y-90 ibritumomab tiuxetan, the I-131 tositumomab therapy dose can be imaged using the 364-keV gamma emissions. The tositumomab regimen uses the same tositumomab monoclonal antibody for pretreatment (in the nonradiolabeled form) as for dosimetry and therapy (in the I-131–labeled form). The I-131 label means that, unlike a pure

beta-emitter, the dose requires shielding. Also, it must be determined before discharging the patient that the exposure to others will not be greater than 500 mrem from the patient. I-131 tositumomab protocols require additional scans to determine dosimetry, which adds to inconvenience compared to Y-90 ibritumomab tiuxetan.

Because the I-131 radiolabel can disassociate from the monoclonal antibody and result in unwanted thyroid exposure, the patient must receive thyroid-blocking medication, such as with SSKI beginning at least 1 day before the studies and continuing for 2 weeks.

The patient is first treated with nonlabeled tositumomab to block excess CD20 sites. This helps decrease nonspecific antibody targeting. Following this, the dosimetry studies are done with a low dose of I-131 tositumomab. Serial scans allow calculation of how fast activity clears from the body (residence time) before calculating the therapy dose, which is also based on the patient's platelet levels.

Toxicity

As with Y-90 ibritumomab tiuxetan, similar significant hematological side effects can occur. Up to 15% of patients may require supportive care such as transfusions and colony-stimulating factor. Long-term side effects are possible, such as the myelodysplastic syndrome and secondary leukemia. Hypothyroidism may occur if proper premedication is not given to block the thyroid from taking up I-131.

HAMA titers are commonly elevated initially, although reports of symptomatic reactions are rare. The patients who had extensive previous chemotherapy became seropositive approximately 10% of the time, whereas patients who received I-131 tositumomab as a first-line therapy had initially elevated titers up to 70% of the time.

Results

Overall, 63% (54%-71%) of patients refractory to rituximab showed response. Of these, 29% of the patients experienced complete response. The median duration of response was 26 months, significantly longer than with Y-90 ibritumomab tiuxetan.

Prostate Cancer

Background

Prostate cancer staging is based on the combination of physical examination, histopathological Gleason score, and serum prostate-specific antigen (PSA). Therapy with radical prostatectomy is not undertaken when evidence shows nodal involvement or distant spread. Lymph nodes are the most common site of metastatic involvement, usually occurring in a stepwise fashion from periprostatic or obturator nodes to internal or external iliac nodes, and

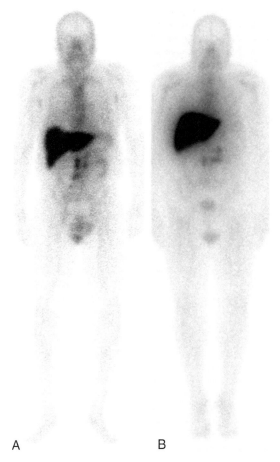

A   B

FIGURE 12-15. Prostate cancer lymph node metastases. **A,** In-111 capromab pendetide whole-body scans 96 hours after dosing reveal multiple abnormal foci in the midabdomen from lymph node metastases. **B,** Images from a different patient show a slightly altered biodistribution. Even though uptake in the liver is more intense, blood pool activity is limited and the study remains diagnostic with visible nodal involvement in the abdomen.

then to common iliac and periaortic nodes. Frequent sites of distant metastases are the skeleton, liver, and lungs.

If the PSA fails to decline after prostatectomy or begins to rise, residual or recurrent tumor is likely. Identification of patients with isolated disease in the prostate bed is important. If disease is localized to the prostate fossa or pelvis, radiation therapy offers the potential for effective treatment. However, if recurrence involves periaortic lymph nodes or other distant sites outside the therapy field, radiation therapy exposes the patient to significant morbidity with no potential for cure.

Staging is often difficult. Bone scans are indicated with a serum PSA greater than 10 to 20 ng/mL or a high Gleason score. CT and MRI have limited value because of their low sensitivity for detecting nodal involvement. In addition, F-18 FDG PET has low sensitivity for prostate cancer and plays no role in staging or detecting early recurrence.

Indium-111 Capromab Pendetide (ProstaScint)
Attempts to target PSA with radiolabeled antibodies proved insensitive and resulted in significant HAMA

reactions. In-111 capromab pendetide (In-111 ProstaScint) is a murine monoclonal antibody that targets prostate-specific membrane antigen (PSMA), a glycoprotein expressed by more than 95% of prostate adenocarcinomas (Fig. 12-15). PSMA expression is higher in malignant than nonmalignant cells and is higher in metastatic lesions than in primary tumors. Unlike PSA, it is not affected by hormone levels. In-111 capromab pendetide has been found useful for detection of soft tissue metastases in two situations: patients with newly diagnosed cancer at increased risk for advanced disease and patients with rising PSA after prostatectomy or radiation.

In-111 capromab pendetide has a biological half-life of 72 hours, with 10% of the dose excreted in the urine within 72 hours and a smaller amount through the bowel. Normal distribution includes the liver, spleen, bone marrow, and blood pool structures. Clearance occurs into the bowel and bladder. Nonspecific binding in blood pool structures is especially problematic because the lymph nodes being evaluated lie in close approximation to the vessels.

The highest radiation dose is received by the liver, followed by the spleen and kidneys. HAMA response has been reported in 8% of patients after one dose and in 19% of those receiving multiple injections. These levels will usually return to normal after a few months. Overall adverse effects were noted in 4% of patients, mostly mild and reversible. Issues included elevated bilirubin, hypertension, hypotension, and injection site reaction.

Acquisition
Planar whole-body images or spot views from skull to mid-femur are useful to assess biodistribution and identify distant metastases. SPECT should be performed from the lower edge of the liver down through the bottom of the pelvis, with attenuation correction if possible. Registering images retrospectively to CT using manual or automated software techniques is time consuming and often limited by differences in positioning. Acquisition with SPECT/CT is preferred where available (Fig. 12-16). Some sites still perform a dual acquisition of a Tc-99m red blood cell SPECT along with the In-111 examination to help map the blood pool background.

Interpretation
The learning curve for interpretation of In-111 capromab pendetide studies is steep. The FDA approved this radiopharmaceutical for clinical use and interpretation only by physicians who have undergone specific training in the acquisition and interpretation of these studies. There are several reasons for the difficulty in addition to the high levels of nonspecific blood pool activity. With SPECT, images are low count and low resolution. Bowel and bladder clearance can complicate interpretation. Increased uptake may be seen in the prostate bed after radiation therapy, although uptake in the prostate bed after surgery or radiation must be regarded with suspicion for residual or recurrent tumor. False positive examination findings have been reported at surgical sites, from arthritis, tortuous vessels, and bowel (Fig. 12-17).

In-111 capromab pendetide has been shown more accurate than CT or MRI for detection of lymph node

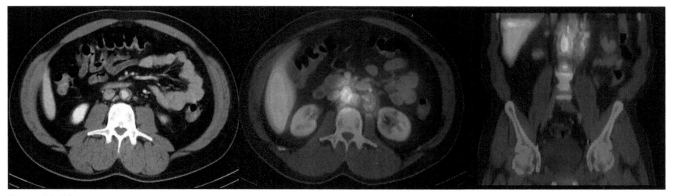

FIGURE 12-16. *Left,* A patient with high clinical suspicion for recurrent prostate cancer but no definite metastases on enhanced CT. Marked uptake was seen in the small retroperitoneal lymph nodes on In-111 capromab pendetide SPECT/CT. *Middle and right,* From metastases. (Courtesy Dr. Leonie Gordon.)

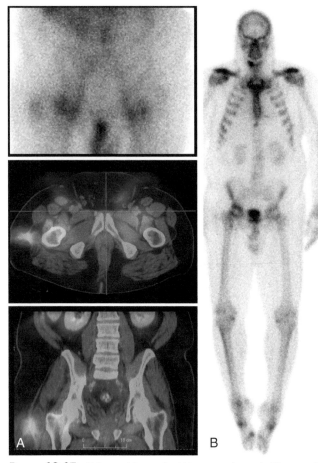

FIGURE 12-17. False positive on In-111 capromab pendetide scan. **A,** Abnormal activity lateral to the right hip on coronal images *(upper)* localizes to stranding along the muscles from prior procedure on fused axial *(middle)* and coronal *(lower)* images. Additional uptake in the femoral neck was also related to the surgery. The bone scan (**B**) done just 2 weeks earlier should show mild nonspecific uptake in the femur and arthritic changes in the hips. No areas suggestive of bone metastasis are seen elsewhere.

metastases. The sensitivity for nodal involvement ranges from 49% to 62%; this compares to sensitivities of 4% for CT and 15% for MRI in one of the same reports. The specificity ranges from 72% to 97%, but negative predictive values are all quite high (94%).

Assessment of the prostate bed varies. While sensitivity maybe as high as 89.6%, specificity can be as low as 18.2%. In addition, the study does not discriminate between prostate and seminal vesicle involvement.

Evaluation of the bone is limited, perhaps because of the low PMSA expression and significant background marrow activity. In general, bone scan is used for identification of osseous metastases.

▬ NONSPECIFIC BINDING TUMOR AGENTS

Technetium-99m Sestamibi

Potential uses of Tc-99m sestamibi (Tc-99m MIBI) generally parallel those of thallium-201 but with superior dosimetry and imaging characteristics (Table 12-10). Known as Cardiolite for cardiac perfusion studies and commonly used to identify parathyroid adenomas, it is also marketed as Miraluma for breast imaging. Cellular uptake occurs as a result of passive diffusion, and it is concentrated in the mitochondria. Like with Tl-201, tumor activity is greater in more active cells, including many tumors (Fig. 12-18).

Breast Imaging Background

A great need exists for noninvasive methods of evaluating the breast for early tumor diagnosis and follow-up. Mammography remains the primary breast cancer screening method, with reported sensitivities ranging from 75% to 95%. Specificity is a known problem with mammography, with many patients undergoing biopsy for benign lesions. In addition, the sensitivity of mammography is much lower in younger women, especially those with dense breasts. Ultrasound is an extremely valuable problem-solving tool, particularly in the breast. However, it is highly user dependent, and low positive predictive values have been reported, on the order of only 10%.

Contrast-enhanced MRI with gadolinium has been shown sensitive for breast cancer detection and is strongly advocated for screening women in high-risk groups such as those with *BRCA1* and *BRCA2* genetic mutations. However, patterns of gadolinium enhancement and clearance are often difficult to interpret, and the specificity of breast MRI is somewhat limited. In addition, many patients cannot

TABLE **12-10** Physical Characteristics of Nonspecific Tumor Binding Agents

Radiotracer	Physical half-life (hr)	Decay	Photopeaks		Injected dose mCi (MBq)	Organ receiving highest dose rad/mCi (mGy/MBq)	Effective dose rem/mCi (mSv/MBq)
			keV	Abundance (%)			
Ga-67	78	EC	93	41	10 (370)	Colon 0.74 (0.2)	0.44 (0.12)
			185	23			
			300	18			
			394	4			
Tl-201	73	EC	69-83	94	3 (111)	Kidneys 1.7 (0.46)	0.85 (0.23)
Tc-99m sestamibi	6	IT	140	88	Varies	Gallbladder 0.14 (0.039)	0.033 (0.009)

Data from Dosimetry: International Commission on Radiological Protection. *Radiation dose to patients from radiopharmaceuticals.* International Commission on Radiological Protection. Publ. No. 53, 1998.
EC, Electron capture; *IT,* isomeric transition.

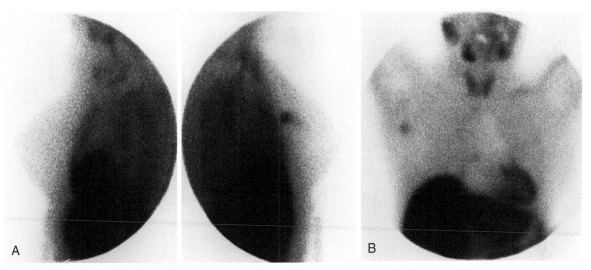

FIGURE **12-18.** Scintimammography. A palpable right breast mass shows obvious accumulation of Tc-99m sestamibi in the upper outer breast on lateral (**A**) and anterior (**B**) images on a routine gamma camera scan.

undergo the examination because of renal failure, claustrophobia, large body habitus, or arthritis.

Fluorine-18 Fluorodeoxyglucose Positron Emission Mammography

F-18 FDG PET/CT is useful for the staging and restaging of locally advanced breast carcinoma. However, the sensitivity of a whole-body scanner is more limited in breast cancer than in many other tumors, particularly in low-grade breast tumors. A dedicated breast positron emission mammography, or PEM, camera has recently entered clinical use. These cameras have very high intrinsic resolution, on the order of 1 to 2 mm and are superior to whole-body scanners for the detection of primary tumors. However, PEM imaging still has many of the disadvantages of whole-body FDG PET imaging, including the same preparation (fasting, controlled serum glucose levels), a 50- to 60-minute delay after injection, and a need for significant dosing room shielding. The 10 mCi (370 MBq) recommended F-18 FDG dose results in a substantial breast radiation dose, over 10 times the effective dose of digital mammography

(Table 12-11). Current PEM research appears promising when F-18 FDG doses half the amount originally recommended are used. F-18 FDG PEM seems well suited to follow the effects of therapy, identify tumor recurrences, and visualize multifocal or synchronous lesions in the ipsilateral and contralateral breast.

Molecular Breast Imaging With Technetium-99m Sestamibi

The ability of Tc-99m sestamibi to detect breast cancers with traditional gamma camera imaging has been well documented over the years. However, imaging the breast with a routine gamma camera is technically challenging, requiring special efforts to position the prone patient with the breast hanging off the table or through a special holder cutout. The recent clinical introduction of dedicated single-head and dual-head dedicated breast imaging cameras that provide molecular breast imaging or breast-specific gamma imaging has resulted in tremendous growth. Single-head, high-resolution gamma cameras with a small field of view first allowed reliable detection of tumors less than 1 cm. Newer commercially available solid-state detector

TABLE 12-11 Comparison of Radiation Doses in Breast Imaging*

Modality	Breast dose mGy/mCi (mGy/MBq)		Effective dose mSv/mCi (mSv/MBq)	
Tc-99m sestamibi	0.141 (0.0038)	25 mCi = 3.5 mGy	0.333 (0.009)	25 mCi = 8.3 mSv
				8 mCi = 2.66 mSv
				4 mCi = 1.33 mSv
				2 mCi = 0.67 mSv
F-18 FDG PET	0.318 (0.0086)	10 mCi = 3.2 mGy	0.703 (0.019)	10 mCi = 7.03 mSv
Digital mammography	1-1.2 mGy/view (4-5 mGy/4 views)		0.48-0.6 mSv/4 views	

*Based on International Commission on Radiological Protection weighting.
FDG, Fluorodeoxyglucose; *PET*, positron emission tomography.

systems, such as cadmium zinc telluride (CZT), show even higher intrinsic spatial resolution and the potential for even greater sensitivity at lower administered doses. In addition, newer dual-head detector cameras may better image tumors at low doses, helping minimize the impact of distance from the detector.

Uptake and Dosimetry

The methoxy-isobutyl-isonitrile lipophilic cation passively diffuses into the cell, and retention results from attraction between the positively charged lipophilic molecule and the negatively charged mitochondria. Up to 90% of Tc-99m sestamibi is concentrated in the mitochondria. Clearance from the cells is slow, allowing more than adequate time for imaging. P-glycoprotein, increased in cases expressing a multidrug resistance gene, pumps cations and lipophilic substances out of cells and may have an impact on the use of Tc-99m sestamibi in following therapy response.

The breast is highly radiation sensitive, and the risk for radiation-induced cancers from imaging studies such as mammography have been calculated. Efforts to bring the effective dose down to at least the level of a mammogram (2-4 mCi [75-150 MBq]) are highly desirable. However, in some patient populations, the risk-to-benefit ratios suggest that even the higher doses of Tc-99m sestamibi may be worthwhile if scans can identify cancers that cannot otherwise be found, such as in high-risk patients with dense breasts.

Methodology

A sample protocol is listed in Box 12-5. However, the dose of Tc-99m sestamibi recommended was based on recommendations from standard cameras with a large field of view. Significantly lower doses are being investigated for molecular breast imaging in which dedicated breast cameras put the breast in close approximation with the detectors. Many sites use 8 mCi (296 MBq), and early studies report success with much lower doses—as low as 2 to 4 mCi (74-148 MBq).

To help prevent false positive examination results, imaging should be done after a delay of 3 to 4 weeks after core biopsy or 2 weeks after fine-needle aspiration. Imaging early in the menstrual cycle (days 2-12) is also recommended.

Interpretation

Normal breast parenchyma shows mild, usually symmetric activity. Small focal areas of uptake are most suggestive of malignancy, and patchy uptake is likely benign.

Box 12-5. Technetium-99m Sestamibi Scintimammography and Breast-Specific Gamma Imaging: Summary Protocol

PATIENT PREPARATION
None

RADIOPHARMACEUTICAL
8 mCi (296 MBq) Tc-99m sestamibi intravenously
*Consider lower doses (2-4 mCi [74-148 MBq]) for dual head cadmium zinc telluride detector small field of view dedicated breast cameras.

INSTRUMENTATION AND ACQUISITION
Small field of view dedicated single-head or dual-head breast camera
  Begin imaging 5 to 10 minutes after injection
  Immobilize breast with light compression
  Image 7 to 10 min/view (craniocaudad [CC] and mediolateral oblique [MLO])
  Image injection site
  Additional views optional: True (90-degrees) lateral, axillary tail, cleavage view, exaggerated CC, implant displacement
Routine gamma camera (not preferred)
  Begin imaging 5 to 10 minutes after injection
  Place patient prone on table with breasts hanging dependent, preferably in holder through cutouts
  10 minutes/view for prone lateral and supine anteroposterior chest, including axilla
  Image injection site
  Obtain marker view of any palpable nodule

However, the intensity of the uptake may not parallel the aggressiveness of the lesion. Uptake in the axilla may represent nodal metastasis, particularly if no dose infiltration is seen.

The sensitivity of breast-specific gamma imaging is high, on the order of 91% to 95%. Lesions larger than 1 cm are generally easily seen. For subcentimeter lesions, sensitivity varies, with reports of 3 to 7 mm routinely visualized, although sensitivity decreases with size. Limited data have shown superior detection of tumors over mammography in patients with dense breasts and higher sensitivity for lobular carcinomas than other breast imaging modalities, including MRI. In addition, early studies show specificity at least similar to that of MRI, although higher (65%-90%)

TABLE 12-12 Tumor Imaging and Other Applications of Non–Positron Emission Tomography Agents

Agent	Historical Uses	Current Applications
Ga-67	Lymphoma Hepatocellular cancer (Lung cancer) *Pneumocystis* pneumonia	Osteomyelitis spine (Infections)
Tl-201	Bone and soft tissue sarcoma Kaposi sarcoma	Recurrent glioma Intracranial lymphoma
Tc-99m sestamibi	Routine gamma camera breast imaging parathyroid adenoma	Parathyroid adenoma BSGI (MBI) Intracranial uses like Tl-201

BSGI, Breast-specific gamma imaging; *MBI,* molecular breast imaging.

in some cases. A 2011 multicenter trial, Weigert et al reported sensitivity of 91%, specificity of 77%, positive predictive value of 57%, and negative predictive value of 96%. The high negative predictive value suggests that Tc-99m sestamibi could be used to evaluate questionable lesions on mammogram. However, with a false negative rate of 6% for breast-specific gamma imaging, biopsy should be performed when mammogram indicates a need but scintigraphic imaging is normal.

Thallium-201 Tumor Imaging

Although the potassium analog Tl-201 chloride is commonly known as a cardiac perfusion radiopharmaceutical, it has long been known to accumulate in many tumors, with some listed in Table 12-12. Multiple factors influence cellular uptake, including blood flow delivery and the membrane sodium-potassium adenosine triphosphatase (ATPase) pumping. Overall, distribution is proportional to blood flow, although activity in tumor relates to cellular activity and viability. Biological clearance is primarily via the kidneys. Given the suboptimal imaging characteristics and poor dosimetry compared to technetium-based agents (Table 12-10), it is not surprising that applications are limited to occasional use, such as in the brain to assess possible recurrent glioma or help differentiate toxoplasmosis from intracranial lymphoma.

Gallium-67 Tumor Imaging

Gallium-67 (Ga-67) was initially used as a bone-imaging agent and is still sometimes used for the assessment of infection. Ga-67 is sensitive for many cancers, including hepatocellular cancer, sarcomas, and lung cancer (Table 12-12). For years, Ga-67 was primarily used in the assessment of lymphoma (Fig. 12-19). Eventually, CT became the primary imaging modality in lymphoma, with Ga-67 used as a problem-solving tool. Recently, Ga-67 has become relatively obsolete for tumor imaging, with the dissemination of F-18 FDG and PET/CT cameras.

Although its biodistribution is complex, Ga-67 has a biological behavior similar to that of iron. It is carried in the blood by iron transport proteins, such as transferrin. Excretion of 15% to 25% of the dose occurs through the

kidneys in the first 24 hours, with the bowel becoming the major route of excretion after that. Radiation dosimetry and imaging characteristics are not optimal (Table 12-10), with high-energy photons and significant background activity. However, sensitivity is high, improved by using a higher injected dose, delaying imaging for 3 to 7 days for background clearance, and performing the routine acquisition of SPECT images of the chest, abdomen, and pelvis.

■ LYMPHOSCINTIGRAPHY: THE SENTINEL LYMPH NODE

Background

Cancers such as melanoma and breast carcinoma tend to metastasize first to regional lymph nodes. Mapping the lymphatic drainage around a tumor has improved staging in patients with early cancer (no clinically evident nodal involvement) by identifying the lymph node (or nodes) most likely to reveal occult metastases. This node, the sentinel lymph node (SLN), directly drains the region of the tumor. Once identified, it can be excised for close histological scrutiny. This process has not only proved more accurate for staging than dissecting larger numbers of nodes in the perceived drainage basin but also has markedly decreased morbidity, such as lymphedema, from lymphadenectomy.

SLN biopsy is indicated for patients at risk for node metastases, especially early stage, with no clinically evident metastatic disease. Although the procedure has been explored in a variety of tumors, such as cancers of the head and neck, cervix, and colon, it has been widely accepted for melanoma and breast cancer (Fig. 12-20).

Radiopharmaceutical and Dosimetry

No particular radiopharmaceutical is approved for lymphoscintigraphy in the United States, and many agents have been used, such as Tc-99m human serum albumin (HSA), Tc-99m dextran, Tc-99m DTPA-mannosyl-dextran, and Tc-99m ultrafiltered sulfur colloid. However, the most commonly used agents are Tc-99m sulfur colloid in the United States, Tc-99m nanocolloid in Europe, and Tc-99m antimony trisulfide in Canada and Australia. Small particles migrate quickly, but show shorter lymph node residence times, and larger particles may not migrate. Because particles sizes for sulfur colloid tend to be large, recommended preparation includes slowly passing the dose through a 0.22-μ millipore filter.

Methodology

SLN biopsy is preferably done before wide local excision of the primary lesion to avoid problems from surgery altering lymph flow. The injection can be performed on the day of surgery, or within 18 hours of surgery on the day before. Various techniques have been used. An intradermal injection, raising a tight wheal, generally results in good dose migration through the lymphatic vessels. For melanoma, the dose is injected in 4 to 6 divided doses within 1 cm around the lesion or scar. Different injection sites have been used for breast

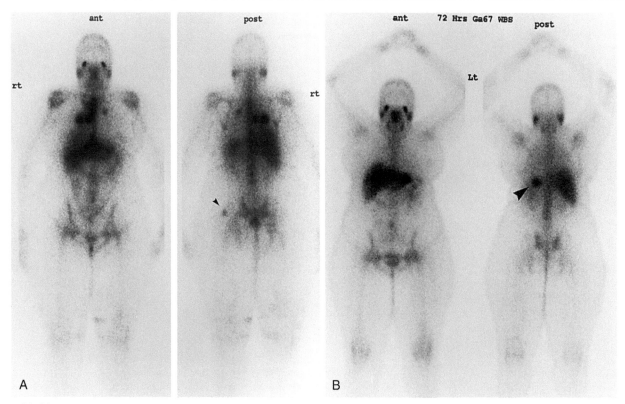

FIGURE 12-19. Ga-67 images from a patient with Hodgkin disease **(A)** revealing tumor in the mediastinum and right perihilar region as well as an injection granuloma in the left buttock *(black arrowhead)*. **B,** Follow-up scan after therapy shows resolution of tumor in the thorax but development of a new area of activity in the left upper quadrant *(white arrowhead)*. SPECT images (not shown) determined this activity was in the region of the stomach and correlated with gastritis reported clinically. *Ant,* Anterior; *Lt,* left; *Post,* posterior; *Rt,* right.

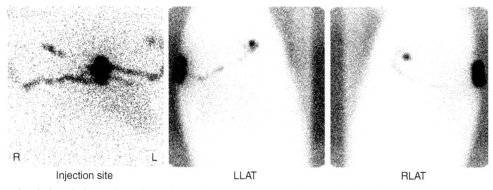

Injection site   LLAT   RLAT

FIGURE 12-20. Lymphoscintigraphy in a patient with melanoma illustrates the value of imaging in detecting unpredictable patterns of drainage. Activity moves from the region of the lesion on the trunk to sentinel lymph nodes in both axilla. *L,* Left; *LLAT,* left lateral; *R,* right; *RLAT,* right lateral.

cancer, including intradermal, subdermal, subcutaneous, peritumoral, periareolar, and subareolar. Although peritumoral injection, using ultrasound guidance if needed, is recommended for deep tumors, subdermal or intradermal injections are sufficient in most cases, resulting in rapid dose migration and very rare visualization of internal mammary nodes. Periareolar injections can be used if the tumor is in the upper quadrant near the axilla, to avoid confusion or crosstalk between the injection site and any nodes. Vigorous massage of the injection site helps promote dose movement.

Imaging should begin immediately, with the patient injected on the camera table, because the sentinel nodes may be visualized in minutes. Sequential images are performed at 5-minute intervals until the node is detected, usually within 60 to 90 minutes. Transmission images using a cobalt-57 sheet source placed between the patient and the camera for 10 to 15 seconds can help provide anatomical landmarks.

Any visualized nodes are marked on the skin. An intraoperative gamma probe is used for detection, with the sentinel node at least 2 times above background, but usually quite a bit more. Nodes removed at surgery are rechecked with the probe to make sure they show increased activity.

Findings

The first "hot spot" seen is considered the sentinel node. If additional sites of increased activity are found, these are also removed. Although intraoperative vital blue dye injection and preoperative radiolabeled colloids have been used independently, together they appear to result in the greatest sensitivity for the SLN. There is no consensus on a procedure if the node cannot be visualized.

Melanoma

Of the many factors influencing prognosis in melanoma, the primary lesion's thickness (depth of tumor invasion measured in millimeters), lesion ulceration, and mitotic rate are the most useful in staging early tumors and predicting occult lymph node involvement. Lymph node involvement is the most important independent predictor of survival.

Currently, the American Joint Committee on Cancer uses lesion thickness cutoffs of 1.0, 2.0, and 4.0 mm, similar to the old Breslow classification, to set the T-stage parameters. Patients with intermediate thickness tumors, greater than 1.0 mm but less than 4.0 mm, may benefit most from SLN biopsy. Of patients with tumors less than 1.0 mm (stage I), the procedure can be considered if there are other high-risk factors such as the presence of a high mitotic rate in the biopsy (≥ 1 mitosis/mm^2) or lesion ulceration (stage IB).

SLN biopsy accuracy is much higher than clinical assessment. False negative rates are reported at 5%, with recurrences of 3% to 6% seen among those who had been found negative for disease initially on SLN assessment. Also, complication rates are much lower than for complete lymph node dissection: 10.1% versus 37.2% in Multicenter Selective Lymphadenectomy Trial I (MSLTI) and 4.6 versus 23.2% in the Sunbelt Melanoma Trial.

Limited data have been reported on survival benefit from SLN biopsy. Preliminary results from the large MSLTI showed no difference in survival between patients who were in an observation group and those who underwent SLN biopsy (86.6% vs. 87.1% $p = 0.58$). However, 5-year survival among patients in the observation group who did develop lymph node metastases was much lower than in patients in the SLN biopsy group who had positive lymph nodes initially (52.4% vs. 72.4%).

Breast Cancer

Axillary node status is a major prognostic factor in early-stage breast cancer. Even in small, T1 tumors (≤ 2 cm), axillary nodes are involved at initial staging 10% to 30% of the time, and this number increases to 45% for T2 lesions (2.1-3.0 cm). Some centers limit SLN biopsy to those with unifocal tumors smaller than 2 to 3 cm; others offer the procedure to patients with large T2 or T3 lesions (>5 cm) and multifocal or multicentric lesions. In breast cancer, use of the sentinel node biopsy has largely replaced axillary lymph node dissection.

Most of the time, the SLN is identified in the axillary region. The presence of internal mammary nodes may be demonstrated with greater frequency with periareolar injections. The significance of internal mammary lymph node visualization is often unclear. Some disagreement exists on surgical management of these nodes, with many not including the findings in their assessment at staging. Clearly, the internal mammary nodes are frequently involved in breast cancer and attention to this region is warranted, particularly in medially located primary tumors, when restaging, such as with PET/CT.

Lymphoscintigraphy detects the SLN in 90% to 98% of cases. False negative rates of 7% to 8.5% are typical, although some significantly higher levels have been reported. Although this is above the 5% target felt to be acceptable, many surgeons do not perform confirmatory axillary dissection if the SLN is free of tumor. The risk for lymphedema is considerable lower after SLN biopsy than from axillary dissection (5% vs. 13%).

Some recent trials have shown low recurrence rates (0.12%-0.6%) in patients initially free of spread on SLN biopsy. This is well within the expected range. However, a clear impact on survival has not been demonstrated. The preliminary results in the National Surgical Adjuvant Breast and Bowel Project trial, for example, showed an 8-year survival rate of 90.3% in SLN biopsy cases compared to 91.8% in the axillary lymph node dissection group.

■ INTRAARTERIAL RADIOACTIVE MICROSPHERES

Background

Tumors, both primary and metastatic, commonly involve the liver. In the case of hepatocellular cancer, surgical resection and liver transplantation are the only methods for cure, but the majority of patients present with unresectable disease. In the setting of liver metastases, additional palliative or adjuvant therapy is frequently needed in addition to chemotherapy to reduce tumor burden or symptoms.

Many new treatments have grown over the past several years, including direct ablation, hepatic arterial chemotherapy pumps, chemoembolization, and most recently, drug-eluting and radioactive microspheres. Procedures such as thermal ablation (microwave and radiofrequency), cryoablation, and percutaneous injections have proved effective but are not suitable for patients with large or multiple lesions.

Transarterial chemoembolization (TACE) has been recommended as a front-line therapy for patients with large or multifocal hepatocellular tumors. TACE involves a combination of a chemotherapy agent with an embolic agent (steel coils, microspheres, particles, sponges) that induces ischemic necrosis and locally delivers chemotherapy. Newer drug-eluting microspheres provide an advantageous sustained chemotherapy agent release in comparison with TACE. Radiolabeled microspheres also can be delivered via the hepatic artery, thereby offering the advantage of delivering a large dose of radiation directly to the region of the tumor, so-called selective internal radiation therapy.

These directed intraarterial therapy techniques take advantage of the fact that 80% of the blood supply to hepatic tumors originates from the hepatic artery and three quarters of the blood perfusing normal liver parenchyma is from the portal venous system. Therefore lesions preferentially take up the dose and do not need to be ablated individually.

Two radioembolization microsphere agents are available clinically: Y-90 SIR-Sphere and Y-90 Therasphere. Y-90 SIR-Sphere has been approved for use with adjuvant chemotherapy in hepatic metastases from colon cancer and Y-90 Therasphere for unresectable hepatocellular carcinoma.

Radiopharmaceutical

Physical characteristics of the two Y-90 microsphere agents are outlined in Table 12-13. The beta emissions from the Y-90 label have a mean penetration length of 2.5 mm and energy of 0.94 MeV, resulting in 100 to 150 Gy intratumoral dose. However, nearby tumor cells are relatively spared. With the physical half-life of Y-90 at 2.68 days, approximately 94% of the dose is delivered by 11 days. Dose calculation is based on many factors, including the tumor burden within the liver (Table 12-14) and the amount of shunting present from the lungs into the liver. The typical doses given are in the range of 40 to 70 mCi (1.5-2.5 GBq). The microspheres will remain in the liver and do not degrade physically.

Methodology

Potential patients must be carefully screened before undergoing radiolabeled microsphere therapy. The functional status of the patient, liver function, and estimated tumor burden are all examined. Patency of the portal vein must be established because portal vein thrombosis has been a contraindication, although some studies suggest it need not be absolute. Arteriography of hepatic vasculature is performed, and anomalous vessels that could result in accidental delivery into stomach, bowel, or other structures may be embolized. With the catheter in the expected position for therapy administration, arteriovenous shunting is assessed with a Tc-99m macroaggregated albumin (MAA) scan (Fig. 12-21). The Tc-99m MAA is administered into the liver. The catheter is removed and the groin stabilized. The patient is then scanned anteriorly and posteriorly. The shunt fraction is calculated using a geometric mean calculation based on counts obtained from regions of interest over the lungs and over the liver. For Y-90 SIR-spheres, the dose is adjusted according to Table 12-15 to help prevent radiation pneumonitis. When using Y-90 Theraspheres, the activity is higher on the glass beads, so a lower level of shunting (<10%) is accepted.

TABLE 12-13 Physical Characteristics of Radiolabeled Microspheres

Agent	Radiolabel	Particle size (microns)	Particle material	Activity (Bq/particle)
SIR-Sphere	Y-90	35	Resin	50
		20-60		
Therasphere	Y-90	25	Glass	2500
		20-30		

TABLE 12-14 Yttrium-90 Microsphere Therapy Calculations

Liver involvement by tumor (%)	Recommended Y-90 dose (GBq)
>50	3
25-50	2.5
<25	2

After these procedures, the patient returns another day for the therapy itself. The catheter is placed in the same position under fluoroscopic guidance. The dose is administered with a very slow push to prevent refluxing the dose into the systemic circulation. The patient can then be taken to the nuclear medicine department and imaged using the bremsstrahlung radiation emitted from the Y-90 to confirm proper localization (Fig. 12-22). SPECT and SPECT allow the best visualization and comparison to the CT findings.

Patients can be discharged to home after the procedure. Some radiation safety precautions are needed concerning urine because a small amount of activity is excreted through the kidneys. The patient should be instructed to flush the toilet twice and use careful hand hygiene in the bathroom for the first 24 hours after the procedure.

Findings

Y-90 microsphere therapy has been shown to be relatively safe and effective. Side effects potentially include gastric ulcers, radiation hepatitis or cholecystitis, and radiation pneumonitis. Myelosuppression is not expected with current agents.

After Y-90 microsphere therapy, significant response can be seen in tumor appearance on CT with a decrease in size

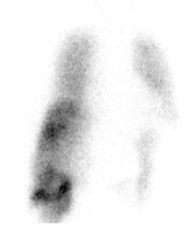

FIGURE 12-21. Intraarterial administration of Tc-99m MAA into the liver allows quantification of any shunt through the liver. Heterogeneous uptake seen above in the liver is not unusual, but the high levels of lung activity indicate a problem, despite all visible accessory vessels having been embolized. The liver-lung shunt was calculated to be 40%, and therapy with the Y-90–labeled microspheres was canceled.

TABLE 12-15 Yttrium-90 SIR-SPHERE Dose Correction Based on Lung Shunting*

Hepatopulmonary shunting (%)	Dose reduction (%)
<10	0
10-15	20
15-20	40
>20	100

*Maximum allowable shunting for Y-90 Therasphere = 10%

and development of necrosis within the lesion. F-18 FDG PET/CT has been done at 1 month and may help monitor response (Fig. 12-23). The majority of patients demonstrate at least partial response. Studies have shown responses in patients who were not responding to chemotherapy, with hepatocellular cancer in some patients becoming resectable. Limited data suggest some improvement in median survival, particularly in those receiving higher doses.

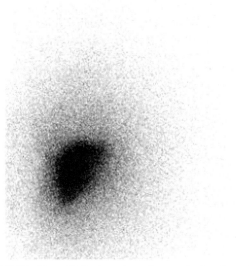

FIGURE 12-22. Planar Y-90 microspheres image after intrahepatic artery injection for therapy using the bremsstrahlung radiation. Although planar images can determine whether the distribution is adequate, SPECT fused with CT provides better correlation.

BONE PAIN PALLIATION

Metastatic disease to the bone is a common problem causing significant pain and disability in patients with cancer. Numerous methods are available for the treatment of bone pain. These include analgesics, chemotherapy drugs, hormonal therapy, bisphosphonates, external beam radiation, and even surgery. Radiopharmaceuticals are an important addition to this list of treatments. Radiopharmaceuticals available for treatment of bone pain are listed in Table 12-16.

Bone-seeking radiopharmaceuticals have been used to treat bone pain from cancer for decades. These agents localize to bone, in areas of bone repair and turnover. Therefore they deposit in areas of metastasis. The therapeutic effects depend on the emission of beta particles. Beta particles are high energy but travel only millimeters from the site of deposition. This ensures the effects are limited to the abnormal bone and normal tissue is spared. These agents are extremely useful because they can be given in addition to other therapies such as external beam radiation or even after external beam therapy has reached maximal limits.

Phosphorus-32

Phosphorus-32 is one of the earliest known bone-seeking radioisotopes. It has been used in intraperitoneal infusion for treatment of tumors such as ovarian cancer and in the treatment of polycythemia vera. It is available for intravenous administration for bone pain palliation. A range of skeletal absorbed doses have been calculated (25-63 rad/mCi [0.68-1.733 cGy/MBq]). However, it appears that the normal marrow receives a high dose relative to the tumor as a result of distribution of P-32 in the inorganic matrix and

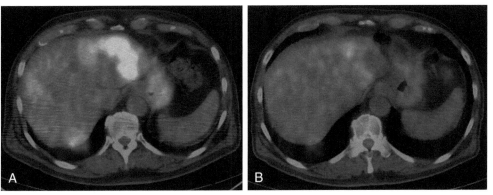

FIGURE 12-23. Monitoring therapy. F-18 FDG PET/CT images of the liver in a patient with unresectable hepatocellular carcinoma (**A**) before and (**B**) 1 month after Y-90 Therasphere administration show marked improvement.

TABLE 12-16 Radiopharmaceuticals for Bone Pain Palliation

Radionuclide	Pharmaceutical	Physical half-life (days)	β Max (MeV)	Beta mean (MeV)	Maximal tissue distance (mm)	Gamma photon (keV)
P-32	Orthophosphate	14.3	1.71	0.695	8	—
Sr-89	Chloride	50.5	1.46	0.583	6.7	—
Sm-153	EDTMP	1.95	0.8	0.224	3.4	103
Re-186	HEDP	3.8	1.07	0.349	4.7	137

EDTMP, Ethylenediamine tetra; *HEDP*, hydroxyethylidene-1, 1-diphosphonic acid.

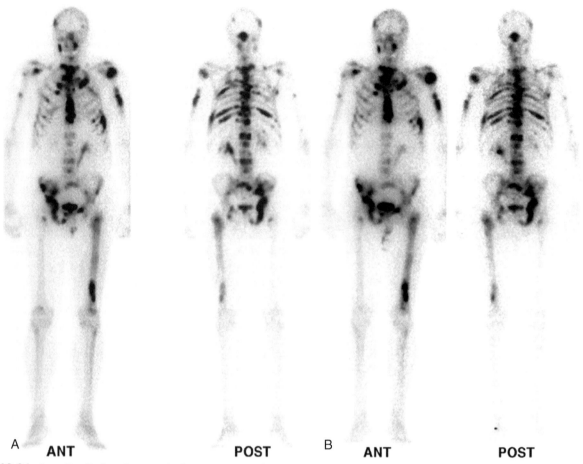

FIGURE 12-24. Sm-153 palliation of metastatic disease bone pain. **A,** The whole-body Tc-99m MDP bone scan before therapy confirms the presence of osseous metastasis that will accumulate the therapy agent. **B,** The whole-body scan done with the Sm-153 therapy dose shows close correlation with the lesions seen on bone scan. *Ant,* Anterior; *Post,* posterior.

cellular regions. Also, the lack of a gamma emission means no external imaging can be done to assess distribution.

Strontium-89

Strontium-89 is a pure beta-emitter approved by the FDA for management of metastatic bone pain under the trade name Metastron. It selectively localizes in areas of bony turnover, predominantly in blastic lesions. It is retained longer in regions of metastasis than normal bone. The pathway of excretion is predominantly through urine, with about one third bowel excretion. Dosimetry is outlined in Table 9-18.

A 4-mCi (148 MBq) dose is administered intravenously slowly over 1 to 2 minutes. An alternative dose of 55 μCi/kg (2.04 MBq/kg) may be used. Repeat dosing is possible, but factors such as initial response, hematological status, and current status must be considered in each case. In general, a repeat administration is not recommended before 90 days have elapsed.

Toxicity
Because toxicity occurs to marrow components, platelets, and white blood cells, the hematological status of each patient must be evaluated before therapy. After obtaining a baseline platelet count, platelets should be measured at least every other week. Typically, platelets will decrease 30% from baseline and reach the nadir 12 to 16 weeks after therapy. Toxicity is generally mild; however, Sr-89 must be used with caution in those with white blood cell counts less than 2400 and platelets less than 60,000. A small number of patients experience transient worsening of symptoms.

Approximately 20% of patients will become pain free. Around 75% of patients will experience some significant decrease in pain, although some series have reported up to 90% of patients experience some symptom relief. Pain relief begins approximately 7 to 20 days after injection and generally lasts 3 to 6 months.

Samarium-153

Samarium-153 (Quadramet) is a beta-emitting radiopharmaceutical that has the added advantage of a gamma emission that can be detected for external imaging. It has been approved for use in patients with osteoblastic metastases that can be visualized on a nuclear medicine bone scan (Fig. 12-24).

Sm-153 is administered in a 1.0-mCi/kg (37 MBq/kg) dose intravenously over the course of 1 minute. Approximately 50% of the dose is localized to bone. It accumulates in metastatic lesions in a 5:1 ratio compared with normal bone. Patients should be well hydrated and void frequently because the primary route of clearance is through the urine. Approximately 35% of the dose is excreted in the first 6 hours.

As in Sr-89, the bone marrow toxicity is a limiting factor. Toxicity is usually mild, although serious side effects and even fatalities have been reported. Platelets decreased on the order of 25% from baseline and white blood cells by 20%.

The short range of the Sm-153 beta particle should be advantageous when considering the dose to normal marrow. A response rate on the order of 83% has been reported. Pain relief is generally noted within 2 weeks, with a duration of 4 to 40 weeks.

Rhenium-186 Hydroxyethylidene Diphosphonate

Rhenium-186 hydroxyethylidene diphosphonate (HEDP) is formed by combining a diphosphonate useful for bone pain therapy, etidronate, with a beta-emitter. Re-186 HEDP is another agent that may be useful for the palliation of bone pain. It emits a gamma ray useful for imaging and lesion identification. It rapidly localizes to bone, with approximately 14% retained in bone. The remainder is rapidly cleared, with approximately 70% of the dose excreted in the urine 6 hours after injection.

■ SUGGESTED READING

Breast

Berg WA, Zheng Z, Lehrer D, et al. Detection of breast cancer with the addition of annual screening ultrasound or single-screening MRI to mammography in women with elevated breast cancer risk. *JAMA.* 2012;307:1775-1877.

Berg WA, Madsen KS, Schilling K, et al. Comparative effectiveness of positron emission mammography and MRI in the contralateral breast of women with newly diagnosed breast cancer. *AJR Am J Roentgenol.* 2012;198:219-232.

Conners AL, Hruska CB, Tortorelli CL, et al. Lexicon for standardized interpretation of gamma camera molecular breast imaging: observer agreement and diagnostic accuracy. *Eur J Nucl Med Mol Imaging.* 2012:Jan 31 [Epub ahead of print.]

Goldsmith SJ, Parsons W, Guiberteau MJ, et al. SNM practice guideline for breast scintigraphy with breast-specific γ-cameras. 2010. Available at: http://snm.org/guidelines.

Hendrick RE. Radiation doses and cancer risks from breast imaging studies. *Radiology.* 2010;257(1):246-253.

O'Connor MK, Hua L, Rhodes DJ, et al. Comparison of radiation exposure and associated radiation-induced cancer risks from mammography and molecular imaging of the breast. *Med Phys.* 2010;37(12):6187-6198.

Rhodes DJ, Hruska CB, Phillips SW, Whaley DH, O'Connor MK. Dedicated dual-head gamma imaging for breast cancer in women with dense breasts. *Radiology.* 2011;258(1):106-118.

Tadwalkar RV, Rapelyea JA, Torrente J, et al. Breast-specific gamma imaging as an adjunct modality for the diagnosis of invasive breast cancer with correlation to tumor size and grade. *Br J Radiol.* 2011;85(1014):e212-e216.

Wahner-Roedler DL, Boughey JC, Hruska CB, et al. The use of molecular breast imaging to assess response in women undergoing neoadjuvant therapy for breast cancer: a pilot study. *Clin Nucl Med.* 2012;37(4):344-350.

Wang CL, MacDonald LR, Rogers JV. Positron emission mammography: correlation of estrogen receptor, progesterone receptor, and human epidermal growth factor receptor 2 status and 18F-FDG. *AJR Am J Roentgenol.* 2011;197(2):W247-W255.

Weigert JM, Bertrand ML, Lankowsky L, Stern LH, Kieper DA. Results of a multicenter registry to determine the clinical impact of breast-specific gamma imaging, a molecular breast imaging technique. *AJR Am J Roentgenol.* 2011;198(1):W69-W75.

Somatostatin Receptor Imaging

Balon HR, Goldsmith SJ, Siegel BA, et al. Society of nuclear medicine procedure guideline for somatostatin receptor scintigraphy with In-111 pentetreotide, version 2.0. 2002. Available at: http://interactive.snm.org/docs/SRS_Final_v2_0.pdf.

Kabasakal L, Demirci E, Ocak M. Comparison of (68)Ga-DOTATAE and (68) Ga-DOTANOC PET/CT imaging in the same patient group with neuroendocrine tumors. *Eur J Nucl Med Mol Imaging.* 2012;39(8):1271-1277.

Kwekkeboom DJ, Krenning EP. Somatostatin receptor imaging. *Semin Nucl Med.* 2002;32(2):84-91.

Adrenal Imaging

Bombardieri E, Giammarile F, Aktolum C, et al. 131I/123I-Metaiodobenzylguanidine (MIBG) scintigraphy-procedure guidelines for tumor imaging. 2010. Available at: http://interactive.snm.org/docs/EANM_guideline_for_I131_I123_MIBG_Scintigraphy.pdf.

Antibody Imaging

Hagenbeek A. Radioimmunotherapy for NHL: experience of 90Y-ibritumomab tiuxetan in clinical practice. *Leuk Lymphoma.* 2003;44(suppl 4):S37-S47.

Rieter WJ, Keane TE, Ahlman MA, et al. Diagnostic performance of In-111 capromab pendetide SPECT-CT in localized and metastatic prostate cancer. *Clin Nucl Med.* 2011;36:872-878.

Taneja SS. ProstaScint® scan: contemporary use in clinical practice. *Rev Urol.* 2004;6(suppl 10):S19-S28.

Wong TZ, Turkinton TG, Polascik TJ, Coleman RE. ProstaScint (capromab pendetide) imaging using hybrid gamma camera-CT technology. *AJR Am J Roentgenol.* 2005;184(2):676-680.

Wyngaert JK, Noz ME, Ellerin B, et al. Procedure for unmasking localization information from ProstaScint scans for prostate radiation therapy treatment planning. *Int J Radiat Oncol Biol Phys.* 2004;60(2):654-662.

Lymphoscintigraphy

Buscombe J, Paganelli G, Burak ZE, et al. Sentinel node in breast cancer procedural guidelines. *Eur J Nucl Med Mol Imaging.* 2007;34(12):2154-2159.

Gershenwald JE, Ross ML. Sentinel-lymph-node biopsy for cutaneous melanoma. *N Engl J Med.* 2011;364(18):1738-1745.

Hindie E, Groheux D, Brenot-Rossi I. The sentinel node procedure in breast cancer: nuclear medicine as a starting point. *J Nucl Med.* 2011;52(3):405-414.

Lyman GH, Giuliano AE, Somerfield MR, et al. American society of clinical oncology guideline recommendations for sentinel lymph node biopsy in early stage breast cancer. *J Clin Oncol.* 2005;23(30):7703-7720.

Intraarterial Microsphere Therapy

Ahmadzadehfar H, Biersack HJ, Ezzidin S. Radioembolization of liver tumors with yttrium-90 microspheres. *Semin Nucl Med.* 2010;40(2):105-121.

Kalva SP, Thabet A, Wicky S. Recent advances in transarterial therapy of primary and secondary liver malignancies. *Radiographics.* 2008;28(1):101-117.

CHAPTER 13

Gastrointestinal System

Radionuclide gastrointestinal imaging studies provide unique noninvasive functional and quantitative diagnostic information not available from anatomical imaging. This chapter will discuss gastrointestinal scintigraphy by starting at the top and moving down the gastrointestinal system.

■ ESOPHAGEAL MOTILITY

The esophagus transports ingested food from the mouth to the stomach, clears regurgitated substances, and prevents acid reflux and tracheobronchial aspiration (Fig. 13-1).

Dysmotility Disorders

Esophageal motility disorders present with symptoms of painful swallowing (dysphagia). They are classified as primary (e.g., achalasia) or secondary (e.g., scleroderma) or alternatively by the type of dysfunction (e.g., amotility, hypomotility, hypermotility) (Box 13-1).

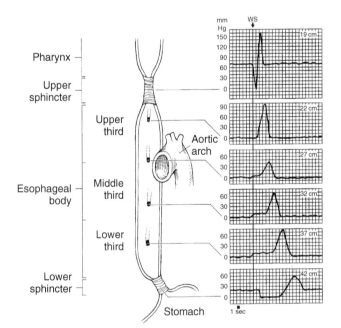

FIGURE 13-1. Esophageal anatomy and motility. Swallowing initiates a coordinated peristaltic contraction that propagates down the esophagus. The esophagus has three distinct regions: the upper esophageal sphincter (UES), which allows food to pass from the mouth to the esophagus and prevents tracheobronchial aspiration; the esophageal body, with striated muscle proximally and smooth muscle distally; and the lower esophageal sphincter (LES), a high-pressure smooth muscle region that prevents gastric reflux but relaxes during swallowing to allow passage of food into the stomach. Manometric pressure changes with a 8-mL bolus water swallow *(WS)* are shown. After swallowing, the UES pressure falls transiently, then the LES pressure falls and remains low until the peristaltic contraction passes aborally through the UES and esophageal body, which closes the LES.

Achalasia is a primary esophageal motor disorder. It manifests as absent or partial relaxation of the lower esophageal sphincter and loss of esophageal body peristalsis, resulting in food retention. Symptoms in addition to dysphagia may include weight loss, nocturnal regurgitation, cough, and aspiration. Its cause is unknown. Contrast esophagrams show retention in a distended column, narrowed sphincter, and delayed clearance. Manometry detects an absence of peristalsis in the distal two thirds of the esophagus, increased lower esophageal sphincter pressure, and incomplete sphincter relaxation with swallowing.

Some motility disorders are manifestations of systemic disease—for example, scleroderma, a connective tissue disorder often involving the smooth muscle of the esophagus. Contrast radiography visualizes a dilated aperistaltic esophagus, barium retention, and reflux. Manometry detects decreased or absent lower esophageal sphincter pressure and reduced contraction amplitude. Systemic lupus erythematosus and polymyositis also may manifest with smooth muscle esophageal motility disorders. Esophageal striated muscle abnormalities occur in patients with muscular dystrophy, myasthenia gravis, and myotonia dystrophica.

Diffuse esophageal spasm presents with symptoms of intermittent chest pain and dysphagia. Barium swallow and manometry detect abnormal nonperistaltic contractions of the esophageal body. The nutcracker esophagus has characteristic high-amplitude prolonged high-pressure peristaltic contractions. It is unclear whether these entities represent real disorders or are manometric abnormalities that may or may not be related to patient symptoms.

Standard Diagnostic Methods

Barium esophagrams detect anatomical lesions and mucosal changes, but provide only qualitative assessment of

---

BOX 13-1. Classification of Esophageal Motility Disorders

PRIMARY
Achalasia, esophageal spasm, nutcracker esophagus

SECONDARY
Scleroderma, lupus erythematosus, polymyositis
Muscular dystrophy, myotonia dystrophica, myasthenia gravis
Diabetic, alcoholic enteropathy

DEGREE OF MOTILITY
Amotility
Achalasia, scleroderma

Hypomotility
Presbyesophagus

Hypermotility
Diffuse esophageal spasm, nutcracker esophagus

motility. Esophageal manometry directly measures esophageal pressure, peristalsis, and sphincter contraction and relaxation.

Scintigraphy

Esophageal transit scintigraphy has been used to screen symptomatic patients before considering more invasive procedures, to diagnose or exclude esophageal motility disorders, and to evaluate effectiveness of therapy in patients with a diagnosis of esophageal dysmotility.

Radiopharmaceuticals

Technetium-99m sulfur colloid or Tc-99m diethylenetriaminepentaacetic acid (DTPA), 200 to 300 µCi (7.4-11.1 MBq), dispersed in a small volume of clear liquid, is commonly used. Semisolid meals are said to be more sensitive for detecting esophageal dysmotility.

Methodology

Typical liquid (Box 13-2) and semisolid (Box 13-3) esophageal motility protocols are described. Acquisition in the posterior view allows for easier administration of the bolus and closer observation of the patient. The supine position may be preferable in some cases because it eliminates the effect of gravity on esophageal emptying. However, gravity is the only mechanism of emptying in achalasia and thus upright positioning is required for serial studies in this disease.

Multiple swallows are often necessary for complete emptying, even in normal subjects, because of a 25% incidence of "aberrant" swallows—that is, extra swallows, occurring between two prescribed swallows. Aberrant swallows inhibit subsequent swallows and delay transit.

Any normal residual remaining after an initial swallow will clear when followed by a dry swallow.

Analysis and Quantification

Image analysis of sequential images in conjunction with cinematic display is often adequate for diagnosis of severe motility abnormalities (Figs. 13-2 and 13-3). Quantification can be helpful for diagnosis of less severe abnormalities and for comparison of serial studies over time to determine therapeutic effectiveness. TACs can be derived for the entire esophagus or selected regions (Figs. 13-3, *C*, and 13-4).

Esophageal transit can be quantified by calculating a transit time or the percent residual activity in the esophagus. *Transit time* is defined as the time from the initial entry of the bolus into the esophagus until all but 10% of peak activity clears (abnormal >15 seconds). *Percent residual esophageal activity* is calculated using the formula ($[E_{max} - E_t]/E_{max}) \times 100$, where E_{max} is maximum esophageal counts and E_t is the counts after dry swallow number t (abnormal, >20%). For a semisolid meal, abnormal retention at 20 minutes is greater than 5%.

Accuracy

The esophageal transit study has high sensitivity for the detection of achalasia, but somewhat lower sensitivity for other disorders, limiting its routine use as a screening test. Its specificity for differentiating the cause of different disorders is not high. The transit studies are most commonly ordered to either screen patients with low suspicion of a motility disorder to avoid invasive manometry or to evaluate therapeutic response.

Dosimetry

Table 13-1 provides the radiation dose to the patient for children of different ages for gastroesophageal scintigraphy. Table 13-2 shows adult dosimetry based on the

---

BOX 13-2. Esophageal Transit Scintigraphy (Liquids): Summary Protocol

PATIENT PREPARATION
Patient should fast overnight.
Place radioactive marker on cricoid cartilage.
Position the patient supine.
Practice swallows with nonradioactive bolus.

RADIOPHARMACEUTICAL
Tc-99m sulfur colloid or DTPA, 300 µCi (11 mBq)
in 10 mL of water

INSTRUMENTATION
Camera setup: Tc-99m 140 keV photopeak with 20% window
Computer setup: 0.8-second frame × 240; byte mode, 64 × 64

SWALLOWING PROCEDURE
Swallow radiopharmaceutical as a bolus.
Dry swallow at 30 seconds, then radiolabeled bolus every 30 seconds × 4.
No swallowing between boluses.

PROCESSING
Time-activity curves, condensed dynamic images

QUANTIFICATION
Time to 90% emptying
Transit time

BOX 13-3. Esophageal Transit Scintigraphy (Semisolid Meal): Summary Protocol

PATIENT PREPARATION
Overnight fast.
Patient position: Seated, posterior camera acquisition

RADIOPHARMACEUTICAL
Tc-99m sulfur colloid or DTPA 1.0 mCi (37 MBq)
mixed with 120 mL milk, 19 g of cornflakes, 1 g sugar

COMPUTER SETUP
Feeding phase: 10-second frames × 12 (64 × 64 matrix)
Spontaneous emptying phase: 10-second frames × 120
Water ingestion phase: 10 seconds × 6
Carbonated beverage phase (150 mL): 10 seconds × 6

PROCESSING
Draw a region of interest around the esophagus.
Display the time-activity curve
Display a condensed image

QUANTIFICATION
Calculate the percent retention (esophageal counts/total counts × 100)
Normal percent retention, less than 5% at 20 minutes

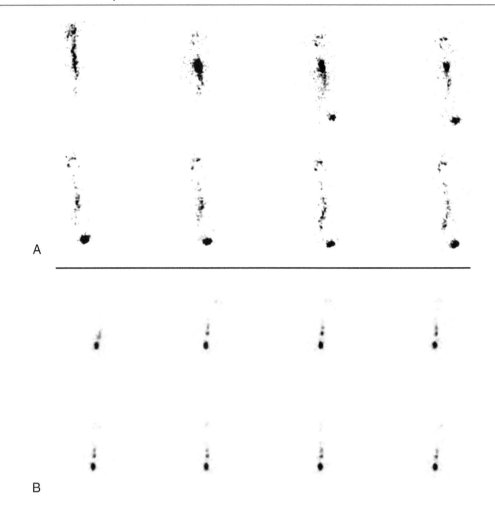

FIGURE 13-2. A, Normal esophageal clear liquid transit. Images obtained supine at 1-second intervals. The initial swallowed bolus travels rapidly down the esophagus. A small amount of diffuse residual activity remains in the distal esophagus. Transit time was 11 seconds (normal, <15 seconds). **B,** Scleroderma. Dysmotility with poor propagation of bolus and retention of the activity in the distal esophagus.

radiopharmaceutical and the particular meal used. The large intestine receives the highest radiation absorbed dose.

GASTROESOPHAGEAL REFLUX DISEASE

Gastroesophageal reflux disease (GERD) is a common and sometimes serious medical disorder. Heartburn is the major symptom in adults. Complications include esophagitis, bleeding, perforation, stricture, Barrett esophagus, and cancer. The symptoms in children are different, usually with respiratory symptoms, iron deficiency anemia, and failure to thrive. Gastroesophageal reflux is a normal physiological event in infants that usually resolves spontaneously by 7 to 8 months of age. In infants, 5% to 10% have persistent symptoms and serious sequelae of strictures, recurrent pneumonia, and inanition.

Symptomatic disease is more likely in patients with an associated esophageal motility disorder, increasing the duration of mucosal exposure to refluxate. Other factors include the efficacy of the antireflux mechanism, the volume of gastric contents, the potency of refluxed material (acid, pepsin), mucosal resistance to injury, and mucosal reparative ability.

Diagnosis

Various tests are used to diagnose GERD. Barium esophagography can detect mucosal damage, stricture, and tumor, but has low sensitivity for detecting reflux. Esophageal endoscopy allows direct visualization of esophageal mucosa and permits biopsy of ulcerations and areas suspicious for malignancy. Hydrochloric acid (0.1 N) infused into the distal esophagus (Bernstein acid infusion test) has been used to reproduce reflux symptoms and confirm their esophageal origin.

The Tuttle acid reflux test is considered the standard for diagnosis of GERD but is technically demanding. A pH electrode is placed in the distal esophagus for 24-hour monitoring. An abrupt drop in pH (<4.0) is diagnostic. However, a second reflux event cannot be detected until acid has cleared the pH probe. Reflux volume clears within seconds, but acid clearance takes several minutes, requiring swallowed saliva, limiting temporal sensitivity for detection of reflux.

Scintigraphy

The radionuclide test for reflux is physiological and quantitative. It is most commonly requested for neonates.

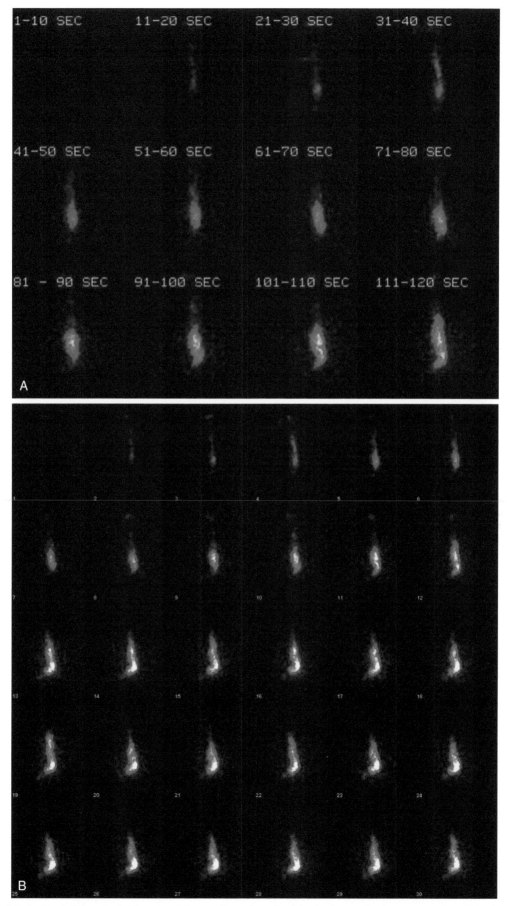

FIGURE 13-3. Achalasia: Semisolid meal. **A,** Ten-second frames. Retention of activity in the esophagus, most prominently in the distal esophagus. **B,** Two-minute frames. Persistent distal esophageal retention with minimal clearance into the stomach.

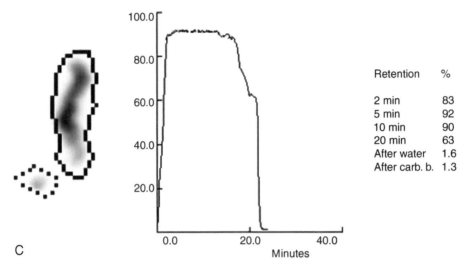

Retention	%
2 min	83
5 min	92
10 min	90
20 min	63
After water	1.6
After carb. b.	1.3

C

FIGURE 13-3, cont'd. C, Quantification of esophageal emptying. TAC. Calculated retention at 20 minutes: 63% (<5% is normal). After ingestion of water and carbonated beverage rapid emptying occurs.

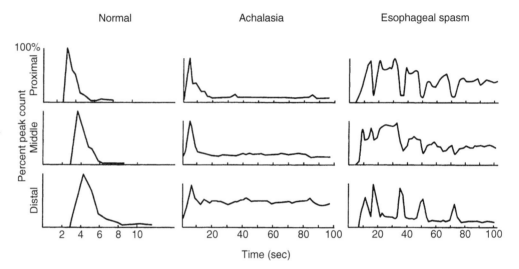

FIGURE 13-4. Esophageal time-activity profiles: Normal, achalasia, and esophageal spasm. Ranges of interests were drawn for the proximal, middle, and distal esophagus and TACs generated. *Left:* Normal subject. Bolus proceeds promptly sequentially from proximal to distal esophagus. *Middle:* Achalasia. Retention most prominent in the lower esophagus. *Right:* Spasm, uncoordinated contraction. Bolus has poor esophageal progression.

TABLE 13-1 Dosimetry for Technetium-99m Sulfur Colloid Gastroesophageal Scintigraphy for Children

	Rad/100 μCi by Age*			
Organ	Newborn	1 Year	5 Years	10 Years
Stomach	0.383	0.093	0.050	0.031
Large intestine	0.927	0.380	0.194	0.120
Ovaries	0.099	0.042	0.033	0.072
Testes	0.018	0.007	0.003	0.011
Whole body	0.020	0.011	0.006	0.004

Data modified from Castronovo FP. Gastroesophageal scintiscanning in a pediatric population: dosimetry. *J Nucl Med.* 1986;27(7):1212-1214.
*Usual dose, 200-300 μCi (7.4-11.1 MBq).

Detection of reflux events is affected by the volume of the ingested meal and the rate of gastric emptying. Sensitivity for detection of reflux decreases as the stomach empties.

Methodology

In the past, the radionuclide reflux study was performed in a manner similar to the barium contrast study, using Valsalva maneuvers and an abdominal binder to progressively increase intraabdominal pressure during each sequential static 30-second image. The method is not physiological and has poor sensitivity. It is no longer recommended. A "milk" study is preferable.

After the infant ingests infant's formula or milk mixed with Tc-99m sulfur colloid, the study is acquired on a computer using a rapid framing rate, 5- to 10-second frames for 60 minutes. The high temporal acquisition rate provides high sensitivity for detection of reflux events compared to longer framing rates. This same methodology is recommended for older children and adults, although mixed with orange juice. Gastric emptying is determined during the same study by acquiring static images immediately after ingestion and at 1 and 2 hours. A protocol is described in Box 13-4.

Image Interpretation

All frames should be reviewed. Cinematic display can be helpful. Reflux is seen as distinct spikes of activity into the esophagus (Fig. 13-5). Various methods of quantification have been used. A simple semiquantitative interpretive method grades each reflux event as high- or low-level

TABLE 13-2 Adult Dosimetry for Esophageal and Gastric Scintigraphy

Agent and meal	Millirads/study meal, by organ					
	Stomach	Small intestine	Large intestine	ovaries	testes	Total body
LIQUID						
300 µCi Tc-99m sulfur colloid	28	83	160	29	2	5
1 mCi Tc-99m DTPA	93	280	520	98	5	20
250 µCi In-111 DTPA	110	490	2000	420	27	60
SOLID						
500 µCi Tc-99m sulfur colloid in ovalbumin	120	120	230	42	2	9
500 µCi Tc-99m in chicken liver	120	120	230	42	2	9

Data modified from Siegel JA, Wu RK, Knight C, et al. Radiation dose estimates for oral agents used in the upper gastrointestinal diseases. *J Nucl Med.* 1983;24(8):835-837.

DTPA, diethylenetriaminepentaacetic acid.

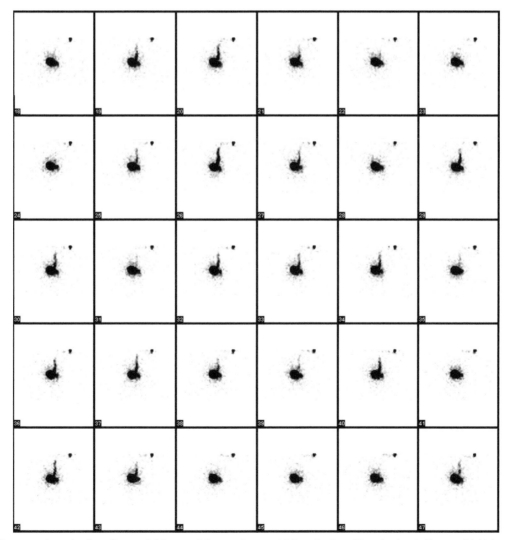

FIGURE 13-5. Gastroesophageal reflux. Sequential 5-second frames show multiple episodes of long-lasting (>15 seconds) high-grade (above mid-esophagus) reflux events.

(≥ or < mid-esophagus), by its duration (10 seconds or longer or less), and by the temporal relationship to meal ingestion (reflux events at low gastric volume carry greater significance). The total number of reflux events can be summed in four categories: low-level, less than 10 seconds; low-level, 10 seconds or longer; high-level, less than 10 seconds; and high-level, 10 seconds or longer.

Alternatively, regions of interest can be drawn for the esophagus and TACs generated. Various quantitative parameters have been used. Peaks greater than 5% are diagnostic of reflux.

Normal values for neonates or young children have not been established. Neonates normally have some reflux. The greater the number of high reflux events, and the longer they last, the more severe is the problem. Reflux events that occur with small gastric volumes have more clinical significance because reflux is occurring without the effect of the increased pressure of a full meal volume and acid buffering.

Pulmonary aspiration should be looked for in reflux studies, although detection sensitivity is poor. Normal gastric emptying for formula or milk at 1 hour is 40% to 50% and at 2 hours is 60% to 75%. The 2-hour emptying value is considered the most reliable.

A salivagram is a more sensitive method of detecting aspiration. It is a variation of an esophageal transit study. A small volume of radiotracer in water is placed in the infant's posterior pharynx. The study is acquired with a rapid framing rate, similar to the reflux study, followed by static images (Fig. 13-6).

Accuracy

Early literature reported a poor sensitivity (60%-70%) for radionuclide gastroesophageal reflux studies. This was due to the long framing rates used. With more rapid framing rates sensitivity is reported to be 75% to 100%, superior to barium studies. The standard is pH monitoring; however, it has limitations—for example, 24-hour monitoring and poor temporal resolution. The highest sensitivity is achieved using both scintigraphy and pH monitoring.

The reported sensitivity for detection of aspiration on gastroesophageal reflux (milk) studies is approximately 25%. The salivagram study can often demonstrate clinically suspected aspiration when the gastroesophageal reflux study is negative.

▬ GASTRIC MOTILITY SCINTIGRAPHY

The radionuclide study is the accepted gold standard for diagnosis of gastric dysmotility. A radiographic contrast study can detect a gross delay in emptying and mechanical obstruction, but is insensitive for detection of gastroparesis and is not quantitative. Many other methodologies have been proposed; however, all have limitations.

The most recent popularized method is the "camera-in-a-pill," which has commercial backing. The patient swallows the devise as a capsule. Gastric emptying is estimated by detecting an increase in pH when it reaches the small bowel. The patient must carry an external detection device, it is relatively expensive, and few data have been published on its value.

Anatomy and Physiology

The stomach is a smooth-muscle hollow viscous with a sphincter at both ends, anatomically divided into the cardia, fundus, body, antrum, and pylorus (Fig. 13-7). The mucosa contains glands that produce hydrochloric acid and digestive enzymes. Gastric motility is produced by neuromuscular gastric activity and small intestinal neuroendocrine feedback.

The proximal and distal portions of the stomach have distinct functions. The fundus (proximal portion) acts as a reservoir, accepting large meals with only minimal increase in pressure (receptive relaxation and accommodation). Its

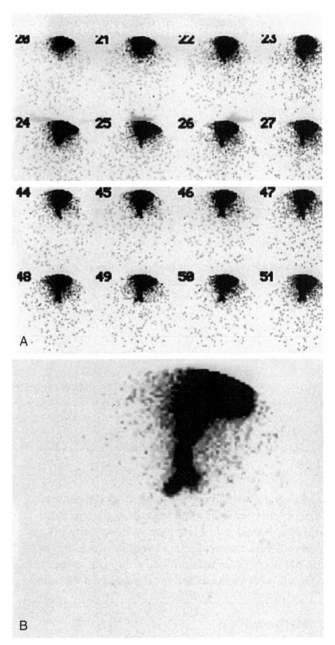

Figure 13-6. Salivagram: Aspiration. Neonate with swallowing and neurological problems. A gastroesophageal reflux study (not shown) revealed numerous reflux events, but no aspiration. **A,** After radiotracer was placed in the posterior pharynx, sequential 5-second frames showed transit into the tracheal bifurcation. **B,** High-count anterior image at one hour shows persistent retention at the tracheal bifurcation.

muscular contraction is tonic, producing a constant pressure gradient between the stomach and pylorus, which is responsible for liquid emptying. Liquids normally empty in a monoexponential pattern—that is, the larger the volume, the more rapid the emptying (Fig. 13-8). Minimal or no delay occurs before emptying begins. Adding calories, salts, or acidity all slow the rate of liquid emptying.

The antrum (distal stomach) has a neural pacemaker that initiates phasic rhythmic contractions that stimulate solid emptying. After meal ingestion, muscular contractions sweep down the antrum in a ringlike pattern,

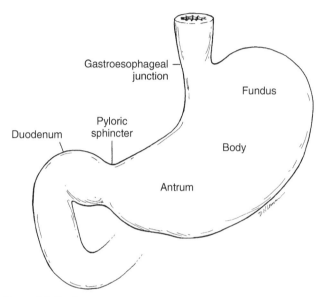

FIGURE 13-7. Gastric anatomy. The proximal stomach (fundus) accommodates and stores food and its tonic contraction is responsible for liquid emptying. The distal stomach (antrum) has phasic contractions responsible for solid food emptying. The antrum mixes and grinds food into small enough particles to pass through the pylorus.

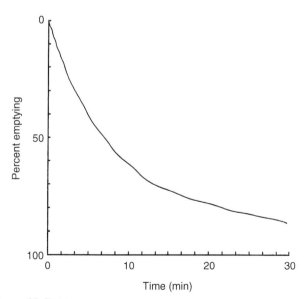

FIGURE 13-8. Normal clear liquid emptying. Ingestion of 300 mL of water mixed with Tc-99m sulfur colloid. One-minute frames for 30 minutes. TAC generated by drawing a whole stomach range of interest. Emptying begins immediately. The clearance curve pattern is monoexponential, with a half-emptying time of 9 minutes (normal <23 minutes).

squeezing food toward the pylorus. Larger food particles are not allowed to pass and are retropelled. The solid material is converted into chyme through contact with acid and peptic enzymes and mechanical grinding. Food particles become progressive smaller, until able to pass through the pyloric sphincter (1-2 mm). The pylorus, at the junction of antrum and duodenal bulb, acts as a sieve, regulating gastric outflow.

The length of time required for grinding solid food into small particles before emptying begins is the lag phase, usually lasting 5 to 20 minutes (Fig. 13-9). Once solid emptying begins, clearance into the duodenum commonly occurs at a constant rate, in a linear pattern. The rate of emptying depends on the size and contents of the meal. Meals with larger volume and weight, more carbohydrates, protein, or fat, empty slower (Box 13-5). Emptying occurs more rapidly when standing compared to sitting and more rapidly sitting compared to lying.

In the fasting state between meals, forceful contractions empty nondigestible debris from the stomach (interdigestive contractions). Motilin, a peptide hormone secreted by the upper small bowel mucosa, initiates this interdigestive event.

Gastric Stasis Syndromes

Indications for a gastric emptying study are listed in Box 13-6. Symptoms suggestive of gastroparesis include postprandial early satiety, nausea, vomiting, and bloating. Most patients with gastroparesis have a functional cause. The radionuclide study cannot differentiate a functional delay in emptying from anatomical obstruction—for example, tumor or pyloric channel ulcer. Endoscopy or contrast barium radiography is required for that purpose. Although most patients with gastroparesis have a chronic emptying problem, temporary reversible causes occur.

Chronic Gastroparesis

The causes for chronic gastric stasis syndromes are diverse and have been categorized in various ways (Box 13-7).

Diabetic gastroenteropathy occurs in patients with long-standing insulin-dependent diabetes mellitus and is caused by vagal nerve damage as part of a generalized autonomic neuropathy. In addition to causing disagreeable postprandial symptoms, abnormal emptying may exacerbate the problem of diabetic serum glucose control because timing of the insulin dose with food ingestion and absorption can be unpredictable with gastroparesis.

Nonulcer dyspepsia, a common disorder, is characterized by upper abdominal symptoms that are ulcerlike or dyspeptic. Some of these patients have gastroparesis.

Reversible Causes for Gastroparesis

Various reversible clinical causes include viral gastroenteritis, trauma, and metabolic derangements (Box 13-7). Hyperglycemia per se, independent of diabetic gastroenteropathy, may delay emptying. Thus gastric motility studies should be performed with patients under optimal diabetes control. For patients with diabetes, a fasting blood sugar should be checked before the study. The study should not be done if the fasting blood sugar is greater than 200 mg/dL.

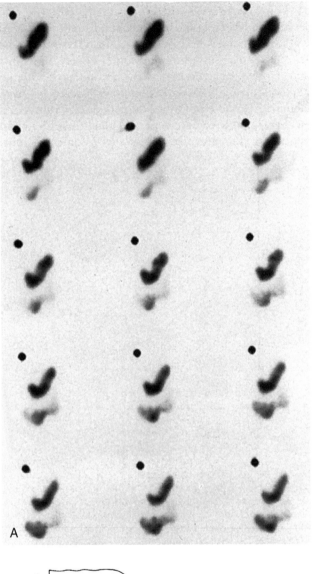

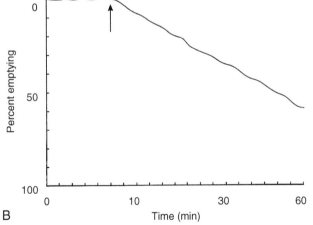

FIGURE 13-9. Biphasic normal pattern of solid gastric emptying. **A,** Five-minute sequential images acquired for 60 minutes. The meal moves normally from the gastric fundus to the antrum and then begins to clear into small intestines. **B,** Computer-generated TAC shows a lag phase of 9 minutes *(arrow)* before emptying begins (normal 5-25 minutes). A linear pattern of normal emptying follows. Radioactive marker on right side.

Box 13-5. Factors That Affect the Rate of Gastric Emptying

Meal content	Time of day
Fat, protein, acid, osmolality	Patient position (standing, sitting, supine)
Volume	Gender
Weight	Metabolic state
Caloric density	Stress
Particle size	Exercise

Box 13-6. Clinical Indications for Radionuclide Gastric Emptying Study

Patients with insulin-dependent diabetics and persistent postprandial symptoms
Diabetics with poor blood glucose control
Nonulcer dyspepsia
Severe reflux esophagitis.
Unexplained nausea and vomiting
Assess response to a motility drug

Box 13-7. Causes of Acute and Chronic Gastric Stasis Syndromes

ACUTE
Trauma
Postoperative ileus
Acute viral infections (e.g., gastroenteritis)
Hyperalimentation
Metabolic: Hyperglycemia, acidosis, uremia, hypokalemia, hypercalcemia, hepatic coma, myxedema
Physiological: Labyrinth stimulation, physical and mental stress, gastric distention, increased intragastric pressure
Hormone increases: Gastrin, secretin, glucagon, cholecystokinin, somatostatin, estrogen, progesterone

CHRONIC
Anatomic
Gastric ulcer
Surgery, vagotomy
Pyloric hypertrophy
Postradiotherapy
Tumors

Functional
Diabetic gastroenteropathy
Nonulcer dyspepsia
Dermatomyositis
Systemic lupus erythematosus
Amyloidosis
Hypothyroidism
Familial dysautonia
Pernicious anemia
Tumor associated gastroparesis
Progressive systemic sclerosis
Fabry disease
Gastroesophageal reflux

Many commonly used therapeutic drugs may delay gastric emptying (Table 13-3).

Rapid Gastric Emptying

Rapid emptying occurs in patients who have had gastric surgery (e.g., pyloroplasty or gastrectomy) and in patients with hyperthyroidism or gastrinoma (Zollinger Ellison syndrome). Some patients with insulin-dependent diabetes have rapid gastric emptying (Box 13-8). Symptoms of rapid emptying include palpitations, diaphoresis, weakness, and diarrhea (dumping syndrome). Sometimes, symptoms of rapid emptying may be similar to those of delayed emptying.

Pharmacological Therapy

Few prokinetic medications are available for therapy of gastroparesis. Metoclopramide (Reglan), the most commonly used, is not effective in all patients, symptom relief is not always accompanied by improvement in emptying, and serious side effects may occur (e.g., tardive dyskinesia occurs in 10% of patients taking the drug for >3 months). Domperidone is not approved for clinical use in the United States because of reports of fatal arrhythmias. Erythromycin, a motilin agonist, is increasingly used therapeutically; however, it has a high incidence of nausea and vomiting. Analogs are in development.

TABLE 13-3 Pharmaceuticals That Delay Gastric Emptying

Drug type	Specific drugs
Cardiovascular	Nifedipine, calcium channel blockers, beta-adrenergic agonists (Inderal)
Respiratory	Isoproterenol, theophylline
Gastrointestinal	Sucralfate, anticholinergics
Reproductive	Progesterone, oral contraceptives
Neuropsychiatric	Diazepam (Valium), Librium, Librax, Ativan, tricyclic antidepressants, levodopa, phenothiazine (Thorazine)
Opiates Alcohol and nicotine	OxyContin, Percodan, Percocet

Box 13-8. Causes of Rapid Gastric Emptying

PRIOR SURGERY
Pyloroplasty
Hemigastrectomy (Billroth I, II)

DISEASES
Duodenal ulcer
Gastrinoma (Zollinger Ellison syndrome)
Hyperthyroidism
Diabetics (subgroup)

HORMONES
Thyroxine
Motilin
Enterogastrone

Surgical Management

Surgical intervention is employed to treat refractory gastroparesis. A common approach is implantation of an electrical gastric stimulator. Its mechanism of action does not involve acceleration of gastric emptying but rather stimulation of vagal pathways that promote fundic relaxation and reduce afferent hypersensitivity. In some patients, gastric resection is required.

Gastric Emptying Scintigraphy

Radiopharmaceuticals

For accurate reproducible quantification of radionuclide solid gastric emptying studies, the radiotracer must be tightly bound to the solid component of the meal. Elution of the radiolabel will result in a part-solid, part-liquid labeled mixture and unreliable results.

Early investigators used a physiologically superb method to ensure high labeling efficiency. Tc-99m sulfur colloid was injected into the wing vein of a chicken. After binding of the agent to Kupffer cells in the liver (15 minutes), the chicken was sacrificed, the liver removed, cooked, and then mixed with stew for palatability and volume. Binding efficiency was 98% and highly stable in gastric juice. This method is not used clinically today for obvious reasons.

Most imaging clinics use radiolabeled eggs for solid gastric emptying studies. When mixed and cooked, Tc-99m sulfur colloid binds to the albumen in egg white. Although whole eggs work well, egg whites and egg substitutes have higher percent binding and are preferable.

For liquid meals, the radiotracer should equilibrate rapidly and be nonabsorbable. Tc-99m sulfur colloid and Tc-99m DTPA meet these criteria. Clear liquids and full liquids have been used.

Dual-phase studies with a radiotracer for the solid meal and another for the liquid phase provide simultaneous solid and liquid emptying information. In these studies, In-111 DTPA is typically used as the liquid marker (171, 247 keV) and Tc-99m sulfur colloid (140 keV) bound to the solid meal (Fig. 13-10). The two components can be detected by their separate photopeaks.

Methodology

Many different methods and protocols have been used for solid gastric emptying studies. Meal composition, patient positioning, instrumentation, framing rate, study length, and quantitative methods have varied. All of these factors affect the rate or amount of gastric emptying. Normal values must be well validated for the meal and methodology used.

Standardization of Solid Gastric Emptying Scintigraphy

Gastroenterologists have had concerns that different meals, gastric emptying protocols, and normal values were used by different referral imaging clinics. They have pushed for a standardized gastric emptying protocol.

In 2008 an expert panel of gastroenterologists and nuclear medicine physicians met and published *Consensus Recommendations for Radionuclide Gastric Emptying Scintigraphy*. The recommendations included a simplified protocol, a

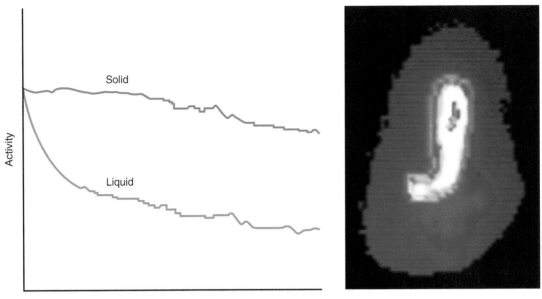

FIGURE 13-10. Dual-phase solid-liquid emptying. Simultaneously acquired solid and liquid study. The solid egg meal is labeled with Tc-99m sulfur colloid and the liquid (water) meal with In-111 DTPA. Images were acquired each minute for 120 minutes.

***Box 13-9.* Standardized Gastric Emptying (Tougas): Summary Protocol**

PATIENT PREPARATION
Referring physician should determine what medications are to be continued before study
A fasting blood sugar is recommended before study, particularly for diabetics
Perform study in the morning after an overnight fast or NPO for 6 hours before study.

RADIOPHARMACEUTICAL AND MEAL
Tc-99m sulfur colloid 1 mCi (37 MBq) bound to 4 oz egg substitute (Egg-Beaters or generic equivalent) by microwaving or scrambling after dispersing Tc-99m sulfur colloid in egg. Stir once or twice while cooking until mixture reaches consistency of omelet. Meal also consists of two slices of white bread, strawberry jam (30 g), and water (120 mL)
Meal should be ingested within 10 to 15 minutes.

INSTRUMENTATION
Gamma camera: Large field of view, dual detector camera
Collimator: Low energy, parallel hole
Tc99m photopeak with a 20% window around 140 keV
Computer setup: 1-minute frames (128 × 128 word mode matrix)

PATIENT POSITION
Position patient either upright or lying with camera heads anterior and posteriorly.
A single-head camera can be used, taking an image anteriorly, then posteriorly.

IMAGING PROCEDURE
Acquire 1-minute frames at time 0 (immediately after ingestion) and 1, 2, and 3 hours.

PROCESSING
Draw region of interest region of interest to outline stomach on all images. Decay correction is mandatory. The geometric mean of the anterior and posterior views should be determined at each time point. The percent retention or percent gastric emptying should be calculated at 1, 2, and 4 hours.

INTERPRETATION
Delayed gastric emptying
1 hour <10% emptying
2 hours <40% emptying
4 hours <90% emptying
Rapid gastric emptying at 1 hour >70%
These values apply to the entire meal and are not valid for different meals or incomplete ingestion of the standard meal.

NPO, Nil per os.

---

standardized meal and protocol, a 4-hour study length, and validated normal values.

The simplified study can be performed at any imaging clinic that has a gamma camera and computer workstation. The protocol published by Tougas and colleagues (Box 13-9) was selected because it required only 1-min images acquired at four time points (immediately after ingestion and at 1, 2, and 4 hours) and calculation of the percent gastric emptying at those time intervals (Fig. 13-11). A 4-hour study has been shown to detect more

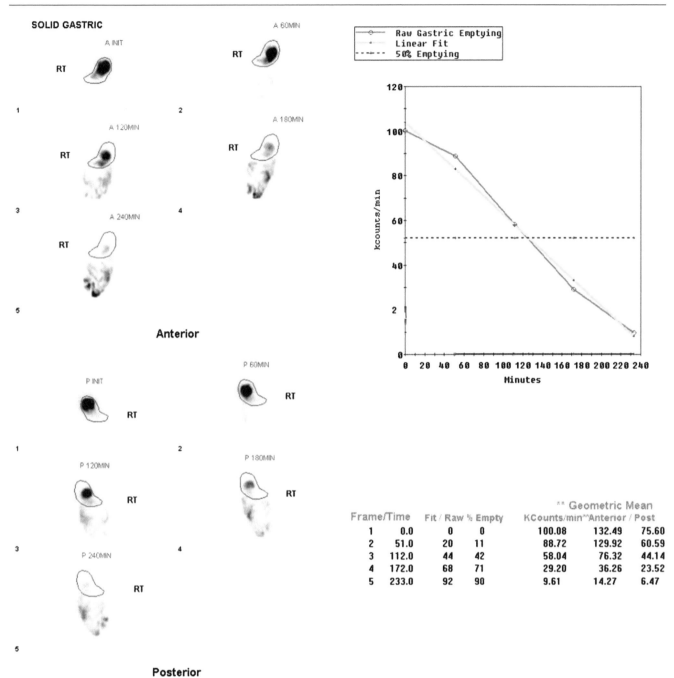

Frame/Time		Fit / Raw % Empty		** Geometric Mean KCounts/min** Anterior / Post		
1	0.0	0	0	100.08	132.49	75.60
2	51.0	20	11	88.72	129.92	60.59
3	112.0	44	42	58.04	76.32	44.14
4	172.0	68	71	29.20	36.26	23.52
5	233.0	92	90	9.61	14.27	6.47

FIGURE 13-11. Normal solid gastric emptying using the standardized-hour Tougas protocol. *Left,* Anterior and posterior images acquired at time 0, 1, 2, 3 (optional), and 4 hours. *Right,* TAC and results shown below. The percent geometric mean gastric emptying at 2 hours (112 min) was 44% (normal >40%) and at 4 hours (233 min) was 90% (normal >90%). The latter borderline value was considered normal.

than 30% more patients with gastroparesis than a 2-hour study. Normal values were established in 123 normal patients, the largest published normal gastric emptying database.

For research or clinical purposes, some centers have added additional time intervals, methodology, or quantification to the standardized protocol—for example, more frequent imaging to calculate a lag phase, generation of a TAC and its analysis, and calculation of other quantitative values. However, using the percent gastric emptying at the time points detailed in the Consensus Recommendations ensures that results are comparable among institutions.

The standardized meal includes an egg substitute (4 oz, equal to two whole eggs), two slices of bread, strawberry jam (30 g), and water (120 mL). After ingestion of the radiolabeled solid meal, images are acquired at ingestion and at 1, 2, and 4 hours.

Although a 4-hour study length might seem demanding on patient clinic flow, the standardized protocol can actually improve it. Multiple patients can be studied using one camera because total imaging time per patient is short—that is, 1-minute images at time 0, 1, 2, and 4 hours. It is not difficult to perform imaging on 5 or 6 patients on a single camera in a morning.

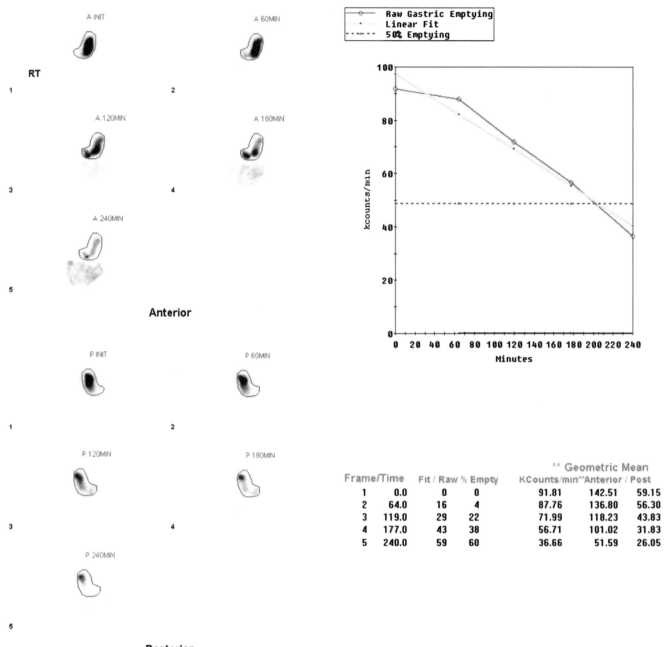

Frame/Time		Fit / Raw % Empty		KCounts/min^^Anterior / Post		^^ Geometric Mean
1	0.0	0	0	91.81	142.51	59.15
2	64.0	16	4	87.76	136.80	56.30
3	119.0	29	22	71.99	118.23	43.83
4	177.0	43	38	56.71	101.02	31.83
5	240.0	59	60	36.66	51.59	26.05

Figure 13-12. Delayed solid gastric emptying using the standardized protocol. At 2 hours (119 min), the percent gastric emptying is 22% (normal >40%) and 60% at 4 hours (240 min) (normal >90%).

Interpretation. A study is judged to be normal if the 2-hour and 4-hour values are greater than 40% emptying (<60% retention) and 90% emptying (<10% retention), respectively. The published protocol by Tougas and colleagues used "percent retention" for their normal values. This textbook uses "gastric emptying".

Normal values imply that the entire meal was ingested. Ingestion of a smaller volume of the meal, whether eggs, bread, jam, or water, would be expected to have more rapid emptying. Normal values have not been published for partial meal ingestion. Thus, a statement to this effect should be added to the interpretation—for example, "No obvious delay in emptying. However, because the patient did not ingest the entire meal, the study likely overestimates the rate of emptying. The normal values apply only to the specific described meal."

Delayed gastric emptying at either 2 or 4 hours is abnormal (Fig. 13-12). Most commonly, emptying is delayed at both 2 and 4 hours or normal at 2 hours and abnormal at 4 hours. However, some patients are abnormal at 2 hours but normal at 4 hours. The latter is not satisfactorily explained, but should be reported, because it is not normal and may be related to the patient's symptoms. The study can be stopped at 2 hours if the 4-hour normal values have been achieved. Some clinics also obtain images at 3 hours and thus can stop at that time if more than 90% emptying has occurred. Rapid emptying is considered to be greater than 70% emptying at 1 hour (Fig. 13-13).

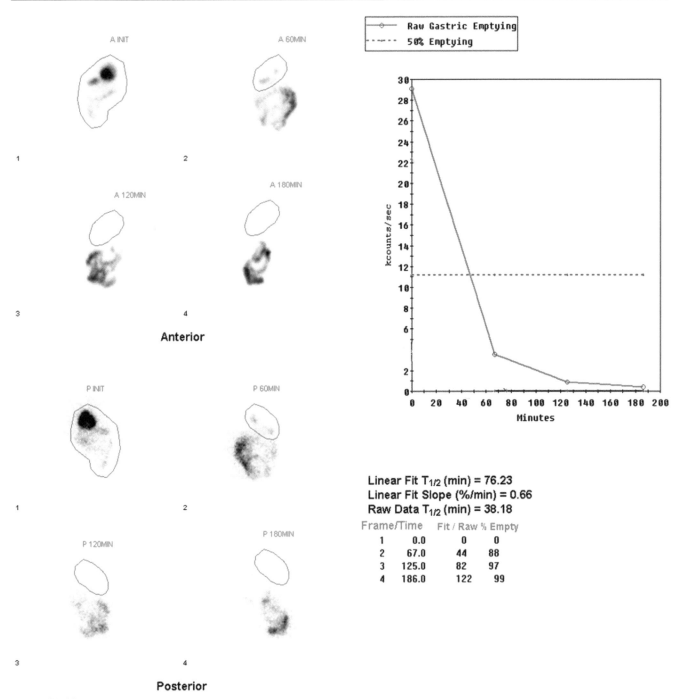

Linear Fit T$_{1/2}$ (min) = 76.23
Linear Fit Slope (%/min) = 0.66
Raw Data T$_{1/2}$ (min) = 38.18

Frame/Time		Fit / Raw % Empty	
1	0.0	0	0
2	67.0	44	88
3	125.0	82	97
4	186.0	122	99

FIGURE 13-13. Rapid solid gastric emptying. At 1 hour (67 min) solid gastric emptying is 88% (abnormal >70%). The initial (time 0) region of interest includes abdominal activity. Because of rapid emptying, there was transit to the small bowel by the first image. For accurate determination of the total ingested radiolabeled meal, the large region of interest is required for the first image only.

One published investigation reported that the 2-hour emptying value can predict 4-hour empting in more than 50% of patients. If at 2 hours gastric emptying is less than 35%, it can be interpreted as delayed and stopped, or if 55% or greater, it can be interpreted as normal, with an accuracy of 0.95 (Bonta et al, 2011).

Alternative Solid Meals

Some patients are allergic to eggs or will not eat them. Oatmeal and full liquids (e.g., milk) have been used; however, limited data exist on normal values for alternative meals. Clear liquids have been well documented, are described in the following section, and may be the best alternative.

Liquid Gastric Emptying

Clear liquid meals have been used, both as an alternative to a solid meal for patients not able to tolerate solids and as part of dual-isotope, dual-phase studies.

In the past, accepted teaching was that liquid studies were less sensitive for detection of gastroparesis than

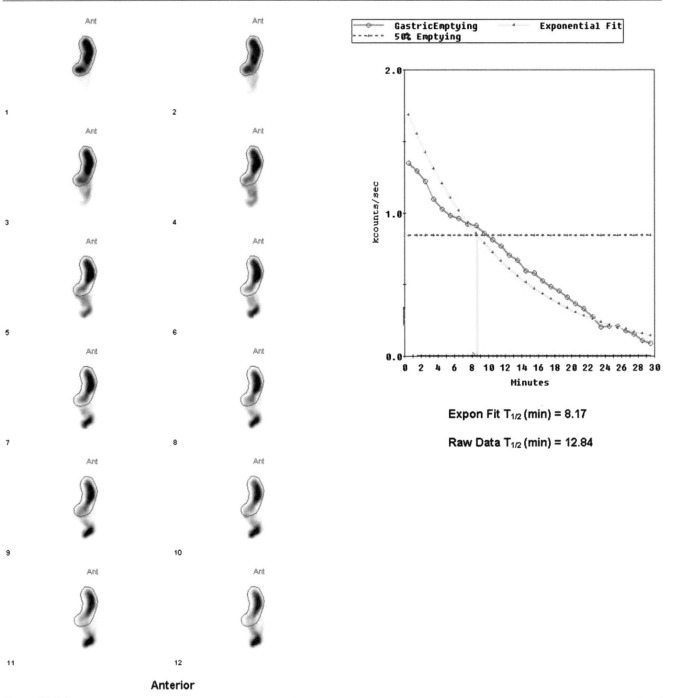

Anterior

FIGURE 13-14. Normal liquid (water) gastric emptying. Only the first 12 of 30 images are shown. A region of interest was drawn around the stomach and a TAC generated. An exponential $T_{1/2}$ fit *(yellow line)* was 8.17 min. The half time of emptying was 12.84 (normal <23 minutes). In theory, they should be the same. However, overlap of the region of interest with small bowel may prolong apparent emptying. Like all nuclear medicine studies quantification must be interpreted in conjunction with the images and regions of interest. In this case both results were in the normal range. *Expon,* Exponential.

solid studies and liquids become abnormal only in late stages of gastroparesis. Thus it has been repeatedly said that only solid gastric emptying is necessary for clinical purposes. This is not well documented and has proved erroneous.

Recent publications comparing clear liquid (water)–only studies with the solid gastric emptying standardized meal surprisingly found that liquid emptying detects more gastroparesis than the solid study. Some patients have normal solid and liquid studies, others delayed liquid and solid, some delayed solids and normal liquids, and, of importance, some patients have normal solid, but delayed liquid emptying. In patients with a normal solid study, 30% to 35% will have delayed liquid emptying.

The methodology for clear liquid–only studies is straightforward. Because liquids normally empty rapidly, only a 30-minute study is required (1-minute framing rate) (Figs. 13-14 and 13-15). Imaging begins immediately after ingestion of 300 mL water with 1 mCi Tc-99m DTPA. The methodology is detailed in Box 13-10. Solid and liquid

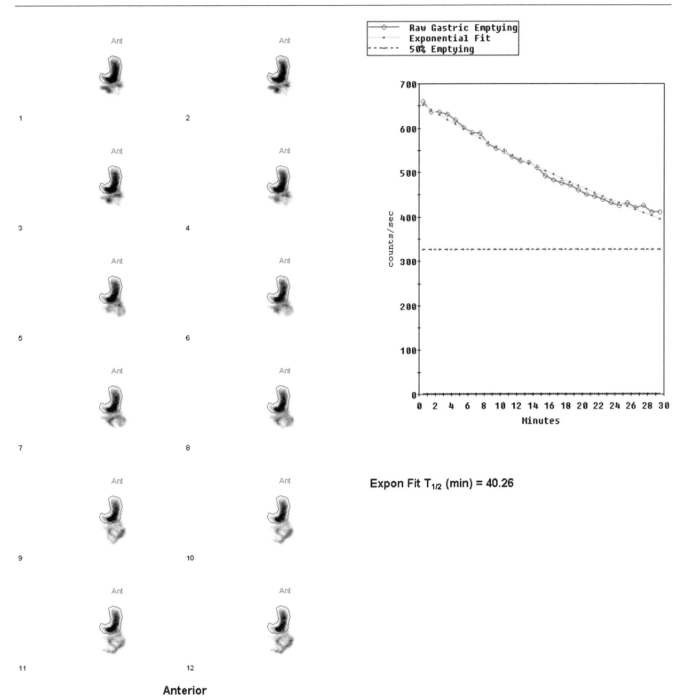

Expon Fit T$_{1/2}$ (min) = 40.26

Anterior

FIGURE **13-15.** Delayed clear liquid gastric emptying. Sequential 1-minute images with delayed emptying of water from the stomach. T$_{1/2}$ of >40 minutes (normal <23). Only the first 12 of 30 images are shown. *Expon*, Exponential.

studies can be performed sequentially on the same day, with the liquid first with In-111 DTPA, followed by the solid study with Tc-99m sulfur colloid.

Dual-Isotope Dual-Phase Gastric Emptying Studies

Simultaneous evaluation of liquid and solid gastric emptying is possible with dual-isotope studies (Fig. 13-10). Normal values are not necessarily identical to solid-only or liquid-only studies because the solid meal slows liquid emptying and the liquid can affect the rate of solid emptying. A recent dual isotope investigation reported delayed liquid emptying in approximately one fourth of patients with normal solid emptying.

Quantification of Gastric Emptying

Decay Correction. Correction for radioactive decay is mandatory for solid meals because of the short half-life of the Tc-99m radionuclide (6 hours) and the relatively long duration of the study (4 hours).

Attenuation Correction. The ingested meal transits the stomach, not only from superior to inferior and from left to right but also posterior to anterior. The latter occurs because the gastric fundus is relatively posterior to the

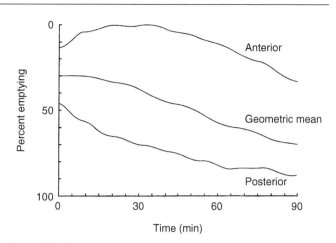

FIGURE 13-16. Geometric mean attenuation correction. The TACs of both anterior and posterior projections show the effect of attenuation. Anterior detector acquisition has a rising TAC before it begins to empty. The posterior detector curve shows decreasing counts from time zero. The geometric mean corrected curve has a normal pattern with an initial lag phase, then linear emptying.

is a mathematical correction for attenuation performed at each data point.

$$\text{Geometric mean} = \sqrt{(\text{Counts}_{\text{anterior}} \times \text{Counts}_{\text{posterior}})}$$

Left Anterior Oblique Method. An alternative to the geometric mean method for attenuation correction is to acquire the study in the left anterior oblique view. This compensates for attenuation because the head of the gamma camera is roughly parallel to the movement of the stomach contents; thus the effect of attenuation is minimized (Fig. 13-18). The advantages of this method are that it requires no mathematical correction, and a single-headed camera can be used. Results correlate well with those of the geometric mean method (Fig. 13-17); however, the geometric mean is the more accurate method.

Scatter Correction. With dual-isotope meals (e.g., In-111 DTPA in water and Tc-99m sulfur colloid as the solid meal marker), correction for downscatter (In-111 into the Tc-99m window) and upscatter (Tc-99m into the In-111 171 keV window) may be necessary. However, the error is inconsequential if the dose ratio of Tc-99m to In-111 is at least 4:1—true with recommended doses of Tc-99m 1 mCi and In-111 200 µCi.

Quantitative Analysis. Various methods for quantifying gastric emptying have been used. From a physiological standpoint, the length of the lag phase and a rate of emptying may be calculated. However, the clinical value of this information is not clear. Furthermore, more data points in addition to the standardized protocol would be necessary to make this accurate. This approach is mainly indicated for research purposes.

Standardized Solid Gastric Emptying Quantification
A stomach region of interest is drawn for all anterior and posterior views at each time point. Decay correction and attenuation correction should be performed. The percent emptying is calculated at each time point. Most commercial computer workstations now use a semiautomated methodology for calculation of the percent gastric

antrum. If a single camera detector is positioned anteriorly, increasing counts will be detected during the early portion of the study as the radiolabeled stomach contents move from the fundus to the antrum because of progressively less soft tissue attenuation. A rising TAC results, even though the amount of food in the stomach is unchanged (Fig. 13-16). This artifact of attenuation adversely affects the accuracy of quantification, resulting in an underestimation of emptying, between 10% and 30%, depending on patient size and anatomy (Fig. 13-17). It is usually more pronounced in obese patients, but it often occurs in nonobese patients and is not predictable before an individual study. Thus, attenuation correction should be routinely performed.

Geometric Mean Method. Although other methods of attenuation correction are possible, the geometric mean method is the gold standard and required by the Consensus Recommendations. Anterior and posterior views are acquired, preferably simultaneously using a dual-headed gamma camera. With a single-headed camera, they can be acquired sequentially. The geometric mean

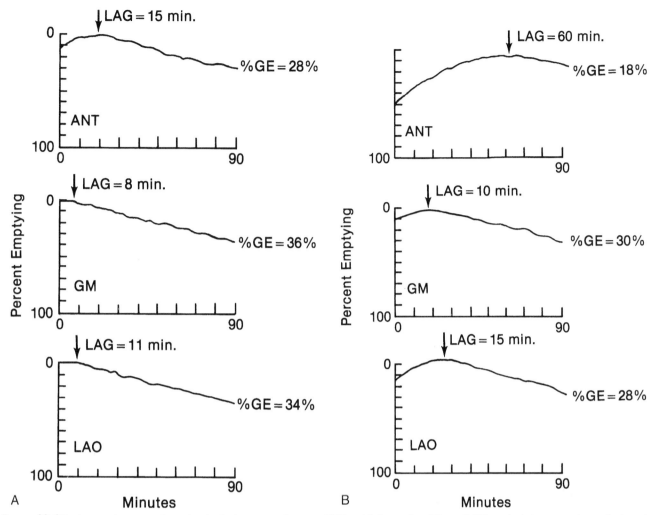

A

B

FIGURE 13-17. Attenuation correction using both the geometric mean *(GM)* and left anterior oblique *(LAO)* methods in two patients. **A,** Anterior detector–only acquisition TAC shows a moderate rise in counts over 15 minutes *(top).* GM correction *(middle)* has a shortened lag phase of 8 minutes and greater gastric emptying. LAO method *(bottom)* results are very similar to GM method. **B,** Anterior-only acquisition shows very long lag phase of 50 minutes *(top).* GM correction shortens the lag phase considerably, although there is still some initial rise, suggesting incomplete correction *(middle).* The percent gastric emptying is improved greatly. The LAO method shows similar results *(bottom).*

emptying (Figs. 13-14 to 13-16). The percent gastric emptying at each time point is calculated.

Liquid Gastric Emptying Quantification

A gastric region of interest is drawn, and a half-time of emptying (time in minutes when counts become half of peak counts) and/or an exponential mathematical fit $T_{1/2}$ is calculated (Figs. 13-17 and 13-18). Small bowel overlap in the region of interest may artificially elevate the emptying time. Excluding this overlap region from the region of interest will more accurately determine the rate of emptying. This will not adversely affect the $T_{1/2}$ because the entire stomach empties liquids at the same rate. Normal values for a clear liquid (water) study alone have been well validated, with a $T_{1/2}$ less than 23 minutes (mean ± 3 standard deviations).

▬ INTESTINAL TRANSIT SCINTIGRAPHY

Small and large intestinal transit scintigraphy are routinely performed at a minority of imaging clinics today, however, this will likely change in the future. A detailed review of

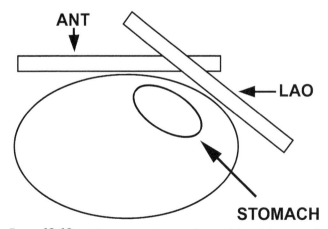

FIGURE 13-18. Left anterior oblique *(LAO)* acquisition. If the camera is placed in the LAO projection, the radiolabeled stomach contents move roughly parallel to the head of the gamma camera, compensating for the effect of varying attenuation. No mathematical correction for attenuation is required. See Figure 13-17. *ANT,* Anterior.

methodologies for intestinal transit studies is referenced. This section will provide a limited subject overview.

Small intestinal dysmotility presents with a wide range of clinical manifestations, including dyspepsia, postprandial epigastric or periumbilical abdominal pain, bloating, nausea, vomiting, and diarrhea. Many of these symptoms overlap with gastric transit abnormalities, although different therapy is required.

Colonic dysmotility symptoms include constipation, diarrhea, fecal incontinence, and lower abdominal pain. Several patterns of have been described, including isolated anal sphincter dysfunction (adult Hirschsprung disease), isolated rectosigmoid dysfunction, slow transit through the entire colon (colonic inertia and chronic intestinal pseudo-obstruction). Although pharmacological therapy may be helpful, differentiation of these patterns is important if a surgical approach is required.

Small Intestinal Transit Methodologies

Nonscintigraphic Methods

Nonradionuclide small bowel transit studies are not quantitative. Mixing barium contrast media with food and plotting its movement is an index of the transit rate. The meal is nonphysiological, and the radiation dosimetry is relatively high compared to scintigraphic methods.

The hydrogen breath test measures the hydrogen produced when a carbohydrate (carbon-14 lactose) is fermented by colonic bacteria. The test measures the transit time of the meal's leading edge from mouth to cecum, not bulk transit. The transit rate is affected by the rate of gastric emptying. Fermentative bacteria in the colon are required but absent in one quarter of the population.

Small Intestinal Scintigraphic Transit Methodology

Scintigraphic measurement of intestinal transit is less straightforward than gastric emptying. The radiolabeled meal must withstand the acid environment of the stomach and the alkaline milieu of the small intestine. With gastric emptying, all of the radiolabeled meal resides within the stomach at the start of acquisition and quantification depends only on how much or how fast it empties. With intestinal transit, a protracted infusion from the stomach occurs, with no identifiable time zero, thus making quantificiation more complex.

Small bowel transit can be measured by direct placement of the radiotracer by intubation at the site of the proximal small bowel. However, this is invasive and not usually practical. Transit is more commonly measured using an ingested liquid marker—for example, In-111 DTPA, with or without a solid meal. Images are acquired for 4 to 5 hours. The radiolabel spreads out as it moves through the small bowel. Identification of first accumulation in the cecum has been used to estimate the rate of small bowel transit (Fig. 13-19, A).

Large Intestinal Transit

Radiographic Methods

Cineradiography and fluoroscopy with radiopaque markers have been used to estimate colonic transit times. Interpretation is limited by the infrequent abdominal images and difficulty in determining the exact location of the markers because of overlap of large and small bowel. The study is not physiological and results in a relatively large radiation dose to the patient.

Large Bowel Transit Scintigraphy

In-111 DTPA is the most commonly used radiotracer. With oral ingestion, the study requires 72 to 96 hours. Gallium-67 citrate has also been used to measure both small and large intestinal transit. It is not absorbed from the bowel, and 98% of the dose is excreted in feces.

Radiopharmaceuticals have been investigated that do not breakdown before reaching the large bowel (e.g., radiolabeled cellulose fiber). An interesting approach is the use of In-111 polystyrene cation-exchange resin pellets placed in a gelatin capsule coated with a pH-sensitive polymer that resists disruption at pH levels of the stomach and proximal small bowel but breaks down at the ileocecal valve because of the increasing pH.

Quantification has been performed in several ways. One method seeks to determine the geometric center—that is, a weighted average of the counts in each region of the large bowel at specific time intervals over several days (Fig. 13-19, B).

▬ PROTEIN-LOSING ENTEROPATHY

Excessive protein loss through the gastrointestinal tract has been associated with a variety of diseases, including intestinal lymphangiectasia, Crohn disease, Ménétrier disease, amyloidosis, and intestinal fistula.

Tc-99m human serum albumin, In-111 transferrin, and Tc-99m dextran have all been successfully used to confirm protein-losing enteropathy. In-111 chloride binds in vivo to serum proteins, most notably transferrin, similar to Ga-67. Abdominal imaging can be used to visualize the protein leak. None of these radiopharmaceuticals are available commercially in the United States. Case reports suggest that Tc-99m methylene diphosphonate (MDP) bone scans can detect protein losing enteropathy.

▬ *HELICOBACTER PYLORI* INFECTION

The Nobel Prize in Medicine was awarded in 2005 for the discovery that ulcer disease is caused by *Helicobacter pylori*, a gram-negative bacterium. Antibiotic treatment often cures or greatly reduces the recurrence of duodenal and gastric ulcer disease. This was a major advance in therapy from the prior chronic medical treatment of symptoms and, in many cases, gastric surgery.

Urea Breath Test for *Helicobacter pylori*

In the presence of the bacterial enzyme urease, orally administered urea is hydrolyzed to carbon dioxide (CO_2) and ammonia. If the urea carbon is labeled with either the stable isotope carbon-13 or radioactive beta-emitter C-14, it can be detected in breath analysis as CO_2. *H. pylori* is the most common urease-containing gastric pathogen; thus a positive urea breath test is equated with infection.

The urea breath test is now widely available. This test is simple to perform, noninvasive, accurate, and inexpensive.

An onsite analyzer is not needed because an expired air-filled balloon can be mailed for breath gas analysis. Overall accuracy is high. False-negative results may occur with recent use of antibiotics or bismuth-containing medications. False-positive results occur in patients with achlorhydria, contamination with oral urease-containing bacteria, and colonization with another *Helicobacter* species, such as *H. felis*.

The initial diagnosis is usually made by gastric biopsy. The urea breath test is mostly used to determine the effectiveness of therapy against *H. pylori*. Serological tests cannot determine the effectiveness of therapy because the antibody titer falls too slowly to be diagnostically useful.

GASTROINTESTINAL BLEEDING

Effective therapy for acute gastrointestinal bleeding requires localization of the site of hemorrhage. History and examination often can distinguish upper from lower tract bleeding (i.e., melena vs. bright red rectal bleeding). Upper-tract hemorrhage can be confirmed with gastric intubation and localized with flexible fiberoptic endoscopy. Lower-tract bleeding is more problematic. Colonoscopy

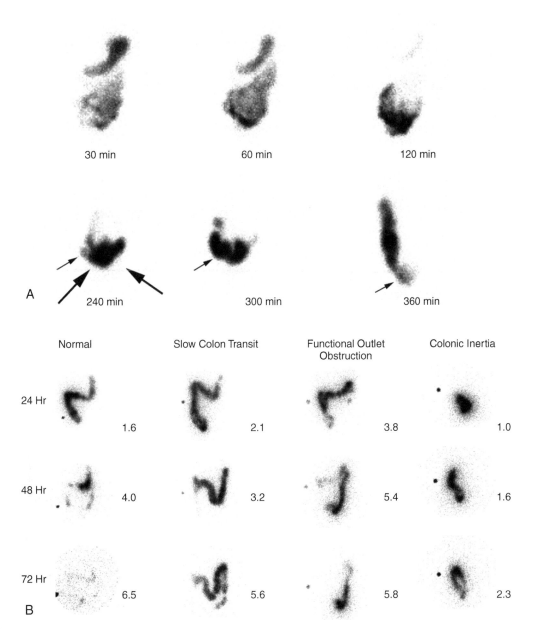

FIGURE 13-19. Intestinal transit scintigraphy. **A,** Small bowel transit. Leading edge transit analysis (In-111 DTPA, anterior view) is based on first visualization of cecum/ascending colon *(small arrows).* If activity does not progress into the cecum or ascending colon by 6 hours the amount of activity that has passed through the small bowel and fills the terminal ileum *(large arrows)* by 6 hours is measured (normal >40% of total administered activity). **B,** Colonic transit. Images at 24, 48, and 72 hours for analysis of segmental transit. Interpretation based on both visual inspection and quantification of the geometric center of activity. Three major abnormal diagnostic patterns are shown: generalized slow colon transit, functional rectosigmoid obstruction, and colon inertia. The geometric center calculation is to the right of each image. (Courtesy Alan Maurer, MD.)

and barium studies are of limited value during active hemorrhage.

Contrast Angiography

When positive, angiography is diagnostic. However, it is not helpful when negative. This means only that the patient is not actively bleeding at the time of the procedure. Because gastrointestinal bleeding is typically intermittent, clinical symptoms and signs of active bleeding are often unreliable for predicting whether the patient is bleeding at any one time point. Clinical signs of active hemorrhage often develop after bleeding has ceased.

Because repeated angiographic studies are not usually practical, angiographers are often the ones who request a radionuclide gastrointestinal bleeding study be performed before the invasive contrast study. The radionuclide study can (1) ensure that the patient is actively bleeding and (2) localize the site of bleeding to its likely vascular origin (e.g., celiac, superior, or inferior mesenteric arteries). This enables the angiographer to inject contrast promptly into the appropriate artery, limiting the duration of the study and the amount of contrast media required.

Radionuclide Scintigraphy

Technetium-99m Sulfur Colloid

Scintigraphy for gastrointestinal bleeding was first described in 1977 with the use of Tc-99m sulfur colloid. After intravenous injection of 10 mCi Tc-99m sulfur colloid, it is rapidly extracted from the blood (3-minute half-life) by reticuloendothelial cells of the liver, spleen, and bone marrow. With active bleeding, the radiotracer extravasates at the bleeding site into the bowel lumen, increasing with each recirculation of blood (Fig. 13-20). Continued extravasation with simultaneous background clearance results in a high target-to-background ratio, permitting visualization of the active bleeding site (Fig. 13-21).

Images are obtained over 20 to 30 minutes. Active hemorrhage is seen in the first 5 to 10 minutes of imaging. Detection of bleeding in the splenic flexure or transverse colon regions is complicated by intense normal liver and spleen uptake. The major disadvantage of the Tc-99m sulfur colloid method is that bleeding must be active at the time of injection, similar to angiography.

Tc-99m red blood cell (RBC) scintigraphy has largely replaced the Tc-99m sulfur colloid method. A large multicenter prospective study and other reports have shown a clear superiority of the Tc-99m RBC method.

Technetium-99m Red Blood Cells

The Tc-99m RBC method was first described in 1979. The major advantage over Tc-99 sulfur colloid is that images

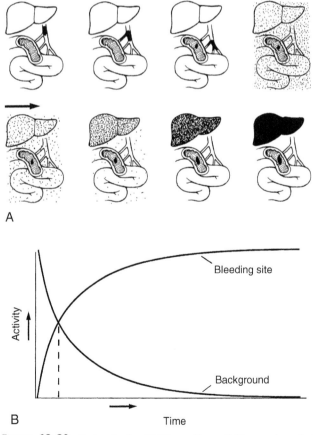

FIGURE 13-20. Rationale for Tc-99m sulfur colloid gastrointestinal bleeding study. **A,** After injection, Tc-99m sulfur colloid is cleared rapidly by the reticuloendothelial system, with a serum half-life of 3 minutes. Tc-99m sulfur colloid extravasates at the site of bleeding with each recirculation. Because of rapid background clearance, a high-contrast image results. **B,** TACs demonstrate rapid clearance of background and increasing activity at the bleeding site.

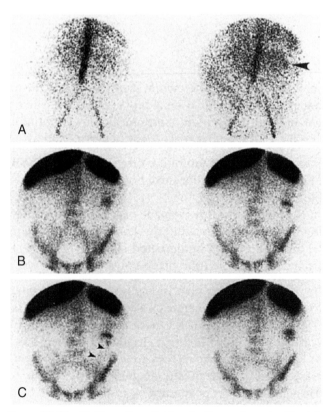

FIGURE 13-21. Tc-99m sulfur colloid study: Descending colon bleed. **A,** Two 3-second flow images; the second image indicates extravasation at the site of bleeding (*large arrowhead*). **B** and **C,** Four sequential 5-minute images confirm the site of bleeding. Images in **C** show movement to the more distal left colon (*small arrowheads*).

can be acquired for a longer length of time, limited only by the physical half-life of Tc-99m and the stability of the radiolabel, thus usually up to 24 hours. This increases the likelihood for detection of intermittent bleeding.

The target-to-background ratio and image quality increase with the increasing percent binding of Tc-99m to the RBCs. Free unlabeled Tc-99m pertechnetate is taken up by the salivary glands and gastric mucosa and secreted into the gastrointestinal tract. This potentially complicates interpretation. Thus good radiolabeling efficiency is important.

Red Blood Cell Radiolabeling Methods
RBC labeling requires that Tc-99m be reduced so that it can bind to the beta chain of the hemoglobin molecule. Stannous ion (tin) in the form of stannous chloride or pyrophosphate is used for this purpose. Various methodologies have been used over the years for labeling of RBCs with

---

Box 13-11. Methods of Technetium-99m Red Blood Cell Labeling

IN VIVO METHOD (LABELING EFFICIENCY, 75% TO 80%)
1. Inject stannous pyrophosphate.
2. Wait 10 to 20 minutes.
3. Inject Tc-99m sodium pertechnetate.

MODIFIED IN VIVO (IN VIVTRO) METHOD (LABELING EFFICIENCY, 85% TO 90%)
1. Inject stannous pyrophosphate.
2. Wait 10 to 20 minutes.
3. Withdraw 5 to 8 mL of blood into shielded syringe with Tc-99m.
4. Gently mix syringe contents for 10 minutes at room temperature.

IN VITRO (BROOKHAVEN) METHOD (LABELING EFFICIENCY, 98%)
1. Add 4 mL of heparinized blood to reagent vial of 2 mg Sn^{+2}, 3.67 mg Na citrate, 5.5 mg dextrose, and 0.11 mg NaCl.
2. Incubate at room temperature for 5 minutes.
3. Add 2 mL of 4.4% EDTA.
4. Centrifuge tube for 5 minutes at 1300 g.
5. Withdraw 1.25 mL of packed red blood cells and transfer to sterile vial containing Tc-99m.
6. Incubate at room temperature for 10 minutes.

IN VITRO COMMERCIAL KIT (ULTRA TAG) (LABELING EFFICIENCY, >97%) (FIG. 13-22)
1. Add 1 to 3 mL of blood (heparin or acid citrate dextrose as anticoagulant) to reagent vial (50-100 µg stannous chloride, 3.67 mg Na citrate) and mix. Allow 5 minutes to react.
2. Add syringe 1 contents (0.6 mg sodium hypochlorite) and mix by inverting four or five times.
3. Add contents of syringe 2 (8.7 mg citric acid, 32.5 mg Na citrate, dextrose) and mix.
4. Add Tc-99m 10 to 100 mCi (370-3700 MBq) to reaction vial.
5. Mix and allow to react for 20 minutes, with occasional mixing.

Tc-99m (Box 13-11). The in vivo and modified in vivo methods depend on biological clearance of undesirable extracellular reduced stannous ion.

In Vivo Method. Stannous pyrophosphate (15 µg/kg body weight) is injected intravenously. After 15 to 30 minutes, Tc-99m pertechnetate is injected. Both diffuse across the RBC membrane. The tin binds to hemoglobin and reduces the Tc-99m intracellularly.

Although the in vivo technique is simple, the labeling yield is not high, on the order of 80% but frequently as low as 60% to 65%. Free Tc-99m pertechnetate results in images with poor target-to-background ratios. In some cases, labeling may fail dramatically because of drug interactions or other causes (Table 13-4). Care should be taken not to inject through heparinized intravenous tubing. This labeling method is usually adequate for cardiac wall motion evaluation and ejection fraction calculation, but it is not adequate for gastrointestinal bleeding studies.

Modified In Vivo (In Vitro) Method. Stannous pyrophosphate is injected intravenously (Box 13-11). After 15 to 30 minutes, 3 to 5 mL of blood is withdrawn through an intravenous line into a shielded syringe containing Tc-99m pertechnetate and a small amount of anticoagulant, ACD solution, or heparin and agitated periodically. The syringe is left attached to the intravenous line during the procedure so that the entire system is closed. The contents of the syringe are then reinjected into the patient after 10 minutes. Labeling efficiency is approximately 85%.

Like with the in vivo method, drugs, intravenous solutions, and various clinical conditions may interfere with labeling efficiency. Heparin is the most common cause. It oxidizes the stannous ion and complexes with pertechnetate, thus reducing binding. Other causes are listed in Table 13-4.

In Vitro Method. As originally described, this method required drawing the patient's blood, centrifuging to separate the RBCs from serum, radiolabeling the RBCs, and then reinjecting. Labeling efficiency was very high. However, today a simple commercial kit method (UltraTag, Mallinckrodt, St. Louis, Mo.) is used (Box 13-11). Labeling efficiency

---

TABLE 13-4 Causes of Poor Technetium-99m Red Blood Cell Labeling

Drug	Mechanism or comment
Stannous ion	Too little or too much will result in poor labeling.
Heparin	A Tc-99m–labeled heparin complex may form when Tc-99m is injected through a heparinized catheter.
Methyldopa, hydralazine	Oxidation of stannous ion, diminution of reduction capacity.
Doxorubicin	Decreased labeling efficiency; effect related to drug concentration.
Quinidine	May increase production of antibodies to red blood cells.
Iodinated contrast	Multiple mechanisms: lowering of stannous reduction capacity, altering stannous distribution, competition for red blood cell binding sites, alterations in Tc-99m binding sites.

is greater than 97%. This method uses whole blood and does not require centrifugation or RBC transfer.

The patient's blood is withdrawn and added to a reaction vial containing stannous chloride (Fig. 13-22). The stannous ion diffuses across the RBC membrane and binds to the hemoglobin. Sodium hypochlorite is added to oxidize extracellular stannous ion to prevent extracellular reduction of Tc-99m pertechnetate. A sequestering agent removes extracellular stannous ion. Tc-99m pertechnetate is then added, which crosses the RBC membrane and is reduced by stannous ion in the cell. The mixture is incubated for 20 minutes before reinjection. This approach is less subject to drug-to-drug labeling interference and problems of excessive or deficient stannous ion, and it is simple for technologists to perform.

Technetium-99m Red Blood Cell Dosimetry

Radiation to the patient is relatively low compared with contrast angiography. The target organs for Tc-99m erythrocytes are the spleen and the myocardial wall. The whole-body dose for labeled erythrocytes is 0.4 rad/25 mCi (0.15 cG/925 MBq) (Table 13-5).

Image Acquisition Methodology

An imaging protocol is described in Box 13-12. The patient is imaged in the supine position and the camera placed

anteriorly. After intravenous injection, a flow study is acquired (1- to 2-second frames). One-minute images are acquired for 60 to 90 minutes. A static left lateral view of the pelvis is then obtained. It can help differentiate activity in the bladder from that in the rectum and occasionally from penile activity.

TABLE 13-5 Dosimetry for Technetium-99m Red Blood Cells and Tc-99m Pertechnetate (Meckel)

	Tc-99m RBCs (UltraTag) rad/20 mCi (cGy/740 MBq)	Tc-99m pertechnetate (Meckel) rad/5 mCi (cGy/185 MBq)
Heart wall	2.0	0.650 (0.130)
Thyroid		
Bladder wall	0.48	0.265 (0.053)
Spleen	2.2	
Blood	0.80	1.250 (0.250)
Stomach wall		
Liver	0.58	
Red marrow	0.30	0.095 (0.019)
Ovaries	0.32	0.110 (0.022)
Testes	0.22	0.045 (0.009)
Large intestine		0.340 (0.068)
Total body	0.3	0.070 (0.014)
Effective dose	0.518	0.390*

*From U.S. Food and Drug Administration–approved package inserts.
RBCs, Red blood cells.

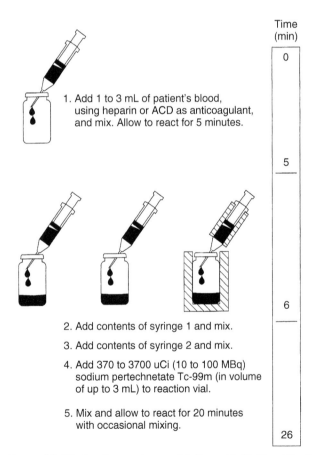

1. Add 1 to 3 mL of patient's blood, using heparin or ACD as anticoagulant, and mix. Allow to react for 5 minutes.

2. Add contents of syringe 1 and mix.

3. Add contents of syringe 2 and mix.

4. Add 370 to 3700 uCi (10 to 100 MBq) sodium pertechnetate Tc-99m (in volume of up to 3 mL) to reaction vial.

5. Mix and allow to react for 20 minutes with occasional mixing.

Time (min): 0, 5, 6, 26

Figure 13-22. In vitro erythrocyte labeling with Tc-99m (UltraTag RBC). Each kit consists of three nonradioactive components: a 10-mL vial containing stannous chloride, syringe 1 containing sodium hypochlorite, and syringe 2 containing citric acid, sodium citrate, and dextrose *(ACD)*. Typical labeling efficiency is greater than 97%.

> ### Box 13-12. Technetium-99m Red Blood Cell Scintigraphy for Gastrointestinal Bleeding: Summary Protocol
>
> **PATIENT PREPARATION**
> None
>
> **RADIOPHARMACEUTICAL**
> Tc-99m–labeled red blood cells
>
> **INSTRUMENTATION**
> Gamma camera: Large-field-of-view
> Collimator: High resolution, parallel hole.
> Computer setup: 1-second frames for 60 seconds;
>   1-minute frames for 60 to 90 minutes.
> As needed up to 24 hours: Delayed image sequence
>   as 1-minute frames for 30 minutes.
>
> **PATIENT POSITION**
> Supine; anterior imaging, with abdomen and pelvis in
>   field of view.
>
> **IMAGING PROCEDURE**
> Inject patient's Tc-99m–labeled erythrocytes intravenously.
> Acquire flow images, followed by static images for 60
>   to 90 minutes.
> Acquire image of neck for thyroid and salivary uptake
>   and left lateral view of pelvis.
> If study is negative or bleeding is recurrent, may
>   repeat 30-minute acquisitions.

If the study is not diagnostic, delayed imaging can be obtained for up to 24 hours. These should always be acquired at the same framing rate and generally for 30 minutes.

Image Interpretation

The purpose of this exam is to determine if bleeding is active as well as the likely site of bleeding. Both are

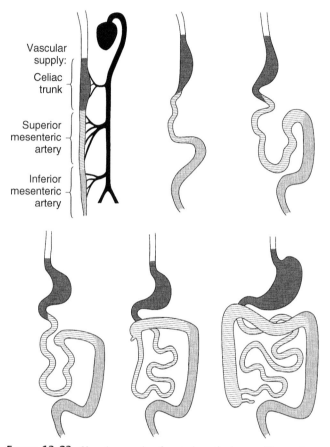

FIGURE 13-23. Vascular supply of gastrointestinal tract. The embryological development of the gastrointestinal tract explains its anatomical configuration and its vascular distribution. This schematic diagram also relates the gastrointestinal anatomy to its arterial supply (celiac, superior mesenteric, and inferior mesenteric arteries).

important to the angiographer. If the scintigraphic study is negative, angiography is likely to be negative as well. Because intestinal anatomy is complex due to its embryological development (Fig. 13-23) and scintigraphic image resolution is limited, review of the 1-minute frames displayed dynamically on computer can aid in pinpointing the vascular origin of the bleed.

Excessive gastric, thyroid, and soft tissue background activity suggests poor labeling. Imaging of the neck (thyroid, salivary glands) and stomach can confirm free Tc-99m pertechnetate. Bladder filling with Tc-pertechnetate or other reduced Tc-99m compound may make it difficult to see adjacent rectal bleeding. This is where the left lateral view can be helpful.

Rapid hemorrhage may occasionally be seen on the flow phase; however, it is most helpful when bleeding is not active—for example, in detection of a vascular blush resulting from angiodysplasia or tumor (Fig. 13-24). Flow can also confirm vascular structures (e.g., kidneys, ectatic vessels, or uterus), thus helping with image interpretation on later images.

More than 80% of bleeding sites are detected during the initial 90-minute study (Figs. 13-25 to 13-27). Because bleeding is intermittent, further delayed imaging may be necessary and can be quite helpful. The timing will depend on the patient's condition and the logistics of the clinic.

Diagnostic Criteria. Specific standard criteria must be used to avoid incorrect interpretations (Box 13-13): Radiotracer activity must appear where there was none before, increase over time, and move in a pattern consistent with intestinal anatomy, antegrade and/or retrograde. Fixed activity should not be diagnosed as an active bleeding site and is likely the result of a vascular structure—for example, hemangioma, accessory spleen, or ectopic kidney.

Large intestinal bleeds typically appear as relatively linear activity moving along the periphery of the abdomen in the expected anatomical pattern (Figs. 13-25 and 13-26). The small bowel is more centrally located, and blood moves rapidly through its curvilinear looping segments (Fig. 13-27). Small intestinal bleeds can sometimes

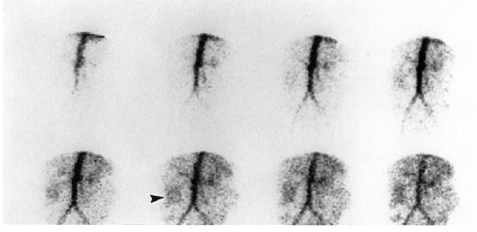

FIGURE 13-24. Positive blood flow: No active bleeding. Increased focal flow (3-second frames) to the region of the ascending colon *(arrowhead).* The 90-minute Tc-99m RBC study was negative, as well as a second acquisition for 30 minutes at 3 hours. Colonoscopy with biopsy diagnosed colon cancer in the ascending colon.

be hard to localize and may be first be detected by pooling of radiotracer in the cecum.

Scintigraphy has limitations in exact anatomical localization; however, a bleeding site can usually be localized to the proximal or distal small bowel, cecum, ascending colon, hepatic flexure, transverse colon, splenic flexure, descending colon, sigmoid colon, or rectum. This information can help the angiographer determine which vessel (celiac, superior mesenteric, or inferior mesenteric artery) to inject first with contrast.

Although the radionuclide bleeding study is not indicated for upper gastrointestinal bleeding, the first indication of such a bleed is sometimes seen on a study ordered for a suspected lower gastrointestinal bleed. Gastric hemorrhage must be differentiated from free Tc-99m pertechnetate. With both, gastric activity will transit to the small bowel and eventually the large bowel. Images of the thyroid and salivary glands can help confirm or exclude free Tc-99m pertechnetate as the likely source of the gastric activity.

Pitfalls. Pitfalls are defined as normal, technical, or pathological findings that could be misinterpreted as active hemorrhage (Box 13-14). The presence of free Tc-99m

pertechnetate caused by poor radiolabeling or dissociation of the label in vivo would be considered a technical pitfall. A common pitfall is focal activity in the genitourinary tract. Urinary renal pelvic or ureteral activity resulting from free pertechnetate or another Tc-99m–labeled reduced compound might be wrongly thought to be active bleeding. Upright positioning and oblique or posterior views may be helpful to clarify the source of activity.

Activity seen in the region of the bladder in the anterior view can be misinterpreted. This can be due to rectal bleeding, uterine activity with menses, and normal penile blood pool. A left lateral or left anterior oblique view is essential for making the correct interpretation (Figs. 13-28 and 13-29).

Intraluminal radioactivity first detected on delayed static images can pose a diagnostic dilemma. Activity in the sigmoid colon or rectum seen on delayed images (e.g., 8 to 24 hours), may have originated from anywhere in the gastrointestinal tract. Misinterpretation can be avoided by acquiring dynamic 1-minute images for 30 minutes when delayed imaging is required. An active bleeding site should be diagnosed only by using the criteria described (Box 13-14).

Other potential pitfalls include abdominal varices, hemangiomas, accessory spleen, arterial grafts, aneurysms,

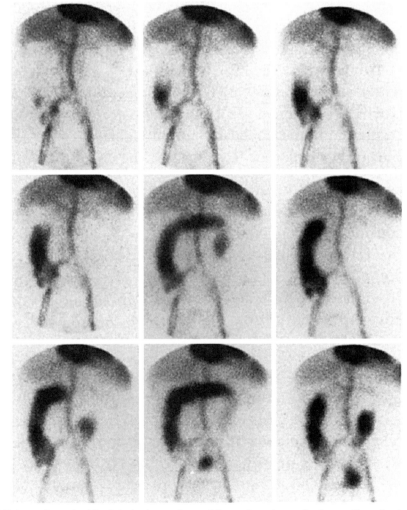

Figure 13-25. Tc-99m RBC: Ascending colon bleed. Active hemorrhage originates from the proximal ascending colon in the region of the cecum, then transits the transverse colon and enters the left colon and rectosigmoid region by the end of the 60-minute study.

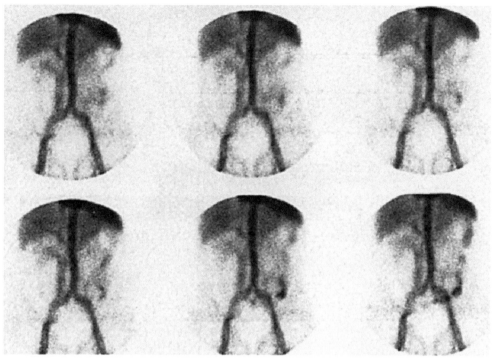

FIGURE 13-26. Tc-99m RBC: Left colonic bleed. Dynamic summed images acquired over 60 minutes show increasing activity in the region of the descending colon, which moves proximally to the splenic flexure and distally to the sigmoid colon.

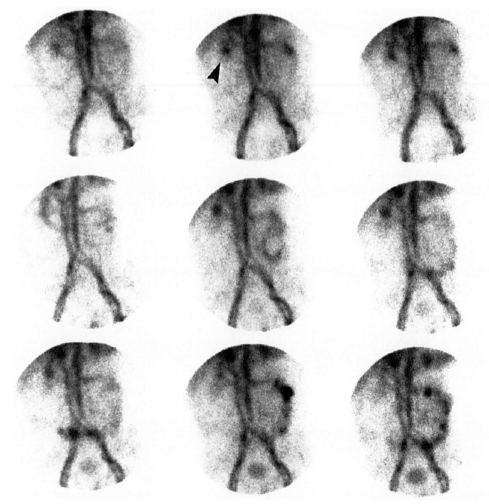

FIGURE 13-27. Tc-99m RBC: Duodenal bleed. Active bleeding is initially seen in the region of the duodenum *(arrowhead)*, and sequential images show transit through the small intestines.

ectopic kidneys, and renal transplants, all of which show fixed and nonmoving activity (Fig. 13-30). Activity clearing through the hepatobiliary system and gallbladder may be related to a rare hemobilia; however, patients with renal failure may have gallbladder visualization as a result of radiolabeled fragmented heme breakdown products (porphyrins). **Accuracy.** Only 2 to 3 mL of extravasated blood is required for scintigraphic detection. In experimental studies, bleeding rates of 0.05 to 0.1 mL/min could be detected, comparing favorably with contrast angiography, which is able to detect bleeding rates of 1 mL/min or greater, a 10-fold difference.

Many investigations over the years have reported high accuracy for radionuclide gastrointestinal bleeding scintigraphy; however, others have reported poorer accuracy

and have not found the study helpful (Table 13-6). Thus controversy exists regarding its clinical utility.

The reasons for this discrepancy in reported accuracy of localization are several. Misinterpretation may be from poor methodology—for example, infrequent image acquisition, described pitfalls, and incorrect localization based on single delayed images. Whether the patients had the radionuclide bleeding study early in the course of their workup or only after hospitalization with extensive negative radiological and endoscopic evaluation is a critical factor for detecting active bleeding. The radionuclide study will have the highest yield when performed as soon as possible after arrival in the emergency room or on admission.

The gold standard has been a problem in these investigations. The majority of patients do not get angiography. False negatives occur because the patient is not actively bleeding at the time of the study. Colonoscopy is often not possible during active bleeding. Detection of pathological abnormalities on radiographic studies or colonoscopy after bleeding has ceased does not necessarily indicate that they were the source of bleeding.

In spite of these factors, the majority of investigations have found the gastrointestinal bleeding study to be accurate in bleeding site localization and clinically useful. A telling point is that angiographers are the ones at many institutions that demand scintigraphy before their invasive procedure. Being readily available and having good communication with referring physicians is critical for success.

■ HETEROTOPIC GASTRIC MUCOSA

Meckel diverticulum is the most common and clinically important form of heterotopic gastric mucosa. The terminology frequently used is *ectopic gastric mucosa;* however, it is not truly correct. *Ectopic* refers to an organ that has migrated—for example, ectopic kidney. *Heterotopic* refers to a tissue at its site of origin. For example, other manifestations of heterotopic gastric mucosa are in gastrointestinal duplications, postoperative retained gastric antrums, and Barrett esophagus.

Radiopharmaceutical

Tc-99m pertechnetate has been used since 1970 to diagnose heterotopic gastric mucosa, most commonly Meckel diverticulum, as the cause of gastrointestinal bleeding in a child. Other types of heterotopic gastric mucosa have been diagnosed and localized with the study.

Mechanism of Uptake

The mucosa of the gastric fundus contains a variety of cell types (e.g., parietal cells, which secrete hydrochloric acid and intrinsic factor, and chief cells, which secrete pepsinogen. The gastric antrum and pylorus contain G cells that secrete the hormone gastrin. Columnar mucin-secreting epithelial cells are found throughout the stomach. They excrete an alkaline juice that protects the mucosa from the highly acidic gastric fluid.

Parietal cells were originally thought to be solely responsible for Tc-99m pertechnetate gastric mucosal uptake and secretion. However, experimental evidence points to the mucin-secreting cells as important. Tc-99m pertechnetate

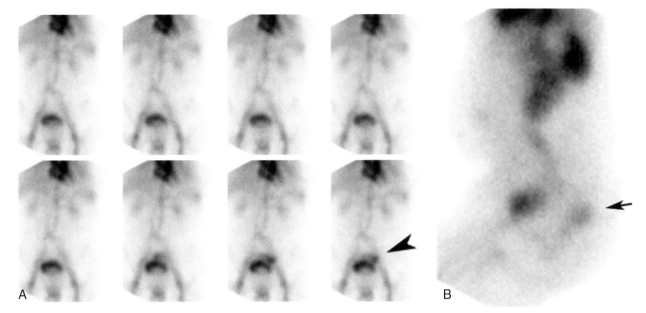

FIGURE 13-28. Tc-99m RBC: rectal bleed. **A,** The last three of the 1-minute images show increasing activity just superior and to the left of the bladder *(arrowhead),* very suggestive of rectosigmoid colon bleed. **B,** Left lateral view. Blood is confirmed to be in the rectum *(arrow).*

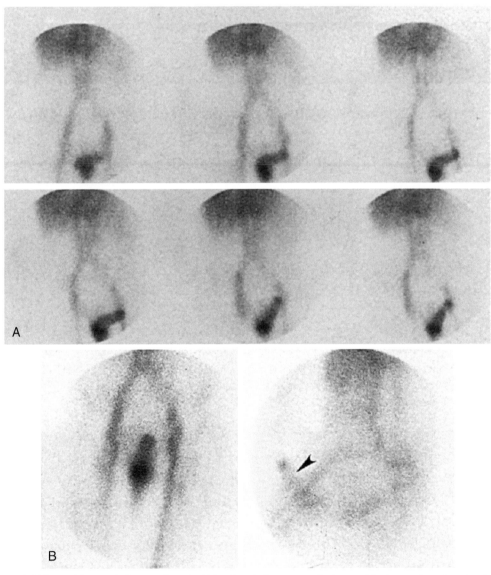

FIGURE 13-29. Potential false positive result for gastrointestinal bleeding. **A,** Images acquired every 10 minutes show changing, increasing activity in the lower left and middle pelvic region. **B,** Anterior *(left)* and left lateral *(right)* images acquired 90 minutes after tracer injection show the activity to be the penile blood pool *(arrowhead).* Left lateral views should be obtained when pelvic activity is seen, to separate rectal, bladder, and penile activity.

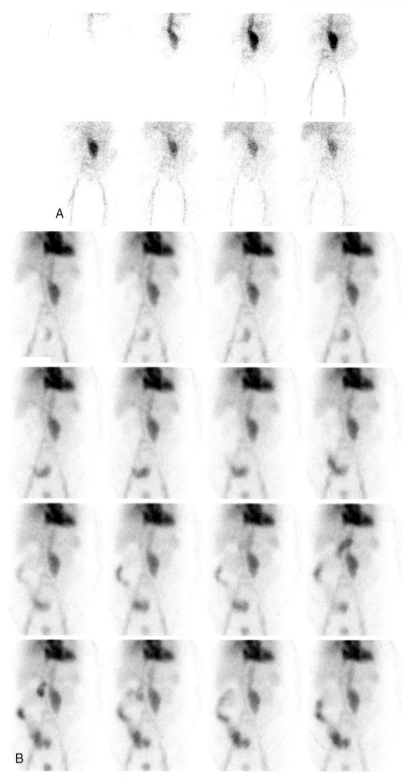

FIGURE 13-30. Aortic aneurysm and acute bleed. **A,** Flow study demonstrates activity retained in the distal aorta in a fusiform configuration. **B,** On dynamic imaging over 60 minutes, an acute bleed is seen to originate in the mid lower pelvis, moving with time to the ascending and transverse colon, most consistent with a cecal bleed. An abdominal aortic aneurysm showed persistent activity throughout the study. The fixed activity suggests that this is not active bleeding.

TABLE **13-6** Correct Localization of Gastrointestinal Bleeding with Technetiumc-99m Red Blood Cells

First author	Year	No. scans	% Positive	% Correct
Suzman	1996	224	51	96
Orechhia	1985	76	34	94
O'Neill	2000	26	96	88
Emslie	1996	75	28	88
Leitman	1989	28	43	86
Bearn	1992	23	78	82
Dusold	1984	74	59	75
Rantis	1995	80	47	73
Van Geelen	1994	42	57	69
Nicholson	1989	43	72	67
Hunter	1990	203	26	58
Bentley	1991	182	60	52
Garofalo	1997	161	49	19
Voeller	1991	111	22	0

uptake has been found in gastric tissue with no parietal cells, and autoradiographic studies have shown uptake in the mucin cell.

Dosimetry

The target organ for Tc-99m pertechnetate is the stomach, followed by the thyroid gland (Table 13-5).

Meckel Diverticulum

The most common congenital anomaly of the gastrointestinal tract is Meckel diverticulum. It occurs in 1% to 3% of the population. It results from failure of closure of the omphalomesenteric duct in the embryo. The duct connects the yolk sac to the primitive foregut through the umbilical cord. This true diverticulum arises on the antimesenteric side of the small bowel, usually 80 to 90 cm proximal to the ileocecal valve. It is typically 2 to 3 cm in size but may be considerably larger.

Heterotopic gastric mucosa is present in 10% to 30% of patients with Meckel diverticulum, in 60% of symptomatic patients, and in 98% of those with bleeding (Box 13-15).

Clinical Manifestations

Gastric mucosal secretions can cause peptic ulceration of the diverticulum or adjacent ileum, producing pain, perforation, or bleeding. More than 60% percent of patients with complications of Meckel diverticulum are under age 2. Bleeding from Meckel diverticulum after age 40 is very unusual, but it does occur.

Diagnosis

Meckel diverticulum can be missed on small bowel radiography because it has a narrow or stenotic ostium, fills poorly, and has rapid emptying. Angiography is useful only with brisk active bleeding and rarely used. The Tc-99m pertechnetate scan is considered the standard method for preoperative diagnosis of a Meckel diverticulum.

BOX **13-15.** Epidemiology of Meckel Diverticulum

1% to 3% incidence in the general population.
50% occur by age 2 years.
10% to 30% have ectopic gastric mucosa.
25% to 40% are symptomatic; 50% to 67% of these have ectopic gastric mucosa.
95% to 98% of patients with bleeding have ectopic gastric mucosa.

BOX **13-16.** Meckel Diverticulum: Summary Protocol

PATIENT PREPARATION
Fasting 4 to 6 hours before study to reduce size of stomach.
No pretreatment with sodium perchlorate; may be given after completion of study.
No barium studies should be performed within 3 to 4 days of scintigraphy.
Void before, during if possible, and after study.

PREMEDICATION
Optional: Cimetidine 20 mg/kg orally starting 24 hours before study and last taken 1 hour before study.

RADIOPHARMACEUTICAL
Tc-99m pertechnetate
   Children: 30-100 uCi/kg (1.1-3.7 MBq/kg)
      Minimum Dose: 200 uCi (7.4 MBq)
   Adults: 5 to 10 mCi (185-370 MBq) intravenously

INSTRUMENTATION
Gamma camera: Large field of view
Collimator: Low energy, all purpose or high resolution.

PATIENT POSITION
Position patient supine under camera with xiphoid to symphysis pubis in field of view

IMAGING PROCEDURE
Obtain flow images: 60 1-second frames.
Obtain static images: 500k counts for first image, others for same time every 5 to 10 minutes for 1 hour.
Erect, right lateral, posterior, or oblique views may be helpful at 30 to 60 minutes.
Obtain postvoid image.

Methodology

A standard protocol is described in Box 13-16. Patient preparation is important. Barium studies should not be performed for several days before scintigraphy because attenuation by the contrast material may prevent lesion detection. Procedures such as colonoscopy or laxatives that irritate the intestinal mucosa can result in Tc-99m pertechnetate uptake and should be avoided. Some drugs (e.g., ethosuximide [Zarontin]) may cause unpredictable uptake.

A full stomach or urinary bladder may obscure a Meckel diverticulum; thus fasting for 2 to 4 hours before the study or continuous nasogastric aspiration to decrease stomach size is recommended. The patient should void before the study and at the end before imaging.

Potassium perchlorate should *not* be used to block thyroid uptake because it will also block uptake of Tc-99m pertechnetate by the gastric mucosa. It may be administered after the study to wash out the radiotracer from the thyroid and thus minimize radiation exposure.

Pharmacological Augmentation

Various pharmacological maneuvers have been used to improve the detection of Meckel diverticulum, including cimetidine, pentagastrin, and glucagon.

Cimetidine. The histamine H_2-receptor antagonist cimetidine increases uptake of Tc-99m pertechnetate by inhibiting its release from the gastric mucosa. No large or controlled studies have been done to validate its overall diagnostic utility; however, many recommend its routine use because of its assumed effectiveness and lack of significant risks or side effects. Others reserve its use for a patient with a suspected false negative Tc-99m pertechnetate scan for Meckel diverticulum. The usual dose is 20 mg/kg orally for 2 days before the study.

Pentagastrin and Glucagon. Pentagastrin increases the rapidity, duration, and intensity of Tc-99m pertechnetate uptake. Glucagon has antiperistaltic effect and is used with pentagastrin to decrease bowel peristalsis to prevent tracer washout from a diverticulum. Pentagastrin is associated with significant side effects and no longer available in the United States.

Image Interpretation

Meckel diverticulum appears as a focal area of increased intraperitoneal activity, usually in the right lower quadrant (Fig. 13-31). Tc-99m pertechnetate uptake is seen within 5 to 10 minutes after injection, and increases over time, usually at a rate similar to that of normal gastric uptake.

Lateral or oblique views can help confirm the anterior position of the diverticulum versus the posterior location of renal or ureteral activity. Upright views may distinguish fixed activity (e.g., duodenum, from ectopic gastric mucosa, which moves inferiorly); this also serves to empty renal pelvic activity. The intensity of activity may fluctuate because of intestinal secretions, hemorrhage, or increased motility washing out radiotracer. Postvoid images can empty the renal collecting system and aid in visualization of areas adjacent to the bladder.

Accuracy

False negative studies can result from poor technique, washout of the secreted Tc-99m pertechnetate, or lack of sufficient gastric mucosa. Small diverticula may not be detectable by scintigraphy. An impaired diverticular blood supply from intussusception, volvulus, or infarction can give false negative study results.

The reported accuracy of Meckel scintigraphy is high. One large study reported results in 954 patients (mostly

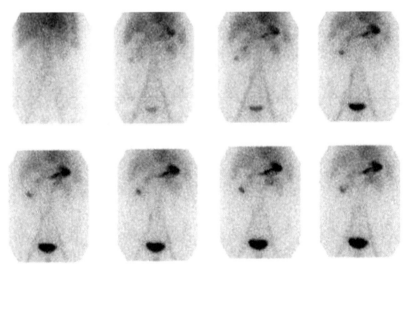

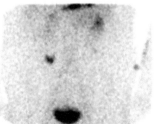

FIGURE 13-31. Meckel diverticulum. Child with rectal bleeding Sequential images show focal accumulation in the right mid to upper abdomen. Surgery confirmed this to be a Meckel diverticulum. Note simultaneous progressive uptake in the stomach and the Meckel diverticulum. Delayed static image *(below)* confirms the diagnosis.

children) who had undergone scintigraphy for suspected Meckel diverticulum using modern imaging methods and found an overall sensitivity of 85% and specificity of 95%. Detection in adults has a somewhat poorer sensitivity than in children.

Causes for false positive study results are listed in Box 13-17. Activity in the genitourinary tract is the most common cause for false positive study results (Fig. 13-32). Other false positives include tumors and inflammatory or obstructive lesions of the intestines.

Gastrointestinal Duplications

Duplications are cystic or tubular congenital abnormalities that have a mucosa, smooth muscle, and alimentary epithelial lining attached to any part of the gastrointestinal tract, but often the ileum. Most are symptomatic by age 2 years. Twenty percent occur in the mediastinum. Heterotopic gastric mucosa occurs in 30% to 50% of duplications.

The diagnosis is usually made at surgery. Rarely, a preoperative diagnosis is made by barium radiography or ultrasonography. Duplications often appear on scintigraphy as

---

Box 13-17. Causes for False Positive Results in Meckel Scan

URINARY TRACT
Ectopic kidney
Extrarenal pelvis
Hydronephrosis
Vesicoureteral reflux
Horseshoe kidney
Bladder diverticulum

VASCULAR
Arteriovenous malformation
Hemangioma
Aneurysm of intraabdominal vessel
Angiodysplasia

OTHER AREAS OF ECTOPIC GASTRIC MUCOSA
Gastrogenic cyst
Enteric duplication
Duplication cysts
Barrett esophagus
Retained gastric antrum

Pancreas
Duodenum
Colon

HYPEREMIA AND INFLAMMATORY
Peptic ulcer
Crohn disease
Ulcerative colitis
Abscess
Appendicitis
Colitis

NEOPLASM
Carcinoma of sigmoid colon
Carcinoid
Lymphoma
Leiomyosarcoma

SMALL BOWEL OBSTRUCTION
Intussusception
Volvulus

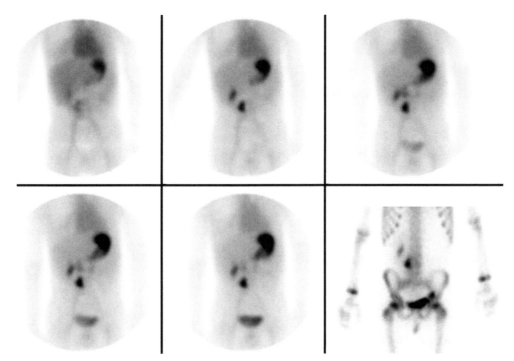

FIGURE 13-32. Meckel scan: False positive. Sequential images show 2 foci of activity to the right of midline that progressively increase with time (and with bladder activity). A bone scan done 6 months before this study showed a similar pattern consistent with renal clearance. This patient has crossed-fused ectopia.

large, multilobulated areas of increased activity. Mediastinal gastrointestinal cysts can be preoperatively confirmed with Tc-99m pertechnetate scintigraphy.

Retained Gastric Antrum

The gastric antrum may be left behind in the afferent loop after a Billroth II gastrojejunostomy. The antrum continues to produce gastrin, no longer inhibited by acid in the stomach because it is diverted through the gastrojejunostomy. The high acid production leads to marginal ulcers.

Endoscopy or barium radiography may demonstrate the retained gastric antrum. A Tc-99m pertechnetate scan can be confirmatory. Uptake in the gastric remnant is seen as a collar of radioactivity in the duodenal stump of the afferent loop. The retained antrum usually lies to the right of the gastric remnant. In one series, uptake was seen in 16 of 22 patients with a retained antrum.

Barrett Esophagus

Chronic gastroesophageal reflux can cause the distal esophagus to become lined by gastric columnar epithelium rather than the usual esophageal squamous epithelium. This condition, known as Barrett esophagus, is associated with complications of ulcers, strictures, and an 8.5% incidence of esophageal adenocarcinoma.

Tc-99m pertechnetate scans show intrathoracic uptake contiguous with that of the stomach but conforming to the shape and posterior location of the esophagus. Today the diagnosis is usually made with endoscopy and mucosal biopsy.

▬ PERITONEAL SCINTIGRAPHY

Peritoneal scintigraphy has been used over the years for various indications, to evaluate peritoneal distribution for planned intraperitoneal chemotherapy, to detect pleural–peritoneal communications (e.g., as cause for pleural effusion), to assess peritoneal shunt patency, and to evaluate problems that occur with peritoneal dialysis.

Peritoneal scintigraphy can diagnose pleura–peritoneal and scrotal–peritoneal communications, hepatic hydrothorax, traumatic diaphragmatic rupture, loculation of chemotherapy or peritoneal dialysis catheter flow, and obstructed Leveen or Denver peritoneal–venous shunts. A typical protocol is described in Box 13-18.

Both Tc-99m sulfur colloid and Tc-99m macroaggregated albumin (MAA) have been used because they do not diffuse through peritoneal surfaces. Tc-99m sulfur colloid is taken up by the liver and Tc-99 MAA by the lungs. Both radiopharmaceuticals will stay below the diaphragm unless

---

Box 13-18. Peritoneal Scintigraphy: Summary Protocol

PATIENT PREPARATION
Place peritoneal catheter access
Patients with minimal ascites may benefit from 500 mL of saline or other fluid infused into the peritoneal cavity before the study
Patients on peritoneal dialysis should have 500 mL dialysate infused before study. They should have 100 mL dialysate with them for infusion after intraperitonal injection of radiotracer

RADIOPHARMACEUTICAL
Tc-99m sulfur colloid or Tc-99m MAA, 3 mCi (111 MBq)

INSTRUMENTATION
Gamma camera: Large field of view
Energy window: 20% window centered at 140 keV
Collimator: Low energy, parallel hole

PATIENT POSITION
Position patient supine under gamma camera

PROCEDURE
Check catheter patency before radiopharmaceutical injection.
Inject the radiopharmaceutical slowly in approximately 10 mL saline followed by fluid flush.

IMAGING
Obtain anterior and lateral static images for 5 minutes (128 × 128) or 500k counts
Have patient ambulate if possible; alternatively turn from side to side.
Repeat imaging 1 hour after injection.

INTERPRETATION
Radiopharmaceutical should normally distribute throughout the peritoneal cavity, although usually inhomogeneously.

MAA, Macroaggregated albumin.

a pleural–scrotal connection or a patent shunt is present (Fig. 13-33). For purposes of chemotherapy, it can confirm good distribution throughout the peritoneum. To judge peritoneal venous shunt patency, Tc-99m MAA has the advantage of being taken up by the lungs, confirming patency.

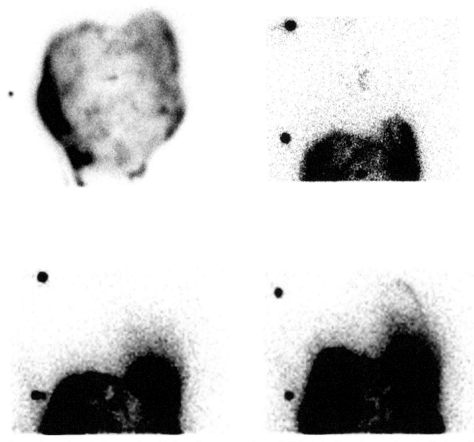

FIGURE 13-33. Anterior peritoneal perfusion studies. Both patients on peritoneal dialysis had persistent pleural effusions. Tc-99m sulfur colloid injected intraperitoneally. *Upper,* Normal intraperitoneal distribution *(left);* only activity above the diaphragm is assumed to be thoracic duct *(right).* *Lower,* Activity seen in left chest, suggestive of pleural distribution at 1 hour *(left);* definite uptake in pleural effusion at 2 hours *(right).*

▬ SUGGESTED READING

Abell TL, Camilleri M, Donohoe K, et al. Consensus recommendations for gastric emptying scintigraphy. A Joint Report of the Society of Nuclear Medicine and the American Neurogastroenterology and Motility Society. *J Nucl Med Technol.* 2008;36(1):44-54.

Bonta DV, Lee HY, Ziessman HA. Shortening the four-hour gastric emptying protocol. *Clin Nucl Med.* 2011;36(4):283-285.

Bunker SR, Lull RJ, Tanasescu DE, et al. Scintigraphy of gastrointestinal hemorrhage: superiority of 99mTc red blood cells over 99m Tc sulfur colloid. *AJR Am J Roentgenol.* 1984;143(3):543-548.

Castronovo Jr FP. Gastroesophageal scintiscanning in a pediatric population: dosimetry. *J Nucl Med.* 1986;27(7):1212-1214.

Diamond RH, Rothstein RD, Alavi A. The role of cimetidine-enhanced Tc-99m pertechnetate imaging for visualizing Meckel's diverticulum. *J Nucl Med.* 1991;32(7):1422-1424.

Emslie JT, Zarnegar K, Siegel ME, et al. Technetium-99m-labeled red blood cell scans in the investigation of gastrointestinal bleeding. *Dis Colon Rectum.* 1996;39(7):750-754.

Fahey FH, Ziessman HA, Collin MJ, et al. Left anterior oblique projection and peak-to-scatter ratio for attenuation compensation of gastric emptying studies. *J Nucl Med.* 1989;30(2):233-239.

Heyman S. Pediatric nuclear gastroenterology: evaluation of gastroesophageal reflux and gastrointestinal bleeding. In: Freeman LM, Weissman HS, eds. *Nuclear Medicine Annual.* New York: Raven Press; 1985.

Klein HA, Wald A. Esophageal transit scintigraphy. In: Freeman LM, Weissman HS, eds. *Nuclear Medicine Annual.* New York: Raven Press; 1985.

Maurer AH, Kevsky B. Whole-gut transit scintigraphy in the valuation of small bowel and colon transit disorders. *Sem Nucl Med.* 1995;25(4):326-338.

Sfakianakis GN, Haase GM. Abdominal scintigraphy for ectopic gastric mucosa: a retrospective analysis of 143 studies. *AJR Am J Roentgenol.* 1982;138(4):7-12.

Tougas G, Eaker EY, Abell TL, et al. Assessment of gastric emptying using a low fat meal: establishment of international control values. *Am J Gastroenterol.* 2000;5(6):1456-1462.

Winzelberg GG. Radionuclide evaluation of gastrointestinal bleeding. In: Freeman LM, ed. *Freeman and Johnson's Clinical Radionuclide Imaging.* Vol. 3. New York: Grune & Stratton; 1986.

Ziessman HA, Fahey FH, Atkins FB, Tall J. Standardization and quantification of radionuclide solid gastric-emptying studies. *J Nucl Med.* 2004;45(5):760-764.

Ziessman HA, Chander A, Ramos A, Wahl RL, Clark JO. The added value of liquid gastric emptying compared to solid emptying alone. *J Nucl Med.* 2009;50(5):726-731.

Zuckier LS. Acute gastrointestinal bleeding. *Sem Nucl Med.* 2003;33(4):297-311.

CHAPTER 14

Infection and Inflammation

Infection imaging has long been an important area for nuclear scintigraphy. Gallium-67 citrate was the first clinical infection-seeking radiopharmaceutical and is still used today, although in a more limited role. Radiolabeled leukocytes (white blood cells [WBCs]) are usually the preferred radiopharmaceutical. Fluorine-18 fluorodeoxyglucose (FDG) is increasingly used (Box 14-1). New radiopharmaceuticals with various mechanisms of uptake are under active investigation.

PATHOPHYSIOLOGY OF INFLAMMATION AND INFECTION

Inflammation is a tissue response to injury that attracts cells of the immune system, specialized serum proteins, and chemical mediators to the site of damage. Infection implies the presence of microorganisms. Although infection is usually associated with inflammation, the reverse is not always true. The inflammatory reaction is triggered by the products of tissue injury. which may result from trauma, foreign particles, ischemia, and neoplasm. Infection without inflammation occurs in severely immunosuppressed patients.

The inflammatory response is associated with increased blood flow, increased vascular permeability, and emigration of leukocytes out of blood vessels into the tissues (chemotaxis). Plasma carries proteins, antibodies, and chemical mediators that modulate the inflammatory response to the site of infection (Fig. 14-1).

RADIOPHARMACEUTICALS

Gallium-67 Citrate

The radiopharmaceutical Ga-67 citrate was originally developed as a bone-seeking radiopharmaceutical, used initially as a tumor-imaging agent and subsequently for its infection-seeking properties.

Gallium is a group III element in the Periodic Table of the Elements (Fig. 1-1) with atomic structure and biological behavior similar to those of iron. The *radionuclide* Ga-67 is produced by cyclotron. It decays by electron capture, emits a spectrum of gamma rays (93, 185, 288, 394 keV), and has a physical half-life of 78 hours (Table 14-1). With each decay, it emits four photopeaks ranging from 93 to 394 keV, all with low abundance (% likelihood of emission with each decay) (Table 14-1). The lower-energy photons cause considerable scatter; the higher-energy photons are difficult to collimate and not efficiently detected by the thin crystal (three-eighth inch) of present-day gamma cameras.

Mechanism of Uptake, Pharmacokinetics, and Distribution

After intravenous injection, Ga-67 citrate circulates in plasma bound to transferrin. The complex is transported to the inflammatory site by locally increased blood flow and vascular permeability (Table 14-2). Its ferric ion–like properties allow it to bind to lactoferrin released from dying leukocytes (higher binding affinity than to transferrin) and bacterial siderophores.

Ga-67 clears slowly from the blood pool. By 48 hours after injection, 10% is still bound to plasma proteins and total body clearance is slow (biological half-life of 25 days). Binding at the site of infection occurs by 12 to 24 hours. Excretion is primarily via the kidneys the first 24 hours. Subsequently, the colon becomes the major route of excretion.

Ga-67 has widespread organ uptake and soft tissue distribution (Table 14-3). Greatest uptake is seen in the liver, followed by bone and bone marrow and spleen (Fig. 14-2). Renal clearance is seen during the initial 24 hours. By 48 hours, the kidneys are only faintly seen.

Sites of variable uptake include the nasopharynx, lacrimal and salivary glands, and breast (Fig. 14-2); all elaborate lactoferrin. Inflammatory or stimulatory processes increase lactoferrin production and uptake, thus increased uptake occurs in the salivary glands in Sjögren's syndrome, in lacrimal glands in sarcoidosis, and breast during lactation. Breast uptake varies according to the menstrual cycle phase and is seen prominently postpartum. Thymic uptake is normal in children.

Postoperative sites may have increased Ga-67 uptake for 2 to 3 weeks. Uptake occurs at healing fractures (Fig. 14-3) and in sterile abscesses associated with frequent intramuscular injections (e.g., insulin or iron-depot injections). Salivary gland uptake is increased after local external beam irradiation or chemotherapy. Normal distribution is altered by whole-body irradiation, multiple blood transfusions (excess ferric ions), or recent gadolinium MRI (Fig. 14-4).

Methodology

An imaging protocol for Ga-67 is described in Box 14-2. Bowel preparation with laxatives and enemas to facilitate more rapid clearance is no longer recommended because it is not usually effective and may cause mucosal irritation and inflammation, producing increased Ga-67 uptake.

Box *14-1*. Radiopharmaceuticals for Infection Imaging Approved for Clinical Use

Ga-67 citrate
In-111 oxine–labeled leukocytes
Tc-99m HMPAO–labeled leukocytes
F-18 FDG
Tc-99m fanolesomab (NeutroSpec) (FDA approved, then withdrawn from U.S. market)
Tc-99m sulesomab (LeuTech) (approved and used in Europe)

FDA, U.S. Food and Drug Administration; *FDG*, fluorodeoxyglucose; *HMPAO*, hexamethylpropyleneamine oxime.

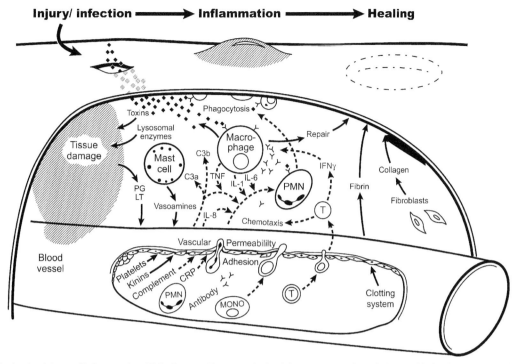

FIGURE 14-1. Pathophysiology of inflammation. This diagram illustrates the body's response to tissue injury and infection. Permeability of the vascular endothelium plays a central role in allowing blood cells and serum components access to the tissues. Antibodies and lymphocytes amplify or focus these primary mechanisms. If inflammation persists beyond a few days, macrophages and lymphocytes play an increasing role. *CRP*, chronic reactive protein; *IFNγ*, interferon gamma; *IL*, interleukin; *LT*, leukotriene; *MONO*, monocyte; *PG*, prostaglandin; *PMN*, polymorphonuclear neutrophil; *T*, t-lymphocyte; *TNF*, tumor necrosis factor. (Modified from Playfair JHL and Chaim BM. *Immunology at a Glance.* 7th ed. Malden, MA: Blackwell Publishing; 2001.)

TABLE 14-1 Physical Characteristics of Gallium-67, Indium-111, and Technetium-99m

Radionuclide	Half-life (hr)	Photopeak (keV)	Relative abundance of photons (%)
Ga-67	78	93	41
		185	23
		288	18
		394	4
In-111	67	173	89
		247	94
Tc-99m	6	140	89

TABLE 14-2 Mechanisms of Localization of Infection-Seeking Radiopharmaceuticals

Radiopharmaceutical	Mechanism
Ga-67 citrate	Binds to lactoferrin and bacterial siderophores
Radiolabeled leukocytes	Diapedesis and chemotaxis
Antigranulocyte monoclonal antibodies	Antibody-antigen binding to activated leukocytes
Chemotactic peptides	Binding to activated leukocytes
Tc-99m ciprofloxacin	Binds to living bacteria

TABLE 14-3 Normal Distribution of Radiopharmaceuticals Used for Infection Imaging

Radiopharmaceutical	Liver	Spleen	Marrow	Bone	Gastrointestinal	Genitourinary	Lung
Ga-67 citrate	***	*	*	*	***	*	
In-111 oxine–labeled leukocytes	**	***	**				*
Tc-99m HMPAO–labeled leukocytes	**	***	**		**	**	*

HMPAO, Hexamethylpropyleneamine oxime.

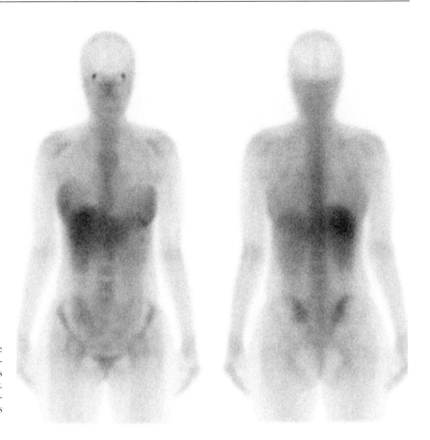

Figure 14-2. Normal Ga-67 distribution. Considerable soft tissue and breast distribution are seen. Prominent lacrimal uptake is noted bilaterally. Highest organ uptake is seen in the liver, followed by bone and bone marrow. Lesser uptake is seen in the spleen, scrotum, and nasopharyngeal region. Some large intestinal clearance is noted.

A medium-energy collimator is indicated. Only the three lower photopeaks (93, 185, 300 keV) are acquired for imaging. The usual administered adult dose is 5 mCi (185 MBq). Although 24-hour images may be diagnostic, whole-body imaging at 48 hours is standard. This ensures adequate background clearance and a good target-to-background ratio. Spot images, single-photon emission computed tomography (SPECT) or SPECT/CT are frequently obtained.

Dosimetry

The highest radiation absorbed dose from Ga-67 is to the large intestine, 3.7 rads/5 mCi (3.7 cGy/185 MBq), followed by the bone marrow, 3.5 rads/cGy. Whole-body effective dose is 1.9 rads/5 mCi (1.9 cGy/185 MBq) (Table 14-4). Radiolabeled leukocytes have now been used for more than three decades for detection of infection and inflammation. Both indium-111 oxine and technetium-99m hexamethylpropyleneamine oxime (HMPAO) labeled WBCs are used clinically. Each has advantages and disadvantages.

Leukocyte Physiology

Leukocytes are the major cellular components of the inflammatory and immune response that protect against infection and neoplasia and assist in the repair of damaged tissue. Nucleated precursor cells differentiate into mature cells within the bone marrow.

Peripheral leukocytes include granulocytes (neutrophils, 55%-65%; eosinophils, 3%; and basophils, 0.5%), lymphocytes (25%-35%), and monocytes (3%-7%). At any one time, only 2% to 3% of neutrophils reside in the circulating blood, using it mainly for transportation to sites of need. The rest are distributed in a "marginated" pool that is adherent to vascular endothelial cells in tissues: 90% are in the bone marrow, the rest are in the spleen, liver, lung, and, to a lesser extent, the gastrointestinal tract and oropharynx. These marginated cells can be marshaled into the circulating pool by various stimuli, including exercise, epinephrine, or bacterial endotoxins.

Neutrophils circulate in the peripheral blood for 5 to 9 hours. They respond to an acute inflammatory stimulus by migrating toward an attractant (chemotaxis) and enter tissues between postcapillary endothelial cells (diapedesis) (Fig. 14-1). They phagocytize the infectious agent or foreign body and enzymatically destroy it within cytoplasmic vacuoles. This process is inhibited by exposure to corticosteroids and ethanol. Leukocytes survive in tissues for only 2 to 3 days.

Lymphocytes arrive at inflammatory sites during the chronic phase. Monocytes act as tissue scavengers, phagocytosing damaged cells and bacteria and detoxifying chemicals and toxins. At sites of inflammation, monocytes transform into tissue macrophages.

Indium-111 Oxine Leukocytes

Since the early 1980s, mixed leukocytes have been radiolabeled with In-111 8-hydroxyquinoline (oxine) and used clinically to detect infection and inflammation.

Indium is a group III element in the Periodic Table of the Elements (Fig. 1-1). It decays by electron capture, emits two gamma photons of 173 and 247 keV (Table 14-1), and has a physical half-life of 67 hours (2.8 days). The *radionuclide* In-111 is cyclotron produced and thus must be ordered the day before cell

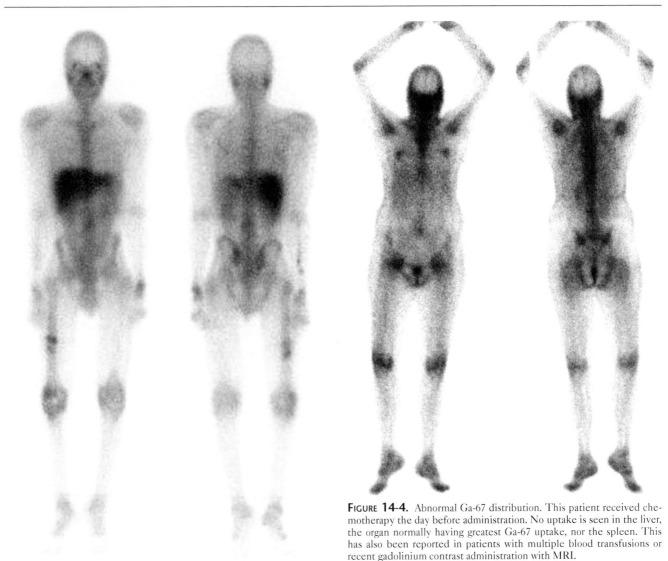

FIGURE 14-4. Abnormal Ga-67 distribution. This patient received chemotherapy the day before administration. No uptake is seen in the liver, the organ normally having greatest Ga-67 uptake, nor the spleen. This has also been reported in patients with multiple blood transfusions or recent gadolinium contrast administration with MRI.

FIGURE 14-3. Ga-67 citrate uptake with fractures. Patient was in accident 2 weeks earlier causing extensive trauma. Scan requested for postoperative fever and concern for possible infection in known fractured L-3 vertebral body. Note very mild uptake in L-3, thought not to be infected, but prominent uptake in known right femur fracture.

labeling. Oxine is a lipid-soluble complex that chelates metal ions (e.g., indium).

Adequate radiolabeling and imaging requires more than 5000/mm³ peripheral leukocytes, although it can sometimes be performed with counts as low as 3000/mm³. Radiolabeling must be performed under a laminar flow hood. The in vitro labeling procedure requires a minimum of 2 hours. Lacking facilities and trained personnel to radiolabel the cells, many hospitals send the patient's blood to an outside commercial radiopharmacy. Thus it takes 3 to 4 hours before the cells are returned and reinfused.

Fifty milliliters of venous blood ensures sufficient numbers of radiolabeled leukocytes for adequate labeling; however, 20 to 30 mL is sometimes acceptable for children. Careful handling is required to avoid damaging the cells, which could adversely affect their migration and viability. Proper labeling does not affect normal physiological

---

Box 14-2. Gallium-67 Citrate Imaging: Summary Protocol

PATIENT PREPARATION
No recent barium contrast studies

RADIOPHARMACEUTICAL
Ga-67 citrate 5 mCi (185 MBq) injected intravenously

INSTRUMENTATION
Gamma camera: Large field of view
Photopeak: 20% window over 93-keV, 185-keV, and 300-keV photopeaks
Collimator: Medium energy

IMAGING PROCEDURE
48-hour images: Whole body anterior and imaging, including head and extremities
High count spot images (e.g., laterals, obliques, etc.)
SPECT or SPECT/CT of the head and neck, chest, abdomen, or pelvis, as indicated

SPECT, Single-photon emission computed tomography.

TABLE **14-4** Radiation Dosimetry for Gallium-67 Citrate, Indium-111 Oxine, and Technetium-99m HMPAO Leukocytes

Organ	Ga-67 citrate rads/5 mCi (cGy/185 MBq)	In-111 oxine WBCs rads/500 µCi (cGy/18.5 MBq)	Tc-99m HMPAO WBCs rads/10 mCi (cGy/370 MBq)
Bladder wall			2.8
Large intestine	3.7		**3.6**
Liver	2.2	2.66	1.5
Bone marrow	**3.5**	1.99	1.6
Spleen	1.8	**20.00**	2.2
Ovaries	1.5	0.20	0.3
Testes	1.0	0.014	1.9
Total body	2.2	0.37	0.3
Effective dose	1.9	0.7	0.4

HMPAO, Hexamethylpropyleneamine oxime; *WBCs,* white blood cells. Target organ dose is in bold.

function. The radiolabel usually remains stable in vivo for more than 24 hours.

Details of the radiolabeling process are detailed (Box 14-3). The patient's blood is drawn, it is allowed to settle, and then the majority of the erythrocytes removed. In-111 oxine labels granulocytes, lymphocytes, monocytes, platelets, and erythrocytes.

Radiolabeling cannot be performed in plasma. It must be separated and retained for later resuspension with the WBCs before reinfusion. The leukocyte pellet is suspended in saline and incubated with In-111 oxine. The lipid solubility of the In-111 oxine complex allows it to diffuse through cell membranes. Intracellularly, the complex dissociates, oxine diffuses back out of the cell, and In-111 binds to nuclear and cytoplasmic proteins.

Pure granulocyte preparations have been radiolabeled and used clinically. However, they require elaborate density gradient separation techniques and have not shown a clinical advantage over mixed leukocytes and thus are not generally used.

Standard quality control measures, such as testing for sterility and pyrogenicity, cannot be performed because of the need for prompt reinfusion after labeling to ensure cell viability. However, the final radiopharmaceutical preparation is routinely examined for abnormal morphology, clumping, excessive red cell contamination, and percent labeling efficiency, which typically ranges from 75% to 90% (Box 14-2). When labeling is less than 50%, the cells should not be reinfused. The final preparation contains radiolabeled granulocytes, lymphocytes, and monocytes, but there will also be 10% to 20% platelets and erythrocytes.

After infusion of the radiolabeled leukocytes, no significant elution of the In-111 from the leukocytes occurs. The effective half-life of clearance from the blood circulation is 7.5 hours. Initial distribution after reinfusion is to the blood pool, lungs, liver, and spleen. Early lung uptake is the

Box 14-3. Radiolabeling Autologous Leukocytes with Indium-111 Oxine

PREPARATION
Patient's peripheral leukocyte count should be greater than 5000 cells/mm³.

PROCEDURE
1. Collect autologous blood
    Draw 30 to 50 mL into an ACD anticoagulated syringe using a 19-gauge needle.
2. Isolate leukocytes:
    Separate red blood cells (RBCs) by gravity sedimentation and 6% hetastarch, a settling agent.
    Centrifuge the leukocyte-rich plasma at 300 to 350 *g* for 5 minutes to remove platelets and proteins.
    A white blood cell (WBC) button forms at the bottom of the tube.
    Draw off and save the leukocyte-poor plasma (LRP) for later washing and resuspension.
3. Label leukocytes
    Suspend WBCs (LRP) in saline (includes neutrophils, lymphocytes, monocytes, some RBCs).
    Incubate with In-111 oxine for 30 minutes at room temperature and gently agitate.
    Remove unbound In-111 by centrifugation. Save wash for calculation of labeling efficiency.
4. Prepare injectate
    Resuspend 500 µmCi In-111–labeled leukocytes in saved plasma (LPP).
    Inject via peripheral vein within 2 to 4 hours.
5. Perform quality control
    Microscopic examination of cells.
    Calculate labeling efficiency:
        Assay the cells and wash in dose calibrator.
        Labeling efficiency = $C/([C+ W] \times 100\%)$ where C is activity associated with the cells and W is activity associated with the wash.

result of cellular activation from in vitro cell manipulation. By 4 hours after reinjection, lung and blood pool activity decrease, although not always completely (Fig. 14-5).

By 24 hours, blood-pool activity is normally no longer present. Persistent blood pool at 24 hours suggests a high percentage of labeled erythrocytes or platelets. The highest uptake is in the spleen, followed by liver and then bone marrow (Fig. 14-5). Neither genitourinary, hepatobiliary, nor intestinal clearance is normally seen (Table 14-3).

The ultimate test of viability of leukocytes is in vivo function manifested by a normal distribution within the body and the ability to detect infection. If the infused leukocytes become nonviable, increased liver and lung uptake may be seen on scintigraphy. With excessive erythrocyte and platelet labeling, blood pool is prominent.

Radiation Dosimetry
The adult spleen receives 15 to 20 rads/500 µCi (15-20 cGy/18.5 MBq); however, in small children the spleen may

4 hours

24 hours

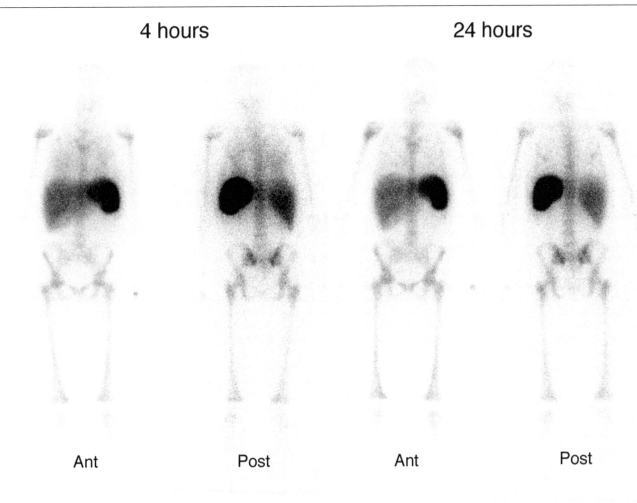

Ant   Post   Ant   Post

FIGURE 14-5. In-111 oxine–labeled leukocytes in normal distribution at 4 and 24 hours. Anterior *(Ant)* and posterior *(Post)* whole-body images. The highest uptake is seen in the spleen, followed by the liver, and then the bone marrow. No intestinal or renal clearance is seen. The 4-hour images show some bilateral lung uptake that resolves by 24 hours. No other apparent change in distribution is seen between 4 and 24 hours. Image quality is superior at 24 hours.

receive 30 to 50 rads/cGy (Table 14-1). For this reason, In-111 labeled leukocytes are rarely used in children.

Imaging Methodology. An imaging protocol for In-111 oxine leukocytes is described in Box 14-4. Images are acquired on the 173- and 247-keV photopeaks (20% window) with a medium-energy collimator. Whole-body imaging is routine. High-count spot images, SPECT, and SPECT/CT are options.

Images are routinely acquired 24 hours after radiopharmaceutical injection, an advantage over Ga-67 (Table 14-5). Further delayed images rarely give additional information. Early imaging (e.g., at 4 hours) is less sensitive than 24-hour imaging for detecting infection; however, it is standard for inflammatory bowel disease. Inflamed mucosal cells slough, become intraluminal, and move distally over time. Thus 24-hour images can be misleading and erroneous as to the site of inflammation. Fixed activity between 4- and 24-hour images in a patient with inflammatory bowel disease suggests an abscess.

Image Interpretation. Scintigraphic images reflect the distribution of WBCs in the body. Activity outside the expected normal leukocyte distribution suggests infection (Fig. 14-6). Focal uptake equal to that in the liver or greater suggests an abscess. Activity equal to that in the liver generally signifies a clinically important inflammatory site; activity less than occurs in bone marrow generally suggests an inflammatory response.

Interpretive pitfalls (i.e., potential false positive and false negative findings) should be kept in mind (Box 14-5). Leukocytes accumulate at sites of inflammation—for example, intravenous catheters; nasogastric, endogastric, and drainage tubes; tracheostomies; colostomies; and ileostomies. Unless very intense, this uptake should not be considered abnormal. Uninfected postsurgical wounds commonly show faint uptake for 2 to 3 weeks. If uptake is intense, persists, or extends beyond the surgical wound site, infection should be suspected (Fig. 14-7). Uptake occurs at healing bone fracture sites, with the degree

Box 14-4. **Indium-111 Oxine Leukocyte Scintigraphy: Summary Protocol**

RADIOPHARMACEUTICAL

In-111 oxine in vitro–labeled leukocytes 500 µCi (18.5 MBq)

INSTRUMENTATION

Camera: Large field of view
Window: 20% centered over 173- and 247-keV photopeaks
Collimator: Medium energy

PATIENT PREPARATION

Draw 50 mL of blood. Radiolabel cells in vitro (Box 14-2).

PROCEDURE

Inject labeled cells intravenously, preferably by direct venipuncture through a 19-gauge needle. Contact with dextrose in water solutions may cause cell damage.

Imaging at 4 hours is critical in localizing inflammatory bowel disease.

Perform routine whole-body imaging at 24 hours.

Acquire anterior abdomen for 500k counts, then other images for equal time. Include anterior and posterior views of the chest, abdomen, and pelvis, and spot images of specific areas of interest (e.g., feet) for a minimum of 200k counts or 20 minutes.

Perform SPECT or SPECT/CT in selected cases.

SPECT, Single-photon emission computed tomography.

TABLE 14-5 Optimal Imaging Time for Infection-Seeking Radiopharmaceuticals

Radiopharmaceutical	Time (hr)
Ga-67	48
In-111 leukocytes	24
Antigranulocyte monoclonal antibodies	1-6
Technetium-99m HMPAO leukocytes	1-4
Chemotactic peptides	1-4
F-18 FDG	1

FDG, Fluorodeoxyglucose; *HMPAO,* hexamethylpropyleneamine oxime.

depending on the time since fracture, its severity, and proper healing.

A major advantage of In-111 leukocytes is the lack of normal intraabdominal activity. However, in addition to infection, abdominal activity may be due to other causes, including accessory spleen, pseudoaneurysm, and noninfected hematomas (Fig. 14-8). Renal transplants normally accumulate leukocytes, probably as a result of low-grade rejection (Fig. 14-9). Intraluminal intestinal activity also can result from swallowed or shedding cells that occur with herpes esophagitis, pharyngitis, sinusitis, pneumonia, or gastrointestinal bleeding.

The sensitivity of leukocyte imaging may be reduced in conditions that alter leukocyte function—for example,

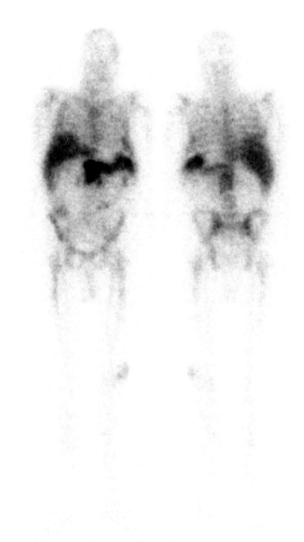

POSTERIOR

FIGURE 14-6. In-111–labeled leukocyte scan with intraabdominal infection. Recent thoracic and abdominal surgery, including splenectomy, with persistent fever. Mid-abdominal and left upper quadrant uptake consistent with infection.

hyperglycemia, steroid therapy, and chemotherapy. Conflicting data exist regarding the sensitivity of In-111 leukocyte scintigraphy for detecting infection in patients receiving antibiotics. The discrepant reports are likely due to the effectiveness of the specific therapy that the patient is receiving. Many patients who have WBC scintigraphy are already on antibiotics.

Concern has been raised that false negative study results might occur with chronic infections. However, most investigations have not found a difference in sensitivity for detection of acute versus chronic infections. Although chronic inflammations attract predominantly lymphocytes, monocytes, plasma cells, and macrophages, they still have significant neutrophilic infiltration. The In-111–labeled mixed-cell population contains many lymphocytes as well as neutrophils. Ga-67 may be advantageous for some patients with low-grade infections—for example, fungal, protozoal.

Technetium-99m Hexamethylpropyleneamine Oxime–Labeled Leukocytes

Tc-99m–labeled leukocytes have advantages over In-111 WBCs (Table 14-6). Being generator produced, Tc-99m is available when needed. The optimal gamma camera Tc-99m photopeak provides superior image quality. Radiation to the patient is considerably lower. Greater activity can be administered, resulting in higher photon yield and better image quality.

The *element* technetium is in group VIIB of the Periodic Table of the Elements (Fig. 1-1). The *radionuclide* Tc-99m is generator-produced from molybdenum-99. Tc-99m decays by isomeric transition, emits 1 gamma photon of 140 keV (Table 14-1) with a physical half-life of 6 hours.

Tc-99m HMPAO (Ceretec, Mediphysics, Princeton, NJ) was originally approved by the U.S. Food and Drug Administration (FDA) for cerebral perfusion imaging. Being lipophilic, it can cross cell membranes. In brain imaging, Tc-99m HMPAO crosses the blood–brain barrier and is taken up by cortical cells, where it changes into a hydrophilic complex and becomes trapped. This experience led to the use of Tc-99m HMPAO to label leukocytes.

The methodology for leukocyte radiolabeling with Tc-99m HMPAO is similar to that used for labeling leukocytes with In-111 oxine. One difference is that Tc-99m HMPAO leukocyte labeling can be performed in plasma. Another is that labeling is primarily of granulocytes, a potential advantage for imaging acute purulent processes, but perhaps less so for more chronic infections. The FDA views Tc-99m HMPAO–labeled leukocytes as an acceptable alternative use of an approved radiopharmaceutical (Tc-99m HMPAO).

Box 14-5. Interpretative Pitfalls in Leukocyte Imaging

FALSE NEGATIVE RESULTS
Encapsulated, nonpyogenic abscess
Vertebral osteomyelitis
Chronic low-grade infection
Parasitic, mycobacterial, or fungal infections
Hyperglycemia
Corticosteroid therapy

FALSE POSITIVE RESULTS
Gastrointestinal bleeding
Healing fracture
Swallowed leukocytes; oropharyngeal, esophageal, or lung disease
Surgical wounds, stomas, or catheter sites
Hematomas
Tumors
Accessory spleens
Renal transplant
Pseudoaneurysm

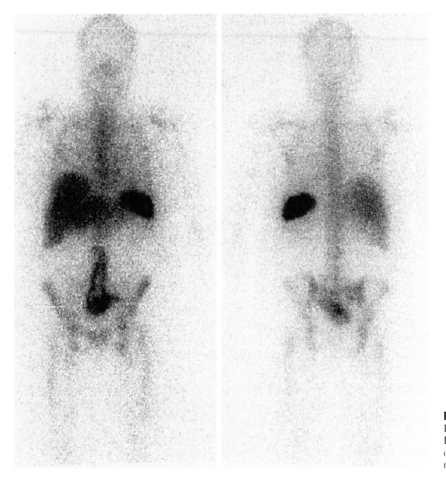

FIGURE 14-7. Postoperative wound infection. In-111 oxine–labeled leukocyte whole-body scan. Dehiscence of the abdominal incision site because of an abscess inferior and deep to incision. Note the more intense uptake inferiorly.

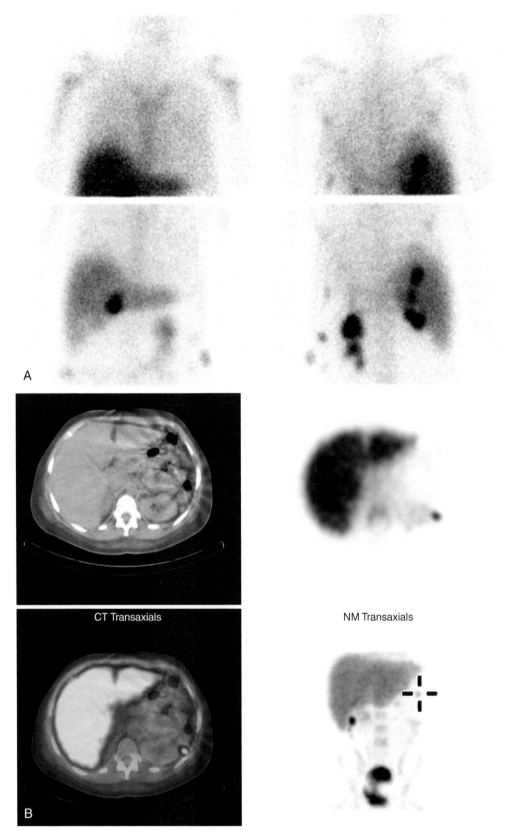

CT Transaxials

NM Transaxials

FIGURE 14-8. False positive In-111–labeled leukocyte scan. The patient presented with recurrent fever. **A,** Static spot images of the chest (anterior and posterior) and abdomen (anterior and posterior). Low-grade subtle uptake occurred in the left lower lobe of the lung consistent with pneumonitis seen on chest radiograph, but poorly seen here. Note that no spleen uptake is seen. Multiple very intense foci of uptake are seen in the abdomen, confirmed as splenules. The patient had splenectomy in the past after trauma. **B,** In-111–labeled leukocyte SPECT/CT and splenules. Patient had fever and bacteremia. History of prior splenectomy and multiple splenules on CT. The study shows the advantage of SPECT/CT for clearly localizing the uptake to splenules seen on CT.

TABLE 14-6 Advantages and Disadvantages of Indium-111 Oxine Versus Technetium-99m Hexamethylpropyleneamine Oxime Labeled Leukocytes

Advantages and disadvantages	In-111 oxine–WBCs	Tc-99m HMPAO–WBCs
Radionuclide immediately available	No	Yes
Stable radiolabel, no elution from cells	Yes	No
Allows labeling in plasma	No	Yes
Dosimetry	Poor	Good
Early routine imaging	No	Yes
Long half-life allows for delayed imaging	Yes	No
Imaging time	Long	Short
Permits dual isotope imaging	Yes	No
Bowel and renal clearance	No	Yes
Image resolution	Good	Fair

HMPAO, Hexamethylpropyleneamine oxime; *WBC,* white blood cell.

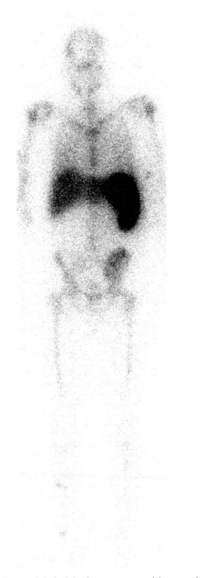

FIGURE 14-9. In-111–labeled leukocyte scan with transplant uptake. Scan obtained for fever of uncertain cause 4 weeks after renal transplant. Uptake in transplant is secondary to moderate rejection and not infection.

The biological half-life of Tc-99m HMPAO–labeled leukocytes in blood is somewhat shorter than that of In-111 oxine leukocytes, 4 versus 6 hours, because of slow elution of the Tc-99m HMPAO from circulating radiolabeled cells.

Tc-99m HMPAO–labeled WBCs distribute in the body similar to In-111–labeled cells, except that the former has hepatobiliary and genitourinary clearance (Fig. 14-10). A secondary labeled hydrophilic complex is excreted, as seen with Tc-99m HMPAO brain imaging. The kidneys and bladder are visualized by 1 to 2 hours after injection. Biliary and bowel clearance occurs as early as 2 hours and is commonly visualized by 3 to 4 hours, increasing with time (Fig. 14-11). Intraabdominal imaging is best performed before 2 hours.

Radiation Dosimetry
The highest radiation dose from Tc-99m HMPAO–labeled leukocytes is the colon, 3.6 rads/10 mCi (3.6 cGy/370 MBq), followed by the bladder and spleen 2.2 rads/10 mCi (2.2 cGy/ MBq) (Table 14-4).

Imaging Methodology. Because of the shorter physical half-life and hepatobiliary and urinary clearance of Tc-99m HMPAO–labeled leukocytes, images are acquired at an earlier time point than In-111 oxine–labeled WBCs (Table 14-5). A detailed protocol is described in Box 14-6. Abdominal imaging should be performed between 1 and 2 hours after reinfusion. For other body regions, such as in the extremities, later imaging is reasonable—for example, 3 to 4 hours. Blood-pool activity is commonly seen compared to In-111–labeled leukocytes because of the earlier imaging time, which can complicate interpretation in the chest or major vessels. The high count rate of Tc-99m provides good SPECT quality.

Image Interpretation. Activity outside the expected normal distribution suggests infection. Care must be used in interpretation of intraabdominal activity, because of the normal genitourinary and hepatobiliary clearance. False positive and false negative results are listed Box 14-5. Delayed imaging may occasionally be helpful (Fig. 14-12), and SPECT/CT can improve localization.

Fluorine-18 Fluorodeoxyglucose

Fluorine-18 fluorodeoxyglucose (F-18 FDG) positron emission tomography (PET), used most commonly for tumor, cardiac, and brain imaging, is increasingly being used to detect infection. Increased FDG uptake occurs with inflammation and infection as a result of activation of granulocytes and macrophages.

F-18 FDG PET has advantages over radiolabeled leukocytes. Problems associated with withdrawing, radiolabeling, and reinfusion of blood products are eliminated. Imaging begins at 1 hour after injection and is completed by 2 hours (Table 14-5). PET image resolution is superior to single-photon imaging. Cross-sectional imaging and PET/CT is standard.

A disadvantage of FDG is that uptake is not specific for infection and may occur from other causes—for example,

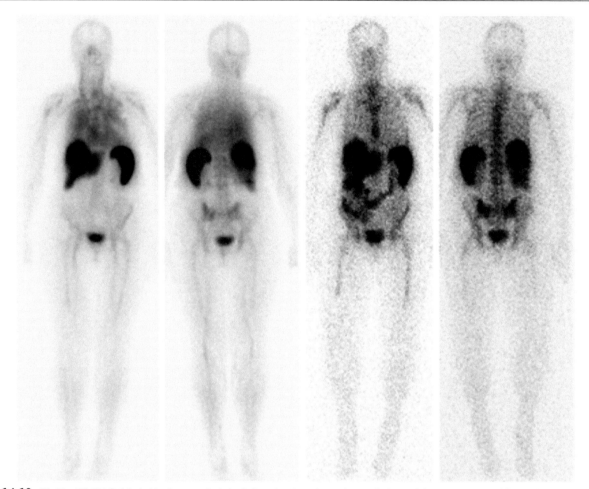

FIGURE 14-10. Tc-99m HMPAO–labeled leukocyte whole-body imaging (anterior and posterior) at 4 *(left)* and 24 hours *(right)*. No intraabdominal activity is seen at 4 hours, except for faint visualization of the renal pelvices. At 24 hours considerable intraabdominal activity is seen, which seems to be in the bowel. Image quality is inferior to that at 4 hours because of the 6-hour half-life of Tc-99m.

fractures, postoperative inflammation, degenerative disease, reaction to orthopedic hardware, and so forth. Published data are limited, although growing. Few accepted diagnostic criteria exist. Reimbursement can be an issue.

Preliminary investigations suggest that F-18 FDG may be useful for diagnosing infection in patients with fever of unknown origin; osteomyelitis, especially in the spine; and vascular grafts (Fig. 14-13). Although investigations have sought to differentiate aseptic from septic hip prostheses, false positive results are not uncommon. For knee prostheses, specificity is poor. FDG has been used to diagnose and localize sarcoidosis, inflammatory bowel disease, and large vessel vasculitis.

Investigational Radiopharmaceuticals

Alternative single-photon radiopharmaceuticals that do not require radiolabeling blood products are desirable. NeutroSpec was thought to be the answer.

Tc-99m fanolesomab (NeutroSpec, Mallinckrodt, St. Louis, MO) is a murine immunoglobulin (Ig)M monoclonal antibody that binds avidly to surface CD15 antigens expressed on human neutrophils and was approved in the United States by the FDA in 2004. Approval was subsequently withdrawn because two patient

deaths were reported after the administration of the radiopharmaceutical.

Technetium-99m sulesomab (LeukoScan), a Tc-99m–labeled antigranulocyte (IgG1) murine antibody Fab′ fragment, is used clinically in Europe. Fab′ fragments have less immunoreactivity than whole antibodies and a better target-to-background ratio because of their rapid renal clearance. Accuracy is similar to that of In-111–labeled leukocytes.

New infection-seeking radiopharmaceuticals are under investigation. Areas of investigation have changed over time, from developing large proteins with nonspecific uptake mechanism (IgG) to receptor-specific proteins of large size (antigranulocyte antibodies) and moderate size (antibody fragments) to small receptor-binding proteins and peptides (cytokines).

Chemotactic peptides, or cytokines (e.g., interleukin-8), interact with specific cell-surface receptors. Produced by bacteria, chemotactic peptides bind to receptors on the cell membrane of neutrophils, stimulating the cells to undergo chemotaxis. Peptide analogs have been synthesized, radiolabeled, and investigated. Localization at sites of infection is rapid because of the small size of these compounds; they easily pass through vascular walls and quickly enter an abscess.

Tc-99m ciprofloxacin (Infecton) is a Tc-99m–radiolabeled fluoroquinolone broad-spectrum antimicrobial agent that binds to DNA of living bacteria. Studies have shown sensitivity similar to that of radiolabeled leukocytes and suggest utility in patients with suspected vertebral infection in which radiolabeled WBCs have reduced sensitivity.

CLINICAL APPLICATIONS FOR INFECTION SCINTIGRAPHY

This section focuses on the most common indications for infection scintigraphy, reviews the pathophysiology of the disease processes, and discusses scintigraphic approaches.

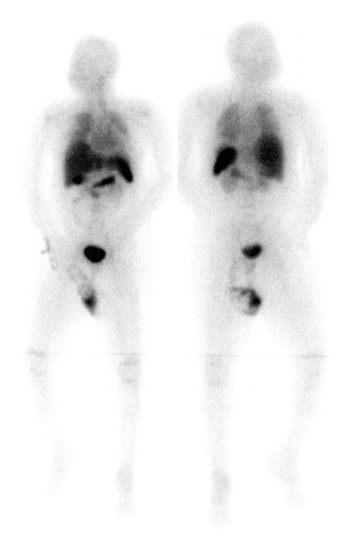

FIGURE 14-11. Whole-body Tc-99m HMPAO images at 4 hours showing radiotracer in the gallbladder, small bowel, and urinary bladder. Urinary contamination is noted.

> ### Box 14-6. Technetium-99m HMPAO Leukocyte Scintigraphy: Summary Protocol
>
> **PATIENT PREPARATION**
> Wound dressings changed before imaging.
>
> **RADIOPHARMACEUTICAL**
> Tc-99m HMPAO in vitro–labeled WBCs 10 mCi (370 MBq)
>
> **INSTRUMENTATION**
> Camera: Large field of view; two-headed camera preferable for whole-body imaging
> Collimator: Low energy, high resolution
> Windows: 20%, centered over 140-keV photopeaks
>
> **PATIENT PREPARATION**
> Draw 50 mL of blood.
>
> **PROCEDURE**
> Radiolabel patient's leukocytes in vitro with Tc-99m HMPAO.
> Reinject labeled cells intravenously, preferably by direct venipuncture through 19-gauge needle. Contact with dextrose in water solutions may cause cell damage.
>
> **IMAGING**
> Imaging between 1 and 2 hours is mandatory for intraabdominal imaging or to localize inflammatory bowel disease.
> Imaging at 4 hours or later may be advantageous for peripheral skeleton (e.g., osteomyelitis of feet).
> Whole-body imaging: Two-headed camera with whole-body acquisition for 30 minutes; 10-minute spot images for regions of special interest.
> SPECT or SPECT/CT in selected cases.

HMPAO, Hexamethylpropyleneamine oxime; *SPECT,* single-photon emission computed tomography.

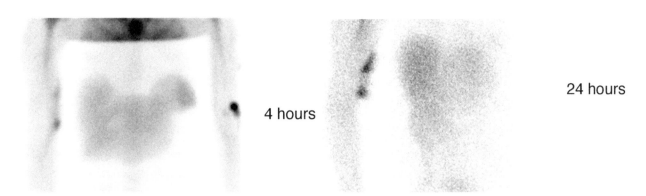

FIGURE 14-12. Infected arteriovenous graft imaged with Tc-99m HMPAO–labeled leukocytes. Image obtained at 4 hours *(above)* shows focal uptake within the graft on the right. Delayed image at 24 hours *(below)* show increasing uptake in the same region.

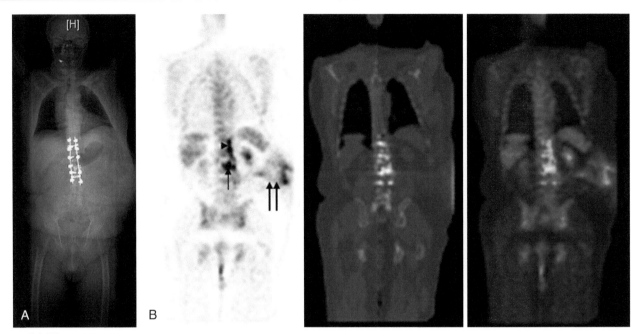

Figure 14-13. Lumbar spine osteomyelitis and infected orthopedic hardware. **A,** A 60-year-old man had spinal hardware implanted more than 8 years previously after a motor vehicle accident. He recently developed a draining left flank wound and was referred for evaluation of possible infected orthopedic hardware. **B,** On the coronal images from the FDG PET/CT study linear left paraspinal hypermetabolism *(arrowhead)* along the metal rod extends from approximately T-11 to L-3 with a standard uptake value (SUV) maximum of 9.3. This activity tracks to an open hypermetabolic wound in the left flank *(double arrow)*, with an SUV maximum of 7.3. Focal hypermetabolism (SUV maximum 8.7) can be seen in an upper lumbar vertebra *(arrow)* consistent with osteomyelitis. (Courtesy Christopher Palestro, MD.)

Osteomyelitis

Osteomyelitis is one of the oldest recorded diseases, first described by Hippocrates in 400 BC.

The histopathology of acute osteomyelitis includes neutrophilic inflammation, edema, and vascular congestion. Because of the bone's rigidity, intramedullary pressure increases, compromising the blood supply and causing ischemia and vascular thrombosis. Over several days, the suppurative and ischemic injury may result in bone fragmentation into devitalized segments called *sequestra*. Infection may spread via haversian and Volkmann canals to the periosteum, resulting in abscesses, soft-tissue infection, and sinus tracts.

With persistent infection, chronic inflammatory cells (e.g., lymphocytes, histiocytes, plasma cells) join the neutrophils. Fibroblastic proliferation and new bone formation occur. Periosteal osteogenesis may surround the inflammation to form a bony envelope, or involucrum. Occasionally a dense fibrous capsule confines the infection to a localized area (Brodie abscess).

Bone infection is usually bacterial in origin. Microorganisms reach the bone by one of three mechanisms: hematogenous spread, extension from a contiguous site of infection, and direct introduction of organisms into bone by trauma and surgery.

The terminology for acute and chronic osteomyelitis is not always consistent and can be confusing. *Acute* usually indicates hematogenous spread. *Chronic* usually indicates an infection starting in overlying soft tissue or introduced at the time of surgery or trauma. It is an active infection, sometimes reactivated, with a neutrophilic inflammatory component.

Acute Hematogenous Osteomyelitis

Hematogenous spread is most commonly seen in children. It involves the red marrow of long bones because of the relatively slow blood flow in metaphyseal capillaries and sinusoidal veins in the region adjacent to the growth plate and the paucity of phagocytes (Figs. 14-14 and 14-15). The bone infection is often secondary to a distant staphylococcal skin or mucosal infection.

In adults, osteomyelitis caused by hematogenous spread most commonly occurs in diabetes. It rarely involves the long bones because red marrow has been replaced by yellow marrow (adipose tissue). It typically occurs in vertebral bodies, where the marrow is cellular with an abundant vascular supply. Infection begins near the anterior longitudinal ligament and spreads to adjacent vertebrae by direct extension through the disk space or by communicating venous channels. Because the adult disk does not have a vascular supply, disk space infection is invariably the result of osteomyelitis in an adjacent vertebra. The initiating event is usually septicemia from urinary tract infection, bacterial endocarditis, or intravenous drug abuse.

Extension From a Contiguous Site of Infection

The most common cause of osteomyelitis is direct extension from overlying soft tissue infection, often secondary to trauma, pressure sores, radiation therapy, or burns. In patients with diabetes and vascular insufficiency, organisms enter the soft tissues through a cutaneous ulcer, usually in the foot, producing cellulitis and subsequently osteomyelitis.

Direct Introduction of Organisms Into Bone

Direct inoculation of infection may occur with open fractures, open surgical reduction of closed fractures, or penetrating trauma by foreign bodies. Osteomyelitis may also arise from perioperative contamination of bone during surgery for nontraumatic orthopedic disorders—for example, laminectomy, diskectomy, or placement of a joint prosthesis.

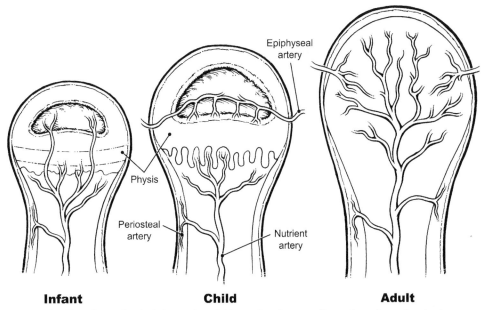

FIGURE **14-14.** Vascular supply of long bones. In the infant and until 18 months of age, small vessels perforate the physis to enter the epiphysis. After 18 months and during childhood, the perforating vessels involute. The epiphysis and metaphysis then have separate blood supplies. Following closure of the physis, branches of the nutrient artery extend to the end of bone (adult) and the principal blood supply to the end of long bones is again from the nutrient artery in the medullary canal. The periosteal artery supplies the outer cortex, whereas branches of the nutrient artery supply the inner cortex.

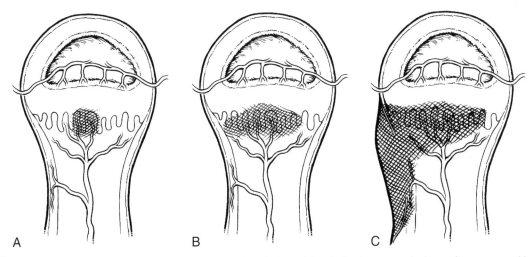

FIGURE **14-15.** Pathophysiology of hematogenous osteomyelitis (child). **A,** Bacterial embolization occurs via the nutrient artery, and bacteria lodge in the terminal blood supply in the metaphysis. **B,** After the infection is established, it expands within the medullary canal toward the cortex and diaphysis. The physis serves as an effective barrier. **C,** The infection then extends through the vascular channels to the cortex to elevate and strip the periosteum from the cortex, and periosteal new bone forms. The bond between the periosteum and perichondrium at the physis prevents extension of the infection into the joint.

Osteomyelitis initially acquired as a child or in adulthood may be manifested years later as recurrent intermittent or persistent drainage from sinus tracts communicating with the involved bone, usually the femur, tibia, or humerus, or as a soft tissue infection overlying it.

Clinical Diagnosis

Biopsy with culture is the definitive test for the diagnosis of osteomyelitis; however, it is invasive and sometimes contraindicated because noninfected bone may become contaminated by overlying soft tissue infection. Risk also exists for pathological fracture in the small bones of the hands and feet. Imaging is often required to confirm or exclude the diagnosis.

Conventional Imaging

Plain film radiographs are indicated when osteomyelitis is suspected. The characteristic changes are permeative radiolucencies, destructive changes, and periosteal new bone formation. These findings can take 10 to 14 days to develop.

Magnetic resonance imaging (MRI) can detect marrow changes of osteomyelitis, such as low-signal intensity on T1-weighted images, high-signal intensity on T2-weighted images, and gadolinium enhancement. Secondary changes such as sinus tracts and cortical interruption increase the diagnostic certainty. Sensitivity and specificity are reported to be high. However, any disease that replaces bone marrow and results in increased tissue

---

Box 14-7. Scintigraphic Diagnosis of Osteomyelitis in Different Clinical Situations

Normal x-ray: Three-phase bone scan
Neonates: Three-phase bone scan; if negative, Tc-99m HMPAO WBCs
Suspected vertebral osteomyelitis: Ga-67 citrate or F-18 FDG
Suspected osteomyelitis in bone marrow-containing skeleton (hips and knees, mid- and hind-foot): Marrow scan + leukocyte study

---

FDG, Fluorodeoxyglucose; *HMPAO*, hexamethylpropyleneamine oxime; *WBC*, white blood cells.

TABLE 14-7 Diagnosis of Osteomyelitis: Accuracy of Different Scintigraphic and Magnetic Resonance Imaging Methods

Type of study	Sensitivity (%)	Specificity (%)
Three-phase bone scan (normal radiograph)	94	95
Three-phase bone scan (underlying bone disease)	95	33
Ga-67	81	69
In-111 oxine–labeled leukocytes	88	85
Tc-99m HMPAO WBCs	87	81
Leukocytes (vertebral)	40	90
Leukocytes + bone marrow	95	90
Magnetic resonance imaging	95	87

HMPAO, Hexamethylpropyleneamine oxime; *WBC*, white blood cell.

water (e.g., healing fractures, tumors, and Charcot joints) may not be distinguishable from infection, and thus MRI is often not specific.

Scintigraphy

The preferred scintigraphic method for diagnosis of osteomyelitis depends on the specific clinical indication (Box 14-7).

Bone Scan

In patients without underlying bone pathology, a three-phase bone scan should be the first scintigraphic study. Sensitivity for the diagnosis of osteomyelitis is high, at greater than 95%; a negative study result excludes osteomyelitis with a high degree of certainty (high negative predictive value). An exception may be neonates who are reported to have false negative study results.

Although the sensitivity of the bone scan is high in patients with underlying bone disease, fractures, orthopedic implants, and neuropathic joints, specificity is poor (30%-50%). Thus by itself it is not usually diagnostic (Table 14-7). Distinguishing soft tissue from bone uptake can be a problem in planar imaging of the feet because of slow soft tissue clearance because of edema. Delayed imaging or particularly SPECT/CT can help distinguish the two (Fig. 14-16).

Gallium-67 Citrate

Because Ga-67 is taken up by bone and bone marrow, increased uptake is often seen at sites of increased bone turnover, similar to that seen on bone scans. Thus false positive interpretations may result in patients with underlying bone disease or orthopedic hardware. Specificity can be increased if interpreted in conjunction with a bone scan.

The criteria for diagnosis of osteomyelitis using Ga-67 scintigraphy in conjunction with a bone scan are (1) if Ga-67 uptake is greater than that seen on the bone scan or (2) if the Ga-67 and bone scan distribution are incongruent (Fig. 14-17). Ga-67 uptake less than on the bone scan is negative for osteomyelitis. A similar degree of uptake on both studies is considered equivocal, and infection cannot be excluded. The accuracy of the combined two studies is still inferior to that of radiolabeled leukocytes, with the important exception of vertebral osteomyelitis (Table 14-7).

Radiolabeled Leukocytes

The reported accuracy of radiolabeled leukocytes for diagnosis of osteomyelitis has varied. Attempts have been made to improve the accuracy by interpreting the study in conjunction with a bone scan, similar to the approach used with Ga-67 (Figs. 14-18 through 14-20). However, this has not appreciably improved the overall accuracy, particularly in the problematic diabetic foot, spine, and hip and knee prostheses. SPECT/CT will likely improve diagnostic accuracy (Fig. 14-21).

Bone Marrow Scan in Conjunction with a Leukocyte Scan

An underlying assumption of leukocyte scintigraphy interpretation for osteomyelitis is that the bone marrow distribution is uniform and symmetric and that an area of focally increased uptake is diagnostic of infection. However, when marrow distribution is altered (e.g., by prior infection, fracture, orthopedic hardware, etc.), radiolabled leukoycte uptake could be misinterpreted as infection.

Tc-99m sulfur colloid can serve as a template for the patient's bone marrow distribution. With infection, the radiolabeled leukocyte study will be discordant with the marrow scan—that is, focal increased uptake on the leukocyte study and decreased or normal uptake on marrow study (Fig. 14-22). With no infection, the leukocyte and marrow scan will have similar distribution.

For Tc-99m HMPAO–labeled leukocytes, the two studies would best be performed on separate days, although subtraction imaging on the same day is feasible. Dual-isotope studies with In-111 oxine–labeled leukocytes and Tc-99m sulfur colloid have advantages but require special attention to methodology. One approach is to perform the Tc-99m scan first because of its shorter half-life. By 24 hours, 94% of the Tc-99m activity will have decayed. Blood required for In-111 leukocyte labeling can be drawn before injection of the Tc-99m tracer and the In-111–radiolabeled cells reinfused after acquiring the Tc-99m scan. The In-111 leukocyte study would be imaged the following day.

An alternative attractive approach is to acquire both studies simultaneously, using a dual-isotope acquisition method. The Tc-99m sulfur colloid is injected immediately before

Immediate Blood Pool

Delayed Imaging

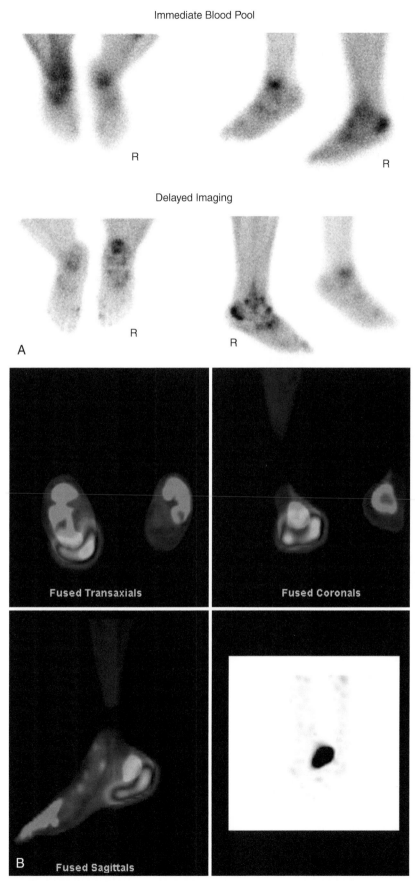

FIGURE 14-16. Heel pain and SPECT CT. **A** *(above)* Blood pool and delayed (plantar and lateral) Tc-99m MDP images show abnormal increased accumulation in the region of the heel. **B.** Tc-99m HMPAO SPECT/CT shows intense uptake in the soft tissue inferior to the calcaneus consistent with soft tissue infection. Osteomyelitis was ruled out.

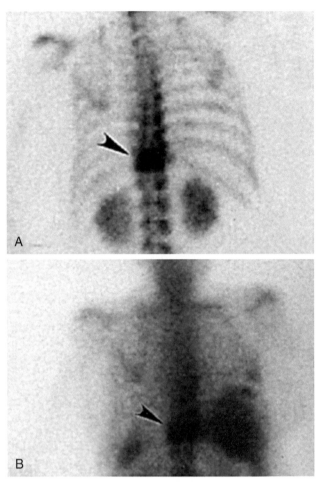

FIGURE 14-17. Ga-67 and bone scan compared to confirm or exclude osteomyelitis of the spine. Fever after laminectomy raised the question of infection. Vertebral Ga-67 uptake **(A)** was judged to be considerably less than that seen on the Tc-99m MDP bone scan **(B)**, and the study was interpreted as negative for vertebral osteomyelitis.

24-hour In-111 leukocyte imaging. This approach ensures identically positioned images for direct comparison. Upscatter from Tc-99m could be minimized by acquiring only the upper 247-keV photopeak of In-111. A narrowed window for the lower 173-keV photopeak could also be used. In-111 downscatter into the Tc-99m window is not usually a problem with the recommended doses because of the low activity of In-111 (500 µCi) compared to Tc-99m (10 mCi).

Fluorine-18 Fluorodeoxyglucose

An increasing number of investigations have shown the value of F-18 FDG for diagnosis of infection. Most of these studies are small, but generally show that FDG imaging can detect infection with high sensitivity and good specificity. Infection in patients with controlled diabetes may be an exception because of the effect of hyperglyemia or hyperinsulinemia on FDG uptake. Nonspecific uptake may be seen with orthopedic hardware, inflammation, and so forth.

Diabetic Foot

Insensitivity of the neuropathic foot to pain can result in asymptomatic trauma, fractures, ulcers, infection, and delay in diagnosis. The diagnosis of osteomyelitis in the

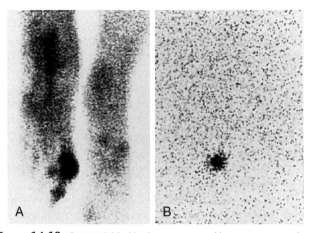

FIGURE 14-18. In-111–labled leukocyte scan and bone scan comparison in osteomyelitis. Suspected osteomyelitis in the region of the first metatarsal in a diabetic. Bone scan **(A)**: Two-hour delayed bone scan shows marked increase in uptake in the distal first metatarsal. Flow and blood pool (not shown) were positive. In-111 oxine–labeled leukocytes **(B)** shows intense uptake in the region of the same distal metatarsal consistent with osteomyelitis. No uptake is noted in other areas of the foot that had increased uptake on the bone scan. Note decreased uptake in many distal digits resulting from peripheral vascular disease.

setting of soft tissue infection is challenging for clinicians and imagers. Radiographs and MRI may not be specific.

Interpretation of the three-phase bone scan can be complicated by the fact that the flow portion of the study may be positive because of overlying soft tissue infection and delayed images may be positive because of fractures, Charcot joints, or degenerative disease. Although sensitivity for diagnosis of osteomyelitis is high, the specificity is poor (Table 14-7).

With In-111–labeled leukocytes for suspected distal foot (toes and metatarsals) osteomyelitis, differentiation of bone uptake from overlying soft tissue infection can be problematic because of the limited anatomical information on the planar WBC scan (Fig. 14-18). The improved resolution of Tc-99m HMPAO–labeled leukocytes can be an advantage because of better bone and soft tissue discrimination. SPECT/CT can be particularly helpful in separating soft tissue and bone uptake. Tc-99m sulfur colloid bone marrow imaging should be used for the mid- and hind-foot in conjunction with radiolabeled leukocytes. A mismatch is consistent with infection (Fig. 14-21).

Although red marrow is not normally present in the distal extremities in adults, neuropathic Charcot joints form marrow and accumulate leukocytes. Fractures may also stimulate marrow formation. Thus Tc-99m sulfur colloid marrow scintigraphy in conjunction with In-111 WBCs is recommended for evaluation of the diabetic mid- and hind-foot.

Vertebral Osteomyelitis

The most common route for vertebral infection is hematogenous spread via the arterial or venous system, although postoperative infection secondary to direct implantation of microorganisms into the intervertebral disk may also occur.

Microorganisms lodge at different sites depending on patient age. Below age 4, end arteries perforate the vertebral

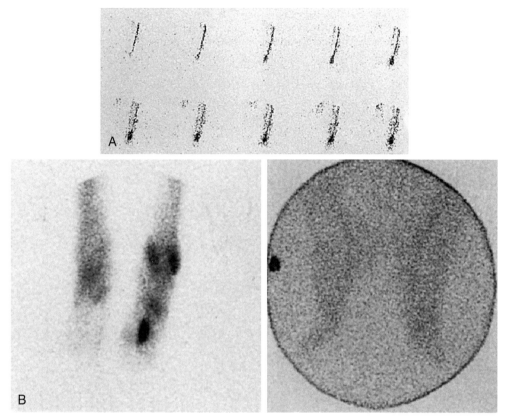

FIGURE 14-19. Suspected metatarsal osteomyelitis. Positive three-phase bone scan, negative In-111–labeled leukocyte results. **A,** Flow study shows increased flow in the region of the distal left midfoot. **B,** *Left,* A 3-hour delayed image shows increased uptake by the third metatarsal. *Right,* The In-111–labeled leukocyte study is negative for infection. Radiograph showed a metatarsal fracture.

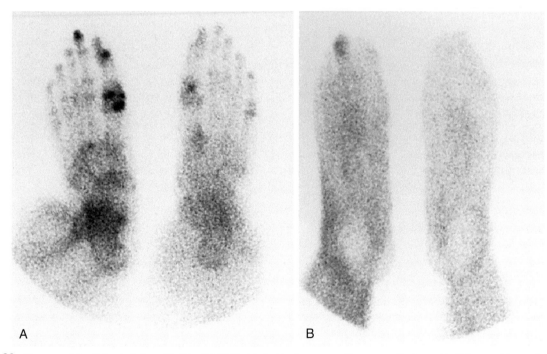

FIGURE 14-20. Osteomyelitis of distal phalanx: Tc-99m HMPAO–labeled leukocytes and bone scan. Patient with diabetes with purulent drainage of the distal second digit of the right foot. **A,** Bone scan shows increased uptake on the distal second digit of the right. The first two phases were also positive. **B,** Tc-99m HMPAO–labeled leukocytes were positive in the distal second digit, consistent with osteomyelitis. Other uptake on the bone scan was negative on the leukocyte study.

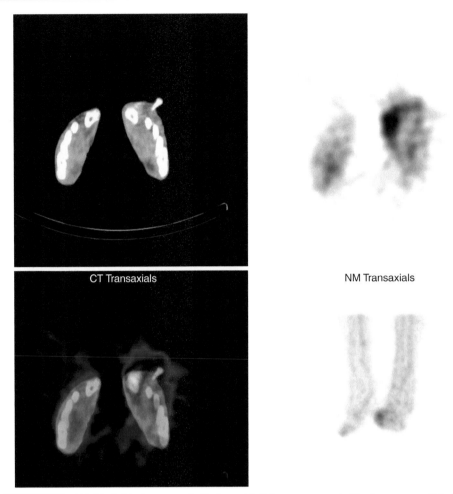

CT Transaxials

NM Transaxials

FIGURE 14-21. SPECT/CT In-111–labeled leukocyte study. Patient with diabetes suspected of having osteomyelitis due to a draining infected large toe ulcer. The maximum intensity projection view (right lower quadrant) shows diffuse uptake in the region of the distal large toe. Soft tissue cannot be differentiated from bone uptake. The fused SPECT/CT image shows *(left lower)* that the uptake is in both soft tissue and bone, consistent with the known overlying soft tissue infection and osteomyelitis.

body end plates and enter the disk space to produce diskitis. In adults, the most common infection site is the subchondral region of the vertebral body, which has the richest network of nutrient arterioles, similar to the vascular tree in the childhood metaphysis. The infection is primarily spondylitis, with secondary spread into the disk space. The infection spreads from the anterior subchondral focus through the vertebral end plate into the intervertebral disk. Later, it destroys the neighboring end plate, involves the opposite vertebral body, and may extend to adjacent soft tissue, resulting in epidural or paravertebral abscess formation.

Bone Scan
The usual scintigraphic pattern of diskitis is increased arterial blood flow, pool, and delayed uptake involving adjacent ends of adjoining vertebral bodies. With localized osteomyelitis, the bone scan will be three-phase positive. Blood flow and pool images can be difficult to evaluate in the thoracic spine because of normal cardiac, pulmonary, and vascular structures.

Leukocyte Scintigraphy
Multiple studies have reported a high false negative rate for vertebral osteomyelitis (40%-50%) using In-111

oxine–radiolabeled or Tc-99m HMPAO–radiolabeled WBCs. Normal or decreased uptake may be seen at the site of infection (Fig. 14-23). This may be due to stagnant blood flow in a bone marrow filled with pus, thrombosis, or infarction.

Gallium-67 Scintigraphy
Ga-67 citrate is superior to leukocyte scintigraphy for vertebral osteomyelitis (Fig. 14-23 and Box 14-8). For best accuracy, Ga-67 should be used in conjunction with a bone scan, using the criteria described previously (Fig. 14-17). An associated paraspinal abscess or disk infection may be also detected with the Ga-67 scan. SPECT and SPECT/CT can be helpful.

Fluorine-18 Fluordeoxyglucose
F-18 FDG is increasingly used as an alternative to Ga-67 for suspected vertebral osteomyelitis. Published data suggest it has good accuracy. Orthopedic hardware and postoperative changes can complicate interpretation. FDG uptake usually normalizes by 3 to 4 months after surgery or fracture (Fig. 14-13). False positive study results can occur. A negative FDG study result is highly predictive.

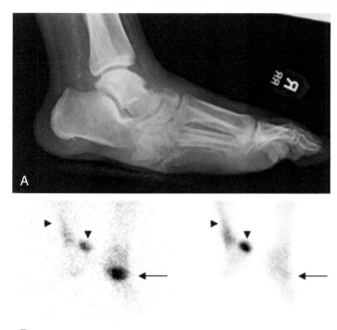

B   In-111 WBCs   Tc-99m SC

FIGURE 14-22. Mismatch of In-111–labeled leukocytes and bone marrow study in osteomyelitis. **A,** The lateral radiograph shows extensive vascular calcifications and midfoot neuropathic joint. Superimposed osteomyelitis could not be excluded. MRI (not shown) was also indeterminate. **B,** On the lateral In–11 WBC scan *(left)*, foci of increased activity are seen in the right midfoot *(arrow)* and the distal left tibia and calcaneus of the left foot *(arrowheads)*. On the lateral Tc-99m sulfur colloid *(SC)* bone marrow image *(right)* no corresponding activity is seen in the right midfoot *(arrow)*, consistent with osteomyelitis. The distribution of activity in the left distal tibia and calcaneus *(arrowheads)* is virtually identical to that with WBCs, confirming that these foci reflect marrow, not infection. Osteomyelitis of the right midfoot was confirmed with a subsequent below-knee amputation. (Courtesy Christopher Palestro, MD.)

Infected Joint Prosthesis

The postoperative infection rate after primary hip or knee replacement is only 1% and after revision surgery is 3%. However, when infection occurs, morbidity can be severe. Because the signs and symptoms are often indolent, diagnosis can be delayed and difficult. Radiographs and even joint aspiration have poor sensitivity for early detection.

Bone Scan

Characteristic bone scan findings can differentiate hip prosthesis loosening from infection. Postoperative uptake usually resolves by 12 months after insertion of a *cemented* total hip prosthesis. Loosening is suggested by uptake at the greater and lesser trochanter and prosthesis tip. Diffuse uptake surrounding the femoral component suggests infection.

A *cementless* or porous coated prosthesis depends on bony ingrowth for stabilization. Ongoing new bone formation is part of the fixation process, causing periprosthetic uptake in a variable pattern for a prolonged period, making interpretation difficult.

Knee prostheses are problematic for bone scintigraphy. More than half of all femoral components and three quarters of tibial components show periprosthetic uptake more

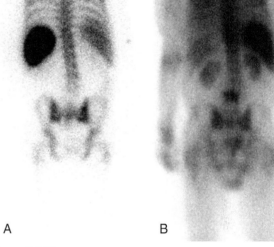

A   B

FIGURE 14-23. False negative result in In-111–labeled leukocyte scan (**A**) and positive Ga-67 scan (**B**) for spinal osteomyelitis. History of past spinal surgery, laminectomy, and fusion, treated successfully for infection; now the patient has recurrent pain. MRI was not diagnostic. Decreased In-111 uptake is seen in the lower lumbar spine. The Ga-67 scan shows intense uptake in the same region. The final diagnosis was osteomyelitis and diskitis in L-4/L-5.

Box 14-8. Gallium-67: Clinical Indications

Severe leukopenia (<3000/m^3 leukocytes)
Sarcoidosis
Idiopathic pulmonary fibrosis
Pulmonary drug reactions (amiodarone, bleomycin)
Pneumocystis jiroveci
Suspected low-grade chronic infections
Immunosuppressed patients
Fever of unknown origin
Malignant external otitis

---

than 12 months after placement. For patients with a cementless hip or total knee replacement, bone scintigraphy is most diagnostic if the scan is normal or if serial studies are available for comparison.

Gallium-67 Scintigraphy

Even in conjunction with bone scintigraphy, Ga-67 is only moderately accurate for the diagnosis of an infected joint prosthesis, reportedly about 80%.

Leukocyte Scintigraphy

The reported accuracy of combined leukocyte and bone scintigraphy for diagnosis of an infected joint prosthesis has varied considerably. Better diagnostic accuracy results from combined interpretation of leukocyte and bone marrow

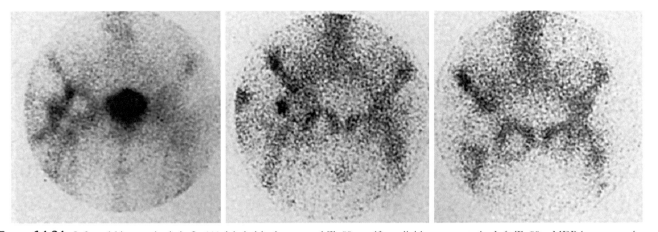

Figure 14-24. Infected hip prosthesis in In-111–labeled leukocyte and Tc-99m sulfur colloid marrow study. *Left*, Tc-99m MDP bone scan shows increased uptake in the region of the right hip prosthesis laterally, consistent with heterotopic calcification. *Middle*, Indium-111–labeled leukocyte study shows focal intense uptake just lateral to the femoral head and more diffuse uptake within the joint space that could be from infection or redistributed marrow. *Right*, Tc-99m sulfur colloid marrow study shows a normal bone marrow distribution with cold head of the femur from the prosthesis. The discordance of the bone marrow and In-111–labeled leukocyte study indicates an infected prosthesis.

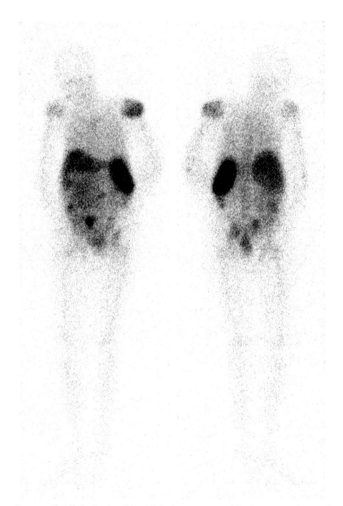

Figure 14-25. Peritonitis. Elderly woman with fever, sepsis, and abdominal pain. The In-111–labeled leukocyte study shows diffuse uptake throughout the abdomen, suggestive of peritonitis, and multiple foci of greater uptake suggestive of abscesses.

scintigraphy. This is because joint prosthesis inevitably results in marrow displacement in an unpredictable manner. Discordance of uptake on leukocyte and marrow scintigraphy is diagnostic of infection (Fig. 14-24). The Tc-99m sulfur colloid marrow study avoids the potential for a false positive study result—that is, interpretation of focal uptake as infection when it is merely displaced marrow. Accuracy is reported to be greater than 90%.

Response to Therapy

Ga-67 and leukocyte scintigraphy can be used to monitor response to therapy—for example, to determine whether an infection has been controlled before surgical replacement of a new prosthesis. Scintigraphic findings revert to normal within 2 to 8 weeks of appropriate antibiotic therapy.

Intraabdominal Infection

Postoperative intraabdominal infection is often confirmed with CT and directed interventional aspiration. However, in patients with nonlocalizing symptoms and negative conventional imaging, the preferred radiopharmaceutical is In-111 oxine–labeled leukocytes (Figs. 14-25 and 14-26) (Table 14-6). There is no intraabdominal intestinal or urinary clearance; thus uptake seen is usually infection. Sensitivity is reported to be approximately 90%.

Early imaging at 4 hours with In-111–labeled WBCs has a lower sensitivity for the detection of infection compared to 24 hours; however, in some urgent situations, early imaging may allow for earlier diagnosis—for example, suspected abscess, acute appendicitis, or diverticulitis.

Tc-99m HMPAO–labeled leukocytes can be used, particularly in children. Early imaging is required because hepatobiliary and renal clearance may be seen by 2 hours. Sensitivity for detecting intraabdominal infection is reported to be high. Delayed imaging can sometimes be helpful to confirm that early detected abnormal activity remains in a fixed pattern. A shifting pattern of activity over time implies intraluminal transit of labeled leukocytes, as seen with inflammatory or ischemic bowel disease, fistula, abscess in communication with bowel, or false

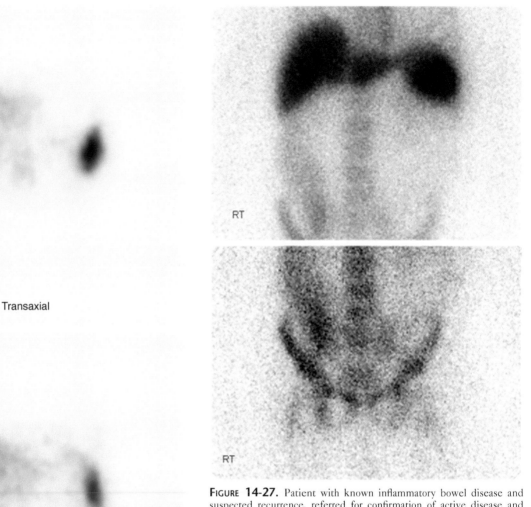

Transaxial

Coronal

FIGURE 14-26. Liver abscess on In-111 oxide–labeled leukocytes. Transverse *(above)* and coronal *(below)* cross-sectional SPECT slices with focal uptake of leukocytes in the right lobe of the liver. An abscess was subsequently drained.

FIGURE 14-27. Patient with known inflammatory bowel disease and suspected recurrence, referred for confirmation of active disease and localization. In-111 oxine–radiolabeled leukocyte study obtained 4 hours after reinfusion of the radiolabeled white blood cells shows localization in the ascending colon adjacent to the cecum. *RT,* Right.

positive causes—for example, swallowed leukocytes from sinus or tracheobronchial infection (Box 14-5).

Abnormal leukocyte uptake is also seen in a variety of noninfectious inflammatory diseases, such as pancreatitis, acute cholecystitis, polyarteritis nodosa, rheumatoid vasculitis, ischemic colitis, pseudomembranous colitis, and bowel infarction.

Inflammatory Bowel Disease

Both ulcerative colitis and granulomatous or regional enteritis or Crohn disease are characterized by intestinal inflammation. Leukocyte scintigraphy can be used to make the diagnosis, determine active disease distribution, and confirm relapse (Figs. 14-27 and 14-28). It can also aid in evaluation of regions hard to see with endoscopy and monitor therapeutic effectiveness.

Comparative studies have indicated that Tc-99m HMPAO–labeled leukocytes are superior to In-111 oxine–labeled leukocytes for diagnosis of inflammatory bowel disease, probably because of the superior image resolution enabling disease localization to specific bowel segments. Crohn disease and ulcerative colitis usually can be distinguished by their distribution. Ulcerative colitis typically has continuous colonic and rectal involvement, whereas Crohn disease involves the small bowel, has skip areas, and spares the rectum.

Leukocyte scintigraphy can differentiate reactivation of inflammatory bowel disease from abscess formation resulting from bowel perforation, a serious complication requiring surgical rather than medical therapy. Radiolabeled leukocyte uptake in an abscess is typically focal, whereas uptake in inflamed bowel follows the contour of the intestinal wall.

If In-111–labeled leukocyte scintigraphy is used, images should be acquired at 4 hours rather than 24 hours because of shedding of the inflamed leukocytes into the bowel lumen from the inflammatory sites and subsequent peristalsis, which can result in incorrect assignment of disease to sites distal to the true lesion. Tc-99m HMPAO imaging should be performed by 2 hours.

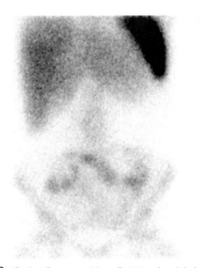

FIGURE 14-28. Crohn disease on 4-hour In-111 oxine–labeled leukocytes. Patient with several-year history of regional ileitis and 2 months of recurrent and worsening symptoms. Scintigraphy confirms active inflammation of ileum.

Renal Disease

Ga-67 has been used to diagnose diffuse interstitial nephritis and localized renal infection. Delayed 48-hour imaging is required because of early urinary tract clearance. Renal parenchymal infection, (e.g., pyelonephritis, diffuse interstitial nephritis, lobar nephronia [focal interstitial nephritis], and perirenal infections) can be diagnosed. Generally, Ga-67 has been superseded by radiolabeled leukocyte imaging (Fig. 14-29) or Tc-99m dimercaptosuccinic acid (DMSA) for pyelonephritis. Radiolabeled leukocytes seem to have similar accuracy. However, radiolabeled WBCs have limited utility for evaluation of renal transplants because all exhibit uptake, regardless of the presence or absence of clinical infection, probably as a result of ongoing low-grade rejection.

Cardiovascular Disease

In-111–labeled leukocytes are not sensitive for detection of subacute bacterial endocarditis. The vegetative lesions contain high concentrations of bacteria, platelets, and fibrin adherent to damaged valvular endothelium, but relatively few leukocytes. However, SPECT and SPECT/CT have improved detection and localization (Fig. 14-30).

Prompt diagnosis of graft infection is critical but often delayed because of its indolent and insidious course. With infection of arterial prosthetic grafts (e.g., femoropopliteal or aortofemoral), ultrasound, CT, and MRI are often unable to distinguish infection from aseptic fluid collections around the graft. Radiolabeled leukocytes can detect

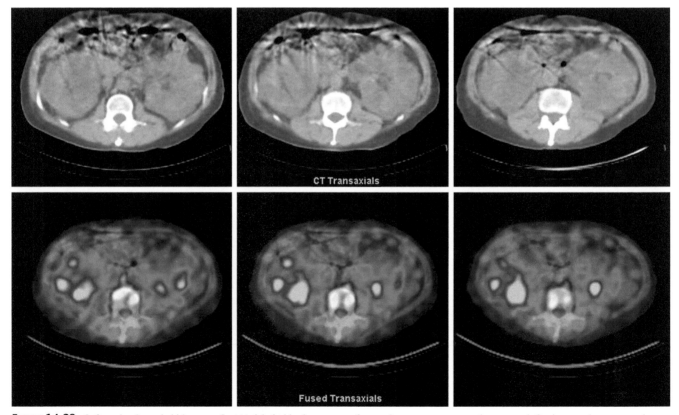

FIGURE 14-29. Infected polycystic kidneys on In-111–labeled leukocyte scan for renal stones, recurrent urinary tract infections, and recent persistent fever of uncertain cause. Low-dose CT *(above)* demonstrates very large multicystic kidneys. Fused SPECT/CT images *(below)* show multiple areas of increased uptake *(yellow)* in the renal cysts diagnostic of infection.

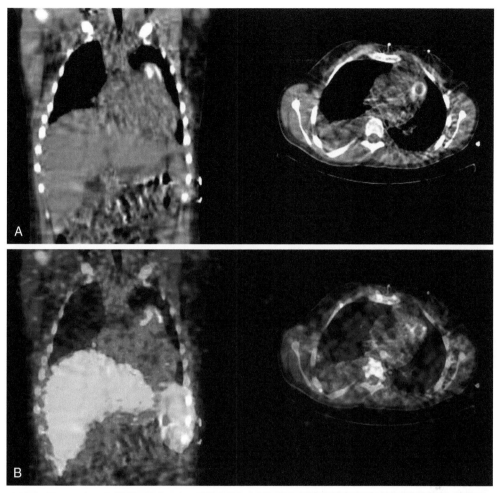

FIGURE **14-30.** A 17-year-old patient with DiGeorge syndrome. truncus arteriosus, and a right ventricular pulmonary artery conduit. He has experienced recent chills and fever and blood cultures positive for *Staphylococcus aureus.* **A,** Coronal and transverse CT shows the pulmonary artery conduit. **B,** Fused SPECT/CT In-111 oxine leukocyte images show uptake that indicates that the conduit is infected.

surgical prosthetic graft infection. In-111 has the advantage of having no blood pool distribution, a limitation of Tc-99m HMPAO. However, early and serial imaging with Tc-99m HMPAO at 5 minutes, 30 minutes, and 3 hours has been shown accurate for confirming the diagnosis (Fig. 14-12).

Pulmonary Infection

Radiolabeled leukocytes are not commonly used to detect pulmonary infection. Low-grade diffuse uptake is seen with a variety of noninfectious inflammatory causes, including acute respiratory distress syndrome, atelectasis, and congestive heart failure, and thus is not diagnostic of infection. Focal intense uptake is likely to be due to infection. Tuberculosis and fungal infections may be detected by In-111–labeled leukocytes, but with poorer sensitivity than Ga-67.

Ga-67 citrate accumulates in many types of acute and chronic pulmonary infections and inflammatory diseases (Box 14-9). It has been used most successfully in the past for detection of chronic diseases such as sarcoidosis (Fig. 14-31), idiopathic pulmonary fibrosis, *Pneumocystis jiroveci* (formerly known as *P. carinii*) (Fig. 14-32), and therapeutic drug-induced pulmonary disease (Boxes 14-8 and 14-9).

BOX 14-9. Gallium-67 Uptake in Interstitial and Granulomatous Pulmonary Diseases

Tuberculosis
Histoplasmosis
Sarcoidosis
Idiopathic pulmonary fibrosis
Pneumocystis jiroveci
Cytomegalovirus
Pneumoconioses (asbestosis, silicosis)
Hypersensitivity pneumonitis

Sarcoidosis

Sarcoidosis is a chronic granulomatous multisystem disease of unknown cause characterized by accumulation of T-lymphocytes, mononuclear phagocytes, and noncaseating epithelioid granulomas in any organ of the body, most commonly the lung, liver, and spleen.

Common systemic symptoms include weight loss, fatigue, weakness, malaise, and fever. Pulmonary manifestations include hilar and mediastinal adenopathy, endobronchial granuloma formation, interstitial or alveolar pulmonary infiltrates, and pulmonary fibrosis.

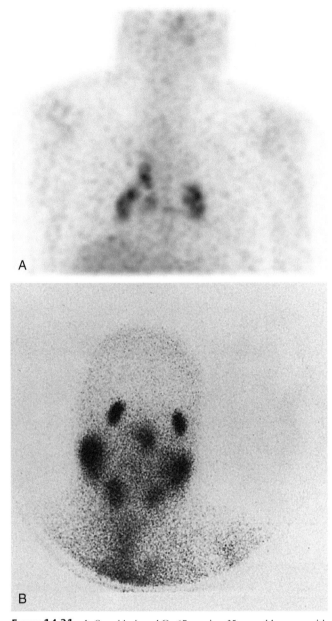

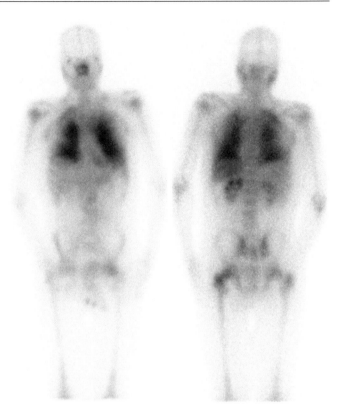

FIGURE 14-32. *Pneumocystis jiroveci* (formerly *P. carinii*) and whole-body Ga-67 scan. A 57-year-old HIV-positive man with bilateral pulmonary pneumonitis. Note characteristic diffuse bilateral Ga-67 uptake.

FIGURE 14-31. A, Sarcoidosis and Ga-67 scan in a 35-year-old woman with new diagnosis of sarcoidosis. Ga-67 scintigraphy demonstrates the "lambda" sign with uptake in paratracheal and hilar adenopathy. **B,** The "panda" sign in a patient with sarcoidosis. Prominent characteristic increased uptake in the lacrimal, parotid, and submandibular salivary glands.

TABLE 14-8 Classification of Chest Radiographic Findings in Sarcoidosis

Type	Radiographic findings
0	Hilar and/or mediastinal node enlargement with normal lung parenchyma
II	Hilar and/or mediastinal node enlargement and diffuse interstitial pulmonary disease
III	Diffuse pulmonary disease without node involvement
IV	Pulmonary fibrosis

Extrapulmonary manifestations of the skin, eyes, heart, central nervous system, bones, and muscle are not rare. Central nervous system and cardiac involvement may lead to death.

The initial presentation is commonly pulmonary, with dyspnea and dry cough, although 20% may be asymptomatic and have only an abnormal chest radiograph. The clinical course is variable. Spontaneous resolution occurs in 30%, 40% have a smoldering or progressively worsening course, 20% develop permanent lung function loss, and 10% die of respiratory failure.

Four categories of radiographic findings identify sarcoidosis (Table 14-8). The alveolitis of sarcoidosis is manifested on radiographs as an infiltrative process. Although patients with radiographs showing type I findings tend to have a reversible form of the disease, those with types II and III usually have chronic progressive disease; these are not necessarily consecutive stages.

Diagnosis is based on a combination of clinical, radiographic, and histological findings. The chest radiograph, although characteristic, is not diagnostic because the typical bilateral hilar adenopathy may be seen with other diseases.

Various diagnostic tests have been used. Bronchoalveolar lavage is an accurate method. An increase in the relative and absolute numbers of T-lymphocytes, monocytes, and macrophages is an indication for therapy. The serum angiotensin-converting enzyme is negative in two thirds of patients, and false positive results are common. The Kveim-Siltzbach test requires intradermal injection of human sarcoid tissue. A nodule develops at the injection site in 4 to 6 weeks in patients with sarcoidosis, and biopsy reveals noncaseating granulomas in 70% to 80%. Biopsy evidence of a mononuclear cell granulomatous inflammatory process is mandatory for definitive diagnosis.

Bronchoalveolar lavage and Ga-67 and F-18 FDG scans have been used as indicators of disease activity. Although many patients require no specific therapy, patients with severe active disease are often treated with glucocorticoids that suppress the activated T-cells at the disease site and the clinical manifestations of the disease.

Gallium-67 Scintigraphy

Ga-67 scans are positive in most patients with active sarcoidosis. The scan has been used to assess the magnitude of alveolitis, guide lung biopsy, and choose the pulmonary segments for bronchoalveolar lavage. It can distinguish active granuloma formation and alveolitis from inactive disease and fibrotic changes. Increased Ga-67 uptake in the lungs is more than 90% sensitive for clinically active disease. Scans are negative in inactive cases.

Ga-67 is more sensitive than a chest radiograph for detecting early disease. Pulmonary uptake on scintigraphy may occur before characteristic abnormalities are present on radiographs (Table 14-8). Patients with a normal Ga-67 scan nearly always have a negative biopsy. Patients with a diagnosis of sarcoidosis and an abnormal chest radiograph, but inactive disease, have negative Ga-67 scans. Ga-67 has been shown to be a sensitive indicator of treatment response, superior to clinical symptoms, chest radiograph, and pulmonary function tests.

Increasingly, F-18 FDG is being used to confirm or exclude the diagnosis of sarcoidosis and determine the extent of disease, its distribution, and disease activity. Although assumed to be at least equal, if not superior, to Ga-67, clinical data are limited.

Scintigraphic Patterns

In early disease, Ga-67 scintigraphy and F-18 FDG often show bilateral hilar and paratracheal uptake (lambda sign) (Figs. 14-31 and 14-33). Pulmonary parenchymal uptake is typically intense and symmetric and may or may not be associated with hilar and mediastinal involvement. Prominent Ga-67 uptake may be seen in the nasopharyngeal region and parotid, salivary, and lacrimal glands (panda sign). The latter is not seen with F-18 FDG.

In contrast to sarcoidosis, patients with malignant lymphoma usually have asymmetric hilar or mediastinal uptake, often involving the anterior mediastinal and paratracheal nodes. Although paraaortic, mesenteric, and retroperitoneal lymph node involvement may be seen in sarcoidosis, this pattern of uptake is considerably more common in lymphoma.

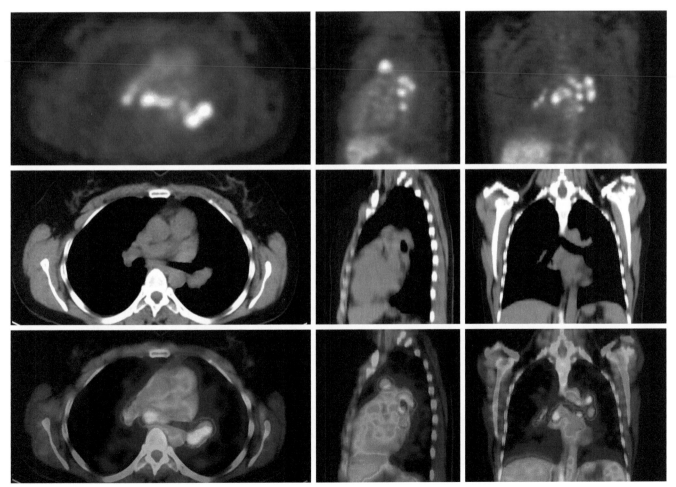

FIGURE 14-33. Sarcoidosis and F-18 FDG. FDG *(above)*, CT *(middle)*, and fused images *(below)*. Mediastinal and bilateral hilar adenopathy.

Idiopathic Interstitial Pulmonary Fibrosis

Idiopathic interstitial pulmonary fibrosis typically follows a progression through stages of alveolitis, with derangement of the alveolar-capillary units and leading to end-stage fibrotic disease. The cause is unknown. Ga-67 uptake occurs in approximately 70% of patients and has been used to monitor disease course and response

---

Box 14-10. Therapeutic Agents Associated with Gallium-67 Lung Uptake

Bleomycin
Amiodarone
Busulfan
Nitrofurantoin
Cyclophosphamide
Methotrexate
Nitrosourea

---

to therapy. The degree of uptake correlates with the amount of cellular infiltration. Limited data show similar findings for F-18 FDG.

Pulmonary Drug Reactions

Common therapeutic drugs known to cause lung injury and result in Ga-67 uptake include cytoxan, nitrofurantoin, bleomycin, and amiodarone (Box 14-10). Ga-67 uptake is an early indicator of drug-induced lung injury, before the radiograph becomes abnormal.

Malignant External Otitis

Malignant external otitis is a life-threatening infection caused by *Pseudomonas* organisms and most commonly seen in patients with diabetes. The three-phase bone scan can be diagnostic, with uptake in the mastoid and temporal bone (Fig. 14-34). Increased Ga-67 can be diagnostic and used to judge response to therapy.

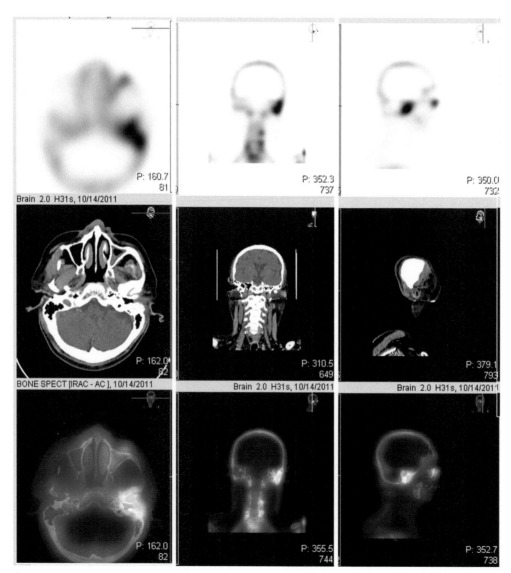

Figure 14-34. Malignant external otitis with osteomyelitis on Tc-99 MDP. SPECT/CT fused images localize uptake to the region of the mastoid and temporal lobes, transverse *(left)*, coronal *(middle)*, and sagittal *(right)*.

Fever of Unknown Origin

Fever of unknown origin has been defined as a temperature of at least 38.3° C (100.9° F) that occurs on more than three occasions, remains undiagnosed for at least 3 weeks, and results in at least 7 days of hospitalization. Ga-67 is a sensitive test for uncovering the source of the fever. In addition to localizing acute infection, Ga-67 can detect chronic, indolent, and granulomatous infections and also tumor sources of fever (Box 14-8). However, postoperative patients with fever are better served with In-111–labeled leukocytes because fever is most commonly caused by an acute infection. F-18 FDG PET/CT is increasingly used for this indication. Early data are promising.

▰ Suggested Reading

Datz FL, Taylor AT Jr. Cell labeling: techniques and clinical utility. *Freeman and Johnson's Clinical Radionuclide Imaging*. 3rd ed. New York: Grune & Stratton; 1986.

Gemmel F, Rijk PC, Collins JMP, et al. Expanding role of F-18 fluoro-d-deoxyglucose PET and PET/CT in spinal infections. *Eur Spine J*. 2010;19(4):540-551.

Glaudemans AW, Signore A. FDG-PET/CT in infections: the imaging method of choice? *Eur J Nucl Med Mol Imaging*. 2010;37(10):1986-1991.

Gotthardt M, Bleeker-Rovers CP, Boerman OC, Oyen WJG. Imaging of inflammation by PET, conventional scintigraphy, and other imaging techniques. *J Nucl Med*. 2010;51(12):1937-1949.

Meller J, Koster G, Liersch, et al. Chronic bacterial osteomyelitis: prospective comparison of F-18 FDG imaging with a dual-headed coincidence camera and In-111 labeled autologous leukocyte scintigraphy. *Eur J Nucl Med*. 2001;29(10): 53-60.

Merkel KD, Brown ML, Dewanjee MK, Fitzgerald RH Jr. Comparison of indium-labeled-leukocyte imaging with sequential technetium-gallium scanning in the diagnosis of low-grade musculoskeletal sepsis. *J Bone Joint Surg Am*. 1985;67(3):465-476.

Oyen WJG, Boerman OC, van der Laken CJ, et al. The uptake mechanism of inflammation- and infection-localizing agents. *Eur J Nucl Med*. 1996;23(4):459-465.

Palestro CJ. 18F-FDG and diabetic foot infections: the verdict is.... *J Nucl Med*. 2011;52(7):1009-1011.

Palestro CJ, Kim CK, Swyer AJ, et al. Total-hip arthroplasty: periprosthetic indium-111-labeled leukocyte activity and complementary technetium-99m-sulfur colloid imaging in suspected infection. *J Nucl Med*. 1990;31(12):1950-1955.

Palestro CJ, Mehta HH, Patel M, et al. Marrow versus infection in the Charcot joint: indium-111 leukocyte and technetium-99m sulfur colloid scintigraphy. *J Nucl Med*. 1998;39(2):346-350.

Peters AM, Danpure HJ, Osman S, et al. Clinical experience with 99mTc-hexamethylpropylene-amineoxime for labeling leucocytes and imaging inflammation. *Lancet*. 1986;2525(8513):946-948.

Van der Bruggen W, Bleeker-Rovers CP, Boerman OC, et al. PET and SPECT in osteomyelitis and prosthetic bone and joint infections: a systematic review. *Semin Nucl Med*. 2010;40(1):3-15.

CHAPTER 15

Central Nervous System

Before the development of computed tomography (CT) in the 1970s, radionuclide brain scans were the only non-invasive method for diagnosing diseases of the brain, including tumors, strokes, and vascular anomalies. The first radionuclide brain scan agents, such as technetium-99m pertechnetate and Tc-99m diethylenetriamine pentaacetic acid (DTPA), did not cross the intact blood–brain barrier (Fig. 15-1). Brain uptake occurred only if there was disruption—for example, with tumor and stroke. The Tc-99m radiopharmaceuticals currently used today are lipophilic and able to readily cross the blood–brain barrier.

Positron emission tomography (PET), which began with the brain decades ago, did not move into widespread clinical use until the advent of PET/CT for oncology and availability of the glucose analog fluorine-18 fluorodeoxyglucose (FDG) without the need for an onsite cyclotron. Although most F-18 FDG imaging is currently done for cancer, use in the brain offers some advantages over single-photon emission computed tomography (SPECT), including better resolution and ease of quantitation. Although magnetic resonance imaging (MRI) and CT are the most commonly used brain-imaging modalities today, nuclear medicine techniques provide unique diagnostic information based on imaging physiology. SPECT and PET can both visualize alterations in function before anatomical changes can be detected.

A list of current clinical indications for brain imaging using scintigraphy is listed in Box 15-1.

Several new compounds have been moving through the approval process. The SPECT agent iodine-123 ioflupane (DaTscan), available in Europe for years, has now been approved for use in the United States to differentiate parkinsonian syndromes from other causes of tremor. Although the only brain PET radiopharmaceutical available for clinical use in the United States for many years was F-18 FDG, an amyloid agent has recently been approved. It is expected that other agents will become available in the future. Many experimental agents are limited by the short, 20-minute physical half-life of their carbon-11 radiolabel. A clear clinical role must be found for other agents. A partial list of some PET agents used for a variety of applications in the brain is listed in Table 15-1.

CEREBRAL ANATOMY

Knowledge of brain anatomy is critical in understanding patterns of disease and image interpretation. The brain consists of the two cerebral hemispheres above the tentorium and the cerebellum below in the posterior fossa. The regions, or lobes, of the brain are illustrated in Figure 15-2. The frontal lobe extends back to the central sulcus, with the parietal lobe just posterior to it. The occipital lobe is most posterior, below the parietooccipital sulcus. The temporal lobes are below the lateral fissure. Within these lobes, key functional centers, or regions, have been identified, that are important when trying to assimilate clinical changes with anatomical and functional images (Fig. 15-3).

Studies such as dynamic radionuclide brain flow and brain death examination allow visualization of the vascular

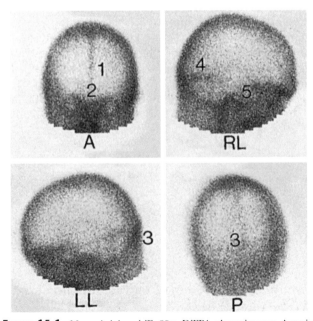

FIGURE **15-1.** Normal delayed Tc-99m DTPA planar images. Anterior *(A)*, right lateral *(RL)*, left lateral *(LL)*, and posterior *(P)* projections. The superior sagittal sinus *(1)* is seen on anterior and posterior views. The floor of the frontal sinus *(2)*, confluence of sinuses *(3)*, transverse sinuses *(4)*, and sphenoid sinus *(5)* are faintly seen.

Box 15-1. Clinical Indications for Central Nervous System Scintigraphy

Dementia diagnosis
Epileptic seizure focus localization
Brain tumor recurrence
Vascular reserve assessment in high-risk patients
Carotid artery sacrifice: Preoperative impact evaluation
Acute stroke: Select thrombolytic agent candidates
Brain death determination
Parkinson disease: Differentiation from essential
 tremor
Cerebrospinal fluid (CSF) evaluation
 CSF shunt function
 Normal-pressure hydrocephalus diagnosis
Investigational uses: Psychiatric disorders and chronic
 effects of head trauma

TABLE 15-1 Positron Emission Tomography Radiopharmaceuticals

Compound	Application
O-15 H$_2$O	Blood flow
O-15 O$_2$	Oxygen metabolism and flow
O-15 or C-11 carboxyhemoglobin	Blood volume
C-11 methionine	Amino acid metabolism
C-11 methylpiperone	Dopamine receptor activity
C-11 carfentanil	Mu opiate receptor activity
C-11 flunitrazepam	Benzodiazepine receptor activity
C-11 scopolamine	Muscarinic cholinergic receptors
C-11 ephedrine	Adrenergic terminals
C-11 PIB	Amyloid deposition
F-18 FDG	Glucose metabolism
F-18 fluoro-L-dopa	Neurotransmitter; peptide synthesis
F-18 AV-45 (F-18 florbetapir)	Amyloid synthesis
F-18 AV-1 (F-18 florbetaben)	Amyloid synthesis
F-18-3′-F-PIB (F-18 flutemetamol)	Amyloid synthesis
F-18 fluorothymidine	DNA synthesis
F-18 MISO	Tumor hypoxia
F-18 FDPN	Opiate receptor (nonspecific) activity

FDG, Fluorodeoxyglucose; *FDPN,* fluoroethyl-6-O-diphrenorphine; *FLT,* fluorothymidine; *F-18 MISO,* fluoromisonidazole; *PIB,* Pittsburgh B compound.

supply of the brain to a limited degree, so understanding the arterial and venous anatomy is important (Figs. 15-4 and 15-5). Even more important for image interpretation is familiarity with the cerebral regions these vessels supply (Fig. 15-6).

■ CEREBRAL BLOOD FLOW AND METABOLISM

Radiopharmaceuticals

Fluorine-18 Fluorodeoxyglucose: Glucose Metabolism

The brain is an obligate glucose user, and F-18 FDG is a glucose analog, allowing accurate assessment of regional cerebral glucose metabolism (rCGM). F-18 FDG is able to cross the blood–brain barrier using glucose transporter systems and enters the neuron. After rapid phosphorylation by hexokinase-1, F-18 FDG is metabolically trapped and cannot proceed further along the glucose metabolism pathway. Approximately 4% of the administered dose is localized to the brain. By 35 minutes after injection, 95% of peak uptake is achieved. Urinary excretion is rapid, with 10% to 40% of the dose cleared in 2 hours. In addition to reflecting regional cerebral blood flow (rCBF), as a marker of glucose metabolism, F-18 FDG can be used to determine tumor viability. With its 110-minute half-life, F-18 FDG does not require an expensive onsite cyclotron.

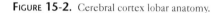

FIGURE 15-2. Cerebral cortex lobar anatomy.

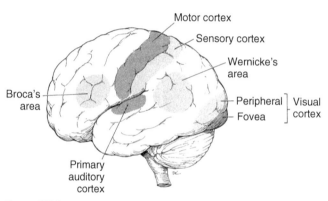

FIGURE 15-3. Motor, sensory, visual, speech, and auditory functional and associative centers of the brain.

Technetium-99m Perfusion Cerebral Blood Flow Radiopharmaceuticals

The two SPECT agents used to assess regional cerebral blood flow are Tc-99m hexamethylpropyleneamine oxime (Tc-99m HMPAO) and Tc-99m ethyl cysteinate dimer (Tc-99m ECD). Favorable characteristics of these two neutral, lipophilic agents include high first-pass extraction across the blood–brain barrier, distribution corresponding to rCBF, and desirable 140-keV gamma photons. However, both slightly underestimate true rCBF, especially at high flow states. The Tc-99m perfusion agents are relatively fixed in the neuron. Therefore, delayed imaging shows what the perfusion pattern looked like at the time of injection. For example, if the agent is injected during an epileptic seizure, images can be performed hours after the seizure.

Technetium-99m Hexamethylpropyleneamine Oxime

Tc-99m HMPAO (Tc-99m exametazime [Ceretec]) was first introduced in the mid-1980s. It was originally available as a kit requiring use within 30 minutes of radiolabeling; however, stabilizers have since been added, allowing a 4-hour shelf life after addition of the radiolabel. Care must be taken

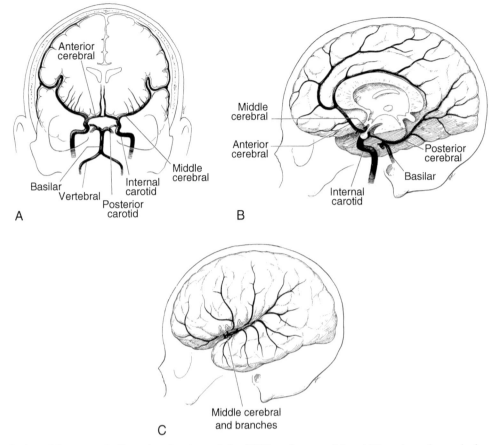

FIGURE 15-4. Cerebral arterial anatomy. **A,** Coronal section shows circle of Willis and course of the middle and anterior cerebral arteries. Internal carotids divide at the base of the brain (circle of Willis) into the anterior and middle cerebral arteries. The middle cerebral artery runs laterally in the sylvian fissure, then backward and upward on the surface of the insula, where it divides into branches to the *lateral* surface of the cerebral hemisphere and to portions of the basal ganglia. **B,** Midline sagittal view shows distribution of anterior, middle, and posterior cerebral arteries. The anterior cerebral artery supplies the cerebrum along its *medial* margin above the corpus callosum and extends posteriorly to the parietal fissure as well as to the anterior portion of the basal ganglia. Vertebral arteries fuse into the basilar artery, which branches at the circle of Willis into the two posterior cerebral arteries supplying the occipital lobe and the inferior half of the temporal lobe. **C,** Left lateral view shows distribution of the middle cerebral artery over the cerebral cortex.

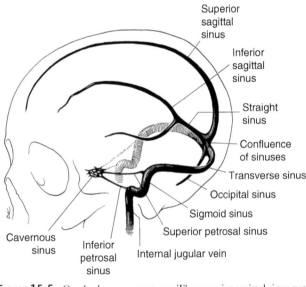

FIGURE 15-5. Cerebral venous anatomy. The superior sagittal sinus runs along the falx within the superior margin of the interhemispheric fissure. The inferior sagittal sinus is smaller, courses over the corpus callosum, and joins with the great vein of Galen to form the straight sinus, which drains into the superior sagittal sinus at the confluence of sinuses (torcular herophili) at the occipital protuberance. Transverse sinuses drain the sagittal and occipital sinuses into the internal jugular vein.

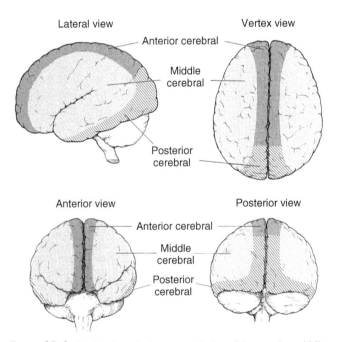

FIGURE 15-6. Regional cerebral cortex perfusion of the anterior, middle, and posterior cerebral arteries.

TABLE **15-2** Dosimetry of Cerebral Imaging Agents

Agent	Organ receiving highest dose	Dose (mGy/MBq)	Effective dose (mSv/MBq)
F-18 FDG	Bladder wall	0.13	0.019
Tc-99m HMPAO	Kidney	0.034	0.0093
Tc-99m ECD	Bladder wall	0.05	0.0077
Tl-201	Kidneys	0.46	0.23
Tc-99m sestamibi	Gallbladder	0.039	0.0085
I-123 ioflupane	Bladder wall	0.053	0.0213
	Striata	0.230	

ECD, Ethyl cysteinate dimer; *FDG*, fluorodeoxyglucose; *HMPAO*, hexamethylpropyleneamine oxime.

that doses from the radiopharmacy have been labeled with fresh generator eluate (<2 hours old) just before delivery. Tc-99m HMPAO has a good first-pass extraction of approximately 80%, with 3.5% to 7% of the injected dose localizing in the brain within 1 minute of injection. Once across the blood–brain barrier, it enters the neuron and becomes a polar hydrophilic molecule trapped inside the cell. However, some of the radiopharmaceutical may be present in different isomeric forms that are not trapped. Although up to 15% of the dose washes out in the first 2 minutes, little loss occurs over the next 24 hours. SPECT images can be acquired from 20 minutes to 2 hours after injection. Excretion is largely renal (40%) and gastrointestinal (15%).

Technetium-99m Ethyl Cysteinate Dimer

Tc-99m ECD (Tc-99m bicisate, Neurolite) is a neutral lipophilic agent that passively diffuses across the blood–brain barrier like Tc-99m HMPAO. Once prepared, the Tc-99m ECD dose is stable for 6 hours. It has a first-pass extraction of 60% to 70%, with peak brain activity reaching 5% to 6% of the injected dose. The blood clearance is more rapid than Tc-99m HMPAO, resulting in better brain-to-background ratios. At 1 hour, less than 5% of the dose remains in the blood, compared to more than 12% of a Tc-99m HMPAO dose.

Once inside the cell, Tc-99m ECD undergoes enzymatic deesterification, forming polar metabolites unable to cross the cell membrane. However, slow (roughly 6% per hour) washout of some labeled metabolites occurs, with almost 25% of the brain activity cleared by 4 hours. Although images may be superior to those with Tc-99m HMPAO 15 to 30 minutes after injection, they may be suboptimal if imaging is delayed.

Dosimetry

The dosimetry for various cerebral radiopharmaceuticals is provided in Table 15-2.

Methodology

Positron Emission Tomography Acquisition

Patient preparation for F-18 FDG brain imaging is similar to that for oncology applications. Patients should fast for

---

Box *15-2.* **Fluorine-18 Fluorodeoxyglucose Positron Emission Tomography Imaging: Summary Protocol**

PATIENT PREPARATION
Patient should fast 4 to 6 hours, avoid carbohydrates, maintain normal blood glucose.
Check blood glucose. If less than 180 to 200, continue.
Elevated glucose: Consider rescheduling, administer insulin, recheck, delay 2 hours.
Inject in quiet, dimly lit room, eyes open.
Wait 30 minutes.

RADIOPHARMACEUTICAL
F-18 FDG 10 to 15 mCi (185-555 MBq)

INSTRUMENTATION
Dedicated PET or PET/CT camera
Coincidence camera

IMAGING
Attenuation correction scan: Gadolinium rods or CT
Acquisition: 7 minutes per bed position for one bed position

PROCESSING
Iterative reconstruction, automated software

CT, Computed tomography; *FDG*, fluorodeoxyglucose; *PET*, positron emission tomography.

4 to 6 hours before injection, should have serum glucose less than 200 mg/dL, should not have had insulin for 2 hours (short-acting insulin) to 6 to 8 hours (long-acting insulin), and should avoid strenuous exercise for a few days before the test. Exercise and insulin will shunt FDG to the muscles and reduce brain uptake.

F-18 FDG should be injected in a quiet, dimly lit room with the patient remaining still and undisturbed during the uptake period (20-30 minutes). Scan acquisition is typically done in a three-dimensional (3-D) mode, although some older systems still allow two-dimensional (2-D) mode acquisition with movable septa to minimize scatter. A sample protocol is listed in Box 15-2.

Single-Photon Emission Computed Tomography Acquisition

As with PET, patients are injected in a quiet, dimly lit room. For the best-quality image, a delay of 30 to 60 minutes for Tc-99m ECD and 30 to 90 minutes for Tc-99m HMPAO should be used to improve the signal-to-noise ratio. Dedicated triple-head gamma cameras are increasingly rare but yield the best results. A dual-head camera creates images superior to those with a single-head SPECT camera. Patient positioning is just as important as the equipment used. The heads of the camera must come as close to the patient as possible, or resolution is reduced. A head-holder attachment extending from the end of the table allows the camera heads to come in closer than the width of a table or the patient's shoulders. In heavy patients and those whose shoulders obstruct the view, the posterior fossa may not be seen. A protocol for Tc-99m cerebral perfusion SPECT imaging is given in Box 15-3. The SPECT images are processed using iterative reconstruction. A filter

---

Box 15-3. **Single-Photon Emission Computed Tomography Cerebral Perfusion Imaging: Summary Protocol**

PATIENT PREPARATION
None

RADIOPHARMACEUTICAL
Tc-99m HMPAO (Ceretec) or Tc-99m ECD (Neurolite) 20 mCi

INSTRUMENTATION
Camera: Dual-head or triple-head SPECT
Head-holder attachment: Head extends beyond table for minimum camera radius
Collimators: High resolution, parallel hole
Computer setup: SPECT acquisition parameters
  Matrix size: 64 × 64
  Zoom: 2
  Rotation: Step and shoot
  Orbit: Circular
  Angle step size: 3 degrees
  Stops: 40 per head
  Time per stop: 40 seconds (total time, 27 minutes)

IMAGING PROCEDURE
Prepare dose according to package insert. Note shelf life.
Begin intravenous access or tape butterfly in place; make patient comfortable in quiet, dimly lit room; inject; patient eyes open; begin scanning in 15 minutes to 2 to 3 hours later.
Position patient so that brain is entirely within field of view of all detectors.
Position collimators as close as possible to patient's head.

PROCESSING
Filtered back projection or iterative reconstruction
Filter: Hamming, 1.2 high-frequency cutoff
Attenuation correction: 0.11 cm^{-1}

ECD, Ethyl cysteinate dimer; *HMPAO,* hexamethylpropyleneamine oxime; *SPECT,* single-photon emission computed tomography.

is applied to smooth the image. In general, filters can be sampled and modified for each patient in the postprocessing stage to achieve an optimal image.

Interpretation

SPECT images generally reflect cortical rCBF, which is determined by oxygen demands of the brain. In addition, blood flow distribution is usually similar to metabolism seen with F-18 FDG. Areas with more synaptic activity require greater blood flow. Activational studies can therefore target areas of the brain showing increased flow when activated by a certain task.

There is a 2:1 to 4:1 differential in blood flow to gray matter compared to white matter seen on SPECT and PET scans. Lesions in the white matter often cannot be detected or even differentiated from cerebrospinal fluid (CSF) spaces on PET or SPECT, so MRI or CT correlation is necessary for identifying white matter changes

and enlarged ventricles. The anatomy seen on CT and MRI is much more detailed than the structures seen with SPECT or PET; however, many structures can be well visualized (Fig. 15-7). Typically, activity is fairly evenly distributed between the lobes of the brain. However, this is dependent on the conditions at the time of injection. For example, bright lights will increase occipital lobes activity, falsely causing the frontal lobes to appear decreased.

The distribution of Tc-99m HMPAO differs only slightly from Tc-99m ECD. Tc-99m HMPAO accumulates more in the frontal lobes, thalamus, and cerebellum, whereas Tc-99m ECD shows higher affinity for the parietal and occipital lobes. Although the differences are not usually noticeable, it would be best to use the same agent for serial examinations. Most clinicians use the agent with which they are most familiar.

The normal distribution of SPECT and PET agents also changes with age. In infants, a relative decrease is seen in frontal lobe perfusion. This increases over time, reaching an adult level by about 2 years of age. In adults, global activity decreases with age, and this decrease is more prominent in the frontal regions. Given these changes, using comparison age-matched normal databases and computer programs that quantitate rCBF may help improve accuracy.

■ CLINICAL APPLICATIONS FOR CEREBRAL PERFUSION IMAGING

Dementia

As our population ages, dementia has an increasing impact on society and health care systems. Clinical symptoms may vary (e.g., short- or long-term memory loss, loss of judgment, personality changes, and loss of other higher cortical functions), and the functional decline can occur rapidly over months or slowly over years. These changes must be differentiated from the normal decline in memory and decreased ability to learn new things that accompany aging.

Dementia is a manifestation of many diseases (Box 15-4). Only about 10% of dementias, such as those caused by vitamin B_{12} or thyroid hormone deficiency, are treatable. However, with better understanding of the disease processes underlying dementia, new therapies are being developed. For example, the cholinesterase inhibitors have some stabilizing effects in patients with Alzheimer disease, occasionally even reversing perfusion trends seen on SPECT scans.

The clinical diagnosis is often difficult and delayed, and anatomical imaging modalities such as CT and MRI may not reveal changes such as atrophy until the end stages of disease. SPECT and PET, on the other hand, have been shown useful in early diagnosis of Alzheimer disease. In addition, these functional modalities show promise for the identification of subjects early before damage is too severe for therapy to have any benefit.

Although PET has higher sensitivity and higher resolution than SPECT, the overall patterns seen in dementia are similar for both rCGM and rCBF. In general, the types of dementia can be characterized as posterior, frontotemporal, or vascular. In addition to a geographic relation, dementias included in each category tend to share some histopathological characteristics. The posterior dementias include

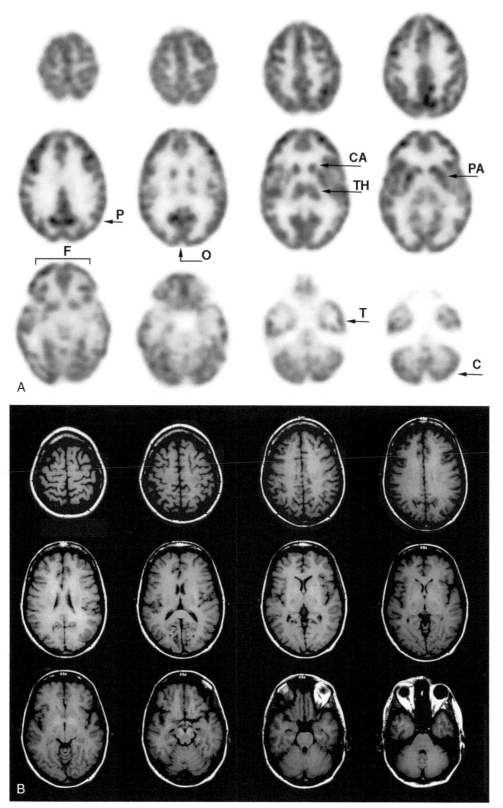

FIGURE 15-7. Normal distribution of F-18 FDG. High-resolution (**A**) transverse PET images with corresponding levels on T1-weighted MRI (**B**).

Continued

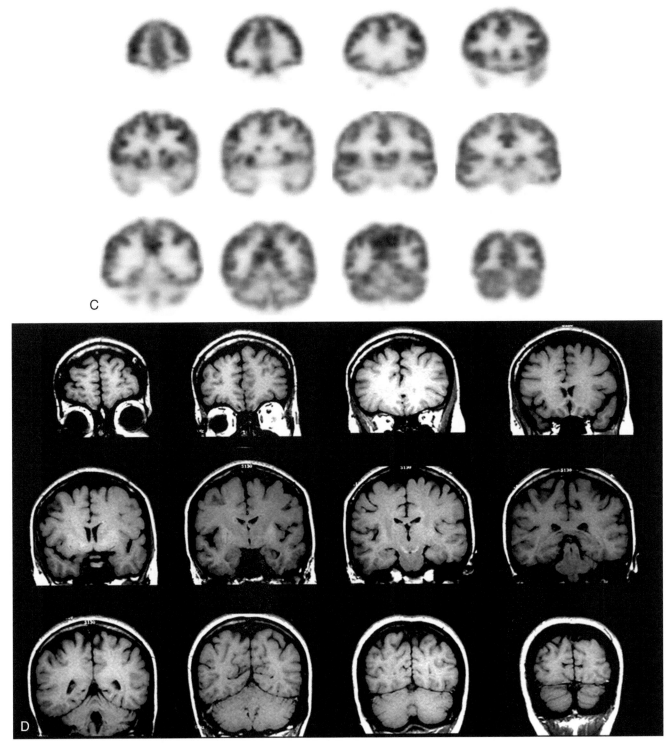

Figure 15-7, cont'd. Coronal PET (**C**) and comparable T1-weighted MRI (**D**). *C,* Cerebellum; *Ca,* caudate; *F,* frontal lobe; *O,* occipital lobe; *P,* parietal lobe; *PA,* putamen; *T,* temporal lobe; *Th,* thalamus.

BOX 15-4. Causes of Dementia

Alzheimer disease	Multiple sclerosis
Parkinson disease	Vitamin B$_{12}$ deficiency
Lewy body disease	Endocrine disorders
Multiinfarct dementia	(hypothyroidism)
Pick disease	Chronic infection
Progressive supranuclear	(tuberculosis, syphilis)
palsy	Human immune
Creutzfeldt-Jacob	deficiency virus
disease	encephalopathy
Huntington chorea	Alcohol and drugs

Alzheimer disease, Lewy body disease, and Parkinson dementia. Pick disease is the classic frontotemporal dementia.

Posterior Dementias
Alzheimer Dementia

Alzheimer disease is the most common of the dementias, estimated to affect nearly 10% of the population over 65 and 50% of those over 85. Diagnosis can be definitively made at autopsy or by the rarely performed brain biopsy, with pathological samples showing characteristic neurofibrillary tangles and amyloid plaques. Originally described as a dementia of a relatively young person (presenile dementia), it is now recognized that many older people originally thought to have multiinfarct dementia actually have Alzheimer disease. On the other hand, 25% of those thought to have Alzheimer disease clinically were found to have other causes of dementia at autopsy.

Imaging findings vary with the stage of disease, but PET and SPECT have both been able to identify cases of Alzheimer disease with a high degree of sensitivity. Studies have shown a higher sensitivity with F-18 FDG PET (up to 94%) than SPECT (78%-91%). The superiority of PET may be most important when trying to identify which patients with mild cognitive impairment will eventually progress on to actual Alzheimer disease. Patients with mild cognitive impairment have deficits on Mini-Mental Status Examination testing but do not meet probable Alzheimer disease criteria. Approximately 15% of patients with mild cognitive impairment progress to Alzheimer disease per year. PET studies have shown that patients with mild cognitive impairment with parietal and temporal hypometabolism were much more likely to go on to Alzheimer disease than those without the pattern. This ability may be crucial in the future for the identification of patients in the presymptomatic or early phases of Alzheimer disease who would benefit from therapy.

The characteristic patterns of Alzheimer disease are well established for both PET and SPECT, with findings present long before atrophy can be detected with MRI. Early disease begins in the posterior cingulate and tends to involve the superior posterior parietal cortex, manifested as bilateral hypometabolism or hypoperfusion (Fig. 15-8, *A*). Temporal lobe involvement is sometimes less reliably seen. Although the classic examples are symmetric, Alzheimer disease is often rather asymmetric, especially in the early stages (Fig.15-8, *B*). As the disease progresses, it involves the frontal cortices, although parietal and temporal lobe involvement usually remains greater. It may be more difficult to diagnose very elderly patients and patients at the end stage of disease because the imaging pattern may be more of a generalized, nonspecific decrease in cortical uptake (Fig. 15-8, *C*). However, sparing of the occipital visual cortex, primary somatosensory and motor cortices, basal ganglia, thalamus, and cerebellum is the norm (Fig. 15-9).

New PET radiopharmaceuticals are being investigated that bind to amyloid, muscarinic receptors, nicotinic receptors, and components of the cholinergic system. Correlation with genetic factors influencing Alzheimer disease will be ongoing. Recent developments have shown a strong link between scintigraphic perfusion patterns and certain genes in Alzheimer disease, including the E4 allele of the apolipoprotein E gene.

Lewy Body Disease

The other diseases that affect the posterior regions of the brain often overlap with each other and with Alzheimer disease. These include Lewy body disease (dementia with Lewy bodies) and dementia of Parkinson disease. Dementia with Lewy bodies is most likely the second most common cause after Alzheimer disease among dementias caused by neurodegenerative disorders. Histopathology shows Lewy body intracellular inclusions (alpha-synuclein) throughout the cortex, brainstem, and limbic system. Clinically, patients with Lewy body dementia often demonstrate a fluctuating dementia, visual hallucinations, falls, and some parkinsonian symptoms, such as tremor. Lewy bodies were originally described in Parkinson disease, and it is likely that dementia with Lewy bodies and Parkinson disease are related as part of a spectrum of disease.

FDG PET and SPECT images can confirm dementia with Lewy bodies by showing changes in the posterior cortical regions. The pattern tends to involve the occipital lobes and cerebellum (Fig. 15-10). The involvement of the primary visual cortex can explain the clinical visual hallucinations. Another deviation from the patterns seen in Alzheimer disease is preservation of hippocampal activity in dementia with Lewy bodies. The imaging findings of dementia in Parkinson disease also can overlap Alzheimer disease, with the exception of occipital involvement and more mesial temporal sparing. It is often important to differentiate patients with Parkinson disease with depression from those with dementia clinically. Depressed patients with Parkinson disease can show decreased prefrontal and caudate activity rather than the posterior pattern so typical of dementia. However, other patterns have been described.

Frontotemporal Dementia

The frontotemporal dementias are a diverse group of diseases. Clinically, patients show varying presentations. Aphasia occurs with temporal lobe abnormalities, and frontal lobe involvement results in personality changes, including loss of judgment and inappropriate behavior. In frontotemporal dementia, memory loss is often secondary or absent as opposed to being the primary problem as in Alzheimer disease. The differential diagnosis of frontotemporal dementia includes Pick disease, semantic dementia, primary progressive aphasia, and familial frontotemporal dementia. Frontotemporal dementia shows frontal and anterior temporal neuronal degeneration. Pick bodies, a type of protein inclusion, are sometimes found, and brain and CSF are sometimes assessed for abnormalities related to tau and ubiquitin proteins. However, concentrated amyloid and Lewy bodies are absent. Understanding the different abnormal proteins found in the dementias may help uncover new diagnostic tests and therapies.

As in the posterior dementias, PET and SPECT have both proved accurate for the detection of frontotemporal dementia (Fig. 15-11). Severe atrophy, seen on MRI, is not visualized until much later than the perfusion and metabolic changes of SPECT and FDG PET.

Decreased perfusion and metabolism in the frontal and temporal lobes may be seen in diseases other than those in the frontotemporal dementia group. These include cocaine abuse, depression, progressive supranuclear palsy, spinocerebellar atrophy, and amyotrophic lateral sclerosis. More commonly, decreased frontal and temporal rCBF and rCGM are secondary to a vascular process. Focal cortical defects, abnormalities on MRI, and areas of scintigraphic asymmetry should raise the level of suspicion for a vascular degenerative process.

Vascular Dementia

Vascular dementia is generally diagnosed through a combination of clinical examination, history, and MRI changes such as focal white matter lesions (subcortical encephalomalacia). However, symptoms may be confusing, and in

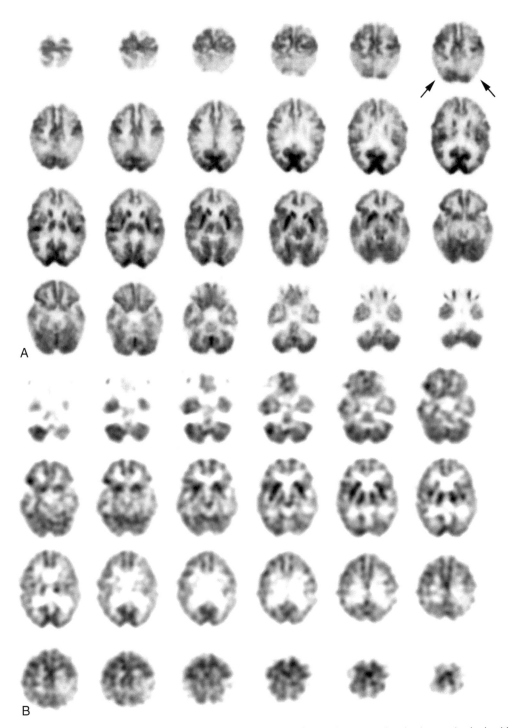

Figure 15-8. Alzheimer disease. **A,** Transaxial PET images reveal decreased metabolism to the temporal parietal cortex beginning high in the posterior parietal region with sparring of the basal ganglia, thalamus, and cerebellum. **B,** Tc-99m HMPAO SPECT shows that although Alzheimer disease is classically described as a symmetric process, it may be quite asymmetric, as seen in the left posterior parietal region.

Continued

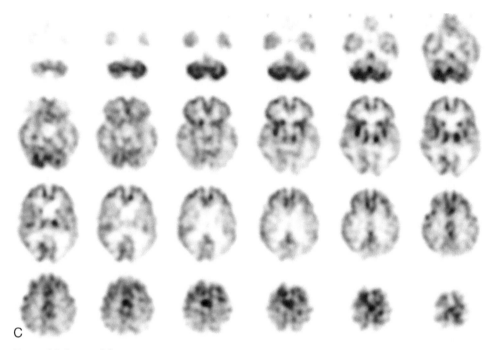

FIGURE 15-8, cont'd. C, As Alzheimer disease becomes more severe it is more diffuse on this SPECT study.

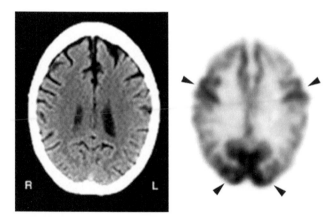

FIGURE 15-9. Alzheimer disease on PET/CT. A patient with moderately advanced Alzheimer disease shows hypometabolism in the posterior parietal and temporal regions but involvement also extends anteriorly. Sparing of the occipital region and sensory motor cortex is clear (arrowheads).

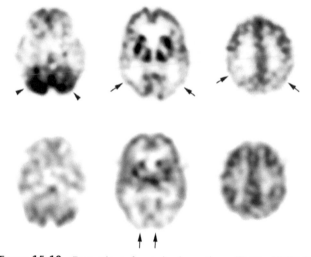

FIGURE 15-10. Comparison of posterior dementias on Tc-99m HMPAO. Top row: Alzheimer disease generally begins near the superior convexity and involves the parietal and temporal regions laterally (arrows), sparing the occiput and cerebellum (arrowhead). Bottom row: Lewy body disease involves the medial occipital region (arrows) and usually has more caudal extension than Alzheimer disease.

15% to 20% of cases, mixed causes are present. Frontal predisposition may be present in vascular dementia, which must be differentiated from expected age-related decreases on scintigraphic examinations. Often, the generalized decrease in rCGM or rCBF seen in the patient with vascular dementia is difficult to differentiate from severe Alzheimer disease (Fig. 15-12). At times, when other causes for dementia such as Alzheimer disease are excluded, vascular dementia may be left as a diagnosis of exclusion.

Epilepsy

Intractable or medically refractory seizures may require surgery for therapy. Precise seizure localization often requires a combination of scalp electroencephalogram (EEG), MRI, magnetoencephalography (MEG), and nuclear medicine imaging for evaluation. These noninvasive studies are important in directing the invasive intracranial EEG grid placement in the operating room and determining therapeutic options. Although MRI often reveals abnormalities at the site of seizure foci, such as mesial temporal hippocampal sclerosis, it is rare for structural imaging to fully visualize the actual extent of the abnormally activated neurons by structural imaging. In addition, although EEG remains critical in seizure localization, it is often inconclusive.

PET and SPECT have very important roles in such seizure evaluation. In the ictal state, activated foci show increased activity, representing increased rCBF and glucose metabolism. Interictal images, however, show normal

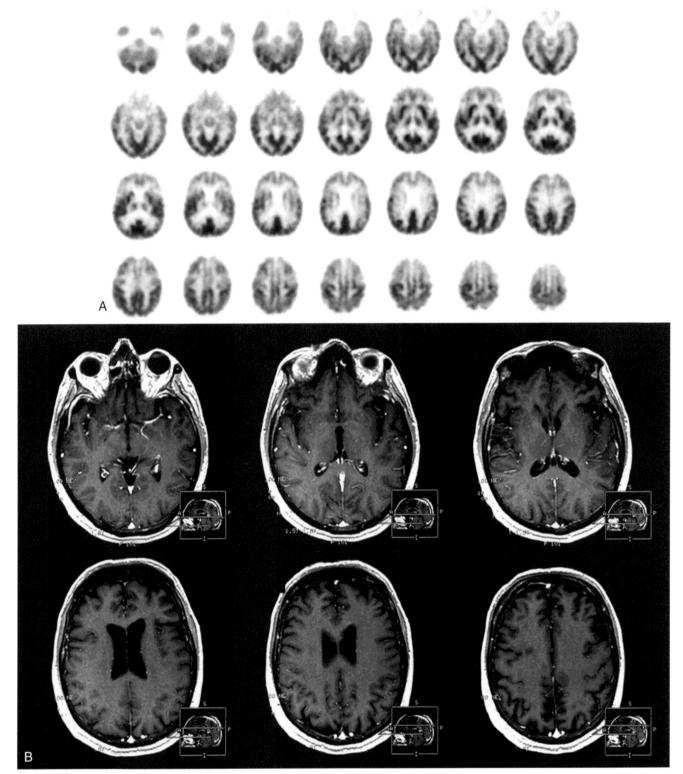

FIGURE 15-11. Frontotemporal dementia sparing posterior parietal regions. **A,** Frontal hypometabolism on PET can be due to many causes and changes visible long before MRI shows atrophy or signal changes. **B,** Postcontrast T1-weighted MRI shows no atrophy, and other MRI sequences were unremarkable.

Continued

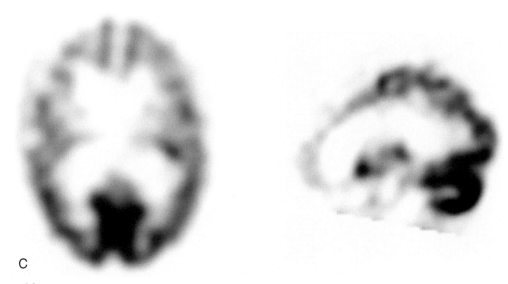

FIGURE 15-11, cont'd. C, Pick disease is rare. It classically shows frontal hypoperfusion with a sharp anterior-to-posterior cutoff, but the findings are somewhat nonspecific and other causes for decreased frontal activity must be considered.

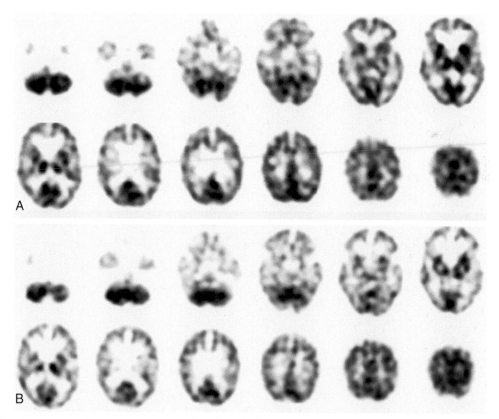

FIGURE 15-12. Vascular dementia often shows a frontal predisposition similar to other frontotemperal dementia. **A,** Vascular dementia may be more diffuse, as seen in this patient, and difficult to differentiate from other causes, including severe Alzheimer disease. **B,** Slow progression was seen in this patient clinically and on a repeat scan 5 years later.

or decreased activity. In the immediate postictal state, activity is changing and may show areas of increased and decreased activity. Clinical knowledge of the seizure status at the time of injection is essential and is best accomplished with continuous monitoring. In addition, because patients may have more than one type of seizure, it must be determined whether the seizure of interest was occurring during the ictal state.

Although ictal studies are most sensitive, they are technically highly demanding and must be done with SPECT (Fig. 15-13). Patients must be admitted and continuously monitored off medication. Once the seizure is identified, trained personnel must inject the radiotracer within seconds of seizure onset. Although imaging can then be delayed, the patient must be able to cooperate with imaging in a reasonable amount of time. Ictal PET would not

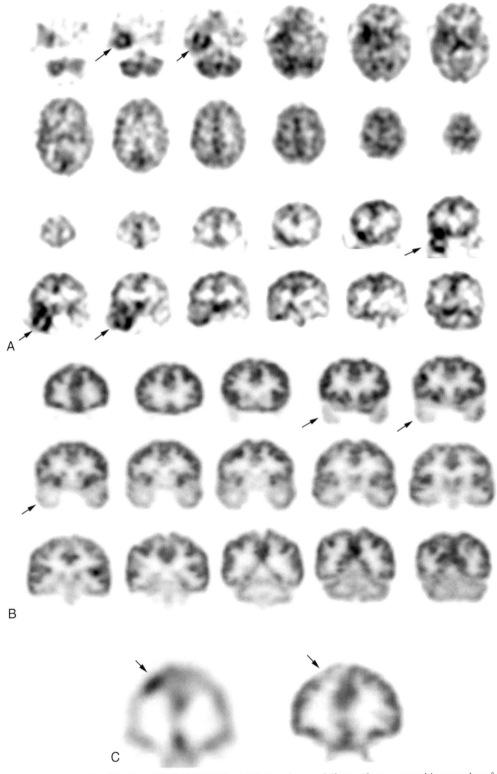

FIGURE 15-13. Seizure imaging. **A,** Ictal Tc-99m HMPAO SPECT axial *(top)* and coronal *(bottom)* images reveal increased perfusion *(arrows)* to the right temporal region from an active seizure. **B,** The abnormal temporal region is a subtle area of hypometabolism *(arrows)* on the interictal FDG PET. **C,** Ictal SPECT in a second patient demonstrates hyperperfusion *(arrow)* in the right parasagittal region *(left)* corresponding to an area of hypometabolism *(arrow)* on interictal PET *(right)* from a seizure focus.

be practical given the half-life of F-18 FDG. Interictal studies are far less sensitive, although interictal PET is superior to interictal SPECT. Clinical knowledge of the most recent seizure is needed to be sure that a study is truly ictal or interictal. Ictal SPECT has a sensitivity of nearly 90% in temporal lobe seizures, and the abnormal areas are generally more extensive than any structural abnormality on MRI. However, sensitivity for extratemporal seizures is much lower, on the order of 50% to 75%. Interictal FDG PET and SPECT is approximately 70%

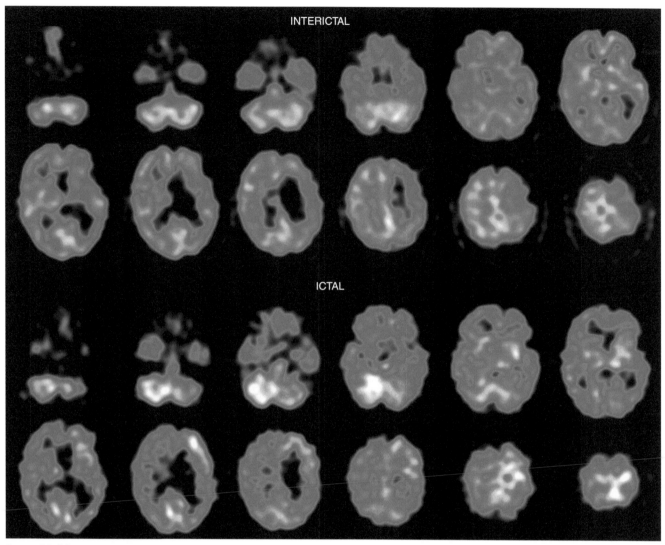

FIGURE 15-14. Interictal Tc-99m HMPAO SPECT reveals extensive hypoperfusion in a congenitally malformed cortex. Ictal images show increased activity throughout much of the frontal and parietal lobes, without a resectable focus, and increased uptake in the right cerebellum from diaschisis.

sensitive for seizure localization. In some cases, extensive or multifocal abnormalities are seen without an excisable lesion (Fig. 15-14).

Cerebrovascular Disease

Background

Although MRI and CT are now preeminent modalities for diagnosing stroke, renewed interest is seen in assessing patients with cerebrovascular disease with PET and SPECT to determine the role of therapeutic intervention. Nuclear medicine studies are frequently positive earlier than CT and may show characteristic cortical defects (Fig. 15-15). Functional imaging offers the ability to visualize and quantitate rCBF and rCGM, which can assess parameters of disease not seen on structural imaging. PET and SPECT can help determine which patients are at risk for stroke, indicate which are most likely to benefit from intervention, and even predict stroke recovery. Relationships such as distant neuronal activity loss (diaschisis), neuron recruitment, and recovery through neuronal plasticity can be studied (Fig. 15-16). In acute stroke, Tc-99m HMPAO SPECT has been used to identify which patients will most likely benefit from thrombolytic therapy, although this can be done with newer MRI techniques.

Carotid Artery Balloon Occlusion Test

Carotid artery balloon occlusion studies are well established in the assessment of vascular reserve. These studies are used in patients who may require permanent internal carotid artery occlusion such as for treatment of intracranial aneurysm. An intravenous injection of Tc-99m HMPAO is done in the angiography suite at the time of internal carotid artery balloon occlusion. The balloon is deflated after 1 minute. Imaging is done once the catheter has been removed. A cerebral arteriogram can show which patients have an intact circle of Willis and cross-filling. Wada neurological testing (also known as the intracarotid sodium amobarbital procedure) is also sometimes possible during the temporary occlusion. Amobarbital infused into the carotid is used to predict speech and memory function. Up to a 20% decrease in morbidity and mortality can be seen by adding a Tc-99m HMPAO

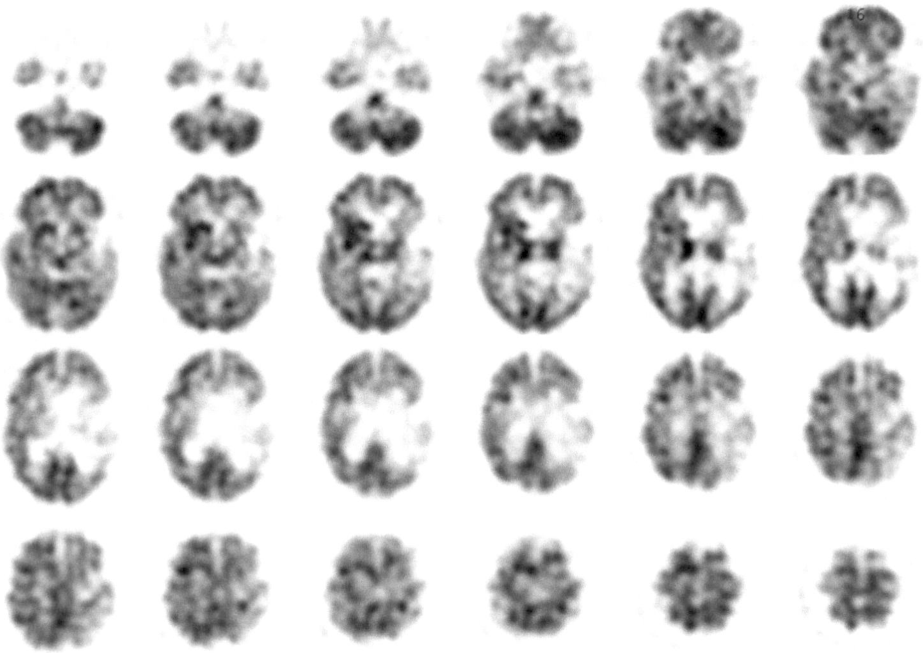

FIGURE 15-15. Left parietal middle cerebral artery cortical stroke. HMPAO SPECT shows significantly decreased perfusion to the region, including subcortical structures.

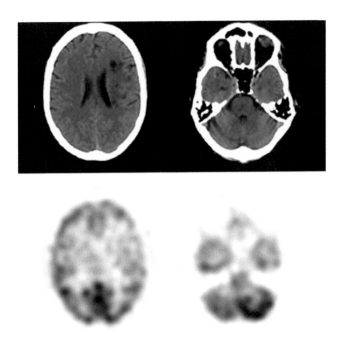

FIGURE 15-16. Crossed cerebellar diaschisis. *Top row,* A subcortical stroke in the left parietal region on CT is subtle on SPECT because the gray matter where HMPAO localizes is not heavily involved. No abnormality is seen in the cerebellum on CT. *Bottom row,* One type of distant stroke effect not seen on CT is revealed on the Tc-99m HMPAO SPECT. Hypoperfusion of the contralateral cerebellum or crossed cerebellar diaschisis is seen.

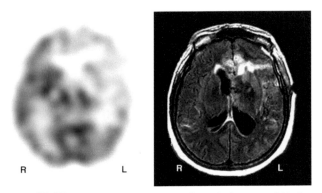

FIGURE 15-17. *Left,* HMPAO SPECT performed after a carotid balloon occlusion injection shows severe left middle cerebral artery territory hypoperfusion identifying a high risk for stroke. The patient underwent permanent left carotid occlusion using gradual occlusion with a Selverstone clamp rather than bypass. *Right,* This gradual occlusion was not sufficient to protect the patient, and the patient had a stroke, seen on CT in the same distribution as the SPECT.

Acetazolamide

SPECT can help assess suspected ischemia and stroke risks in the cases of transient ischemic attacks (TIAs) and vascular diseases such as atherosclerosis and moyamoya. The vascular reserve of patients can be assessed by a pharmacological stress test by imaging after vasodilatory response to increased carbon dioxide caused by acetazolamide (Diamox), a carbonic anhydrase inhibitor and antihypertensive agent. Vasodilation after intravenous administration of 1 g of Diamox leads to an increase in rCBF. Although global blood flow is increased, abnormal vessels cannot dilate and blood is shunted away. This will accentuate any abnormality and better demonstrate territories at risk for infarction (Fig. 15-18). It is important to compare the resting state to the stress state. Change may be best assessed with semi-quantitative analysis of cortical activity.

SPECT scan to the preoperative workup. Patients at risk for stroke after a planned permanent arterial occlusion are easily identified with a significant drop in perfusion to the occluded side on SPECT images. Carotid bypass is generally warranted in these patients, because the remaining vessels cannot meet the needs of the side that will be occluded (Fig. 15-17).

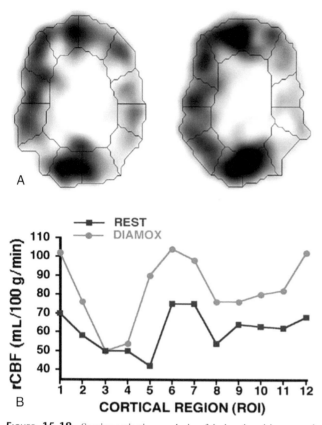

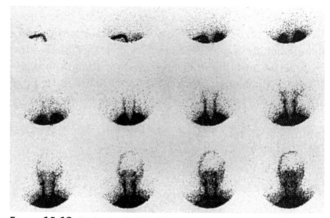

FIGURE **15-19**. Brain death. This Tc-99m DTPA brain blood flow study shows radiotracer transiting the internal carotids; however, there is no intracerebral blood flow. Only external carotid blood flow to the scalp is seen.

FIGURE **15-18**. Semiquantitative analysis of ischemia with acetazolamide (Diamox) SPECT. **A**, Tc-99m HMPAO SPECT before acetazolamide *(left)* shows mild left parietal hypoperfusion. After acetazolamide *(right)*, the brain shows increased activity in response to vasodilation, with the exception of the left parietal defect and the decreased activity from ischemia is even more apparent. **B**, Cortical region of interest (ROI) boxes are drawn like a clock numbered from 1 o'clock to 12 o'clock to generate regional cerebral blood flow (rCBF curves). In this patient, the curves after acetazolamide administration are increased relative to rest perfusion with the exception of a dip from 2 o'clock to 4 o'clock. This signifies an area at high risk for infarction because it is unable to respond to the vasodilation.

Brain Death

Accuracy and speed in making the diagnosis of brain death become critical when organ donation is considered, and life support systems must be used. Although the diagnosis of brain death is by definition a clinical one, clinical diagnosis may be difficult. The specific criteria necessary to make the diagnosis of brain death are as follows:

1. The patient must be in deep coma with total absence of brainstem reflexes or spontaneous respiration.
2. Potentially reversible causes such as drug intoxication, metabolic derangement, or hypothermia must be excluded.
3. The cause of the brain dysfunction must be diagnosed (e.g., trauma, stroke).
4. The clinical findings of brain death must be present for a defined period of observation (6-24 hours).

Although confirmatory ancillary tests are used by clinicians to increase certainty, they cannot themselves establish the diagnosis of brain death. An isoelectric EEG by itself does not establish brain death, and at least one repeat study is required. In the patient with intoxication from barbiturates or other depressive drugs or with hypothermia, the EEG may be flat, even though cerebral perfusion is still present and recovery is possible.

Lack of blood flow to the brain is diagnostic of brain death. Edema, softening, necrosis, and autolysis of brain tissue lead to increased intracranial pressure. As pressure rises, eventually it prevents intracranial perfusion. This can be demonstrated with four-vessel arteriography, but the test is invasive and unnecessary.

The radionuclide brain death study is usually performed when the EEG and clinical criteria are equivocal. It is simple and rapid, and it can be performed at the bedside. Scintigraphy is not affected by drug intoxication or hypothermia. An abnormal radionuclide angiogram showing no cerebral perfusion is more specific for brain death than an isoelectric EEG.

Radiopharmaceuticals

Brain death can be diagnosed using a radionuclide flow study alone because the lack of intracerebral blood flow is diagnostic. Technetium-labeled radiopharmaceuticals are used to assess dynamic flow. Tc-99m DTPA was often used in the past because it is cleared rapidly from the blood, allowing a repeat study if necessary. However, optimal technique is mandatory and interpretation may be difficult (Fig. 15-19).

Tc-99m HMPAO and Tc-99m ECD studies are easier to interpret and are now preferred (Fig. 15-20). Flow images can be obtained but are not necessary, because delayed images showing the fixed presence or absence of brain uptake require flow to the brain. If no CBF is present, no cerebral uptake will occur. Planar images are adequate, and SPECT is not necessary to diagnose brain death.

Methodology

Tc-99m DTPA examinations are more difficult to perform and interpret than Tc-99m HMPAO. An adequate radiopharmaceutical bolus is required to ensure a diagnostic flow study. Images of the injection site can be performed to ensure the dose was adequate and not infiltrated. The radionuclide angiogram protocol for CBF is used in brain death (Box 15-5).

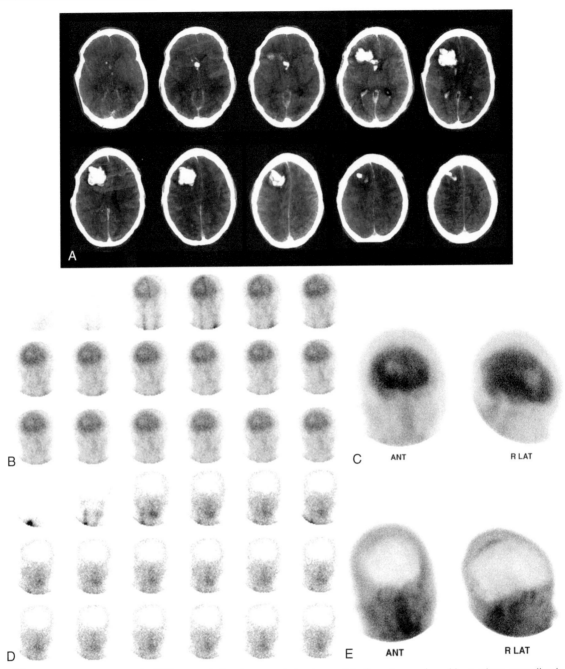

FIGURE 15-20. Brain death evaluation. **A,** CT images of a head trauma victim show a right frontal parenchymal hemorrhage extending into the ventricles. **B,** Tc-99m HMPAO examination to evaluate for brain death. The examination does not show the early arterial phase of perfusion but good cortical perfusion and venous drainage into the superior sagittal sinus and **(C)** good delayed cortical uptake, although with a defect from the hemorrhage. **D,** A follow-up study 3 days later shows internal carotid arterial flow terminating below the head from brain death. **E,** This is confirmed with absent delayed cortical uptake. Any peripheral activity is due to external carotid flow. *ANT,* Anterior; *R LAT,* right lateral.

Image Interpretation

With brain death, flow to both common carotid arteries is seen extending up only to the level of the base of the skull. No visualization of the brain is seen with Tc-99m HMPAO, making it the easiest test to interpret.

A secondary finding, the "hot nose" sign is often seen. This reportedly has been due to increasing intracranial pressure diverting intracranial blood flow into external carotid circulation, resulting in relatively increased flow to the face and nose. However, lateral views show the activity lies far posteriorly, along the brainstem and posterior fossa region. This pattern is nonspecific and also can be seen in internal carotid artery occlusion without brain death.

Tumor Imaging

PET Imaging. F-18 FDG PET has long been used to evaluate brain tumors, showing increased glucose metabolism (Fig. 15-21). F-18 FDG uptake is related to metabolic activity and therefore to tumor grade. Because of this, PET can help direct biopsy to the most aggressive region of a tumor. Low-grade gliomas (World Health Organization [WHO] grades I and II) typically show uptake similar to that of white matter, whereas high-grade tumors (WHO grade III) are similar or increased compared to gray matter. Grade IV (glioblastoma multiforme) shows markedly increased activity compared to normal cortical gray matter. Interestingly, low-grade pilocytic astrocytomas and benign pituitary tumors can show increased F-18 FDG accumulation.

F-18 FDG PET also can be used to identify malignancy in cases in which the MRI is inconclusive. This includes differentiating lymphoma presenting as a ring enhancing lesion from toxoplasmosis infection in immunocompromised patients. However, the most common use of F-18 FDG PET is to determine whether abnormal MRI signal and enhancement after radiation or surgery represents recurrent glioma. PET images show absent or decreased activity in the normal postoperative brain and any area of

increased uptake most likely represents tumor. High levels of background F-18 FDG activity complicate evaluation. Direct, side-by-side comparison with the MRI is critical for image interpretation, and actual fusion of PET images to the MRI is even better. In the case of high-dose radiation therapy, increased F-18 FDG activity can be seen and may persist. Although this activity is generally mild and not greater than normal cortical uptake, serial images to look for any areas of increasing activity may be necessary to exclude early recurrence. Recurrences are typically aggressive with intense radiotracer accumulation.

Although F-18 FDG PET is a valuable clinical tool in the workup of many types of malignancy outside of the CNS, nearly two thirds of intracranial metastatic lesions are not seen on PET because of the high background activity (Fig. 15-22). Therefore MRI remains the standard for metastatic lesion detection.

Numerous other PET radiopharmaceuticals have been used to evaluate tumors with aspects of cellular activity other than glucose metabolism. Evaluating DNA synthesis with F-18 fluorothymidine (FLT) appears superior to F-18 FDG with cases of aggressive, enhancing tumors. Evaluating protein synthesis, such as with C-11 methionine or F-18 fluorodopa, has been shown accurate even in low-grade tumors.

Box 15-5. **Brain Death Scintigraphy: Summary Protocol**

PATIENT PREPARATION
None

RADIOPHARMACEUTICAL
Tc-99m HMPAO or Tc-99m DTPA 20 mCi (740 MBq)

INSTRUMENTATION
Gamma camera setup: Large field of view
Collimator: High resolution, low energy
Window: 15% over 140-keV photopeak
Camera formatter setup: 2- to 3-second flow images for 30 seconds, and then immediate and delayed static images in multiple views
Computer setup: 1-second flow images for 60 seconds (64 × 64 byte mode), and then static images (128 × 128 frame mode)

IMAGING PROCEDURE
1. Inject radiopharmaceutical as an intravenous bolus.
2. Acquire dynamic flow study.
3. *Immediate* 750k static images in the anterior, posterior, right lateral, and left lateral views (optional). Image injection site.

DTPA, Diethylenetriaminepentaacetic acid; *HMPAO*, hexamethylpropyleneamine oxime.

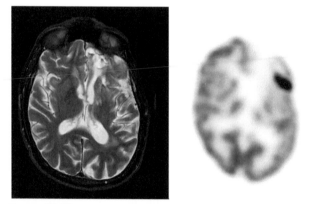

FIGURE 15-21. Recurrent gliomas may be difficult to detect on MRI. T2-weighted MRI shows posttherapy signal changes *(left)*. The recurrent tumor is seen as an intense focus on the FDG PET *(right)*.

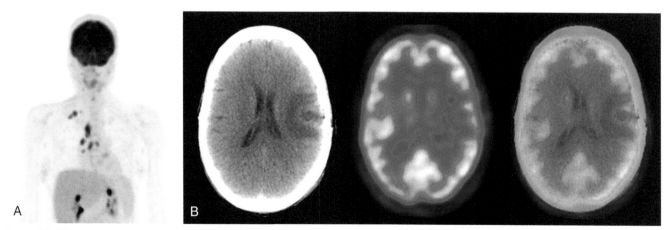

FIGURE 15-22. F-18 FDG images from a patient with metastatic lung cancer show **(A)** avid uptake in disease within the chest on the maximal intensity projection image, but PET/CT images of the brain **(B)** show a left cerebral metastasis with surrounding edema on CT *(left)* with little FDG accumulation on PET *(center)* or fused *(right)* images.

Single-Photon Emission Computed Tomography Tumor Imaging. The SPECT agents Tc-99m HMPAO and Tc-99m ECD are generally not useful for detection of intracranial malignancies. Although increased uptake might be seen in tumors, slightly more commonly with Tc-99m ECD, both agents often show normal or decreased activity.

SPECT evaluation of recurrent gliomas and differentiating intracranial lymphoma can be done with the cardiac imaging agents thallium-201 and Tc-99m sestamibi (Fig. 15-23), which have both shown accumulation in several tumor types. The potassium analog Tl-201 depends on blood flow and blood–brain barrier breakdown for distribution and on metabolic activity with uptake through the Na^+/K^+ pump. Tc-99m sestamibi is transported by the endothelial cell and localizes in active mitochondria. Some accumulation of Tc-99m sestamibi occurs in the choroid plexus, which may make it less than ideal in some tumors.

The procedure for SPECT tumor imaging involves imaging approximately 20 to 30 minutes after injection of 2 to 4 mCi (74-148 MBq) of Tl-201 or 20 mCi (740 MBq) Tc-99m sestamibi. Occasionally, a 2-hour delayed Tl-201 acquisition may be helpful, because the abnormal tumor tissue would be expected to wash out more slowly than normal brain or areas of blood–brain barrier disruption. Visual analysis typically shows uptake equal to or greater than the scalp or the contralateral side in tumors. There is some overlap in the appearance of malignant and infectious processes. An intracranial abscess, for example, often has increased activity. Because infections usually have lower uptake than malignancies, quantitative analysis may help improve specificity. A region of interest is drawn around the abnormal uptake and compared to the contralateral normal. Delayed images may improve sensitivity as the tumor retains activity and the background clears.

■ MOVEMENT DISORDERS

Parkinson disease is the most common of the movement disorders, affecting approximately 1.5% of people over 65 years and 2.5% of those over the age of 80. As the dopaminergic neurons in the substantia nigra degenerate, patients experience resting tremor, rigidity, and bradykinesia. The three groups of parkinsonian syndromes are idiopathic Parkinson disease, secondary Parkinson disease (caused by disease such as Wilson disease or other extrinsic agents such as carbon monoxide poisoning and neuroleptic drugs), and neurodegenerative syndromes such as multisystem atrophy and progressive supranuclear palsy. Clinical differentiation of idiopathic Parkinson disease from causes such as multisystem atrophy may be difficult when patients do not respond to L-dopa therapy. In addition, early in the course of the disease, it may be difficult to determine if patients are suffering from essential tremor rather than Parkinson disease.

The ability of PET to image the dopaminergic system in patients with Parkinson disease and other movement disorders has been known for decades. Imaging involves the corpus striatum, which consists of the lentiform nucleus (putamen and globus pallidus) and caudate nucleus. It is estimated that there is a 2% to 10% decrease in striatal activity per year in Parkinson disease. As the dopaminergic striatal neurons degenerate, effects downstream in the globus pallidus occur.

Radiopharmaceuticals

PET has largely been a research tool in movement disorders, using agents such as F-18 6-fluorodopa (F-18 dopa). New agents can now study different components of the dopamine neurotransmitter system (Fig. 15-24). These radiopharmaceuticals are grouped based on the location or mechanism of dopamine metabolism they image. The classic agent, F-18 dopa, enters the dopamine metabolism pathway early as an analog of L-dopa and measures dopamine neuron integrity and loss. However, F-18 dopa tends to underestimate loss. Other agents target the vesicular monoamine transporter type 2 (VMAT2), presynaptic membrane dopamine transporter (DAT), and postsynaptic dopamine receptors (D2 and D1). New tropane agents derived from cocaine have been developed to image DAT activity. These include F-18/C-11 β-CIT and SPECT agents such as I-123 FP-CIT (I-123 ioflupane or DaTscan).

I-123 ioflupane, which has been used in Europe for over a decade, recently gained approval in the United States for the differentiation of essential tremor from parkinsonian syndromes. After injection, uptake in the brain is 7% at 10 minutes but decreases slightly to 3% after 5 hours. Activity accumulates in the striata, remaining fairly stable for 3 to 6 hours. The main route of excretion is through the urine, with 60% of the injected dose excreted by 48 hours. Fecal

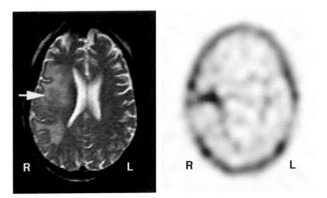

FIGURE 15-23. Intracranial lymphoma. A mass is seen in a patient with acquired immune acquired immune deficiency syndrome on the T2-weighted MRI *(left, arrow)* with the Tl-201 SPECT showing intense tumor uptake *(right).*

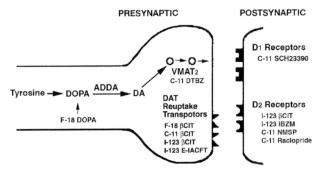

FIGURE 15-24. Dopamine neuron production and metabolism. The sites of PET and SPECT agent uptake are shown. *AAAD,* Aromatic amino acid decarboxylase; *DAT,* dopamine reuptake transporter; *VMAT₂,* vesicular monoamine transporter type 2.

excretion accounts for roughly 14% of the dose. Dosimetry of I-123 ioflupane is listed in Table 15-2.

Method

A protocol for I-123 ioflupane is presented in Box 15-6. One of the most difficult things concerning I-123 ioflupane use is the ordering process as the U.S. Federal Drug Administration (FDA) approval hinged on meeting Drug Enforcement Agency (DEA) insistence that it be treated as a Schedule II controlled substance. Patient medications should be reviewed for any drug that might interfere with

---

Box 15-6. Iodine-123 Ioflupane Imaging: Summary Protocol

PATIENT PREPARATION
Patient should stop interfering medications.
Thyroid blocking: Lugol solution or potassium iodide thyroid at least 1 hour before injection.

RADIOPHARMACEUTICAL
I-123 ioflupane 3 to 5 mCi (111-185 MBq) intravenously
Delay to scan: 3 to 6 hours

INSTRUMENTATION
SPECT camera: Dual-head or triple-head
Collimators: Low energy, high resolution
Energy window: Peak 159 keV ± 10%
Matrix and zoom to a 3.5 to 4.5 mm pixel size

POSITIONING
Supine with off the table head holder to extend head beyond bed and allow tight orbit (11-15 cm)

ACQUISITION
At least 120 views over 360 degrees, minimum 1.5 million counts for optimal image. Iterative reconstruction.

Box 15-7. Medications Potentially Interfering with Iodine-123 Ioflupane

Amoxapine
Amphetamine
Benztropine
Bupropion
Buspirone
Cocaine
Mazindol
Methamphetamine
Methylphenidate
Norepinephrine
Phentermine
Phenylpropanolamine
Selegiline
Sertraline

EFFECTS UNCERTAIN
Dopamine agonists and antagonists
Serotonin reuptake inhibitors: paroxetine, citaopram

---

the examination (Box 15-7). Patient preparation consists of blocking thyroid uptake with potassium iodide (400 mg) or Lugol solution (equivalent 100 mg iodide) at least 1 hour before injection. The patient should be well hydrated and void frequently in the first 48 hours after the examination. After radiotracer injection a 3- to 6-hour delay is needed before SPECT imaging.

Image Findings

Significant uptake is seen in the basal ganglia with low background in the surrounding brain with agents such as I-123 ioflupane (Fig. 15-25). Generally, it is not possible to separate the components of the lentiform nucleus into the putamen and globus pallidus by PET or SPECT. Over the course of the disease, decreased uptake occurs in the posterior striatum initially that then moves anteriorly—posterior putamen first, then anterior putamen, and then finally the caudate nucleus. In patients with early parkinsonian syndromes, the abnormality is often asymmetric. Decreased radiotracer binding corresponds to the symptomatic side, as well as often detecting preclinical disease on the contralateral side (Fig. 15-26). It is not

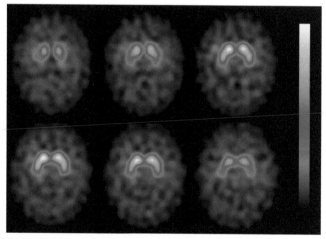

FIGURE 15-25. Normal distribution of the dopamine transporter agent, I-123 ioflupane showing high striatal uptake relative to cortex.

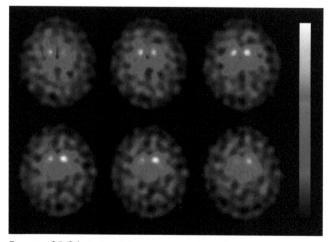

FIGURE 15-26. I-123 ioflupane SPECT images show abnormal decreased activity in the posterior striatum with some sparing anteriorly. Although symmetric here, abnormalities are often asymmetric, especially early on.

possible to differentiate Parkinson disease from other true parkinsonian syndromes such as multisystem atrophy and progressive supranuclear palsy because they all show similar decreases in the substantia nigra. Interobserver variability is good for positive and negative examinations. Although only 78% of patients with Parkinson disease had a positive scan, a negative scan (NPV) effectively excludes the diagnosis of Parkinson disease, with 97% of patients with a non-Parkinson disease, such as essential tremor, showing a normal examination.

AMYLOID IMAGING

Amyloid and Alzheimer Disease

Neurodegenerative dementias appear to involve increased production or abnormal folding of proteins such amyloid β (Aβ). Aβ is a peptide cleaved by various secretases (e.g., gamma secretase) from an amyloid precursor protein. The role of Aβ is unclear, but growing evidence suggests it normally modulates presynaptic activity and neuronal survival. In patients with Alzheimer disease, along with neurofibrillary tangles, Aβ plaque accumulates in extracellular spaces and the walls of small vessels (Alzheimer angiopathy). One theory is that the amyloid causes neuronal damage, resulting in Alzheimer disease through a cascading series of downstream effects. Although the causal relationship of Aβ in the development of Alzheimer disease is not actually known, a relationship exists between the presence of Aβ and the severity of the dementia. As treatments are developed for Alzheimer disease, it is critical to identify patients early, because amyloid accumulation likely begins years before the dementia is evident.

Radiopharmaceuticals
Carbon-11 Pittsburgh B Compound

Several PET radiopharmaceuticals have been developed that bind to Aβ. The first and most studied of these is C-11 Pittsburgh B compound (PIB), developed from thioflavin T, a fluorescent dye used to evaluate amyloid. C-11 PIB has high-affinity binding to insoluble fibrillary Aβ but not to neurofibrillary plaques or amorphous Aβ. Binding of C-11 PIB is seen in more than 90% of patients with Alzheimer disease, but cortical uptake is similar to that in the cerebellum, the usual reference, in normal volunteers. However, Aβ accumulation occurs in asymptomatic elderly patients, increasing from 10% in those younger than 70 years of age to 30% to 40% by age 80. The binding of C-11 PIB does not always mirror areas of abnormality seen with F-18 FDG. C-11 PIB uptake is high in the frontal, temporal, parietal, and occipital cortices and the striatum early on. The high levels of uptake do not significantly change over time, even as F-18 FDG shows growing areas of metabolic decline with disease progression.

Fluorine-18 Amyloid Agents

For an amyloid agent to be widely used, the half-life of the C-11 label is impractically short. A significant development in amyloid imaging was the formulation of an F-18 6-dialkylamino-2-naphthyethylidene derivative, F-18 FDDNP, a lipophilic agent that binds to Aβ. However, many studies have shown that F-18 FDDNP shows less

specific binding than C-11 PIB, with uptake in Aβ, neurofibrillary tangles and other proteins.

Clinical trials since have shown promise with three other F-18–labeled amyloid binding agents: F-18 AV-45 (Florbetapir), F-18 AV-1 (Florbetaben), and F-18-3′-F-PIB (Flutemetamol). Interpretation is made more difficult by the presence of Aβ in cognitively normal elderly patients and high levels of nonspecific white matter binding (Fig. 15-27). However, each of the agents is able to cross the blood–brain barrier, shows high-affinity binding for Aβ, and is able to identify patients with Alzheimer disease compared with controls or patients with frontotemoral lobar degeneration (FTLD). Positive examinations demonstrate high levels of cortical uptake (Fig. 15-28). Because early deposition of amyloid occurs in the deeper cortical levels, the amount of white matter binding seen in these radiopharmaceuticals may cause diagnostic

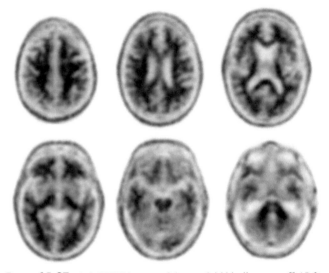

FIGURE 15-27. Axial PET images of the amyloid binding agent F-18-3′-F-PIB in a control patient shows the expected nonspecific white matter binding but no significant cortical accumulation. (Courtesy Dr. Kirk Frey.)

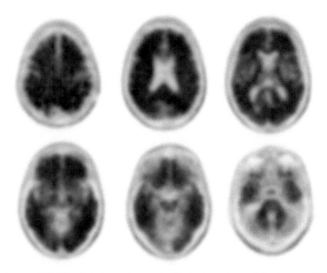

FIGURE 15-28. Alzheimer dementia. Marked cortical activity is seen diffusely on axial PET images of F-18-3′-F-PIB in addition to nonspecific white matter binding in a patient with clinical Alzheimer disease. (Courtesy Dr. Kirk Frey.)

difficulties. New agents, such as C-11/F-18 AZD4694, are being investigated that show lower nonspecific binding.

The potential role of these amyloid agents will need to be determined. At this point, they should be able to confirm the diagnosis of Alzheimer disease. Additional trials looking at factors such as drug therapy impact and early diagnosis in the prodromal mild cognitive impairment stage of disease need to be performed.

CISTERNOGRAPHY

CSF dynamics using radiotracers has been employed for many years to diagnose a site of CSF leakage, determine shunt patency, and manage hydrocephalus. Although CT and MRI are now often used, radionuclide cisternography still plays an important role because of the unique physiological information it provides. To be effective, close coordination with structural imaging studies and detailed knowledge of the clinical problem are necessary.

An understanding of normal CSF dynamics is important for image interpretation. CSF is secreted by the ventricular choroid plexus and, to a lesser extent, from extraventricular sites. Normally, CSF drains from the lateral ventricles through the interventricular foramen of Monro into the third ventricle (Fig. 15-29). With the additional CSF produced by the choroid plexus of the third ventricle, it then passes through the cerebral aqueduct of Sylvius into the fourth ventricle and then leaves the ventricular system through the median foramen of Magendie and the two lateral foramina of Luschka. The CSF then enters the subarachnoid space surrounding the brain and spinal cord. Along the base of the brain, the subarachnoid space expands into lakes called *cisterns*. The

subarachnoid space extends over the surface of the brain. The CSF is absorbed through the pacchionian granulations of the pia arachnoid villi into the superior sagittal sinus.

Radiopharmaceuticals

Radiopharmaceuticals injected intrathecally into the lumbar subarachnoid space must meet strict standards for sterility and apyrogenicity. They should follow the flow of the CSF without affecting the dynamics, and they should rapidly clear through the arachnoid villi. In-111 DTPA is ideal because it is non–lipid soluble, not metabolized, and not absorbed across the ependyma before reaching the arachnoid villi. Imaging in cisternography studies may extend over a period of days; thus In-111 is the radiotracer of choice because of its long half-life (67 hours) and reasonable imaging characteristics. Studies looking for CSF leaks may be done with Tc-99m DTPA because its superior imaging characteristics may improve sensitivity and these studies do not require prolonged imaging.

Methods

Proper sterile lumbar puncture technique is critical and should be done by an experienced clinician to ensure subarachnoid injection. An initial image of the injection site ensures that the radiotracer was delivered to the correct location. Early evaluation confirms dose migration up the vertebral column and a lack of excessive renal activity. Serial imaging is needed, as described in the protocol in Box 15-8.

Pharmacokinetics

Radiotracer injected into the intrathecal space normally reaches the basal cisterns by 1 hour, the frontal poles and

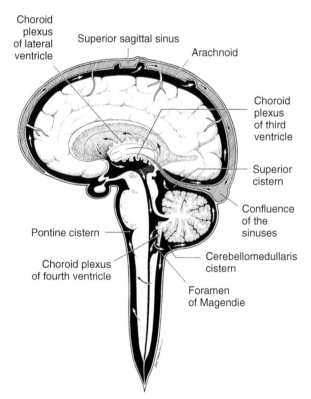

FIGURE 15-29. Flow dynamics of cerebrospinal fluid (CSF). Originating in lateral ventricle choroid plexus, CSF flows through the third and fourth ventricles into the basal cisterns, moves over the convexities, and finally is reabsorbed in the superior sagittal sinus.

Choroid plexus of lateral ventricle
Superior sagittal sinus
Arachnoid
Choroid plexus of third ventricle
Superior cistern
Confluence of the sinuses
Pontine cistern
Cerebellomedullaris cistern
Choroid plexus of fourth ventricle
Foramen of Magendie

Box 15-8. Cisternography: Summary Protocol

PATIENT PREPARATION
None

RADIOPHARMACEUTICAL
In-111 DTPA 250 µCi (9.3 MBq)

INSTRUMENTATION
Gamma camera: Large field of view
Collimator: Medium energy

IMAGING PROCEDURE
Inject slowly into lumbar subarachnoid space using a 22-gauge needle with the bevel positioned vertically.
Instruct patient to remain recumbent for at least 1 hour after injection.
All images should be obtained for 50k counts.

IMAGING TIMES
1 hour: Thoracic-lumbar spine for evaluation of injection adequacy.
3 hour: Base of the skull to visualize basilar cisterns.
24 and 48 hours: Evaluation of ventricular reflux and arachnoid villi resorption.
3, 24, and 48 hours: Obtain anterior, posterior, and both lateral views of the head.

DTPA, Diethylenetriaminepentaacetic acid.

sylvian fissure area by 2 to 6 hours, the cerebral convexities by 12 hours, and the arachnoid villi in the sagittal sinus by 24 hours. Flow to the parasagittal region occurs through both central and superficial routes. The radiotracer does not normally enter the ventricular system because physiological flow is in the opposite direction.

Dosimetry

To some extent, the radiation absorbed dose depends on the clearance dynamics of a particular patient. The spinal cord receives the highest dose, followed by the kidney and bladder, because the radiopharmaceutical undergoes renal excretion (Table 15-3).

Clinical Applications

Hydrocephalus

Hydrocephalus is abnormal enlargement of the CSF spaces resulting from abnormalities of CSF production, circulation, or absorption (Table 15-4). MRI and CT are most often used to select patients who might benefit from intervention, whereas radionuclide cisternography is generally reserved for situations that remain unclear. When assessing hydrocephalus, it must first be known whether the process is noncommunicating or communicating. Then the route of radiopharmaceutical administration and expected pattern during cisternography can be predicted and evaluated.

In noncommunicating causes of hydrocephalus, flow from the ventricular system into the basal cisterns and

TABLE 15-3 Dosimetry of Technetium-99m DTPA and Indium-111 DTPA

Agent	Injection technique	Exposure organ receives highest dose (mGy/MBq)	Effective dose (mSv/MBq)
In-111 DTPA	Lumbar	Spinal cord 0.95	0.14
		Bladder 0.20	
	Cisternal	Spinal cord 0.57	0.12
		Bladder 0.18	
Tc-99m DTPA	Lumbar	Spinal cord 0.046	0.011
	Cisternal	Brain 0.055	0.0066

Data from International Commission on Radiological Protection. Publication 53. Ontario.
DTPA, Diethylenetriaminepentaacetic acid.

TABLE 15-4 Classification of Hydrocephalus

Classification	Site of obstruction
OBSTRUCTIVE	
Noncommunicating	Intraventricular between lateral ventricles and basal cistern
Communicating	Extraventricular, affecting basal cisterns, cerebral convexities and arachnoid villi
NONOBSTRUCTIVE	
Generalized atrophy	None
Localized atrophy	None

subarachnoid space is obstructed. This is commonly due to a mass or congenital abnormality at or above the fourth ventricle, and the diagnosis is usually made by MRI.

In communicating hydrocephalus, CSF is free to flow from the intraventricular region into the subarachnoid space. The obstruction to CSF flow is extraventricular, in the basal cisterns, cerebral convexities, or arachnoid villi. Common causes include previous subarachnoid hemorrhage, chronic subdural hematoma, leptomeningitis, and meningeal carcinomatosis, all leading to poor CSF movement and reabsorption. On anatomical imaging, the ventricular system is dilated out of proportion to the prominence of cortical sulci and the basal cisterns. It may be difficult to differentiate this extraventricular obstruction from nonobstructive hydrocephalus ex vacuo, a secondary expansion of the ventricles to fill the void after neuronal tissue loss from atrophy or stroke.

In the past, radionuclide studies were commonly used to help assess communicating hydrocephalus patients with normal-pressure hydrocephalus to determine whether the patient would be likely to benefit from CSF shunting. Normal-pressure hydrocephalus manifests clinically with progressive dementia, ataxia, and incontinence. Surgical shunting of CSF can potentially cure this cause of dementia, but not all patients improve with surgery.

Cisternography Image Interpretation

Several patterns of flow can be observed after introduction of radiopharmaceutical into the intrathecal space. Normal flow should not reflux into the ventricles and should move over the convexities by 24 hours (Fig. 15-30).

In patients with noncommunicating hydrocephalus, cisternography usually shows a normal pattern of flow up to the basal cisterns, over the convexities. No ventricular reflux is seen. However, if activity is injected into the ventricles through a ventriculostomy rather than via lumbar puncture, serial images show minimal activity in the basal cisterns.

In communicating hydrocephalus, including patients with normal-pressure hydrocephalus, cisternography can show a spectrum of CSF flow patterns (Figs. 15-31 and 15-32). The common denominator is absent flow or a marked delay of activity flow up over the convexities of the brain. Ventricular reflux of activity may occur transiently or persist. Atrophy alone will cause delayed tracer movement through the enlarged subarachnoid space, sometimes with transient ventricular reflux. However, normal clearance over the hemispheres is seen by 24 hours. It has been suggested that patients with communicating hydrocephalus with persistent ventricular activity and no activity over the convexities (the type IV cisternographic pattern) are most likely to benefit from shunting.

Surgical Shunt Patency

A variety of diversionary CSF shunts (ventriculoperitoneal, ventriculoatrial, ventriculopleural, lumboperitoneal) have been used to treat obstructive hydrocephalus. Complications may include catheter blockage, infection, thromboembolism, subdural or epidural hematomas, disconnection of catheters, CSF pseudocyst, bowel obstruction, and bowel perforation.

The diagnosis of shunt patency and adequacy of CSF flow often can be made by examination of the patient and inspection of the subcutaneous CSF reservoir. When this assessment is uncertain, radionuclide studies with In-111

4-Hour Images

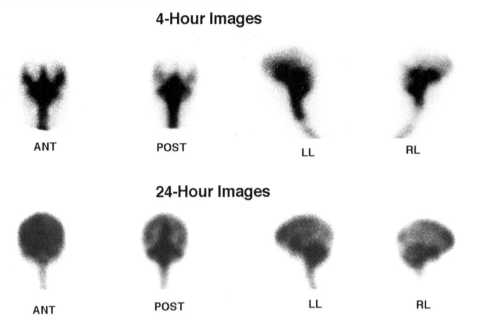

ANT   POST   LL   RL

24-Hour Images

ANT   POST   LL   RL

FIGURE 15-30. Normal cisternogram. Anterior and lateral images 4 and 24 hours after intrathecal radiotracer injection show normal transit up over the convexities with no ventricular reflux. *ANT,* Anterior; *LL,* left lateral; *POST,* posterior; *RL,* right lateral.

Type	Cerebrospinal fluid movement	Causes
I	Basal cistern 2-4 hr Sylvian fissure 6 hr Over convexities 24 hr Decreased activity 48 hr	Normal Intraventricular obstructive hydrocephalus (noncommunicating)
II	No ventricular activity Delayed migration over convexities	Cerebral atrophy Advanced age
IIIA	Transient ventricular activity Clearance by usual migration (often)	Intraventricular obstruction Cerebral atrophy Evolving or resolving communicating hydrocephalus

IIIB	Transient ventricular activity
	Clearance but not by usual migration
	  to convexity
		Communicating hydrocephalus with
		  alternative reabsorption pathway
		  (transependymal)

IV	Persistent ventricular activity Inadequate clearance	Communicating hydrocephalus

FIGURE 15-31. Normal and abnormal patterns of cerebrospinal fluid flow.

DTPA or Tc-99m DTPA are useful for confirming the diagnosis. Familiarity with the specific shunt type and its configuration is helpful. For example, the valves may allow bidirectional or only unidirectional flow. A proximal shunt limb consists of tubing running from the ventricles into the reservoir, and the distal limb carries CSF away from the reservoir into the body.

Shunt injection should be performed with aseptic technique by a physician familiar with the type of shunt in place, preferably the neurosurgeon (Box 15-9). Patency of the proximal shunt limb can sometimes be evaluated before checking distal patency. In patients with certain types of variable or low-pressure two-way valves, the distal catheter is initially occluded by manually pressing on the neck. The pressure may cause injected tracer to flow into the proximal limb.

Images should show prompt flow into the ventricles, followed by spontaneous distal flow through the shunt

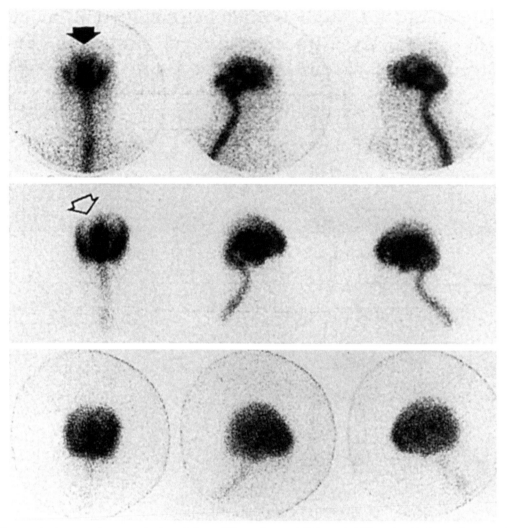

FIGURE 15-32. Communicating normal-pressure hydrocephalus at 24 hours *(top row)*, 48 hours *(middle row)* and 72 hours *(bottom row)* in anterior *(left)*, right lateral *(middle)*, and left lateral *(right)* projections. Ventricular reflux *(closed arrowhead)* is present, as is very delayed flow over the convexities *(open arrowhead)*. The intracerebral activity at 72 hours was caused by transependymal uptake.

Box 15-9. Shunt Patency: Summary Protocol

PATIENT PREPARATION
None

RADIOPHARMACEUTICAL
Tc-99m DTPA 0.5 to 1 mCi (18.5-37 MBq) or In-111 DTPA 250 µCi (93 MBq)

INSTRUMENTATION
Gamma camera: Wide field of view
Collimator: All purpose
Computer and camera setup: 1-minute images for 30 minutes

IMAGING PROCEDURE
Using aseptic technique. Clean the shaved scalp with povidone-iodine.
Penetrate the shunt reservoir with a 25- to 35-gauge needle.

Once the needle is in place, position the patient's head under the camera with the reservoir in the middle of the field of view.
Inject the radiopharmaceutical.
Take serial images for 30 minutes.
If no flow is seen, place the patient in an upright position and continue imaging for 10 minutes.
If still no flow is seen, obtain static images of 50k after 1 and 2 hours.
If flow is demonstrated at any point, obtain 50k images of the shunt and tubing every 15 min until flow to the distal tip of the shunt tubing is identified or for 2 hours, whichever is first.
To determine proximal patency of the reservoir, the distal catheter can be manually occluded during the procedure so that the radiotracer will reflux into the ventricular system.

DTPA, Diethylenetriaminepentaacetic acid.

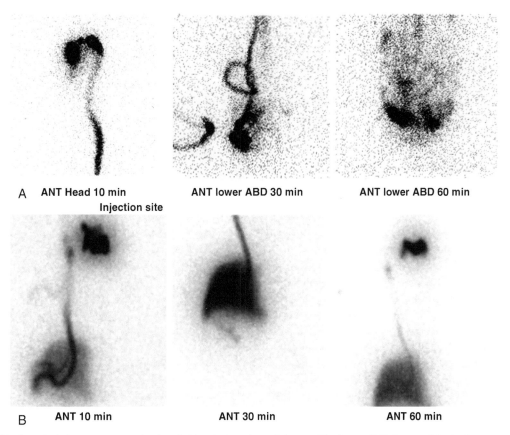

A **ANT Head 10 min**
Injection site   **ANT lower ABD 30 min**   **ANT lower ABD 60 min**

B **ANT 10 min**   **ANT 30 min**   **ANT 60 min**

FIGURE 15-33. Cerebrospinal shunt patency evaluation. **A,** Ventriculoperitoneal shunt at 10 minutes *(left)* shows activity in the reservoir port and distal limb of the shunt moving down the neck and chest. Intraventricular activity is also seen. By 30 minutes *(middle),* activity is in the abdomen with free flow in the peritoneum *(right).* **B,** Ventriculopleural shunt with normal radiotracer flow through the shunt into the pleural space that decreases over time. *ANT,* Anterior.

catheter (Fig. 15-33). The shunt tubing is usually seen. Catheters draining into the peritoneum show accumulation of radiotracer freely within the abdominal cavity. In cases of obstruction, activity does not move through the distal limb on delayed images or may pool close to the tip of the catheter in a loculated collection (Fig. 15-34).

Cerebrospinal Fluid Leak

Trauma and surgery (transsphenoidal and nasal) are the most common causes for CSF rhinorrhea. Nontraumatic causes include hydrocephalus and congenital defects. CSF rhinorrhea may occur at any site, from the frontal sinuses to the temporal bone (Fig. 15-35). The cribriform plate is most susceptible to fracture, which can result in rhinorrhea. Otorrhea is much less common. Accurate localization of CSF leaks can be clinically difficult.

Radionuclide studies are sensitive and accurate methods of CSF leak detection. To maximize the sensitivity of the test, nasal pledgets are placed in the anterior and posterior portion of each nasal region by an otolaryngologist and then removed and counted 4 hours later (Fig. 15-36). A ratio of nasal-to-plasma radioactivity greater than 2:1 or 3:1 is considered positive. The radiotracer is injected intrathecally via aseptic lumbar puncture (Box 15-10).

The site is most likely to be identified during a time when heavy leakage is occurring. Often, the patient position associated with greatest leakage is reproduced during imaging. Imaging in the appropriate projection is important for identifying the site of leak; lateral and anterior imaging

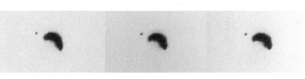

FIGURE 15-34. Obstructed cerebrospinal shunt. After injection of Tc-99m DTPA into the reservoir, refluxing into the ventricles, consistent with patency of the proximal limb of the shunt. However, no distal drainage occurs over 60 minutes from obstruction.

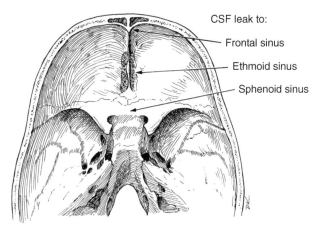

CSF leak to:
— Frontal sinus
— Ethmoid sinus
— Sphenoid sinus

FIGURE 15-35. Common sites of cerebrospinal fluid *(CSF)* leakage.

are used for rhinorrhea and posterior imaging for otorrhea. In cases in which no reason is known for low CSF pressure or when leak around the lumbar region is suspected, additional views should be made of the lumbar region.

Scintigraphic studies show CSF leaks as an increasing accumulation of activity at the leak site (Fig. 15-37). However, counting the pledgets is more sensitive than imaging for detecting CSF leaks. Pledgets are also helpful in determining the origin of the leak (anterior vs. posterior).

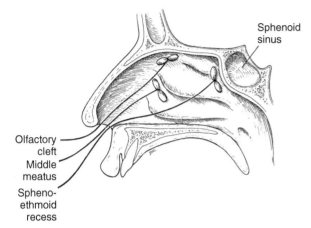

FIGURE 15-36. Placement of pledgets for cerebrospinal fluid leak study. The labeled cotton pledgets are placed by an otolaryngologist at various levels within the anterior and posterior nares to detect leakage from the frontal, ethmoidal, and sphenoidal sinuses.

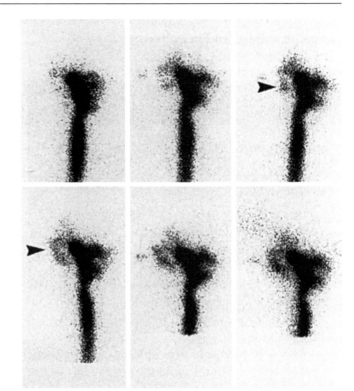

FIGURE 15-37. Positive radionuclide cerebrospinal fluid leak study. In-111 DTPA left lateral views show increasing radioactivity over time originating from the nares and leaking into the nose and mouth *(arrowheads)*.

Box 15-10. Cerebrospinal Fluid Leak Detection: Summary Protocol

PATIENT PREPARATION

Nasal pledgets are placed and labeled as to location. Pledgets should be weighed before placement.

After intrathecal injection, place patient in Trendelenburg position to pool the radiotracer in the basal regions until imaging begins.

Once radiotracer reaches basal cisterns, position patient in a position that increases cerebrospinal fluid leakage.

Rhinorrhea: Incline patient's head forward and against camera face with the camera positioned in the lateral position.

Otorrhea: Obtain posterior images instead of lateral views.

RADIOPHARMACEUTICAL

In-111 DTPA 250 μCi (9 MBq)

INSTRUMENTATION

Gamma camera: Large field of view
Collimator: Medium energy

IMAGING PROCEDURE

Setup

In-111 DTPA 500 μCi (18 MBq) of in 5 mL dextrose 10% in water intrathecally.

Begin imaging when activity reaches the basal cisterns (1-4 hours).

ACQUISITION

Acquire 5 minutes per frame for 1 hour in the selected view, then acquire anterior, left lateral, right lateral, and posterior views.

Obtain 50k images every 10 minutes for 1 hour in the original view.

Remove pledgets and place in separate tubes. Draw a 5-mL blood sample.

Count pledgets and 0.5-mL aliquots of plasma.

Repeat views may be indicated at 6 and 24 hours.

Calculate the ratio of pledgets-to-plasma activity: pledget counts/pledget capacity divided by serum counts/0.5 mL.

INTERPRETATION

Positive for cerebrospinal fluid leakage if the pledget-to-plasma activity ratio is greater than 2-3:1.

DTPA, Diethylenetriaminepentaacetic acid.

▬ SUGGESTED READING

Carmago EE. Brain SPECT in neurology and psychiatry. *J Nucl Med.* 2001;42(4):611.

Devous MD. Functional brain imaging in the dementias: role in early detection, differential diagnosis, and longitudinal studies. *Eur J Nucl Med Imaging.* 2002;29(12):1685-1687.

Herholz K, Herscovitch P, Heiss WD. *NeuroPET.* Berlin: Springer; 2004.

Marshall VL, Reininger CB, Marquardt M, et al. Parkinson's disease is over diagnosed clinically at baseline in diagnostically uncertain cases: a 3-year European multicenter study with repeat [123I] FP-CIT. *Mov Disord.* 2009;24(4):500-508.

Mountz JM, Liu HG, Deutsch G. Neuroimaging in cerebrovascular disorders: measurement of cerebral physiology after stroke and assessment of stroke recovery. *Semin Nucl Med.* 2003;33(1):56-76.

Osorio RS, Berti V, Mosconi L, et al. Evaluation of early dementia (mild cognitive impairment). *PET Clin.* 2005;5:15-31.

Van Heertum RL, Tikofsky RS, Masanori I. *Functional Cerebral SPECT and PET Imaging.* 4th ed. New York: Lippincott Williams & Wilkins; 2009.

CHAPTER 16

Cardiac System

Many cardiac diagnostic studies are available to the cardiologist, including electrocardiography (ECG), echocardiography, computed tomography (CT), CT angiography (CTA), and magnetic resonance imaging (MRI). The continuing value of cardiac nuclear studies stems from their noninvasiveness and accurate portrayal of a wide range of functional and metabolic parameters that predict prognosis and risk.

■ MYOCARDIAL PERFUSION SCINTIGRAPHY

The instrumentation, radiopharmaceuticals, and methodology used for myocardial perfusion scintigraphy have evolved over the years. Multiview planar imaging was followed by single-photon emission tomography (SPECT), gated SPECT, SPECT/CT, positron emission tomography (PET), and PET/CT. The underlying physiological principles that make myocardial perfusion imaging an important diagnostic tool remain unchanged.

Myocardial perfusion scintigraphy depicts sequential physiological events. First, the radiopharmaceutical must be delivered to the myocardium. Second, a viable metabolically active myocardial cell must be present to extract the radiotracer. Finally, a significant amount of the radiopharmaceutical must remain within the cell to allow for imaging. The scintigraphic images are a map of regional myocardial perfusion. If a patient has reduced regional perfusion as a result of hemodynamically significant coronary artery disease (CAD) or a loss of cell viability as a result of myocardial infarction, a perfusion defect or cold region is seen on the images. All diagnostic patterns in the many diverse applications follow from these observations.

Single-Photon Radiopharmaceuticals

Technetium-99m sestamibi and Tc-99m tetrafosmin have supplanted thallium-201 chloride as the most commonly used single-photon myocardial imaging agents, because of their superior image quality and the lower effective radiation dose to the patient.

Technetium-99m Sestamibi

Tc-99m sestamibi (Cardiolite) was the first technetium-labeled cardiac perfusion agent to be approved by the U.S. Food and Drug Administration (FDA) for clinical use in 1990. Generic Tc-99m sestamibi became available late September 2008.

Chemistry

Sestamibi is a lipophilic cation and member of the chemical isonitrile family. The radiopharmaceutical is composed of six isonitrile ligands (chemical name: hexakis 2-methoxyisobutyl isonitrile) surrounding the Tc-99m radionuclide. The radiopharmaceutical is prepared for the patient from a manufacturer-provided kit.

Mechanism of Localization and Uptake

Because it is lipid soluble, Tc-99m sestamibi diffuses from the blood into the myocardial cell. It is retained intracellularly in the region of mitochondria because of its negative transmembrane potential. First-pass extraction fraction is 60% (Table 16-1). Extraction is proportional to coronary blood flow, underestimated at high flow rates and overestimated at low flow (Fig. 16-1).

Pharmacokinetics

After the agent rapidly clears from the blood, myocardial uptake is prompt, surrounded by high lung and liver uptake. The radiopharmceutical remains fixed within the myocardium. This allows for an imaging time window of several hours after administration, based on the radiotracer half-life. Because of renal and biliary excretion, the liver and lungs progressively clear, improving the myocardium-to-background activity ratios with time. Imaging acquisition begins 45 to 60 minutes after tracer administration for resting studies and at 30 minutes for exercise stress studies because of more rapid background clearance.

Dosimetry

The colon is the critical radiation target organ, receiving 5.4 rems/30 mCi (5.4 cGy/1110 MBq) (Table 16-2). The radiation effective whole body dose is 0.9 rem/30 mCi or 0.9 cGy/1110MBq.

Technetium-99m Tetrofosmin

Tc-99m tetrofosmin (Myoview) was approved by the FDA in 1996. It is similar to Tc-99m sestamibi, although not identical. An advantage over Tc-99m sestamibi is its more rapid liver clearance.

Chemistry

Tetrofosmin is a member of the diphosphine chemical class (chemical name: 6,9-bis [2-ethoxyethyl]-3,12-dioxa-6,9 diphosphatetradecane). It is prepared from a commercial kit.

Mechanism of Localization and Uptake

Similar to sestamibi, Tc-99m tetrofosmin is a lipophilic cation that localizes near mitochondria in the myocardial cell and remains fixed at that site.

Pharmacokinetics

After intravenous injection, Tc-99m tetrofosmin is cleared rapidly from the blood and myocardial uptake is prompt. First-pass extraction is slightly less than that of sestamibi (50% vs. 60%), with 1.2% of the injected dose taken up in the myocardium by 5 minutes after injection (Table 16-1).

TABLE 16-1 Physiology and Pharmacokinetics of Thallium-201, Sestamibi, and Technetium-99m Tetrofosmin

Physiology	Thallium-201	Tc-99m sestamibi	Tc-99m tetrofosmin
Chemical class/charge	Elemental cation	Isonitrile cation	Diphosphine cation
Mechanism of uptake	Active transport Na/K ATPase pump	Passive diffusion, negative electrical potential	Passive diffusion, negative electrical potential
Myocyte localization	Cytosol	Mitochondria	Mitochondria
Intracellular state	Free	Bound	Bound
Preparation	Cyclotron	Generator/kit	Generator/kit
First-pass extraction fraction (%)	85	60	50
Percent cardiac uptake (%)	3	1.5	1.2
Myocardial clearance	4-hr $T_{1/2}$	Minimal	Minimal
Body clearance	Renal	Hepatic	Hepatic
Imaging time after injection			
Stress	10 min	15-30 min	5-15 min
Rest	3-4 hr	30-90 min	30 min

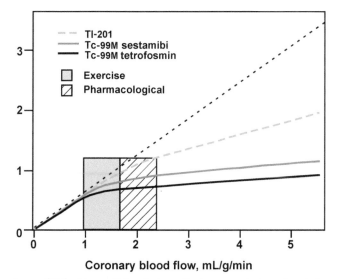

FIGURE 16-1. Myocardial perfusion radiopharmaceutical uptake relative to coronary blood flow. An ideal myocardial perfusion tracer would show a linear relationship to blood flow over a wide range of flow rates (straight diagonal dark dashed line). Tc-99m sestamibi and Tc-99m tetrofosmin all have extraction that is proportional to blood flow but underestimate flow at high flow rates. At rest, the normal myocardial coronary low rate is 1 mL/g/min. With exercise, it can increase to 2 mL/g/min. With pharmacological vasodilation, flow may exceed 2 mL/g/min. Tl-201, Tc-99m sestamibi, and Tc-99m tetrofosmin all have extraction that is proportional to blood flow but underestimate flow at high flow rates.

Extraction is proportional to blood flow, but underestimated at high flow rates (Fig. 16-1).

Heart-to-lung and heart-to-liver ratios improve with time because of physiological clearance through the liver and kidneys. Heart-to-liver ratios are higher for Tc-99m tetrofosmin than sestamibi because of faster hepatic clearance, allowing for earlier imaging. After exercise stress, imaging at 15 minutes is feasible. Rest studies can be started 30 minutes after injection.

Dosimetry
The radiation absorbed dose is similar to that of Tc-99m sestamibi (Table 16-2), although the package insert states

TABLE 16-2 Patient Radiation Dose from Thallium-201, Technetium-99m Sestamibi, Technetium-99m Tetrofosmin

Dose	Tl-201+ rems/3 mCi (cGy/111 MBq)	Tc-99m sestamibi rems/30 mCi (cGy/1110 MBq)	Tc-99m tetrofosmin rems/30 mCi (cGy/1110 MBq)
Heart wall	0.3	0.5	0.5
Liver	1.1	0.8	0.5
Kidneys	**5.1**	2.0	1.4
Gallbladder	0.9	2.8	**5.4**
Urinary bladder	0.6	2.0	2.1
Colon	0.8	**5.4**	3.4
Thyroid	30.0	0.7	0.6
Testes	0.9	0.3	0.4
Ovaries	1.1	1.5	1.1
Total effective dose	1.8	0.9	0.8

Target organ (highest radiation absorbed dose) in **boldface** type.

that the gallbladder receives the highest dose (5.4 rems/20 mCi [5.4 cGy/1110 MBq]), rather than the colon for sestamibi. The reason for the difference may be due to whether the studied subjects ate and had gallbladder contraction. The whole-body radiation effective dose is 0.8 rem/30 mCi (0.8 cGy/1110 MBq).

Thallium-201 Chloride
Radiolabeled potassium (K+) was considered for possible use for myocardial perfusion imaging because it is the major intracellular cation. Sodium (Na+)/K+ homeostasis is maintained via an energy-dependent process involving the Na+/K+ ATPase (adenosine triphosphatase) pump in the myocardial cell membrane. However, neither K+ nor its analogs, cesium and rubidium, were found suitable for

TABLE 16-3 Physical Characteristics of Thallium-201 and Technetium-99m

Physical characteristic	Tl-201	Tc-99m
Mode of decay	Electron capture	Isomeric transition
Physical half-life	73 hours	6 hours
Principal emissions (abundance)*	Mercury x-rays	Gamma rays
	69-83 keV	140 keV (89%)
	Gamma rays	
	167 keV (10%) 135 keV (2.5%)	

*Abundance is the percent likelihood of an emission type occurring with each decay

single-photon imaging because of their high-energy photons. Rubidium-82 is used today for dual-photon imaging with PET.

Tl-201 chloride behaves physiologically similar to K+, although it is not a true K+ analog in a chemical sense. First used for myocardial scintigraphy in the mid-1970s, it was the only perfusion agent available until the 1990s, when Tc-99m–labeled radiotracers were introduced. Tl-201 is less commonly used today because of its poorer image quality, although at some imaging clinics it is used for the rest study in dual-isotope studies or for viability studies.

Chemistry

Thallium is a metallic element in the IIIA series of the Periodic Table of the Elements (Fig. 1-1). In pharmacological doses, thallium is a poison, but is nontoxic in the subpharmacological tracer doses used. It is administered to the patient in the chemical form of thallium chloride.

Physics

The radionuclide Tl-201 is cyclotron produced. It decays by electron capture to its stable mercury-201 daughter, with a physical half-life of 73 hours. The photons available for imaging are mercury K-characteristic x-rays ranging from 69 to 83 keV (95% abundant) and gamma rays of 167 keV (10%) and 135 keV (3%) (Table 16-3). For gamma-camera imaging, a 20% to 30% window is centered at 69 to 83 keV and a 20% window at 167 keV.

Mechanism of Localization and Pharmacokinetics

After intravenous injection, Tl-201 blood clearance is rapid (Fig. 16-2). It is transported across the myocardial cell membrane via the Na+/K+ ATPase pump. More than 85% is extracted by the myocardial cell on first pass through the coronary capillary circulation (Table 16-1). Peak myocardial uptake occurs by 10 minutes. Approximately 3% of the administered dose localizes in the myocardium. Extraction is proportional to relative regional perfusion over a range of flow rates. At high flow rates, extraction efficiency decreases; at low rates, it increases. It can only be extracted by viable myocardium, but not in regions of infarction or scar.

Scintigraphy obtained after Tl-201 uptake reflects capillary myocardial blood flow. It then undergoes redistribution, a continual dynamic exchange between the myocardial cell and the vascular blood pool. As it leaves

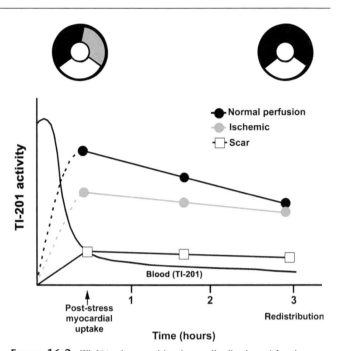

FIGURE 16-2. Tl-201 pharmacokinetics: redistribution. After intravenous injection, Tl-201 clears rapidly from the blood pool. Normal stress peak myocardial uptake occurs by 10 minutes. Redistribution begins promptly after initial uptake. This is a constant dynamic exchange of thallium between the myocytes and blood pool. Normal myocardium progressively clears over 3 hours. In the presence of ischemia, uptake is delayed and reduced and clearance is slow. With infarction, there is little uptake and very little change over time. The schematic diagram relates thallium pharmacokinetics (*below*) to scintigraphic findings (*above*). The ischemic region, although initially hypoperfused compared to the normal region equalizes scintigraphically at 3 hours. (Modified with permission from Dilsizian V, Narula J. *Atlas of Nuclear Cardiology.* Philadelphia: Current Medicine; 2003.)

the myocardial cell, it is replaced by Tl-201 circulating in the systemic blood pool, which also undergoes redistribution. Several hours after injection, the images depict an equilibrium reflecting regional blood volume. With normal perfusion, initial capillary blood flow and delayed regional blood volume images are similar.

These unique pharmacokinetic characteristics of Tl-201 are the basis for the "stress-redistribution" Tl-201 imaging strategy used for the detection of CAD (Fig. 16-2). Regions of decreased perfusion on early poststress images are due to either decreased blood flow (ischemia) or lack of viable cells to fix the tracer (infarction). If an initial perfusion defect persists on delayed images, it depicts infarction. Defects showing "fill-in" of Tl-201 between stress and rest are viable myocardium rendered ischemic during stress.

Dosimetry

The kidneys receive the highest radiation dose at 5.1 rem/3 mCi (5.1 cGy/111 MBq). The whole-body effective dose is 2.4 rem/4 mCi (2.4 cGy/1480 MBq) (Table 16-2).

Tl-201 has relatively high-radiation absorbed dose because of its long biological and physical half-life, limiting the maximum allowable administered dose to 3.5–4.0 mCi (130-150 MBq). Myocardial image quality of Tl-201 is not as good as with Tc-99m–labeled radiopharmaceuticals to a large extent because of the low administered dose.

ANT   LAO   RAO

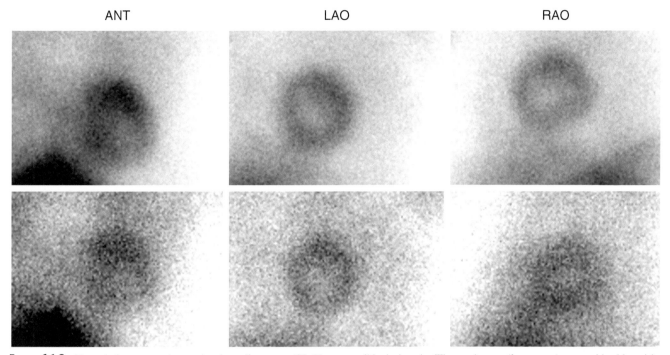

FIGURE 16-3. Normal planar stress *(top row)* and rest *(bottom row)* Tc-99m sestamibi scintigraphy. The rest images *(bottom row)* are considerably noisier because of the lower administered dose (8 mCi) and resulting lower count rates compared to the stress images (25 mCi). Images are acquired so that the three views are at the same angle, between stress and rest, for optimal comparison. *ANT,* Anterior; *LAO,* left anterior oblique; *RAO,* right anterior oblique.

In addition, the range of mercury x-ray emissions of Tl-201 have relatively low photoenergies (69-83 keV), rather than a single optimal energy photopeak, making it less well suited for gamma camera imaging. A high Compton scatter fraction also diminishes image quality. Low count rates makes gated SPECT imaging more difficult compared to Tc-99–labeled agents, especially for large patients.

Other Single Photon Perfusion Agents

Tc-99m teboroxime (CardioTec), approved by the FDA in 1990, has not yet found clinical utility. Dedicated cardiac cameras with a high count rate capability, now starting to become available, may make this radiopharmaceutical potentially more attractive.

This neutral lipophilic radiopharmaceutical comes from a class of compounds called boronic acid adducts of Tc-99m dioxime (BATO). The extraction fraction is higher than that of Tl-201. Uptake is proportional to flow but decreases with increasing flow. Blood clearance half-time is less than 1 minute. Myocardial clearance is very rapid ($T_{1/2}$ 5-10 minutes). Washout is proportional to regional blood flow. Redistribution does not occur. The rapid uptake and clearance dictate a very narrow window for imaging—2 to 6 minutes, resulting in relatively poor-quality SPECT images using standard gamma camera methods because of low counting statistics and rapidly changing distribution.

Imaging Methodologies

Planar Myocardial Perfusion Imaging

Two-dimensional (2-D) planar imaging was the standard imaging method for years. Overall accuracy for diagnosis of CAD was good, although accurate localization of regional perfusion abnormalities had only moderate predictive success for the coronary bed involved.

Image interpretation is limited by high background and overlapping structures in the standard three views (left anterior oblique, right anterior oblique, left lateral) (Figs. 16-3 and 16-4). Stress and rest images must be acquired in the same projection for optimal interpretation.

More accurate assessment of regional perfusion became increasingly important as myocardial perfusion scintigraphy was less frequently used for diagnosis and increasingly used for prognosis, risk stratification, and patient management.

In current practice, planar imaging is limited to patients who are severely claustrophobic and for those who exceed weight restrictions on the SPECT imaging table.

Single-Photon Emission Computed Tomography

SPECT is the standard method for myocardial perfusion scintigraphy. The cross-sectional images have high-contrast resolution and are displayed three-dimensionally along the short and long axis of the heart (Figs. 16-5 and 16-6), providing good delineation of the various regional myocardial perfusion beds supplied by their individual coronary arteries.

SPECT instrumentation, image reconstruction, and quality control are discussed in the section on basic principles. Acquisition and processing parameters depend to some extent on the specific camera and computer software. Variations include the number and position of camera detector heads (Fig. 16-7), continuous acquisition versus step and shoot, the number of camera stops, acquisition time at each angle, and shape of orbit (e.g., elliptical, body contour, circular). Because the heart lies in the anterior lateral chest and considerable cardiac attenuation occurs in

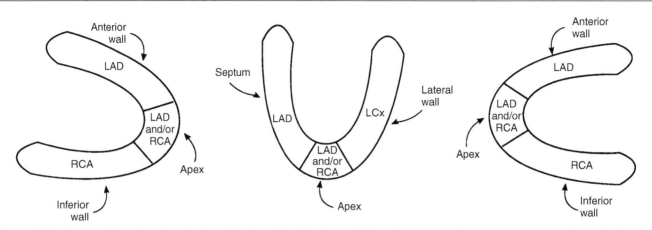

FIGURE 16-4. Planar scintigraphy schematic illustrating the relationship of ventricular wall segments to the coronary artery vascular supply. Anterior, left anterior oblique, left lateral projections. *LAD*, Left anterior descending artery; *LCX*, left circumflex artery; *RCA*, right coronary artery.

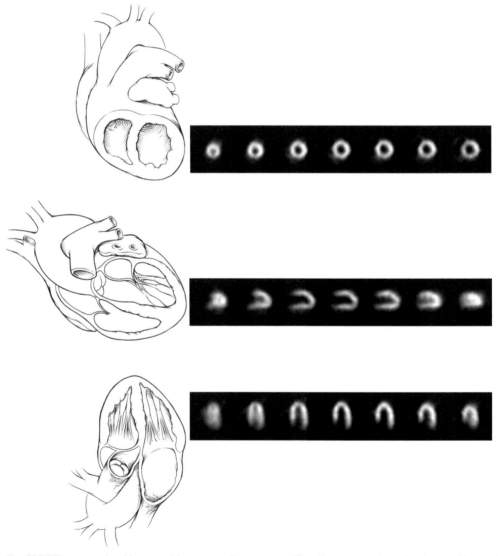

FIGURE 16-5. Cardiac SPECT cross-sectional images with corresponding anatomy. The slices are cut along the short and long axis of the heart: *top* (short-axis), *middle* (vertical long axis), *bottom* (horizontal long axis). The left ventricle is best seen because of its greater myocardial mass; the right ventricle is normally much less well seen. Atria are never visualized.

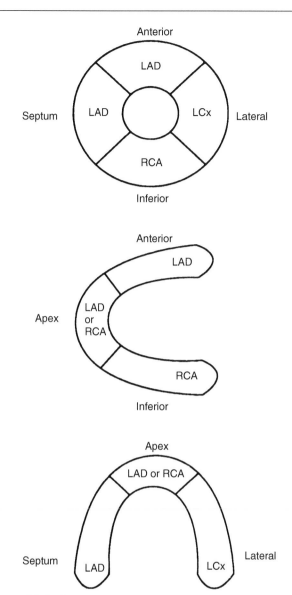

FIGURE **16-6.** SPECT processed to obtain cross-sectional slices cut along the short and long axis of the heart.

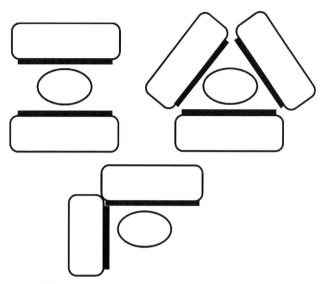

FIGURE **16-7.** Two-head and three-head detector gamma camera configurations for cardiac imaging. A common configuration with the two-head systems is with the heads at right angles to each other *(lower)*. Thus maximal count rate is achieved over a 180-degree rotation. Three-heads are typically acquired over a 270- to 360-degree rotation.

TABLE **16-4** Scintigraphic Patterns by Vascular Distribution: Stenosis and Obstruction

Coronary arteries	Scintigraphic perfusion defects
Left anterior descending	Septum, anterior wall, apex
Left circumflex	Lateral wall, posterior wall, posterior inferior wall, apex
Right coronary	Inferior wall, posterior inferior wall, right ventricular wall
Left main coronary	Anterior wall, septum, posterolateral wall
Multivessel disease	Multiple vascular bed perfusion defects
	Poststress ventricular dilation, increased Tl-201 lung uptake

the posterior projections, SPECT is often acquired over a 180-degree arc from the left posterior oblique to the right anterior oblique projection. The left arm is positioned above the head to minimize attenuation.

Using a two-head camera with the detectors at 90 degrees is a common approach that maximizes sensitivity and minimizes acquisition time. Three-head detectors have added value but are costly and not widely available. High-resolution collimators are used to take advantage of the higher counts obtained from multiple detectors. Good image quality requires the acquisition time be as short as possible while acquiring sufficient counts. Image acquisition with standard SPECT systems requires 20 to 30 minutes. New dedicated cardiac cameras can acquire adequate counts with good image resolution in a shorter period.

Filtered backprojection was the standard method used for cross-sectional image reconstruction; however, with faster computers today, iterative reconstruction techniques are often used, particularly with CT attenuation correction. Software filters are chosen to optimize the trade-off between high-frequency noise and low-frequency oversmoothing. Attenuation correction uses an attenuation map generated by a rotating gamma source or CT.

Cardiac SPECT software reconstructs cross-sectional cardiac images along the short and long axes of the heart—that is, transaxial (short axis), coronal (horizontal long axis), and sagittal (vertical long axis) (Figs. 16-5 and 16-6). This also has become the standard for CT, MRI, and echocardiography. The SPECT cross-sectional images depict the regional perfusion of the myocardium as it relates to the coronary artery supplying blood to that region (Table 16-4) and permits visual estimation of the degree and extent of the perfusion abnormality (Figs. 16-8 and 16-9).

Gated Single-Photon Emission Computed Tomography

The high count rate available from 20 to 30 mCi (740–1110 MBq) of Tc-99m sestamibi or tetrofosmin and two detectors makes ECG gating feasible and common practice today. ECG gated SPECT provides a cinematic three-dimensional display of contracting myocardial slices from summed beats over the acquisition time. Data collection is

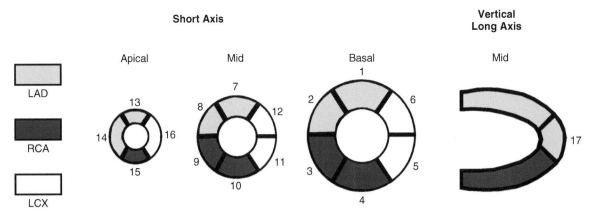

Short Axis

Vertical Long Axis

Apical   Mid   Basal   Mid

LAD

RCA

LCX

FIGURE 16-8. Standardization of SPECT myocardial segments. This method divides the myocardium into 17 regions and has been recommended for all cardiac imaging. The diagram also correlates coronary artery anatomy with regional perfusion. Some computer software systems use a different number of regions. *LAD*, Left anterior descending artery; *LCX*, left circumflex artery; *RCA*, right coronary artery. (Modified with permission from Cerqueira MD, Weissman J, Dilsizian V, et al. Standardized myocardial segmentation and nomenclature for tomographic imaging of the heart: a statement for healthcare professionals from the Cardiac Imaging Committee of the Council on Clinical Cardiology of the American Heart Association. *J Nucl Cardiol.* 2002;2[2]:240–245.)

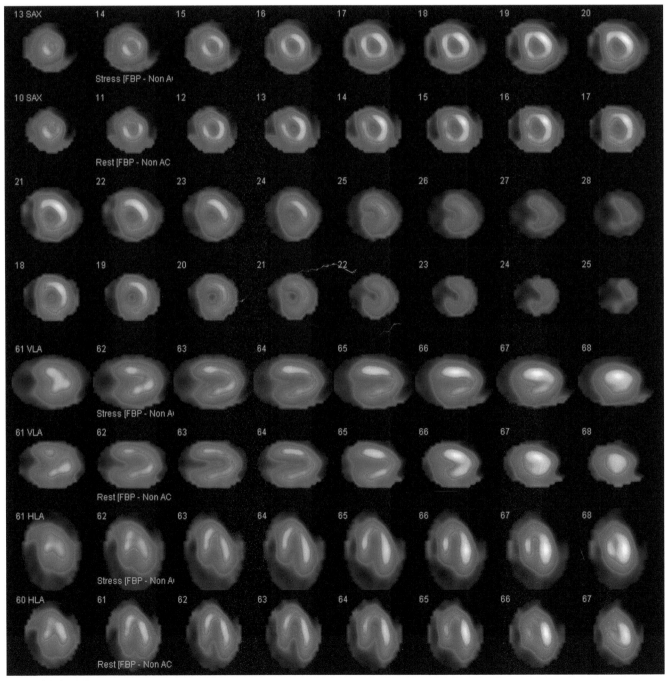

FIGURE 16-9. Normal myocardial SPECT perfusion study. Top *four* rows display the short-axis transaxial images (stress *above*, rest *below*), *fifth and sixth rows* display the horizontal long-axis (sagittal) stress and rest views, and the *seventh and eighth* rows display the vertical long-axis (coronal) views.

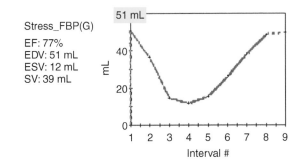

Stress_FBP(G)

EF: 77%
EDV: 51 mL
ESV: 12 mL
SV: 39 mL

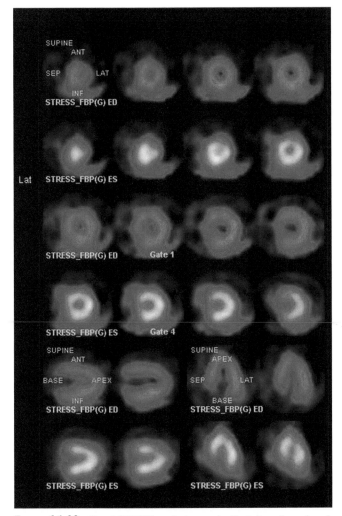

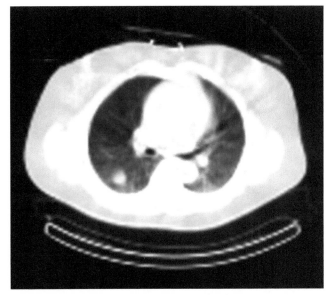

FIGURE 16-11. Incidental CT finding on SPECT/CT. Low-resolution CT scan from hybrid SPECT/CT system shows nodule in the left posterior lung field.

Single-Photon Emission Computed Tomography with Computed Tomography

Hybrid SPECT/CT systems are becoming increasingly available. The CT is used primarily for attenuation correction and coronary artery calcium scoring. Review of the limited-field lung CT images sometimes reveals incidental unknown disease—for example, a lung mass (Fig. 16-11). The potential exists to perform combined contrast CTA and SPECT studies that provide both functional and anatomical imaging presented in a combined three-dimensional (3-D) volume display.

Diagnosis and Evaluation of Coronary Artery Disease

Physiology of Ischemia

Ischemic perfusion abnormalities are usually absent at rest (Fig. 16-12). Under resting conditions, high-grade stenosis (≥90%) in a given epicardial coronary artery produces a downstream decline in the coronary perfusion pressure to the affected vascular territory. Blood flow at rest is maintained by autoregulatory dilation of the coronary arterioles over a wide range of perfusion pressures. By increasing cardiac work, exercise stress increases the demand for oxygen and thus blood flow increases. In the absence of epicardial coronary artery disease, maximum exercise increases coronary flow 3 to 5 times by means of autoregulatory dilation of the coronary arterioles.

Coronary flow reserve across a fixed mechanical stenosis is limited because most coronary arteriolar vasodilator reserve has already been used to maintain resting flow. With exercise, myocardium in the watershed of a coronary artery with a hemodynamically significant stenosis becomes ischemic. Reduced regional blood flow results in less delivery and localization of the perfusion radiopharmaceutical. This hypoperfusion is seen on scintigraphic images as a perfusion defect (i.e., "photopenic" or cold in the ischemic region) surrounded by normal blood flow in the adjacent nonischemic regions of the heart (Fig. 16-13).

FIGURE 16-10. Gated SPECT perfusion study. End-diastolic and end-systolic images of the short-axis views (*top four rows* of images) and vertical and horizontal long-axis views *(bottom two rows)* are shown. The TAC for all eight slices is shown at the *top. ANT,* Anterior; *EDV,* end-diastolic volume; *EF,* ejection fraction; *ESV,* end-systolic volume; *FBP(G),* filtered back projection (gated); *INF,* inferior; *Lat,* lateral; *SEP,* septal; *SV,* stroke volume.

triggered from the R-wave of the ECG. The cardiac cycle is divided usually into 8 frames, less than the 16 frames used for count-rich Tc-99m–labeled red blood cell (RBC) ventriculograms. The 8 frames limit to only a mild degree the temporal resolution (pinpointing end-diastole and end-systole) and accuracy of left ventricular ejection fraction (LVEF) calculation. Edge-detection software programs automatically draw the endocardial surface and delineate the valve plane for LVEF calculation and wall motion and thickening analysis (Fig. 16-10).

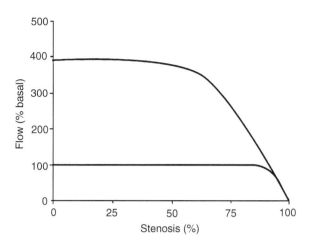

FIGURE 16-12. Relationship between blood flow and severity of coronary stenosis. At rest, myocardial blood flow is not reduced until a coronary stenosis approaches 90%. It then begins to drop off. However, with increased rates of coronary blood flow produced by exercise or pharmacological stress, less severe stenoses (50%-75%) result in reduced coronary flow.

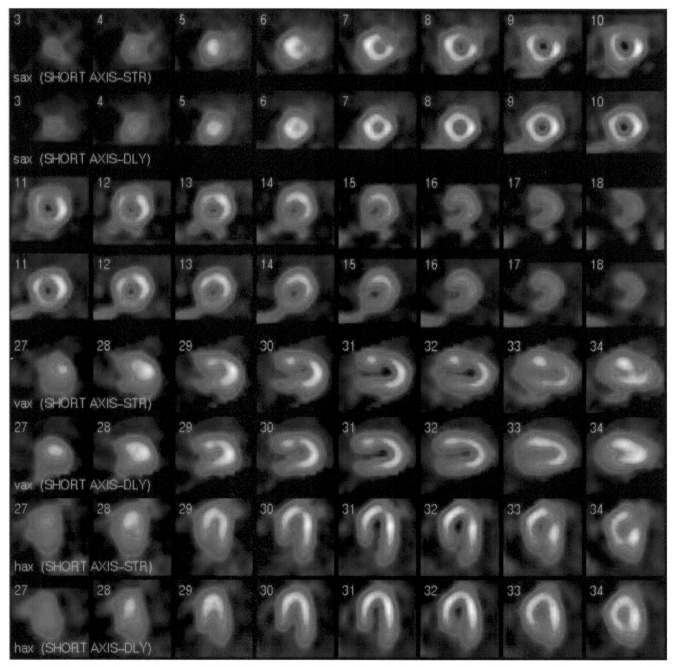

FIGURE 16-13. Ischemia on Tc-99m sestamibi SPECT myocardial perfusion scintigraphy. Reduced perfusion (cold, photopenic) at stress in the anterior lateral left ventricle; normal perfusion at rest. *DLY,* Delay; *hax,* horizontal long axis; *sax,* short axis; *STR,* stress; *vax,* vertical long axis.

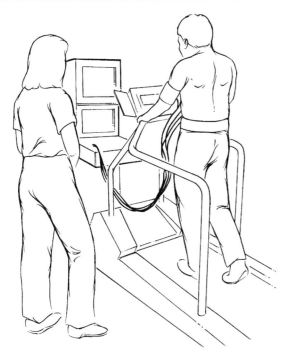

FIGURE **16-14.** Treadmill graded patient exercise with ECG, blood pressure, heart rate, and symptom monitoring.

Box 16-1. Exercise Testing: Rationale and Endpoint Measures

PHYSIOLOGICAL RATIONALE
Physical exercise increases cardiac work
Increased work increases myocardial oxygen demand
Normal coronary arteries dilate and flow increases
Stenotic vessels cannot dilate and flow reserve is limited
Myocardial ischemia is induced

MANIFESTATIONS OF MYOCARDIAL ISCHEMIA
Electrocardiogram: Ion flux across cell membrane is impaired, produces ST segment depression
Perfusion scintigraphy: Decrease in regional flow produces cold defect area on scintigraphy
Radionuclide ventriculography: Regional wall motion abnormality or fall in left ventricular ejection fraction

---

Coronary artery stenoses of more than 70% are generally considered clinically significant based on the rapid fall-off in flow reserve augmentation above this level (Fig. 16-12). However, the anatomical degree of stenosis has a poor correlation with flow reserve and the degree of ischemia. Factors that may affect the functional significance of an anatomical circumferential narrowing include the length, shape, and location of a stenotic lesion. Functional imaging with myocardial perfusion scintigraphy is often needed to evaluate the clinical significance of a known stenosis, particularly in the range of 50% of 70%.

Cardiac Stress Testing
Cardiac stress testing with ECG monitoring has long been used by cardiologists to diagnose ischemic coronary disease. Graded treadmill exercise is the standard method (Fig. 16-14).

Box 16-2. Contraindications for Stress Testing

Acute myocardial infarction
Unstable angina
Severe tachyarrhythmias or bradyarrhythmias
Uncontrolled symptomatic heart failure
Critical aortic stenosis
Acute aortic dissection
Pulmonary embolism
Poorly controlled hypertension

The degree of stress must be sufficient to unmask underlying ischemia (Box 16-1). Exercise increases cardiac workload and oxygen demand. The treadmill study allows for assessment of the patient's functional cardiac status by directly monitoring exercise tolerance, heart rate, blood pressure, and ECG response to graded exercise. Contraindications for cardiac stress testing are listed in Box 16-2.

Exercise-induced myocardial ischemia produces characteristic ST-T segment depression on ECG (Fig. 16-15) caused by alterations in sodium and potassium electrolyte flux across the ischemic cell membrane. The adequacy of exercise is judged by the degree of cardiac work. Heart rate and blood pressure provide such an indication. Patients achieving more than 85% of the age-predicted maximum heart rate (220 − age = maximum predicted heart rate) are considered to have achieved adequate exercise stress. The heart-rate × blood pressure product, metabolic equivalents (METS), and exercise time (minutes) also can be used to judge the adequacy of exercise. Failure to achieve adequate exercise is the most common reason for a false negative stress test result (Box 16-3).

The cardiac treadmill exercise test that cardiologists perform in their offices provides clinically useful functional diagnostic information to help manage patients. However, the overall accuracy of the cardiac treadmill exercise test for the diagnosis of CAD is modest, at approximately 75%, with many false negative and false positive results. Specificity is particularly poor in women; in patients with resting ECG ST-T abnormalities, left ventricular hypertrophy, or bundle branch block; and for those on digoxin. These patients often require myocardial perfusion scintigraphy to confirm or exclude the diagnosis of CAD. Sensitivity and specificity will change according to the diagnostic criterion used—for example, ST segment depressions ≥1 versus ≥2 mm.

Stress Myocardial Perfusion Scintigraphy
The SPECT study provides valuable information on the extent and severity of coronary artery disease useful for risk assessment, prognosis, and patient management.

Exercise Stress with Myocardial Perfusion Scintigraphy
Patients fast for 4 to 6 hours before the test to prevent stress-induced gastric distress and minimize splanchnic blood distribution. Cardiac medications may be held depending on the indication for the stress test—that is, whether for diagnosis or to determine the effectiveness of therapy (Table 16-5). The decision is left to the discretion of the referring physician.

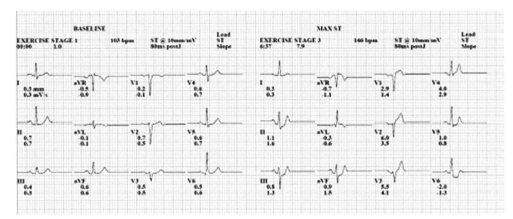

FIGURE 16-15. Treadmill ECG ischemia. Baseline *(left) and* maximal stress *(right)* 12-lead ECG demonstrates ST-T wave depression in II, III, aV$_F$, and V$_6$, consistent with stress induced ischemia.

Box 16-3. Reasons for Failing to Achieve Adequate Exercise

Poor general conditioning, low exercise tolerance
Poor motivation
Arthritis, other musculoskeletal problems
Lung disease
Peripheral vascular disease
Medications (beta blockers)
Angina
Arrhythmia
Cardiac insufficiency

TABLE 16-5 Drugs That Interfere with Stress Testing: Recommended Withdrawal Interval

Drugs	Withdrawal Interval
EXERCISE	
Beta blockers	48-96 hr
Calcium channel blockers	48-72 hr
Nitrates (long acting)	12 hr
PHARMACOLOGICAL	
Theophylline derivatives	48 hr
Caffeine	24 hr

TABLE 16-6 Treadmill Graded Exercise Stress Test

Stage (min)	Total time (min)	Speed (mile/h)	Grade (%)
STANDARD BRUCE PROTOCOL			
1 (3)	3	1.7	10
2 (3)	6	2.5	12
3 (3)	9	3.4	14
4 (3)	12	4.2	16
5 (3)	15	5.0	18
6 (3)	18	6.0	20
MODIFIED BRUCE PROTOCOL			
1 (3)	3	1.7	0
2 (3)	6	1.7	5
3 (3)	9	1.7	10
4 (3)	12	2.5	12
5 (3)	15	3.4	14
6 (3)	18	4.2	16
7 (3)	21	5.0	18

The modified Bruce starts with the same speed as the standard Bruce, but with no slope, followed by slight increase in slope, and then in speed. This protocol is suited for elderly patients or when one anticipates difficulties with physical performance.

Beta blockers may prevent achievement of maximum heart rate and nitrates, and calcium channel blockers may mask or prevent cardiac ischemia, limiting the test's diagnostic value. Assessment of drug therapy effectiveness requires the patient to remain on medication.

In addition to a standard 12-lead baseline ECG, an intravenous line is kept open. The patient is continuously monitored during the study. Graded treadmill exercise is performed according to a standardized protocol (e.g., the Bruce protocol) (Table 16-6). When the patient has achieved maximal exercise or peak patient tolerance, the radiopharmaceutical is injected. Exercise is continued for another minute to ensure adequate uptake. Early discontinuation of exercise may result in tracer distribution reflecting perfusion at submaximal exercise levels. Indications for terminating exercise are listed in Box 16-4. Many of these are manifestations of ischemia; others are due to underlying medical, cardiac, or pulmonary conditions.

Pharmacological Stress with Myocardial Perfusion Scintigraphy

Approximately 50% of patients receive pharmacological stress because it is anticipated that they will not be able to achieve adequate exercise due to concurrent medical problems—for example, pulmonary disease or lower extremity musculoskeletal problems.

Coronary Vasodilating Drugs

Dipyridamole, Adenosine, and Regadenoson. Dipyridamole (Persantine) and adenosine (Adenoscan) are coronary vasodilating drugs that have long been used for stress myocardial perfusion imaging. Regadenoson (Lexiscan) was approved by the FDA in 2009. The vasodilators increase coronary blood flow in normal vessels 3 to 5 times. Because coronary arteries with significant stenoses cannot increase blood flow to the same degree as normal vessels, vasodilator stress results in vascular regions of relative hypoperfusion on myocardial perfusion scintigraphy similar to that seen with exercise-induced ischemia.

This is not a test of ischemia, because cardiac work is not involved, but rather a test of coronary flow reserve (maximum increase in blood flow through the coronary arteries above normal resting flow). Comparative studies have shown similar scintigraphic patterns and overall diagnostic accuracy for exercise and pharmacological stress.

Mechanism of Pharmacological Effect. When endogenously released by the coronary endothelial cells, adenosine activates four coronary receptor subtypes, A1, A2A, A2B, and A3. Only A2A activation produces coronary vasodilation. Activation of the other receptors is responsible for the drug's side effects. The adenosine analog used for stress testing has similar effect. Dipyridamole exerts its pharmacological effect by blocking the reuptake mechanism of adenosine and raising endogenous adenosine blood levels. Regadenoson is a selective A2A receptor agonist.

Patient Preparation. Because vasodilators are antagonized by drugs and food containing chemically related methylxanthines (e.g., theophylline, caffeine) (Fig. 16-16), the drugs must be discontinued before the study because they will counteract vasodilator effectiveness (Table 16-5). Adenosine and dipyridamole may cause bronchospasm in patients with asthma and chronic obstructive pulmonary disease. This is less of a problem with regadenoson, which is now widely used in these patients.

Methodology. The technical details for dipyridamole, adenosine, and regadenoson infusion protocols differ (Fig. 16-17)

Box 16-4. Indications for Terminating a Stress Test

Patient request
Inability to continue because of fatigue, dyspnea, or faintness
Moderate to severe chest pain
Dizziness, near syncope
Pallor, diaphoresis
Ataxia
Claudication
Ventricular tachycardia
Atrial tachycardia or fibrillation
Onset of second- or third-degree heart block
ST-segment depression greater than 3 mm
Decrease in systolic blood pressure from baseline
Increase in systolic blood pressure above 240 mm Hg or diastolic above 120 mm Hg

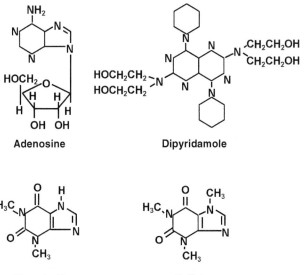

FIGURE 16-16. Close chemical relationship between adenosine and dipyridamole to theophylline and caffeine.

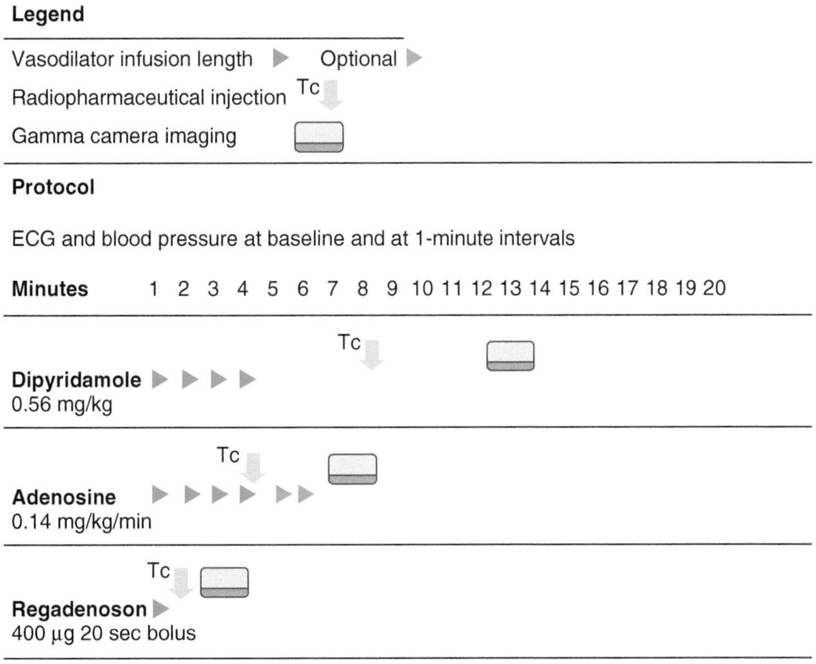

Legend

Vasodilator infusion length ▶	Optional ▶
Radiopharmaceutical injection	Tc ⬇
Gamma camera imaging	▭

Protocol

ECG and blood pressure at baseline and at 1-minute intervals

Minutes   1 2 3 4 5 6 7 8 9 10 11 12 13 14 15 16 17 18 19 20

Dipyridamole ▶ ▶ ▶ ▶
0.56 mg/kg

Adenosine ▶ ▶ ▶ ▶ ▶ ▶
0.14 mg/kg/min

Regadenoson ▶
400 µg 20 sec bolus

FIGURE 16-17. Coronary vasodilation stress protocol.

because of their different pharmacokinetics (Table 16-7). Unlike adenosine and dipyridamole, which are given as constant infusions, regadenoson is given as an intravenous bolus in a fixed dose. A mild to moderate increase in heart rate and reduction in blood pressure confirm the drug's pharmacological effect.

Side Effects. Nausea, dizziness, headache, and flushing are not uncommon. Approximately 20% to 30% of patients experience chest pain; however, it is not usually caused by ischemia. Rarely, a coronary steal syndrome may produce true ischemia. If ECG ST-T depression occurs during infusion, it is highly suggestive of significant coronary disease. Dyspnea and atrioventricular conduction blocks occur predominantly with adenosine.

Regadenoson is relatively safer to use in patients with mild to moderate reactive airway disease and may have fewer other side effects. Because of adenosine's short half-life (<10 seconds), side effects resolve promptly when the infusion is stopped. Because the effect of dipyridamole and regadenoson is prolonged after stopping the infusion (long serum half-lives), aminophylline may be required to reverse the side effects.

Accuracy. Comparative studies have reported similar accuracy for detection of significant coronary disease for adenosine, dipyridamole, and regadenoson compared to exercise-stress SPECT myocardial perfusion scintigraphy. The disadvantage of vasodilator stress is the lack of functional cardiac information provided by exercise.

Dobutamine. For patients unable to exercise but with contraindications for vasodilator therapy (e.g., active symptomatic asthma), dobutamine can be used as an alternative.

Mechanism of Action. Dobutamine is a synthetic catecholamine that acts on alpha- and beta-adrenergic receptors producing inotropic and chronotropic effects that increase cardiac work. In normal coronary arteries, increased blood flow results. In the face of significant stenosis, regional flow does not increase, producing scintigraphic patterns similar to that seen with exercise and pharmacological stress.

Methodology. Initial infusion rate is 5 µg/kg/min over 3 minutes, then increased to 10 µg/kg/min for another 3 minutes and further increased by that amount every 10 minutes until a maximum of 40 µg/kg/min is achieved. The radiopharmaceutical is injected 1 minute after the maximal tolerable dose and the dobutamine infusion is continued for 1 minute.

Accuracy. Dobutamine perfusion imaging has accuracy similar to that of exercise or pharmacological stress. The major limitation is the frequent occurrence of side effects, including chest pain and arrhythmias and inability of many patients to tolerate the maximum required dose.

Imaging Protocols

Various stress and rest perfusion imaging protocols are used, depending on the logistics of the clinic, radiopharmaceutical, patient size, and individual physician preference (Table 16-8). Tc-99m radiopharmaceuticals are usually preferred for myocardial perfusion scintigraphy. Advantages and disadvantages of Tc-99m sestamibi or tetrofosmin over Tl-201 are listed in Box 16-5.

Technetium-99m Sestamibi and Technetium-99m Tetrofosmin

Separate injections are required for the rest and stress studies. It is usually performed as a 1-day protocol, but 2-day protocols are sometimes used (Table 16-8 and Box 16-6).

Single-Day Protocol. The patient receives a lower administered dose of the Tc-99m radiopharmaceutical for the initial study (8-10 mCi [266-370 MBq]) and a several-fold higher dose (25-30 mCi [925-1110 MBq]) for the second study. The second study commences approximately 1.5 hours later to allow time for background

TABLE 16-7 Adenosine and Regadenoson Pharmacokinetics

Pharmacokinetics	Adenosine	Regadenoson
Administration	Intravenous infusion	Intravenous bolus
Dose	140 µg/kg/min	400 µg
Mode of action	Nonselective agonist	Selective A2A agonist
Duration of infusion	4-6 min	10 sec bolus
Radiotracer injection	3rd min after infusion start	30 sec after bolus
Time to peak	30 sec	33 sec
Duration of action	6 sec after infusion stopped	2.3 min
Elimination	Cellular uptake/ metabolism	Renal (57%)

TABLE 16-8 Protocols for Stress Myocardial Perfusion Scintigraphy

Method	Radiopharmaceutical	Rationale
2-Day	Tc-99m sestamibi/tetrofosmin	Obesity, image quality
1-Day	Tc-99m sestamibi/tetrofosmin	Image quality, efficiency
1-Day	Tl-201	Time tested, viability
Dual-isotope	Tl-201 and Tc-99m sestamibi/ tetrofosmin	Image quality, viability, logistics

---

***Box 16-5.* Advantages and Disadvantages of Technetium-99m Sestamibi and Tetrofosmin**

ADVANTAGES

Higher count rates; better quality SPECT images and gated SPECT possible
Higher-energy photons; fewer attenuation artifacts
Simultaneous assessment of perfusion and function
First-pass assessment of right and left ventricular function possible

DISADVANTAGES

No redistribution
Lung uptake not diagnostic
Less extraction at hyperemic flows
Less sensitive than Tl-201 for viability assessment

SPECT, Single-photon emission computed tomography.

Box 16-6. Technetium-99m Sestamibi and Tetrofosmin Myocardial Perfusion Imaging: Summary Protocol

PATIENT PREPARATION
Patient should fast for 4 hours

RADIOPHARMACEUTICAL
10 to 30 mCi (370-1110 MBq) intravenously; see individual protocols below

SPECT IMAGING PROTOCOL
1-Day rest/stress imaging
Rest: 10 mCi (370 MBq); imaging at 30 to 90 minutes
Stress: 30 mCi (1110 MBq); imaging at 15 to 30 minutes
2-Day rest/stress or stress/rest imaging: 30 mCi (1110 MBq)

SPECT ACQUISITION PARAMETERS
Patient position: supine, left arm raised (180-degree arc)
Rotation: counterclockwise
Matrix: 128 × 128 word mode
Image/arc: 64 views (180-degree, 45-degree right anterior oblique, 135-degree left posterior oblique)

SPECT RECONSTRUCTION PARAMETERS*
Ramp filter
Convolution filter: Butterworth
Attenuation correction: Review images with and without correction
Oblique angle reformatting: Short-axis, vertical long-axis, and horizontal long-axis gated SPECT
Electrocardiogram synchronized data collection: R wave trigger, 8 frames/cardiac cycle

PLANAR IMAGING PROTOCOL
Collimator: High resolution
Window: 20% centered at 140 keV
For 1-day rest and stress studies give 10 mCi (370 MBq) at rest and image at 30 to 60 minutes
Rest studies: Begin imaging at 60 to 90 minutes after tracer injection
Obtain anterior, 45-degree left anterior oblique, and left lateral images
Obtain 750,000 to 1 million counts per view
Wait 4 hours and give 30 mCi (1110 MBq) with repeat imaging at 15 to 30 minutes
Stress studies: Begin imaging at 15 to 30 minutes after tracer injection
Obtain stress and rest images in identical projection

SPECT, Single-photon emission computed tomography.
*Choice of SPECT acquisition and reconstruction parameters is highly influenced by the equipment used. Protocols should be established in each nuclear medicine unit for available cameras and computers.

Box 16-7. Thallium-201 Myocardial Perfusion Imaging Protocol

PATIENT PREPARATION AND FOLLOW-UP
Fasting for 4 hours

RADIOPHARMACEUTICAL
Tl-201 chloride 3 to 3.5 mCi (111-120 MBq) intravenously

TIME OF IMAGING
10 minutes after radiopharmaceutical administration and 3 hours later

INSTRUMENTATION
Collimator: Low energy, parallel hole
Photopeak: 30% window centered at 80 keV and 20% at 167 keV Arc and framing: 64 views, 180 degrees (45 degrees right anterior oblique, 135 degrees left posterior oblique), 20 seconds per view

PATIENT POSITION
Position patient supine, with left arm raised.

SPECT RECONSTRUCTION PARAMETERS*
Reconstruction technique: Filtered backprojection or iterative reconstruction
Attenuation correction: Rotating transmission source or computed tomography
Image format: Transaxial short axis, horizontal, and vertical long axis

Planar Imaging
Collimator: Low-energy, general purpose, parallel hole collimator
Photopeak: 20% window centered at 80 and 167 keV
Image acquisition: Anterior, 45 degrees, left anterior oblique (LAO), and left lateral for 10 min each Acquire rest and stress images in identical projections

SPECT, Single-photon emission computed tomography.
*Choice of SPECT acquisition and reconstruction parameters is influenced by the equipment used.

administration of the maximum dose (25-30 mCi) for both studies on separate days. This approach is most commonly used in obese patients.

Thallium-201
Although a 2-day protocol with separate rest and stress injections has been used in the past, Tl-201 redistribution allows for assessment of both stress and rest perfusion after a single injection on the same day. After stress, initial images are obtained at 10 to 15 minutes and delayed images acquired at 3 hours (Box 16-7 and Fig. 16-18).
Dual Isotope. This approach takes advantage of the different photopeaks of Tc-99m (140 keV) and Tl-201 (69-83 keV). Simultaneous acquisition (rest Tl-201 and stress Tc-99m sestamibi and tetrofosmin) is desirable for efficiency reasons; however, it is not practical because downscatter of Tc-99m into the Tl-201 window is significant. Thus the Tl-201 rest study is performed first with 3 to 3.5 mCi (110-130 MBq), followed by the stress study, using 20 to 30 mCi (740-1110 MBq) of the Tc-99m

activity biological clearance and decay. The usual approach is to do the rest study first, followed by the stress study.
Two-Day Protocol. Tissue attenuation can be marked in large patients and result in poor image quality and interpretative difficulties, particularly with the lower dose rest study. A 2-day approach reduces this problem by allowing

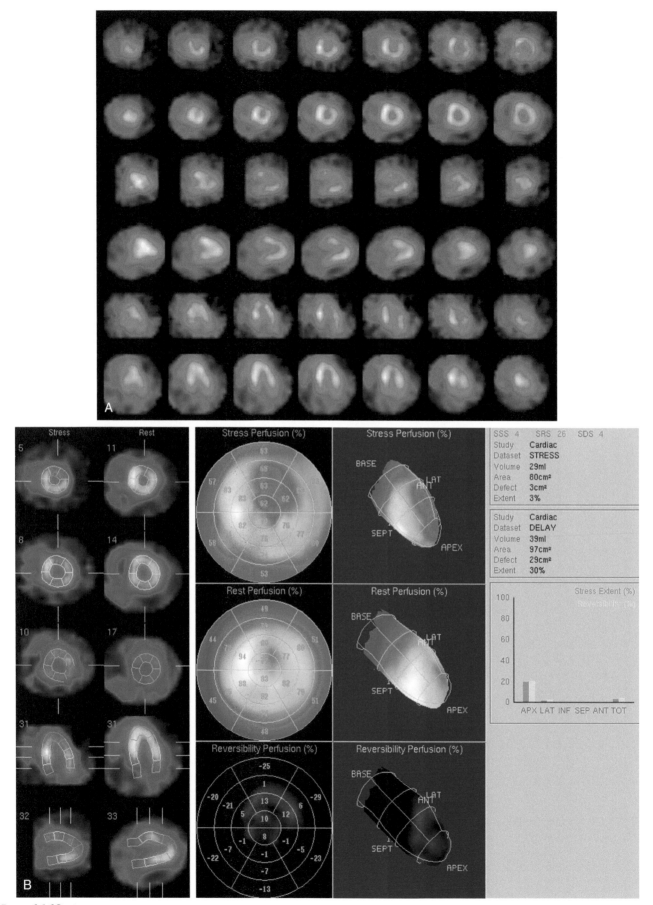

FIGURE 16-18. **A,** Tl-201 1-day protocol shows hypoperfusion in the anterior apical wall 10 minutes after stress *(above)* and complete redistribution *(below)* 3 hours later. **B,** Sestamibi images in another patient *(left)* and polar map and quantitative display *(middle and right)* confirming anterior wall ischemia see in **A.** *ANT,* Anterior; *LAT,* lateral; *SEPT,* septal.

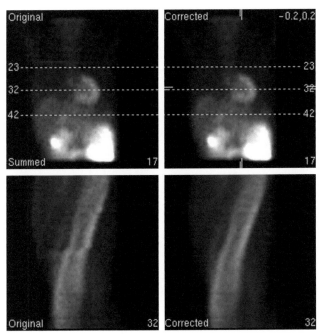

FIGURE 16-19. Sinogram used to detect for patient motion. The projection images are stacked vertically. Because the heart is not in the center of the camera radius of rotation, the position of the left ventricle in the stacked frames varies sinusoidally. Any significant motion is seen as a break in the sinogram. There is a horizontal break in the midsinogram *(left)*. The repeat acquisition shows no break and thus no significant motion *(right)*.

radiopharmaceutical. Upscatter of the higher energy Tl-201 photons (167 keV) is minimal because of their low abundance (10%).

The dual-isotope protocol has advantages. It can be completed more rapidly than Tc-99m protocols because imaging begins earlier, 10 minutes after the stress study and immediately after the rest study. Also Tl-201 provides information on viability (hibernating myocardium). The downside is the poor image quality of Tl-201.

Quality Control
Camera quality control is mandatory for obtaining good-quality images and is discussed in detail in the instrumentation chapters. Image quality may be poor because of insufficient counts in the myocardium, either caused by a low administered dose (e.g., inadvertent subcutaneous injection) or the result of soft tissue attenuation. The latter will be discussed in detail later. Image quality also can be degraded by scatter from activity in the liver or bowel.

Patient Motion. Patient motion during acquisition degrades image quality. Review of the acquisition data before processing should be routine. The projection 2-D planar images acquired every few degrees as the camera moves around the patient should be reviewed by displaying in an endless loop rotating cine display.

A method for confirming motion is to review the "sinogram." Each projection image is stacked vertically and compressed, with maintenance of the count density distribution in the x-axis but minimization of the count density distribution in the y-axis. Because the heart is

not in the center of the camera radius of rotation, the position of the left ventricle in the stacked frames varies sinusoidally. Motion is seen as a break in the sinogram (Fig. 16-19).

Movement of more than two-pixel deviation can adversely affect image quality. If there is significant motion, the study should be reacquired. If that is not possible (e.g., because of patient cooperation problems), software motion correction programs are available with most camera computer systems. These programs usually do not correct in all three axes.

Image Interpretation
Coronary Anatomy and Myocardial Perfusion
Although the anatomy of the coronary circulation varies in detail, the distribution of the major vessels is reasonably predictable (Fig. 16-20, Table 16-4). The left anterior descending coronary artery serves most of the septum and the anterior wall of the left ventricle. Its diagonal branches course over the anterior lateral wall, and septal perforators penetrate into the septum. The left circumflex coronary artery (LCX) and its marginal branches serve the lateral wall and the inferior segment of the lateral wall. The right coronary artery (RCA) and its branches serve the right ventricle, the inferior portion of the septum, and the inferior wall of the left ventricle. The artery that supplies the posterior descending artery (PDA) determines coronary dominance. In approximately 70% of the general population, the PDA is supplied by the RCA (right dominant), 10% of the times by the LCX (left dominant), and the remaining 20% are codominant.

Planar Imaging. The heart has a variably circular or ellipsoid shape in different views (Figs. 16-3 and 16-4). The configuration depends on patient habitus and the orientation of the heart in the chest—that is, vertical versus horizontal. The right ventricle is not usually seen on planar studies with Tl-201 but is often seen with Tc-99m radiopharmaceuticals. Abnormal increased lung uptake is easiest appreciated on planar imaging or in the cine display of preprocessed projection images (Fig. 16-21).

Single-Photon Emission Computed Tomography Rest Images. Normal myocardial perfusion rest images have uniform uptake throughout the left ventricular myocardium (Fig. 16-9). On short-axis SPECT views, the left ventricle has a doughnut appearance. The lateral wall usually has more uptake than the anterior or inferior wall. Decreased uptake is seen near the base of the heart in the region of the membranous septum. The valve planes have an absence of uptake, giving the heart a horseshoe or U-shaped appearance on vertical and horizontal long-axis SPECT slices. The myocardium appears thinner at the apex (apical thinning).

Although some normal lung uptake may often be seen, increased rest uptake occurs in heavy smokers and patients with underlying lung disease and heart failure. Increased uptake with exercise is suggestive of three-vessel disease. This pattern has been better validated with Tl-201. The right ventricle has less uptake than the left ventricle because of its lesser myocardial muscle mass. Right ventricular hypertrophy has increased uptake (Fig. 16-22). Atria are not visualized.

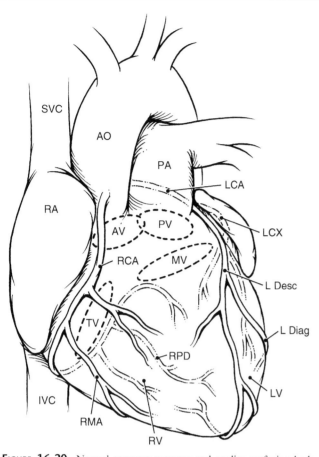

Figure 16-20. Normal coronary anatomy and cardiac perfusion beds. The left main coronary artery is only 0 to 15 mm in length before dividing into the left anterior descending and left circumflex arteries. Major branches of the left anterior descending artery are the diagonal and septal branches. The left circumflex artery *(LCX)* has obtuse marginal branches. The right coronary artery (RCA) originates separately and has important branches that include the posterior right ventricular branches, the posterior descending artery. "Dominance" refers to which coronary artery (RCA or LCFx) supplies the diaphragmatic surface of the left ventricle and posterior septum by giving rise to the posterior descending and posterior left ventricular branches. Right posterior descending *(RPD)*, right marginal branch artery (RMA). The apex may be perfused by branches from any of the three main vessels. *AO*, Aorta; *AV*, aortic valve; *IVC*, inferior vena cava; *LCA*, left coronary artery; *LCX*, left circumflex; *L Desc*, left anterior descending; *L Diag*, left diagonal; *LV*, left ventricle; *MV*, mitral valve; *PA*, pulmonary artery; *PV*, pulmonary valve; *RA*, right atrium; *RMA*, right mesenteric artery; *RV*, right ventricle; *SVC*, superior vena cava; *TV*, tricuspid valve.

Single-Photon Emission Computed Tomography Stress Images. Normal myocardial perfusion images after exercise or pharmacological stress are not strikingly different in distribution from those at rest, although there are differences. The stress image cardiac-to-background ratio is higher because of the increased myocardial blood flow and thus radiotracer uptake. Right ventricular uptake is often increased, but still considerably less than the left ventricle. With good treadmill exercise, reduced activity is seen in the liver because of diversion of blood flow from the splanchnic bed to leg muscles. Pharmacological stress with any vasodilator results in considerable liver activity.

Attenuation Artifacts. The effects of soft tissue attenuation can be seen on most cardiac images and are worse with large patients. Males typically have decreased activity in the inferior wall (Fig. 16-23). This is called *diaphragmatic attenuation*, meaning attenuation by subdiaphragmatic organs interpositioned between the heart and gamma camera. The amount of attenuation effect is dependent on patient size, shape, and internal anatomy.

Women often have relatively decreased activity in the anterior wall, apex, or anterior lateral portion of the heart, secondary to breast attenuation, depending on the size and position of the breasts (Fig. 16-24). Women also may have subdiaphragmatic attenuation, but breast attenuation is dominant and most commonly noted. Anterior and lateral wall attenuation can be seen occasionally in large males with excessive adipose tissue or muscle hypertrophy. Attenuation will also be seen in patients who are not able to elevate their arms during imaging

The cinematic rotating raw data should be reviewed for the presence of attenuation and motion. Regions of reduced myocardial activity from breast or subdiaphragmatic attenuation at both stress and rest could potentially be misinterpreted as myocardial infarction. If attenuation is noted on the cine display, this might suggest an alternative cause for the finding. If the breasts are in different positions for the two studies, this could be misinterpreted as ischemia (Fig. 16-24).

Attenuation Correction. Many SPECT/computer systems have attenuation correction capability. A transmission map is acquired by rotating a gadolinium-153 gamma source around the patient. Hybrid SPECT/CT systems use the CT data for this purpose (Figs. 16-23 and 16-25).

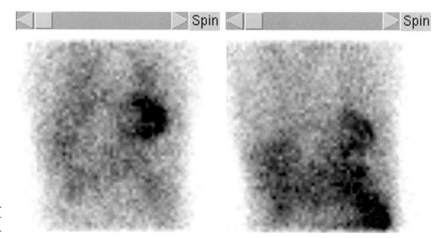

Figure 16-21. Stress-induced Tl-201 lung uptake. This is most commonly seen in patients with three-vessel coronary artery disease. Stress *(left)*, rest *(right)*.

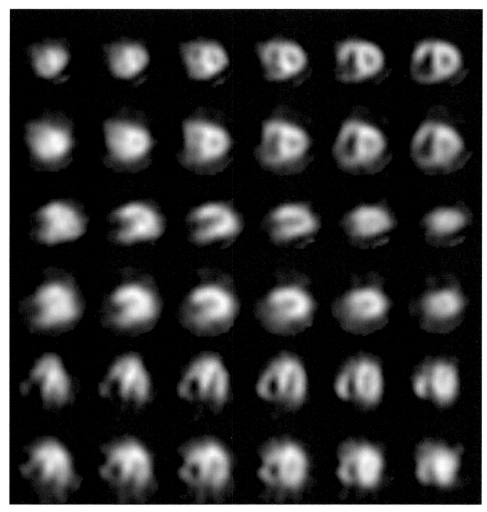

FIGURE 16-22. Right ventricular hypertrophy. Patient has severe pulmonary hypertension secondary to interstitial pulmonary fibrosis. Stress and rest Tc-99 sestamibi show prominent uptake in the hypertrophied right ventricle.

Both non–attenuation-corrected and attenuation-corrected images should always be reviewed. Misregistration of the emission and transmission images can potentially result in artifacts. This is a particular problem for hybrid SPECT/CT systems. The SPECT images are acquired during tidal volume breathing, whereas a rapid CT acquisition is acquired during a very limited phase of respiration. Checking for image fusion should be part of image quality control.

Gated SPECT has become routine (Fig. 16-10) and is usually performed after the stress test. In addition to analyzing global and regional myocardial wall motion, it can help differentiate the decreased fixed activity of an attenuation artifact from myocardial infarction. Good wall motion and myocardial thickening suggest that the decreased counts are due to attenuation and not infarction.

Extracardiac Uptake

Myocardial perfusion radiopharmaceuticals are taken up in all metabolically active tissues in the body except for the brain. They do not cross the normal blood–brain barrier. Structures accumulating Tc-99m–labeled cardiac radiopharmaceuticals that are often in the field of view are the thyroid, salivary glands, skeletal muscle, and kidneys. Prominent liver uptake is seen with rest and pharmacological stress studies. Gallbladder and intestinal activity are routinely seen.

Activity from the liver and bowel adjacent to the heart may cause scatter of counts into the inferior wall and adjacent walls of the heart, increasing apparent uptake, which can complicate interpretation. Focal intense subdiaphragmatic radioactivity adjacent to the heart can sometimes produce cold defects caused by reconstruction artifacts. All cardiac radiopharmaceuticals are taken up by many benign and malignant tumors—for example, parathyroid adenoma and lung cancer. This incidental finding must not be missed (Fig. 16-26).

Diagnostic Patterns in Coronary Artery Disease

Diagnosis of Ischemia and Infarction. Terms used to characterize the status of myocardium (e.g., ischemia, infarction, hibernating, stunning) are defined in Table 16-9. A diagnostic schema (Table 16-10) uses the appearance of the scans on the stress and rest studies for scan interpretation. After initial assessment of the presence or absence of perfusion defects, a complete evaluation of the stress study includes assessment of the location, size, severity, and likely vascular distribution of the visualized

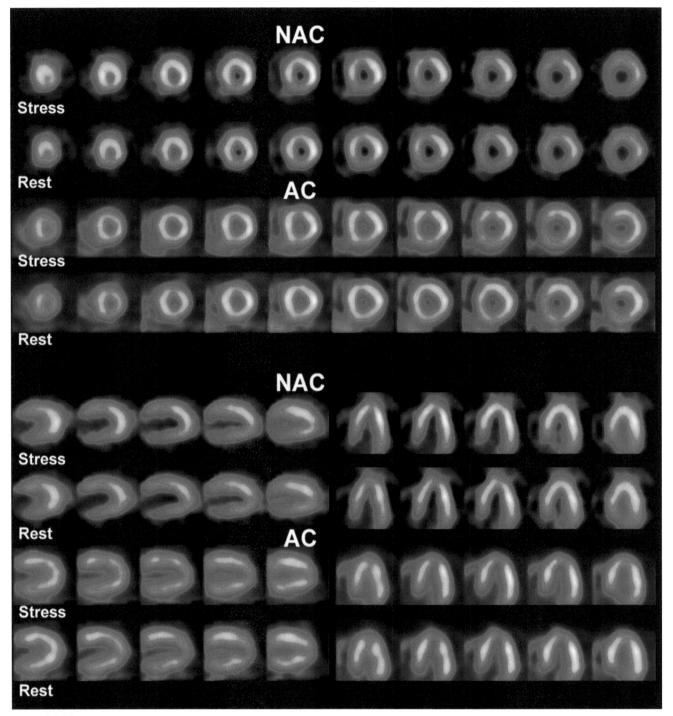

FIGURE 16-23. Inferior wall attenuation correction. Dipyridamole (Persantine) stress and rest Tc-99m sestamibi SPECT/CT study. Noncorrected *(NAC)* stress and rest images and the attenuation-corrected images *(AC)*. Note the improvement in inferior wall perfusion with attenuation correction. The study was interpreted as normal.

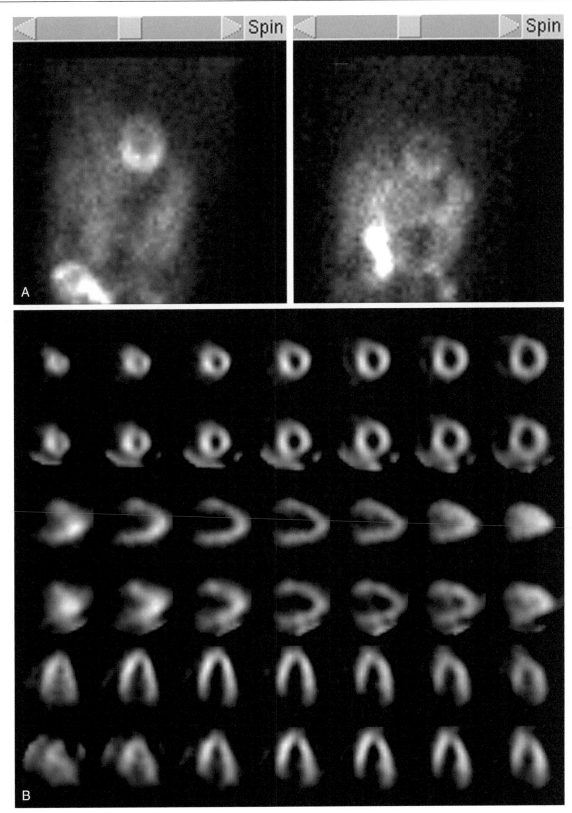

FIGURE 16-24. Breast attenuation. **A,** Single projection image from a cinematic display at stress *(left)* and rest *(right)* illustrates breast attenuation artifacts. Note the decreased activity in the upper portion of the heart. **B,** The patient's SPECT cross-sectional slices show moderately reduced activity in the anterior wall, best seen in the short axis and sagittal views and likely due to attenuation.

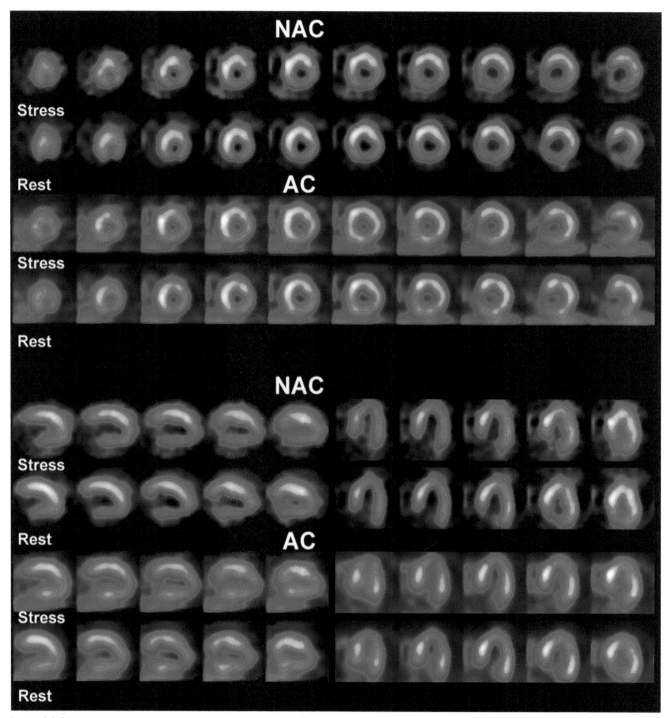

FIGURE **16-25.** Attenuation correction for inferior wall defect in infarction. Uncorrected images shown reduced activity in the inferior wall. Corrected images continue to show reduced uptake. The patient had a history of inferior wall infarction. *AC,* Attenuation-corrected images; *NAC,* noncorrected images.

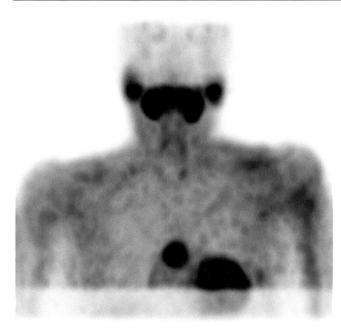

FIGURE 16-26. Incidental tumor diagnosed on myocardial perfusion scintigraphy. This midline mass was diagnosed as a thymoma.

TABLE 16-9 Definitions Describing the Status of the Myocardium

Term	Definition and scan appearance
Myocardial ischemia	Oxygen supply below metabolic requirements because of inadequate blood circulation caused by coronary stenosis
	Hypoperfusion (cold defect) on stress perfusion scintigrams
Myocardial infarction	Necrosis of myocardial tissue, as a result of coronary occlusion
	Hypoperfusion on rest–stress perfusion and decreased uptake with metabolic imaging
Transmural infarction	Necrosis involves all layers from endocardium to epicardium
	High sensitivity for detection by perfusion imaging
Subendocardial infarction	Necrosis involves only muscle adjacent to endocardium
	Lower sensitivity for detection on perfusion imaging
Myocardial scar	Late result of infarction; hypoperfusion on scintigraphy
Hibernating myocardium	Chronic ischemia with decreased blood flow and down regulation of contractility; reversible with restoration of blood flow
	No perfusion on rest imaging, poor ventricular contraction
	Improved perfusion given a long recovery between rest–rest imaging or delayed reinjection Tl-201
	Increased uptake by FDG metabolic imaging mismatched to reduced uptake on perfusion scan
Stunned myocardium	Myocardium with persistent contractile dysfunction despite restoration of perfusion after a period of ischemia; usually improves with time
	Normal by perfusion imaging, poor ventricular contraction
	Uptake by FDG metabolic imaging

FDG, Fluorodeoxyglucose.

TABLE 16-10 Diagnostic Patterns: Stress Myocardial Perfusion

Stress	Rest	Diagnosis
Normal	Normal	Normal
Defect	Normal	Ischemia
Defect	Defect (unchanged)	Infarction
Defect	Some normalization with areas of persistent defect	Ischemia and scar
Normal	Defect	Reverse redistribution*

*The term reverse redistribution was first described with Tl-201 and thus the reason for the terminology. It signifies a larger defect at rest than stress.

abnormalities. Computer quantitative methods are routinely used in conjunction with image analysis (Fig. 16-27). Perfusion defects caused by CAD are more commonly distal, rather than at the base of the heart. A true perfusion defect should be seen on more than one cross-sectional slice and in other cross-section planes. Certainty increases with lesion size and the degree or severity of photon deficiency.

Left Bundle Branch Block. Exercise-induced reversible hypoperfusion of the septum can be seen in patients with left bundle branch block (LBBB) in the absence of coronary disease. Typically, the apex and anterior wall are not involved, as would be expected with left anterior descending (LAD) coronary artery disease. The stress-induced decreased septal blood flow is thought to be caused by asynchronous relaxation of the septum, which is out of phase with diastolic filling of the remainder of the ventricle when coronary perfusion is maximal. This scan abnormality is not seen with pharmacological stress, and thus the latter is indicated in patients with LBBB or ventricular pacemakers.

Poor Prognostic Findings on Perfusion Scintigraphy
Multiple Perfusion Defects. Perfusion defects in more than one coronary artery distribution area indicate multiple vessel disease. Prognosis worsens with increasing number and size of perfusion defects (Fig. 16-28). Not all significant coronary artery stenoses are always seen on stress perfusion scans. Stress-induced ischemia of the most severe stenotic lesion limits further exercise, and thus other stenoses may not be seen and multiple vessel disease may be underestimated. Three-vessel balanced disease may not be seen at all.

Transient Ischemic Dilation. The normal cardiac response is to dilate during stress and return to normal size promptly with cessation of exercise. Poststress ventricular dilation is abnormal and suggests multivessel disease. One explanation for this finding is myocardial *stunning* during stress (Fig. 16-29, Table 16-10). Another is widespread subendocardial ischemia.

Thallium-201 Lung Uptake. Exercise-induced Tl-201 lung uptake is a poor prognostic sign caused by stress-induced ventricular dysfunction, elevated left ventricular end-diastolic pressure, and pulmonary capillary wedge pressure (Fig. 16-21). Lung-to-myocardial activity ratios greater than 0.5 are abnormal. Lung uptake

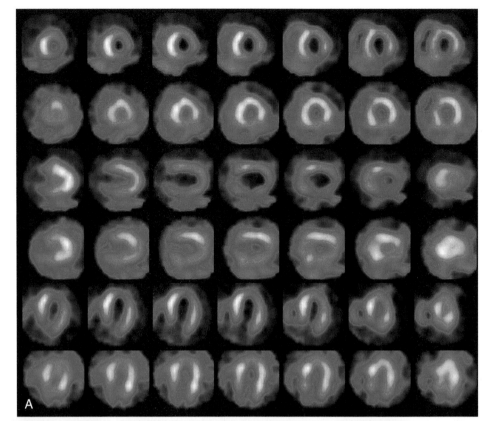

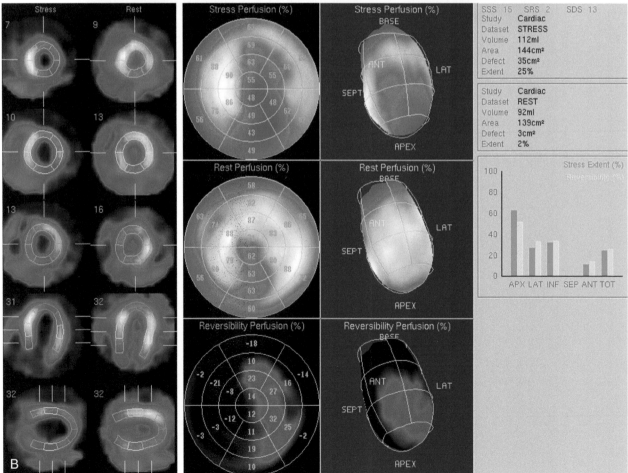

Figure 16-27. Anterior lateral and inferior lateral wall ischemia. Dipyridamole (Persantine) stress and rest study. **A,** Stress images *(top)* show hypoperfusion of the anterior lateral wall and no perfusion to the inferior wall. Rest images *(bottom)* show definite redistribution to the anterior lateral wall but incomplete redistribution to the inferior wall. **B,** Polar map display in 2-D and 3-D of patient study in **A.** Reversibility percentage is as high as 23% to 32% in the anterior lateral and inferior lateral walls.

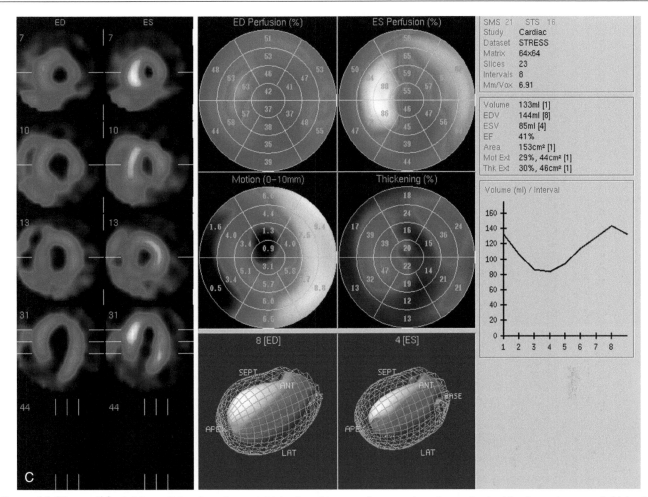

FIGURE 16-27, cont'd. C, Myocardial wall motion and thickening of images of same patient. Images in the *left* column show septal thickening (manifested by brightening) and to a lesser degree anterior lateral wall thickening. Reduced thickening is seen in the inferior wall. The cardiac volume curve and calculated LVEF (41%) show diffuse hypokinesis. *ANT,* Anterior; *LAT,* lateral; *SEPT,* septal.

with Tc-99m agents is less reliable because of normal lung activity.

Accuracy of Myocardial Perfusion Scintigraphy. Sensitivity for the diagnosis of CAD is considerably greater for stress myocardial perfusion scinitigraphy than the exercise treadmill study alone (88% vs. 75%). Specificity is similar (77 %). The accuracy of vasodilator versus exercise stress is very similar.

Myocardial Viability (Hibernating Myocardium). Although the scintigraphic findings of regional hypoperfusion at stress and rest associated with regional myocardial dysfunction are usually due to myocardial infarction, up to 20% of patients with these findings do not have infarction, but rather severe chronic ischemia or *hibernating myocardium* (Fig. 16-30, Table 16-10). Although severely underperfused, the myocytes have preserved cell membrane integrity and sufficient metabolic activity to maintain cellular viability but not contractility. Echocardiography, multiple gated acquisitions (MUGAs), and gated SPECT cannot make the distinction because these regions do not have normal myocardial contraction. These segments are "hibernating" in a functional and metabolic sense. Patients with viable but hypoperfused myocardium can benefit from coronary revascularization

with improvement in cardiac function and reduction in annual mortality.

Tc-99m sestamibi and tetrofosmin underestimate myocardial viability and are not used to diagnose hibernating myocardium. F-18 fluorodeoxyglucose (FDG) is the gold standard for making the diagnosis and is discussed in the section on cardiac PET. Tl-201 has been successfully used.

Thallium-201 Protocols for Assessing Myocardial Viability. Uptake is an energy-dependent process requiring intact cell membrane integrity; thus uptake implies preserved myocardial cell viability. The degree of uptake correlates with the extent of tissue viability. Tl-201 redistribution by 3 hours after injection depends on viable myocytes, the severity of the initial defect after stress testing, and the concentration and rate of decline of Tl-201 in the blood (Fig. 16-2). Various protocols have been used to diagnose viability based on these thallium pharmacokinetics.

Thalliuml-201 Late Redistribution. One approach is to image beyond 3 hours for delayed redistribution—for example, 8 to 24 hours after the stress Tl-201 injection (Fig. 16-31). Severely ischemic myocardium, with slow uptake and clearance, requires more time to redistribute. Delayed uptake has good positive predictive value for

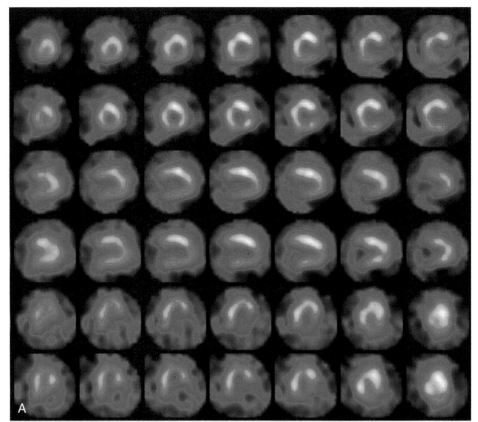

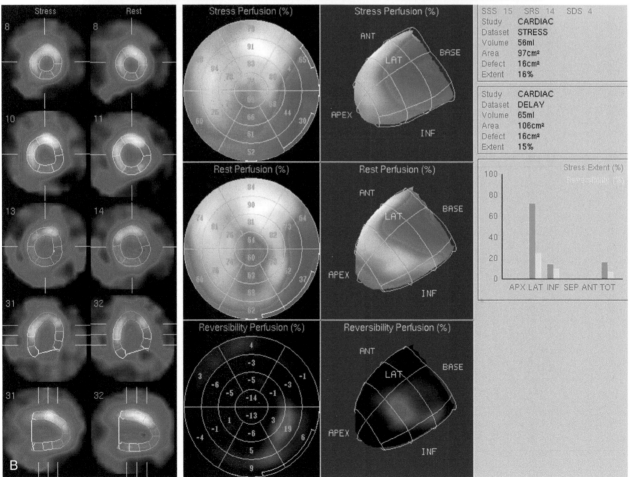

FIGURE 16-28. Multivessel disease. **A,** Lateral wall infarction and inferior lateral ischemia. Dipyridamole (Persantine) stress images show no perfusion of the lateral wall and reduced perfusion to the inferior wall. Rest images show no improvement in the lateral wall but improved perfusion to the inferior wall. **B,** Polar map and quantitative volume display from this patient. The reversibility percentage shows at least one inferior wall region with 19% reversibility. The graph in the right column shows the discrepancy between the stress extent and the reversibility extent, representing the infracted lateral wall. *ANT,* Anterior; *INF,* inferior; *SEPT,* septal.

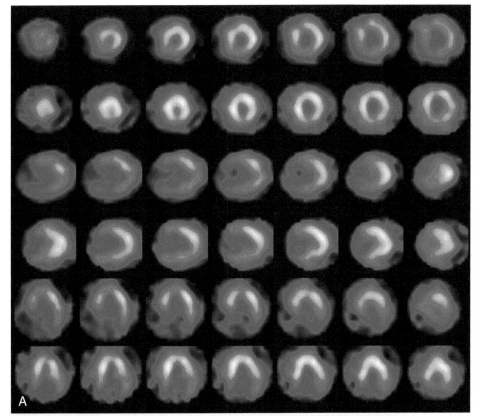

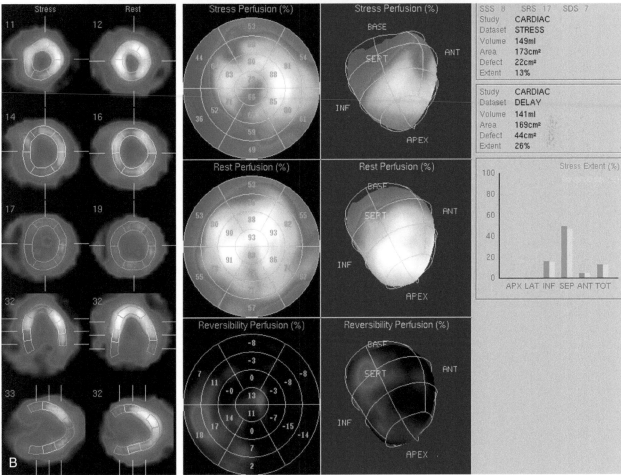

FIGURE 16-29. Multivessel ischemia. **A,** Exercise stress Tl-201 *(top)* and reinjection rest Tl-201 *(bottom)* studies. With stress, there is reduced perfusion to the anterior, septal, and inferior walls. On delayed imaging, there is redistribution to these regions. There is stress induced dilation (TID). **B,** Quantitative polar 2-D and 3-D displays of the patient study in A show reperfusion primarily to the apex, inferior-septal and septal regions of 11% to 17%. This likely underestimates the degree of ischemia, when interpreted in light of submaximal exercise and post-stress dilatation.

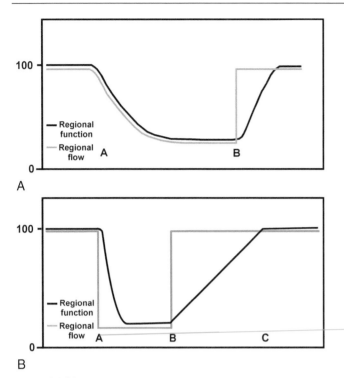

Figure 16-30. Hibernating versus stunned myocardium. **A,** Hibernating myocardium (chronic ischemia) develops over time as a result of chronic hypoperfusion, causing regional wall motion dysfunction. When perfusion is reestablished by surgical intervention, myocardial function gradually returns. **B,** Stunned myocardium is often due to an acute ischemic episode such as thrombosis, which when relieved (e.g., with angioplasty) results in prompt reperfusion. Functional recovery is considerably delayed. (Modified with permission from Dilsizian V, Narula J. *Atlas of Nuclear Cardiology.* Philadelphia: Current Medicine; 2003.)

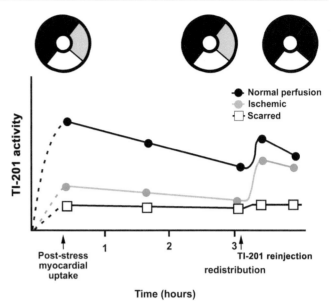

Figure 16-31. Pharmacokinetics of the Tl-201 reinjection method for diagnosing hibernating myocardium. During routine Tl-201 imaging, delayed images may show a persistent fixed perfusion defect in a region of severe or chronic ischemia. Low blood levels of Tl-201 do not allow for adequate redistribution of Tl-201 to the myocardium. Augmenting the Tl-201 blood levels permits greater myocardial uptake and scintigraphic evidence for redistribution and thus viable myocardium. (Modified with permission from Dilsizian V, Narula J. *Atlas of Nuclear Cardiology.* Philadelphia: Current Medicine; 2003.)

identifying regions with the potential for functional improvement after intervention. The negative predictive value is not high because of poor image quality resulting from the low count rate from decay and biological clearance from the body.

Thallium-201 Reinjection. The reinjection of Tl-201 assumes that the lack of redistribution is the result of a low Tl-201 blood level. To increase the blood level, Tl-201 is reinjected (50% of initial dose) after the redistribution images and repeat imaging performed 15 to 20 minutes later (Fig. 16-31). Uptake is predictive of improvement in regional left ventricular function after revascularization. A severe, persistent Tl-201 defect after reinjection suggests a low likelihood for improvement. A rationale for using Tl-201 for the rest study in dual-isotope studies is the opportunity to obtain next-day imaging, with or without reinjection, to determine viability of a fixed defect.

Rest–Rest Thallium-201 Redistribution. When viability, not inducible ischemia, is the clinical question, a rest–rest study may be adequate. Typically such patients have known coronary disease, prior myocardial infarction, and ventricular dysfunction. In the region of infarction, considerable viable but chronically ischemic myocardium may exist. In patients being considered for bypass surgery, the surgeon wants to know whether enough viable myocardium exists to justify revascularization. After Tl-201 injection at rest, images are obtained at 15 minutes. Uptake on

repeat images 3 to 4 hours later reflects viability and likely benefit from revascularization (Fig. 16-32).

Stunned Myocardium

After a transient period of severe ischemia followed by reperfusion, delayed recovery of regional left ventricular function may occur. This is referred to as *stunned myocardium* (Fig. 16-30). The ischemic episode may be a single event, multiple, brief, or prolonged, but not severe enough to cause necrosis. This is seen after thrombolysis or angioplasty in patients who have had acute coronary occlusion. Tissue in the affected perfusion watershed is viable and accumulates the radiopharmaceutical immediately after reperfusion. Tracer uptake indicates viability, but the myocardial segment is akinetic. If it is only stunned and not infarcted, wall motion will improve with time. Stress-induced transient ischemic dilation, stress-induced Tl-201 lung uptake, and poststress gated SPECT ventricular dysfunction may be manifestations of stunned myocardium.

Reverse Redistribution

Worsening of a perfusion defect on rest compared to stress tests or only seen on rest is termed *reverse redistribution*. Various pathological conditions have been suggested; however, the cause is often technical.

Quantitative Analysis

Relative perfusion is often presented in a 2-D *polar map* or *bull's-eye* display generated with circumferential slice count profiles obtained from the short-axis SPECT slices, with the apex at the center of the display and the base of the ventricle at the periphery (see Figs. 16-27, *B,* and 16-28, *B*). Three-dimensional displays are now available as well.

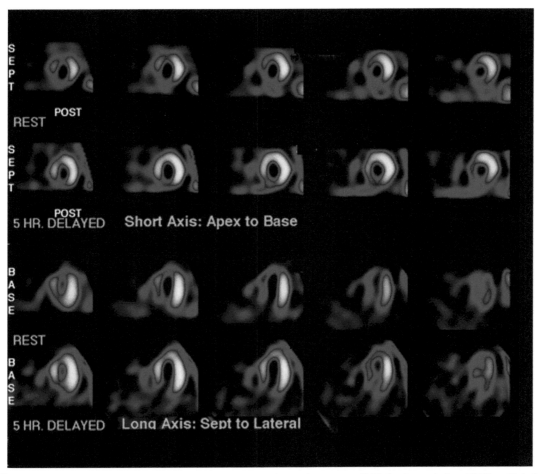

FIGURE 16-32. Rest–rest Tl-201 redistribution. The patient has a history of a previous myocardial infarction and a low LVEF and is being considered for revascularization. The initial rest study shows hypoperfusion of the inferior and anterior septal wall at rest; however, 5-hour delayed images show evidence of viability in the septum and adjacent anterior wall. *POST,* Posterior.

Stress–rest difference polar maps are commonly used to analyze for reversible ischemia.

Gated SPECT analysis of wall motion and thickening is standard (Fig. 16-27, *C*). Calculation of a LVEF is obtained by measuring the change in size of the ventricular cavity during the cardiac cycle using edge detection algorithms.

Sensitivity and Specificity of Myocardial Perfusion Single-Photon Emission Computed Tomography

Coronary angiography has been used as the gold standard for establishing myocardial perfusion scintigraphy accuracy. The angiographic estimated percent coronary stenoses often do not correlate well with their functional severity determined by coronary flow reserve. The amount and degree of coronary disease is often underestimated by angiography.

A true physiological decrease in blood flow may sometimes be seen in the absence of a fixed coronary stenosis because of small vessel disease or metabolic abnormalities.

The reported sensitivity of stress myocardial perfusion imaging has ranged from 70% to 95% and the specificity from 50% to 90%. This wide range is due in part to differences in study populations. Results of studies over the years suggest that myocardial perfusion scintigraphy has an approximate sensitivity of 87% and specificity of 80%.

Because true specificity often cannot be easily determined due to referral bias, the concept of "normalcy rate" has been

---

Box 16-8. Indicators of Adverse Outcome and Prognosis: Single-Photon Emission Computed Tomography Perfusion Imaging

Increased lung-to-heart ratio after stress
Transient left ventricular cavity dilatation after exercise
Multiple and large reversible defects
Multiple and large irreversible defects
Reversible perfusion defects at low level exercise

---

proposed. The normalcy rate is defined as the frequency of normal test results in patients with a low likelihood of CAD, based on Bayesian analysis using age, sex, symptom classification, cholesterol, and results of noninvasive stress testing. Normalcy rates of 90% or greater have been reported for SPECT myocardial perfusion scintigraphy.

An important observation is that persons with normal stress perfusion scans have a better prognosis than those with scintigraphic evidence of ischemia.

Prognosis and Risk Stratification

Diagnosis is an important indication for SPECT myocardial perfusion imaging; however, risk stratification and prognosis have become its primary role (Box 16-8).

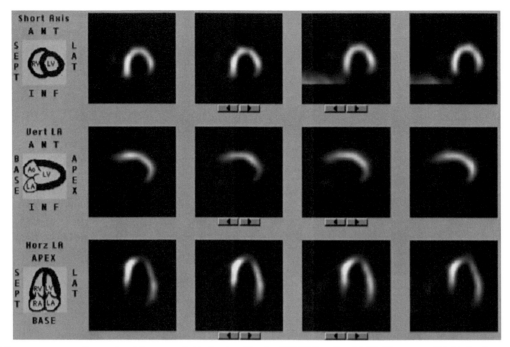

FIGURE 16-33. Emergency room chest pain with myocardial infarction. Resting SPECT study with Tc-99m sestamibi. Radiopharmaceutical injection was given in the emergency room and imaging delayed until the patient was stabilized. The large defect involving the inferior wall of the heart was diagnostic of infarction and the patient was admitted. *ANT,* Anterior; *Ao,* aorta; *Horz LA,* horizontal long axis; *INF,* inferior; *LA,* left atrium; *LAT,* lateral; *RA,* right atrium; *RV,* right ventricle; *SEPT,* septal.

Acute Ischemic Syndromes

Emergency Room Chest Pain. More than 5 million patients go to the emergency room with chest pain each year in the United States. Half are admitted to the hospital. Ultimately only 5% are diagnosed with myocardial infarction. Clinical decision-making requires triage of patients into risk categories based on the probability of infarct or unstable angina and risk assessment. SPECT perfusion imaging can provide information critical to this decision-making process (Fig. 16-33). The accuracy of diagnosis is highest when the radiopharmaceutical is injected during pain, although good accuracy is obtainable for several hours thereafter.

Tc-99m sestamibi or tetrofosmin can be injected in the emergency room and the patient transferred for imaging when initial evaluation and stabilization is complete. Because the radiopharmaceutical is fixed and does not redistribute, delayed imaging reflects blood flow at the time of injection. Negative SPECT studies are highly predictive of a good prognosis. Cardiac events occur in less than 1.5% of patients compared to a 70% incidence in those with a positive study. SPECT perfusion scintigraphy has a high sensitivity (>90%) for detection of transmural infarction immediately after the event. Diminished or absent uptake may be seen in the region of periinfarct ischemia and edema. Sensitivity decreases with time as the edema and ischemia resolve. By 24 hours, small infarctions may not be detectable and the overall sensitivity for larger ones decreases. Sensitivity is lower for nontransmural infarctions.

Acute Myocardial Infarction with ST Elevation. Infarct size, LVEF, and residual myocardium at risk provide important prognostic management information. Submaximal exercise (achieving less than target heart rate)

SPECT perfusion scintigraphy after infarction can detect the presence and extent of stress-induced myocardial ischemia. Pharmacological stress can be safely done as early as 2 to 5 days after infarction, earlier than the submaximal exercise study. Evidence for ischemia warrants aggressive management—for example, coronary angiography or revascularization. If negative, the patient can be treated conservatively.

Unstable Angina and Non-ST Elevation Myocardial Infarction. Early invasive interventional therapy is recommended for patients with high-risk indicators—for example, positive myocardial perfusion scintigraphy. SPECT is used for predischarge risk stratification of patients with unstable angina. Ischemia is seen in a high percentage (90%) of patients who develop subsequent cardiac events compared to those who do not have evidence of ischemia (20%).

Chronic Ischemic Syndromes

Patient Management. Identification of patients at high risk but with minimal symptoms can reduce mortality by coronary artery bypass grafting (CABG) or angioplasty. High risk and low risk are defined as greater than 3% and less than 1% cardiac mortality rate per year, respectively. Many factors assessed by SPECT determine patient prognosis—for example, extent of infarcted myocardium, amount of jeopardized myocardium supplied by vessels with hemodynamically significant stenosis, and severity of ischemia. A normal stress SPECT perfusion study predicts a good prognosis, with less than 1% annual risk for cardiac death or infarct. With abnormal SPECT, the risk for cardiac death or infarction increases. Multivessel disease is associated with high risk. Reduced LVEF is a strong negative prognostic predictor.

TABLE **16-11** Cardiac Positron Radiopharmaceuticals

Mechanism	Radionuclide	Pharmaceutical	Physical Half-life	Production
Perfusion	N-13	Ammonia	10 min	Cyclotron
	Rb-82	Rubidium chloride	76 sec	Generator
	O-15	Water	110 sec	Cyclotron
Glucose metabolism	F-18	Fluorodeoxyglucose	110 min	Cyclotron
Fatty acid metabolism	C-11	Acetate	20 min	Cyclotron
	C-11	Palmitate	20 min	Cyclotron

Assessment of Coronary Bypass Surgery and Angioplasty. Because 40% to 60% of angiographically detected stenotic lesions (50%-75%) are of uncertain significance, myocardial perfusion scintigraphy can stratify risk and assess which patients require revascularization. Those with no ischemia have low risk for cardiac events, even with left main or three-vessel disease on angiography. Those with evidence of ischemia will be aided by successful intervention.

After Percutaneous Coronary Intervention. Symptom status and exercise ECG are unreliable indicators of restenosis. Of patients with recurrent chest pain within a month of intervention, 30% have restenosis. Stress SPECT can identify recurrent ischemia.

After Coronary Bypass Surgery. Abnormal perfusion suggests bypass graft disease in the native coronary arteries beyond the distal anastomosis, nonrevascularized coronaries or side branches, or new disease. SPECT can determine the location and severity of ischemia and has prognostic value early and late after coronary bypass surgery. Ischemia occurring less than 12 months after surgery is usually caused by perianastomotic graft stenosis. Ischemia developing later than 1 year postoperatively is usually caused by new stenoses in graft conduits or native vessels.

Heart Failure: Assessment for Coronary Artery Disease. Heart failure in the adult can be due to various causes, including hypertrophic cardiomyopathy, hypertensive or valvular heart disease, and idiopathic cardiomyopathy. Determining whether left ventricular dysfunction is due to the consequences of CAD or other causes is critical for patient management. If it is the result of coronary disease, revascularization can reverse the dysfunction.

Left ventricular dysfunction resulting from ischemic cardiomyopathy is the result of either large or multiple prior myocardial infarctions with subsequent remodeling or moderate infarction associated with considerable inducible ischemia or hibernation. SPECT sensitivity is high for detection of CAD in patients with cardiomyopathy, although specificity is poor. False positive study findings are due to perfusion abnormalities seen in many patients with nonischemic cardiomyopathy—that is, without epicardial coronary artery disease. Some have regions of fibrosis and decreased coronary blood flow reserve, resulting in both fixed and reversible defects. More extensive and severe perfusion defects are likely to be due to coronary disease, whereas smaller and milder defects are likely to occur in patients with nonischemic cardiomyopathy.

Calcium Screening. Coronary artery calcium scoring has become routine at some centers, particularly those with SPECT/CT and PET/CT. The risk for cardiac events is low with coronary calcium scores of 100 or less. Stress SPECT myocardial perfusion tests are positive in less than 1% of these patients. With scores of 101 to 399, risk for future cardiac events is moderate, with 12% having abnormal stress SPECT perfusion studies. Scores greater than 400 identify patients at high risk, and 50% of these patients have abnormal SPECT studies. Age-based calcium risk data are also available.

Sarcoidosis

Myocardial involvement of the heart with sarcoidosis manifests as dysrhythmias, conduction defects, heart failure, and sudden death. Pathologically any region of the heart can become the site of granuloma deposition. Diagnosis of cardiac involvement can be difficult. Endomyocardial biopsy is confirmative; however, it is an insensitive method because of sampling error.

SPECT myocardial perfusion scintigraphy can detect myocardial involvement in patients with sarcoidosis. Perfusion defects are seen in the right and the left ventricle. In many patients with cardiac sarcoidosis, stress SPECT studies demonstrate a fixed defect. Ga-67 has poorer sensitivity. F-18 FDG PET may be useful to diagnose active cardiac sarcoidosis.

■ POSITRON EMISSION TOMOGRAPHY OF THE HEART

PET for cardiac perfusion imaging has grown once PET/CT scanners and Rb-82 has become widely available. Efforts to develop F-18 labeled perfusion agents continues to move forward. PET affords superior spatial resolution and superior attenuation correction compared to SPECT, and the radiation exposure received from clinical protocols with currently available myocardial perfusion PET tracers is substantially lower than that of SPECT protocols.

Radiopharmaceuticals for Myocardial Perfusion

Nitrogen-13 Ammonia

Nitrogen-13 ammonia would be the preferred PET myocardial perfusion radiopharmaceutical because of its superior imaging characteristics, except that it has a very short physical half-life (10 minutes) requiring onsite cyclotron production.

N-13 decays 100% by positron (beta+) emission (Table 16-11). At physiological pH, the major form of ammonia is NH_4^+. When injected intravenously, it clears rapidly from

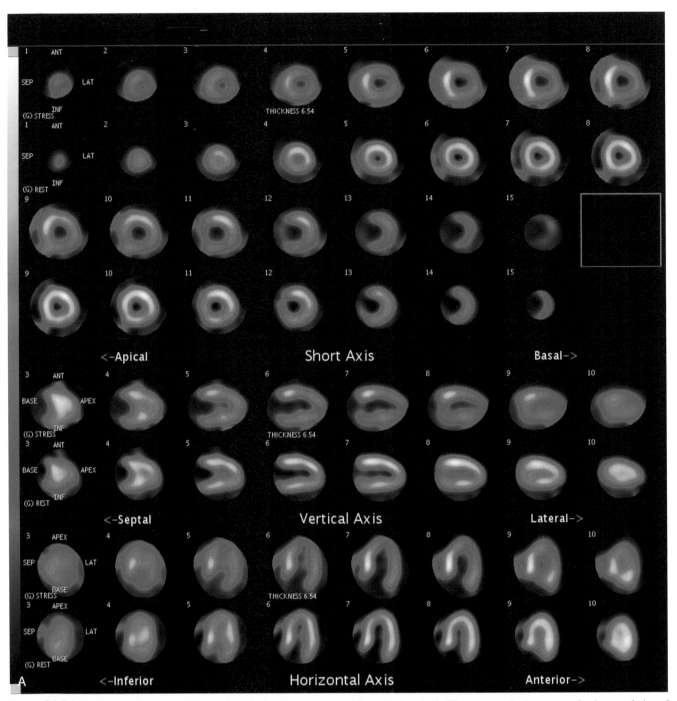

FIGURE 16-34. N-13 ammonia myocardial perfusion scintigraphy in severe multivessel ischemia. **A,** The stress study shows extensive hypoperfusion of the anterior lateral, lateral, inferior-lateral, and inferior wall. The rest study shows normal perfusion. In comparison with rest, stress images suggest dilatation.

Continued

the circulation, with 85% leaving the blood in the first minute and only 0.4% remaining after 3.3 minutes. It diffuses across the myocardial cell capillary membrane, then is converted to N-13 glutamine by glutamine synthetase, and subsequently is trapped within tissues by incorporation in the cellular pool of amino acids. Myocardial uptake is proportional to coronary blood flow.

N-13 ammonia has a 70% to 80% extraction rate by myocardial cells at normal coronary flow rates. As with other perfusion tracers, its extraction efficiency drops at higher flow rates. The N-13 label remains within the heart with a relatively long biological residence time, although its physical half-life is short. The radiotracer is also taken up by the brain, liver, and kidneys. Its positron range of 5.4 mm in tissue contributes to its good imaging characteristics.

Technique

N-13 ammonia 10 to 20 mCi (370-740 MBq) is administered intravenously. Imaging begins 4 minutes after injection, allowing time for pulmonary background activity clearance. In the diagnosis of CAD, a second study is performed after pharmacological stress with protocols similar to those described for SPECT myocardial perfusion scintigraphy (Fig. 16-34).

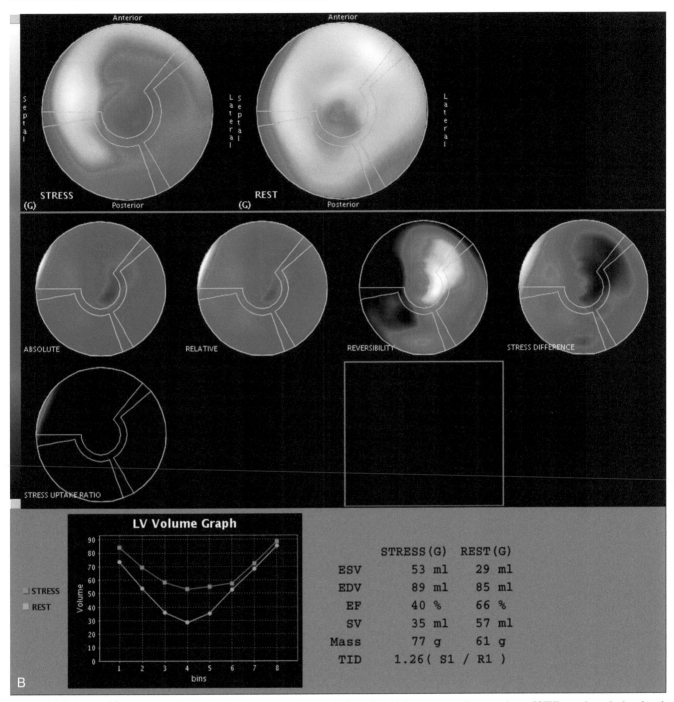

FIGURE 16-34, cont'd. B, Bulls-eye display showing significant reperfusion of multiple segments. Stress and rest LVEF are also calculated and shown. *ANT,* Anterior; *EDV,* end-diastolic volume; *EF,* ejection fraction; *ESV,* end-systolic volume; *LAT,* lateral; *LV,* left ventricle; *SEPT,* septal; *SV,* stroke volume; *TID,* transischemic dilatation.

Radiation Dosimetry

The radiation absorbed dose to the patient from N-13 ammonia is quite low compared to most clinically used radiopharmaceuticals (Table 16-12). The highest radiation dose is to the bladder and the whole body effective dose is 0.2 rem/20 mCi (0.2 cGy/740 MBq).

Rubidium-82 Chloride

PET for cardiac imaging is increasing. The major reason is commercial availability of a strontium-82/Rb-82 generator system (CardioGen-82, Bracco Diagnostics, Princeton, NJ)

(Table 16-11). The half-life of the Sr-82 parent is 25 days; thus facilities using Rb-82 must receive one new generator system each month. They are expensive, and a sufficient volume of cardiac studies is needed to make it financially feasible. Some regional radiopharmacies now transport a single generator to multiple sites on specified days, reducing the high cost for low-volume centers.

Rb-82 is a monovalent cation and true analog of potassium. Like Tl-201, Rb-82 is taken up into the myocardium by active transport through the Na$^+$/K ATPase pump. Its extraction is somewhat lower than that of N-13 ammonia

TABLE 16-12 Radiation Dosimetry for Fluorine-18 Fluorodeoxyglucose, Rubidium-82, and Nitrogen-13 Ammonia

Dose	Fluorine-18 FDG rads/10 mCi (cGy/370 MBq)	Rubidum-82 rads/40 mCi (cGy/1480 MBq)	N-13 Ammonia rads/20 mCi (cGy/740 MBq)
Heart wall	2.5	0.4	0.2
Liver	0.8	0.16	0.3
Kidneys	0.8	**2.8**	0.2
Brain	1.7		0.3
Urinary bladder	3.0		
Colon		0.4	
Thyroid	0.4	**5.6**	0.2
Ovaries	0.4	0.04	0.2
Red marrow		0.16	0.2
Effective dose	1.0	0.8	0.2

Target organ (highest radiation absorbed dose) in **boldface** type.

(60%). The relative myocardial extraction and localization of Rb-82 are proportional to blood flow.

The short half-life of Rb-82 (76 seconds) allows sequential myocardial perfusion studies before and after pharmacological interventions (Fig. 16-35). Rb-82 decays 95% by positron emission and 5% by electron capture. In addition to 511-keV annihilation photons, it emits a 776-keV gamma (15% abundance) and 1395-keV gamma (0.5% abundance). It has a 13- to 15-mm range in soft tissue before undergoing annihilation, resulting in inferior resolution and image quality compared to those of other positron emitters such as N-13. In spite of this, image quality is superior to that of SPECT and has less attenuation effect and subdiaphragmatic scatter.

Technique
Rb-82 (40-60 mCi) is infused intravenously over 30 to 60 seconds. Imaging is delayed for approximately 90 seconds in individuals with normal left ventricular function or 120 seconds in patients with low LVEF (e.g., <30%) to allow time for blood pool clearance. The study is completed 8 minutes after injection. Imaging time is short because of rapid decay and need to minimize reconstruction artifacts. About 80% of the useful counts are acquired in the first 3 minutes and 95% in the first 5 minutes. Sequential studies can be performed within 10 minutes.

Dosimetry
The kidneys, heart, and lungs receive the highest radiation dose. The whole-body effective dose for Rb-82 scan is 0.8 rads/40 mCi (0.8 cGy/1480 MBq).

Oxygen-15 Water
Oxygen-15 water is an excellent radiotracer for quantitative regional myocardial flow measurements (milliliters per minute per gram) because it is a freely diffusible perfusion tracer with 95% extraction by the myocardium that is not affected by metabolic factors. Unlike other perfusion agents, extraction remains linear at very high flow rates; therefore myocardial distribution reflects regional perfusion. Image quality is inferior to that of other PET myocardial perfusion agents. Tracer circulating in the blood pool remains within the ventricular chamber and must be subtracted to visualize the myocardium. Its half-life of 2.2 minutes requires onsite cyclotron production.

Diagnosis of Coronary Artery Disease

Cardiac PET stress tests use pharmacological stress rather than exercise because of the short half-life of the radiopharmaceuticals and because, unlike with SPECT, images are acquired during stress testing. After a resting baseline study, pharmacological stress is used to challenge coronary flow reserve, similar to single-photon protocols.

The scintigraphic appearance of the heart and the diagnostic criteria for Rb-82 and N-13 ammonia studies are the same as for SPECT perfusion scans (Table 16-9). Normal subjects have homogeneous uptake of the tracer throughout myocardium at rest and stress. Perfusion defects seen after pharmacological stress that normalize on rest studies suggest ischemia (Fig. 16-35). Areas of myocardial infarction appear cold on both baseline and poststress images. Patients with hibernating myocardium demonstrate persistent perfusion defects on both phases.

Accuracy of Positron Emission Tomography Versus Single-Photon Emission Computed Tomography
The sensitivity and specificity of PET to detect coronary luminal stenotic lesions of 50% or greater is 92% and 85%, respectively, compared to 85% and 80% for SPECT. The improved PET diagnostic accuracy is due to instrumentation and radiopharmaceutical advantages over SPECT.

PET instrumentation provides higher spatial resolution than SPECT (5-7 mm vs. >15 mm), superior ability to detect tissue radiotracer concentration, better temporal resolution allowing for data acquisition in dynamic sequences to delineate radiotracer kinetics for quantification of absolute myocardial blood flow, and improved correction methods for photon scatter, random events, and photon attenuation. For obese patients and females, this translates into higher image quality, interpretive certainty, and diagnostic accuracy compared to SPECT.

PET myocardial perfusion tracers have superior pharmacokinetic properties because of their higher myocardial net uptake rates at higher coronary flows than their SPECT counterpart, translating into higher PET sensitivity for diagnosis of single-vessel or multivessel coronary disease.

Future Cardiac Positron Emission Tomography Radiopharmaceuticals
N-13 ammonia and Rb-82 are currently the only FDA-approved myocardial perfusion PET tracers for the evaluation of suspected or known CAD. Limits to the widespread use of PET include the high cost of onsite cyclotrons

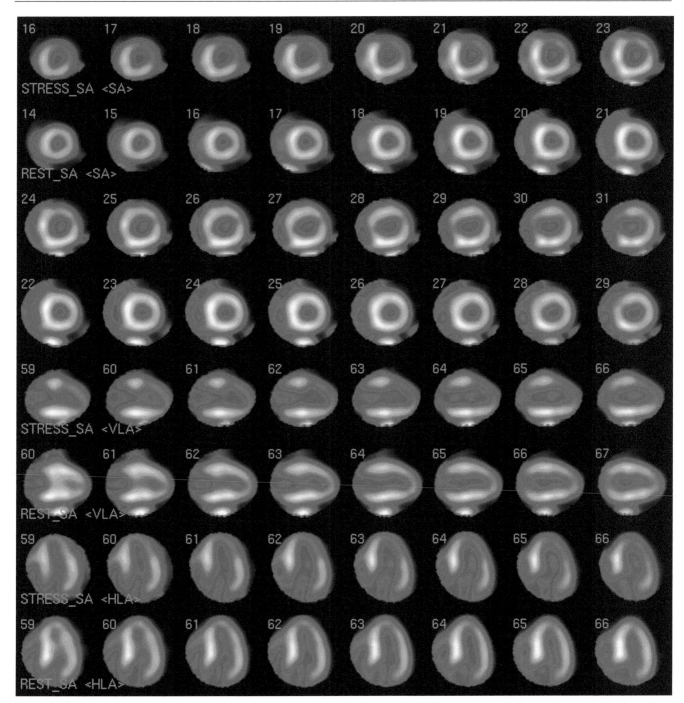

FIGURE 16-35. Rb-82 stress myocardial perfusion study. Reversible ischemia is seen in the anterior lateral and apical myocardium. *HLA*, horizontal long axis; *SA*, short axis; *VLA*, vertical long axis.

required for N-13 ammonia and of generators for Rb-82 and their short half-lives, which impose logistical difficulties.

These issues may be overcome in the future with the development of cyclotron-produced fluorinated perfusion tracers. Their longer half-life (110 min) will allow imaging clinics to have these radiopharmaceuticals shipped from off-site cyclotron facilities, similar to F-18 FDG, and will also make possible exercise stress protocols.

Absolute Myocardial Blood Flow Quantification
In addition to qualitative assessment of the regional distribution, PET allows in vivo dynamic quantitative

measurement of radiotracer distribution in the heart so that estimation of absolute myocardial blood flow at baseline and during vasodilator-induced hyperemia is possible.

Evidence suggests that a low coronary flow reserve (ratio of the hyperemic and resting myocardial blood flow) may be an independent predictor of adverse cardiovascular events, even in the presence of normal regional myocardial perfusion imaging. Patients with severe triple-vessel coronary disease may occasionally demonstrate no perfusion abnormalities on rest–stress PET imaging because of balanced three-vessel ischemia; however, if measured by PET, coronary flow reserve will be depressed or blunted in these patients,

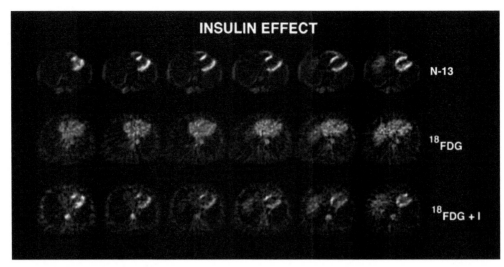

INSULIN EFFECT

N-13

^{18}FDG

^{18}FDG + I

FIGURE 16-36. Importance of glucose loading for FDG cardiac imaging. N-13 ammonia images *(top row)* and two sets of F-18 FDG images of a patient with diabetes. The N-13 ammonia images show a large perfusion defect at the cardiac apex. The initial F-18 FDG images show uptake in blood pool but essentially no myocardial uptake *(middle row)*. After insulin (I) administration *(bottom row)*, FDG accumulates in the myocardium and reveals a matched defect at the apex.

TABLE 16-13 Diagnostic Patterns: Positron Emission Tomography Metabolic and Perfusion Imaging

Diagnosis	Perfusion (N-13 ammonia, Rb-82)	Glucose metabolism (FDG)
Normal myocardium	Present	Present
Ischemic myocardium	Absent or decreased	Present
Myocardial infarction	Absent	Absent

FDG, Fluorodeoxyglucose.

providing the opportunity to detect this high-risk population missed by standard myocardial perfusion imaging.

Positron Emission Tomography Metabolic Radiopharmaceutical

Fluorine-18 Fluorodeoxyglucose
F-18 FDG is a marker of myocardial glucose metabolism. It has a physical half-life of 1.8 hours (110 minutes). Only 1% to 4% of the injected dose is trapped in the myocardium; however, the target-to-background ratio is high. Blood clearance of FDG is multicompartmental and takes considerably longer than the perfusion agents. Imaging begins 45 to 60 minutes after tracer injection (10-15 mCi [370-555 MBq]), allowing for maximal myocardial uptake and blood and soft tissue background clearance. F-18 has the highest resolution of clinically used positron emitters, approximately 2 mm, because the emitted positrons travel only 1.2 mm before annihilation.

Dosimetry
The organ receiving the highest radiation absorbed dose is the urinary bladder (3.0 rads/40 mCi [3.0 cGy/1480 MBq]) (Table 16-12). The whole body effective dose is 1.1 rem/15 mCi [1.1 cGy/575 MBq].

Clinical Indication
Under normal conditions, most of the energy needs of the heart are met through fatty acid metabolism. However, areas of ischemia switch preferentially to glucose

metabolism and have increased uptake of F-18 FDG relative to perfusion. Regional myocardial uptake of F-18 FDG reflects regional rates of glucose usage. In the myocardial cell, after F-18 FDG is phosphorylated to FDG-6-phosphate, no further metabolism takes place and it is trapped.

The state of glucose metabolism in the body highly influences the amount of FDG taken up in the heart. Myocardial glucose uptake is increased by administering glucose to stimulate insulin secretion, which increases cardiac glucose metabolism. High serum glucose and insulin levels and low free fatty acids promote uptake (Fig. 16-36).

Detection of Myocardial Viability
The combination of perfusion imaging and metabolic imaging with FDG can be of great benefit for correctly diagnosing and assessing the potential therapeutic outcome in patients with severely ischemic or hibernating myocardium (Table 16-13).

Hibernating myocardium refers to a state of persistent left ventricular dysfunction secondary to chronically compromised resting myocardial blood flow in patients with obstructive CAD, in whom a revascularization procedure may result in partial or complete recovery of cardiac function. If flow is not restored, the jeopardized myocardium eventually dies.

The rationale for using FDG is that severely ischemic, dysfunctional, but viable myocardium switches from fatty acid metabolism to glucose metabolism. FDG uptake can be greater in severely hypoperfused hypokinetic or akinetic myocardial segment(s) than in the remainder of the heart, a phenomenon referred to as *metabolic-perfusion mismatch*, considered the landmark for hibernating myocardium (Fig. 16-37) In contrast, the combination of matched markedly reduced or absent perfusion and FDG uptake is indicative of scar formation (Fig. 16-38).

For evaluation of myocardial viability with FDG, the substrate and hormonal levels in the blood need to favor utilization of glucose over fatty acids by the myocardium. This is usually done by loading the patient with glucose after a fasting period of at least 6 hours to induce an endogenous insulin response. The temporary increase in plasma glucose levels stimulates insulin production, which in turn reduces fatty acid levels and normalizes glucose levels.

A common method of glucose loading is an oral load of 25 g to 100 g, but intravenous loading is also used. The intravenous route avoids potential problems due to variable gastrointestinal absorption times or inability to tolerate oral administration. Most clinics use the the oral glucose-loading approach, with supplemental insulin administered as needed.

Diabetic patients pose a challenge, either because they have limited ability to produce endogenous insulin or because their cells are less able to respond to insulin stimulation. Thus the fasting/oral glucose-loading method is often not effective. Use of insulin along with close monitoring of blood glucose yields satisfactory results (Box 16-9.)

FDG in the presence of a metabolic-perfusion mismatch is accurate in predicting improvement of regional wall motion and global left ventricular ejection fraction after revascularization. Sensitivity and specificity predicting improvement of regional function after revascularization is approximately 92% and 63%, respectively.

RADIONUCLIDE VENTRICULOGRAPHY

Tc-99m–labeled red blood cell (RBC) radionuclide ventriculography (RVG), alternatively called multigated acquisition (MUGA) study, has been used since the 1970s to analyze global and regional ventricular function. Two methods have been used, the first-pass method, in which all data collection occurs during the initial transit of a tracer bolus through the central circulation, and the equilibrium method, in which data are collected over many cardiac cycles using ECG gating and a tracer that remains in the blood pool. The gated equilibrium study has become the standard method at most centers.

A major advantage of the radionuclide method is that calculation of LVEF is not dependent on mathematical assumptions of ventricular shape. Emitted counts in the ventricle are proportional to its volume.

Radiopharmaceuticals

Equilibrium Blood Pool Radiopharmaceutical
Radiolabeled human serum albumin was originally used; however, radiolabeled RBCs have been the standard technique for decades. Labeling of RBCs can be performed by any of three approaches: in vivo, modified in vivo, or in vitro, described in the Chapter 13 (Box 13-11). The modified in vivo or the in vitro method (Ultra-Tag RBC,

---

Box 16-9. Fluorine-18 Fluorodeoxyglucose Positron Emission Tomography Cardiac Viability: Summary Protocol

PATIENT PREPARATION
Patient should fast after midnight
Obtain rest myocardial perfusion scan
Serum fasting blood sugar (BS)

Nondiabetic
If BS ≤150 mg/dL: 50 g oral glucose solution + regular insulin 3 units intravenously
If BS 151 to 300 mg/dL: 25 g oral glucose solution + regular insulin 3 units intravenously
If BS 301 to 400 mg/dL: 25 g oral glucose solution + regular insulin 5 units intravenously
If BS >400 mg/dL: 25 g oral glucose solution + regular insulin 7 units intravenously
At least 45 minutes after glucose loading and when BS <150 mg/dL, inject F-18 FDG

Diabetic
If BS <150 mg/dL: 25 g oral glucose solution
If BS 151-200 mg/dL: Regular insulin 3 units intravenously
If BS 201-300 mg/dL: Regular insulin 5 units intravenously
If BS 301-400 mg/dL: Regular insulin 7 units intravenously
If BS 401 mg/dL or greater: Regular insulin 10 units intravenously
Obtain BS every 15 minutes for 60 minutes. If BS elevated, administer additional insulin per scale. At least 45 minutes after glucose loading and when BS ≤150 mg/dL, inject F-18 FDG.

RADIOPHARMACEUTICAL
F-18 FDG 0.22 mCi/kg (100 µCi/lb)

TIME OF IMAGING
After 60-minute uptake phase

PROCEDURE
PET acquisition: Cardiac field of view

PROCESSING
Reconstruct along the short and long axis of the heart similar to the perfusion study.

FDG, Fluorodeoxyglucose; *IV*, Intravenously; *NPO*, nil per os; *PET*, positron emission tomography; *SPECT*, single-photon emission computed tomography.

Mallinckrodt, St. Louis, MO) are preferred because of their higher binding efficiency, 85% to 90% and greater than 97%, respectively. Causes for poor RBC labeling are listed in Table 16-14, although these are uncommon using the in vitro method.

Dosimetry
The spleen receives the highest radiation absorbed dose, 2.2 rads/20 mCi (2.2 cGy/740 mBq), followed by the heart wall, 2.0 rads/20 mCi (2.0 cGy/740 mBq). The whole-body effective dose is 0.777 rem/30 mCi (0.777 cGy/1110 MBq).

Equilibrium Gated Blood Pool Studies

The limited counting statistics available during a cardiac cycle and the desirability of linking phases of the cardiac cycle to image data underlie the equilibrium gated blood pool method. ECG leads are placed on the patient, and a gating signal triggered by the R wave of the ECG is sent to the computer (Fig. 16-39). The R wave occurs at the end of diastole and the beginning of systole. Being the largest electrical signal in the ECG, it is relatively easy to detect.

The cardiac cycle is usually divided into 16 frames by computer processing software (Fig. 16-40). Individual frame duration is 40 to 50 msec. This framing rate is a compromise between optimal temporal and statistical data sampling. Sufficient frames are needed to catch the peaks and valleys of the cardiac cycle (temporal sampling), but too many frames reduce counting statistics available in any single frame (statistical sampling).

During each heartbeat, data are acquired sequentially into 16 frames (bins) spanning the cardiac cycle. With imaging of 100 to 300 cardiac cycles, sufficient counting statistics are obtained for valid quantitative analysis and reasonable spatial resolution. Typically 250,000 counts per frame are acquired. An equilibrium gated MUGA protocol is detailed (Box 16-10).

The underlying assumption of R-wave gating is that there is a normal sinus rhythm so that data are added

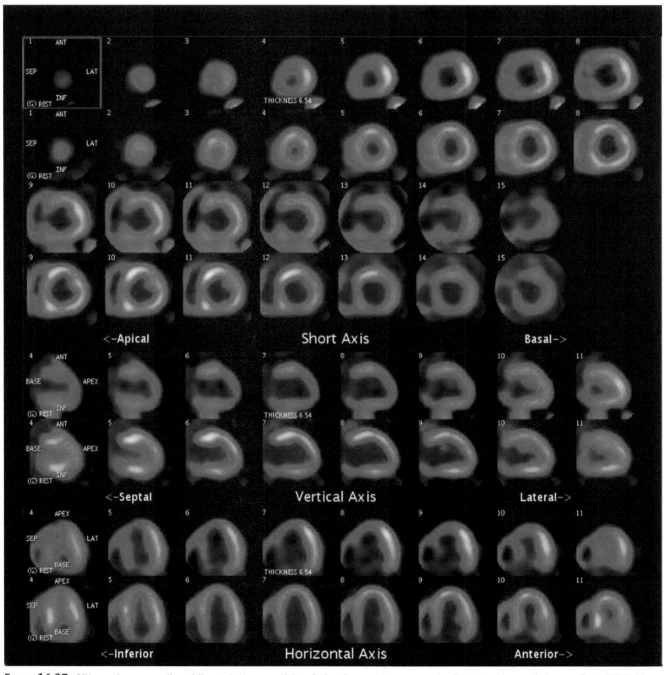

FIGURE 16-37. Hibernating myocardium. Mismatched myocardial perfusion. Images above are resting Rb-82 and images below are F-18-FDG. There is a perfusion metabolic mismatch in the anterior, septal, and apical walls. *ANT,* Anterior; *INF,* inferior; *LAT,* lateral; *SEP,* septal.

together from corresponding segments of the cardiac cycle over the entire study period. Any significant arrhythmia degrades the quality of the data and reduces the accuracy of quantitative analysis. Frequent premature ventricular contractions or rapid atrial fibrillation with an irregular ventricular response is a contraindication to the study (Fig. 16-41). Quantitative error may result if there are greater than 10% premature ventricular contractions or

rapid atrial fibrillation with irregular ventricular response. A rhythm strip should be obtained for every patient before the injection of a radiotracer. Reviewing the beat histogram display is also helpful for analyzing whether the rhythm is regular (Fig. 16-40, *B*). Gating problems may include spurious signals from skeletal muscle activity, giant T waves triggering the gating device, and artifacts from pacemakers.

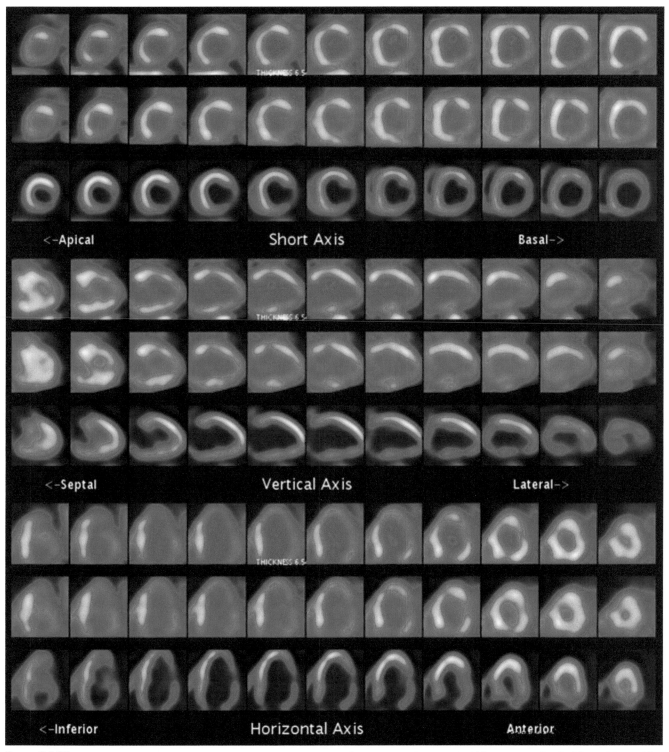

FIGURE 16-38. Negative for hibernating myocardium. Rb-82 myocardial perfusion stress *(above)*, rest *(middle)*, and F-18 FDG *(below)* with matching defects consistent with myocardial infarction and nonviable myocardium.

Computer techniques have been used to filter rhythm data (e.g., exclude premature contractions and postextrasystolic beats); however, this increases the time needed to perform a study, and the specialized buffering software is not widely available. The standard method is to automatically exclude the post-premature beat. Gated list mode, in which all beats are acquired in sequence and the timing recorded for each, allows for data acquisition techniques that can analyze separately the normal sinus beat, the premature contraction, and the postextrasystolic beat. However, this method is not commonly used clinically.

For studies at rest, multiple views (anterior, left anterior oblique, left lateral) are often obtained to evaluate regional ventricular wall motion. The exact camera angle for the left anterior oblique view is determined by moving the head of the gamma camera to find the view that best separates left and right ventricles, usually 35% to 45% left anterior oblique. This permits accurate calculation of the LVEF.

First-Pass Study

Tc-99m diethylenetriaminepentaacetic acid (DTPA) is most commonly used because of its rapid renal excretion

TABLE 16-14 Causes of Poor Technetium-99m Red Blood Cell Labeling

Drug–drug interactions	Heparin, doxorubicin, methyldopa, hydralazine, contrast media, quinidine
Circulating antibodies	Prior transfusion, transplantation, some antibiotics
Too little stannous ion	Insufficient to reduce Tc (VII)
Too much stannous ion	Reduction of Tc (VII) outside of red blood cell before cell labeling
Carrier Tc-99	Buildup of Tc-99m in the Mo-99/Tc-99m generator resulting from long interval between elutions
Too short an interval for "tinning"	Not enough time for stannous ion to penetrate the red blood cells before addition of Tc-99m
Too short an incubation time	Not enough time for reduction of Tc (VII)

and background clearance. However, using Tc-99m–labeled RBCs allows combining a first-pass evaluation of the right ventricle and equilibrium analysis of the left ventricle.

First-pass studies are performed by injecting a compact bolus of the radiopharmaceutical intravenously via a proximal vein, preferably the jugular vein. Injections directly through central catheters placed in the superior vena cava provide the most compact boluses.

Data may be acquired in rapid *frame* mode or in *list* mode, with or without ECG gating. The goal is to obtain 16 to 30 frames per second while the bolus passes through the central circulation. In most patients, the total data acquisition time required is 30 to 60 seconds. A right anterior oblique view at 20- to 30-degree camera position best separates the right atrium and the right ventricle and is also the standard during cardiac catheterization (Fig. 16-42). Quantitative and qualitative analysis of biventricular function are possible.

The major advantage of the first-pass approach is that data are collected rapidly over very few cardiac cycles. Ventricular function can be measured at peak stress during exercise ventriculography or other intervention. Right ventricular function quantification is more accurate than with equilibrium gated blood pool studies because there is no overlap of the two ventricles. The disadvantage of the first-pass approach is that counting statistics are low in each frame because of the count rate limitations of most gamma cameras.

Data Analysis and Study Interpretation

Qualitative Analysis

Comprehensive analysis and interpretation of MUGA studies require both qualitative and quantitative assessments. Wall motion is analyzed by viewing a repetitive cinematic closed loop display of the 16 frames on the computer monitor. Ventricular contraction is inferred from reduction in size of the ventricular cavity activity from diastole to systole and evidence of normal wall motion (Fig. 16-40, *A*). Septal contraction is often less than other wall motion.

Complete absence of wall motion is termed *akinesis;* diminished contraction is *hypokinetic* (Fig. 16-43); paradoxical

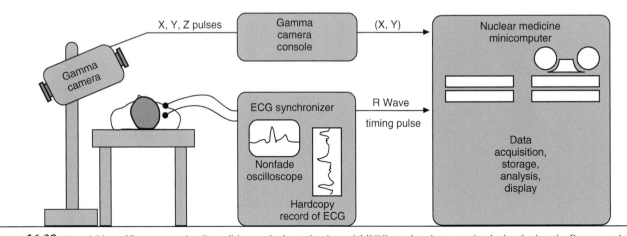

FIGURE 16-39. Acquisition of R-wave gated radionuclide ventriculography. A special ECG synchronizer or *gating* device depicts the R-wave and sends a timing pulse to the nuclear medicine computer system. This timing pulse is used to sort incoming scintillation events into a sequence of frames that spans the cardiac cycle.

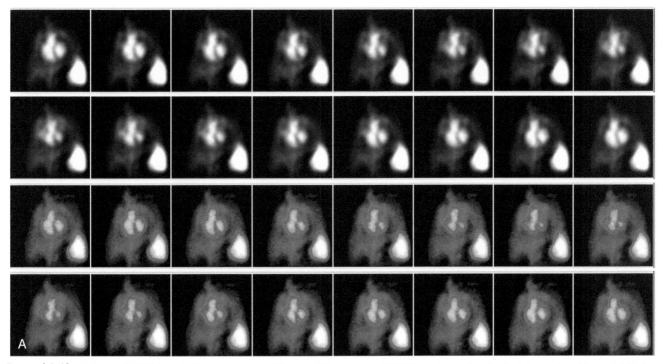

FIGURE 16-40. A, Normal MUGA study. Sixteen sequential frames of R-wave gated MUGA study acquired in the left anterior oblique *(LAO)* view. Displayed in gray scale and a color scale. Note the change in size and count density of the cardiac chambers during the cardiac cycle. End diastole is the first image and end systole the seventh frame. The gray scale and four-color images are from the same date.

wall motion (i.e., an actual outward bulge during systole) is *dyskinetic*. If motion is present but delayed compared with adjacent segments, this is termed *tardokinesis*. In normal subjects, all wall segments should contract, with the greatest incursion seen in the left ventricular free wall and apex. Areas of ventricular scar are typically akinetic or dyskinetic. Tardokinesis is seen with conduction abnormalities such as bundle branch block.

The complete qualitative or visual analysis includes an assessment of cardiac chamber size, assessment of overall biventricular function and regional wall motion, and assessment of any extracardiac abnormalities such as aortic aneurysms or pericardial effusions that are in the detector's field of view. Only portions of the ventricles not overlapped by other cardiac structures should be assessed on any given view—for example, on the anterior view the right ventricle usually overlaps the septum and inferior wall of the left ventricle.

Quantitative and functional or parametric images have been used to detect abnormalities in regional wall motion—for example, calculation of regional ejection fractions. Fourier phase analysis and other parametric image analysis techniques have been used (Fig. 16-40, *B*).

Quantitative Data Analysis
Ejection Fraction
The most frequently calculated quantitative parameter of ventricular function is the LVEF, defined as the fraction of the left ventricular end-diastolic volume expelled during contraction. The underlying principle is that the left ventricular count rate at each point in the cardiac cycle is proportional to ventricular volume. The ventricular counts are determined by drawing a region of interest

over the left ventricle for end-diastole and end-systole and a background region, typically taken as a crescent adjacent to the left ventricular apex (Fig. 16-40, *B*). A background-corrected ventricular time-activity curve (TAC) is generated. End-diastole is the frame demonstrating the highest counts and end-systole the frame with the fewest counts.

The ejection fraction is calculated as follows, with each count corrected for background:

$$\text{Ejection fraction} = \frac{\text{End diastolic counts} - \text{End systolic counts}}{\text{End diastolic counts}}$$

The LVEF in normal subjects ranges from 50% to 75%. The accuracy of the LVEF calculation by RVG is considered superior to that of most nonnuclear techniques because it is volume based. The number of counts is directly proportional to volume.

The time-activity (time-cardiac volume) curve should be inspected as a quality control measure. The count values at the beginning and end of the curve should be identical. The trailing frames in late diastole may have fewer counts, owing to variations in cardiac cycle length, even in patients with normal sinus rhythm. In patients with frequent premature ventricular contractions and rapid atrial fibrillation with an irregular ventricular response, the fall-off in counts at the end of the curve is much greater. Premature or more rapid beats are placed in earlier frames, resulting in fewer counts in the later frames. Thus quantitative analysis of gated data in patients with major dysrhythmias can be inaccurate. On cine display, a fall-off in counts in later frames is seen as a flicker.

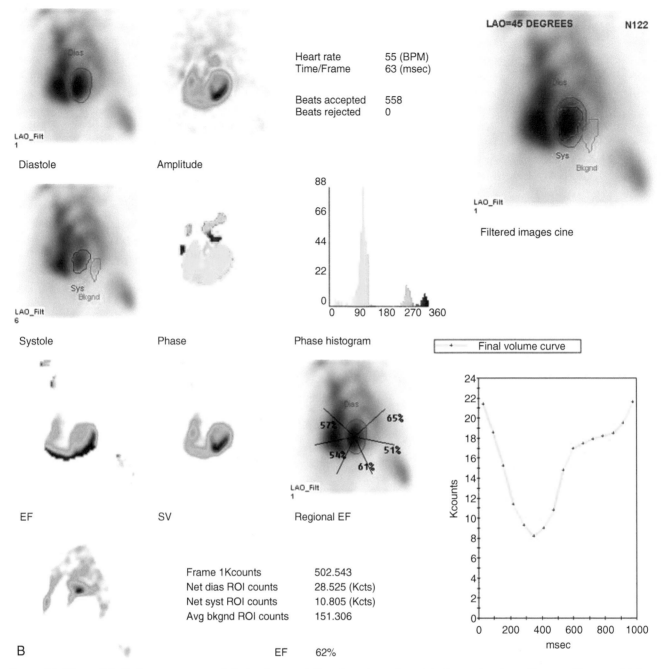

Diastole   Amplitude

Heart rate   55 (BPM)
Time/Frame   63 (msec)

Beats accepted   558
Beats rejected   0

Filtered images cine

Systole   Phase   Phase histogram

Final volume curve

EF   SV   Regional EF

Frame 1Kcounts   502.543
Net dias ROI counts   28.525 (Kcts)
Net syst ROI counts   10.805 (Kcts)
Avg bkgnd ROI counts   151.306

B   EF   62%

FIGURE **16-40,cont'd. B,** Computer processed display shows end-diastolic, end-systolic, and background regions of interest. The normal left ventricular TAC is shown with the atrial kick during the later phase. Phase and functional images are shown and the rate histogram. LVEF is 62%. *Avg,* Average; *bkgnd,* background; *EF,* ejection fraction; *filt,* filter; *Kcts,* kilocounts; *ROI,* region of interest; *SV,* stroke volume.

Box 16-10. **Equilibrium Gated Blood Pool Ventriculography: Summary Protocol**

PATIENT PREPARATION
Rhythm strip to confirm normal sinus rhythm (<10% premature ventricular contractions)

RADIOPHARMACEUTICAL
Tc-99m red blood cells 20 mCi (740 MBq) intravenously

INSTRUMENTATION
Collimator: low-energy general purpose collimator and a
Window: 15% to 20% centered at 140 keV

Imaging: Anterior, left anterior oblique (LAO) (best septal view), and left lateral views.
Gamma camera persistence scope to determine optimal LAO view for separating left and right ventricular activity
Sixteen frames per cardiac with frame duration of 50 msec or less
250k counts per frame for studies performed at rest
100k counts per frame in the optimum LAO view for studies obtained during an intervention

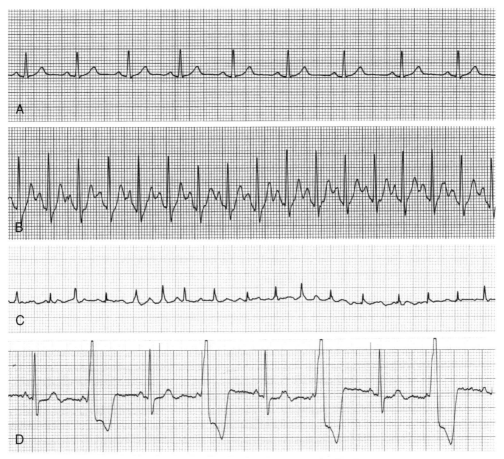

FIGURE 16-41. ECG rhythm strips. **A,** Normal sinus rhythm. **B,** Sinus tachycardia. **C,** Atrial fibrillation with irregular ventricular response. **D,** Premature vascular contractions with bigeminy.

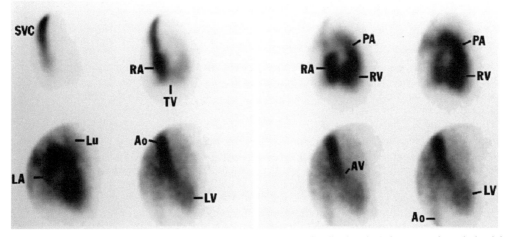

FIGURE 16-42. First-pass radionuclide angiogram. Cardiac structures are sequentially visualized as the bolus passes through the right side of the heart into the lungs and then returns to the left side. *Ao,* Aorta; *AV,* aortic valve; *LA,* left atrium; *Lu,* lung; *LV,* left ventricle; *PA,* pulmonary artery; *RA,* right atrium; *RV* right ventricle; *SVC,* superior vena cava; *TV,* tricuspid valve.

Calculation of a right ventricular ejection fraction (RVEF) from equilibrium data can be performed similarly, however, the regions of interest are more difficult to draw because of overlap of the right atrium and right ventricle and right ventricle and its outflow tract. Thus the results are subject to error. The RVEF is normally lower than the LVEF. The stroke volume is the same for both, but right ventricular volume is larger than left ventricular volume.

A complete analysis and interpretation of the RVG includes a qualitative visual assessment of the cardiac chambers and great vessels to assess their size and relationships. Visual assessment of the dynamic cinematic display is also used to analyze regional wall motion.

Fourier Phase Analysis

Fourier phase analysis reduces 4-D data to a pair of 2-D images. Images portray cardiac contractility (amplitude) and contraction sequence (phase) (Fig. 16-40, *B*). Each pixel in the cardiac image has its own cycle, having an amplitude and a characteristic temporal relationship (phase) with respect to the R wave. The amplitude image portrays the maximum net count variation for each pixel during the cardiac cycle. The phase image portrays the relative time delay from the R wave to the start of the cardiac cycle for that pixel.

If the complete cardiac cycle encompasses 360 degrees, the atria and ventricles are normally 180 degrees "out of phase." Areas of the ventricle that contract slightly earlier in the cardiac cycle owing to the pattern of the electrical conduction down the septum and through the bundle branches are seen as out of phase with adjacent ventricular areas. Wall motion abnormalities are portrayed on phase images as low-amplitude areas. Regions of paradoxical motion resulting from left ventricular aneurysms are 180 degrees "out of phase" with the ventricle. Abnormal conduction patterns (e.g., Wolff-Parkinson-White syndrome, bundle-branch block) cause affected areas to be out of phase with adjacent portions of the ventricle as a result of premature or delayed contraction.

Amplitude and phase maps are often displayed in color to highlight the temporal sequences of cardiac chamber emptying. A dynamic color display mode can be used to demonstrate the propagating wavefront that sweeps across the ventricle during contraction, linking pixels with similar phase angles together. The studies require exceptionally well-synchronized data to be most useful for localizing abnormal conduction pathways.

Functional Images

The intensity of the computer display at each point in an image is determined by the number of counts recorded at that point and proportional to the amount of radioactivity in the corresponding location. By subtracting the end-systolic image from the end-diastolic image point by point, a derived functional image is created. This image may be further processed by dividing it point-by-point by the end-diastolic frame to create an ejection fraction image (Fig. 16-40, *B*). Akinetic wall segments correspond to areas of diminished or absent intensity. For the paradox image, the end-diastolic frame is subtracted from the end-systolic frame. With normal ventricular function, this leaves a void. In patients with areas of paradoxical ventricular wall motion, the systolic bulge is readily detected as an area of unsubtracted activity.

Clinical Applications

The MUGA study is most commonly used to calculate a LVEF in patients receiving cardiotoxic drugs (e.g., doxorubicin).

Coronary Artery Disease

In the past, stress MUGA studies were performed for other indications—for example, to detect myocardial infarction and ischemia. Patients with significant ischemia may have a normal rest LVEF but have a fall in the LVEF or regional motion abnormalities with exercise. The hallmark of

---

Box 16-11. Guidelines for Monitoring Doxorubicin Cardiotoxicity

Baseline evaluation: Before the start of therapy or at least before 100 mg/m^2 has been given

Subsequent evaluations: 3 weeks after the last dose at recommended intervals

1. Patients with normal baseline LVEF (>50%)
   a. Obtain second study after 250 to 300 mg/m^2.
   b. Obtain a repeat study after 400 mg/m^2 in patients with heart disease, hypertension, radiation exposure, abnormal electrocardigram, cyclophosphamide therapy or after 450 mg/m^2 in the absence of risk factors.
   c. Obtain sequential studies thereafter before each dose. Discontinue therapy if >10% decrease in LVEF to <50%.
2. Patients with abnormal baseline LVEF (<50%).
   a. With baseline LVEF <30%, do not start therapy
   b. With baseline LVEF >30% and <50%, perform a study before each dose

Discontinue drug in patients with an absolute decrease in LVEF ≥30% or final LVEF ≤30%.

LVEF, Left ventricular ejection fraction.

---

myocardial infarction on RVG is that of a resting wall motion abnormality in the region of the infarct and commonly reduced global LVEF.

Assessment of Cardiac Toxicity

The most common indication for RVG today is to assess the potential cardiotoxic effects of noncardiac drugs. Anthracycline drugs, used most commonly in the treatment of breast cancer and malignant lymphoma (e.g., doxorubicin [Adriamycin]), produce a cumulative dose-dependent depression of left ventricular function. Acute cardiotoxicity is transient and without permanent consequences. Chronic toxicity leads to progressive left ventricular dysfunction and heart failure. Considerable variability exists in individual susceptibility. Trastuzumab (Herceptin), used for treatment of breast cancer, is also cardiotoxic. The dose is not cumulative, and there is high likelihood of reversal of new dysfunction within 2 to 4 months if medication is discontinued.

Doxorubicin doses of more than 450 to 500 mg/m^2 result in increased occurrence of cardiotoxicity and heart failure. Endocardial biopsy is diagnostic but invasive and not commonly performed. Overt failure is preceded by a progressive fall in the LVEF. Serial monitoring can detect a change in cardiac function, and the drug can be stopped or reduced when a reduction in LVEF is observed. Complete recovery may occur if therapy is discontinued at an early stage.

In patients with a normal baseline LVEF (>50%), moderate toxicity is defined as decline of more than 10% in absolute LVEF, with a final LVEF of less than 50% (Box 16-11). In patients with abnormal baseline (>30% and <50%) (Fig. 16-43), a study is performed before each dose. Doxorubicin is discontinued with an absolute decrease in LVEF of 10% or greater or final LVEF of 30% or less. Trastuzumab should

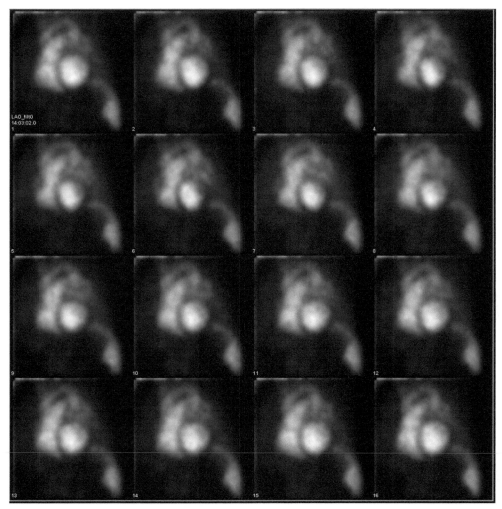

FIGURE 16-43. Abnormal MUGA scan. Sixteen sequential frames shows diffuse hypokinesis of both the right and left ventricle. LVEF was 25%. *LAO,* Left anterior oblique.

be discontinued at least temporarily if LVEF falls by more than 10% to a level of less than 50%.

Pulmonary Disease

Right ventricular enlargement can be seen with RVG. In patients with a new onset of dyspnea, the RVG can help differentiate left ventricular from pulmonary dysfunction. Normal wall motion, LVEF, and chamber size strongly suggests a pulmonary cause.

Congenital Heart Disease

Right-to-left shunts result from a variety of congenital cardiac diseases. They can be confirmed and quantified with Tc-99m–labeled macroaggregated albumin (MAA). With right-to-left shunts, images show uptake with the cerebral cortex and other organs (Fig. 16-44, *A*). However, uptake in other organs (e.g., kidneys) can be due to free Tc-99m pertechnetate. Cerebral cortex uptake is diagnostic. Quantification is best done with whole-body imaging. Regions of interest can be drawn for the lungs and total body (Fig. 16-44, *B*). The calculated percent shunt does not accurately reflect the real percent shunt but correlates with its severity. Greater than 10% is usually abnormal. Right-to-left shunts are a relative contraindication to the use of Tc-99m MAA, because of the theoretical risk for embolizing the capillary bed of the brain. In practice, this is not a problem, although it is recommended that the number of particles be reduced.

■ MYOCARDIAL INFARCT AND AMYLOIDOSIS IMAGING

Tc-99m bone scan radiopharmaceuticals are taken up by the heart in the region of a recent myocardial infarction (Fig. 16-45). Tc-99m pyrophosphate has been used to diagnose infarction because it had higher soft tissue uptake. This test is no longer required by cardiologists to confirm the diagnosis. Several other conditions result in diffusely increased myocardial uptake of bone tracers. The most dramatic is amyloidosis. Myocarditis, postradiation injury, and doxorubicin cardiotoxicity may also have diffusely increased uptake.

Mechanism of Localization

After cell death in acute myocardial infarction, an influx of calcium occurs and calcium phosphate complexes are formed. These microcrystalline deposits act as sites for bone tracer uptake. Some binding also may occur on denatured macromolecules. Some residual blood flow is necessary to deliver the tracer to the infarct area and surrounding tissue. The tracer then diffuses into the necrotic tissue and is

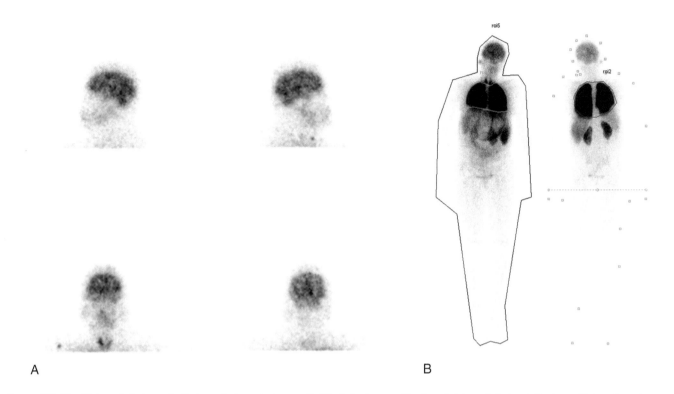

FIGURE 16-44. Right-to-left shunt. **A,** Brain cortical uptake is seen. **B,** Whole-body quantification of right-to-left shunt. Regions of interest are drawn for the whole body and lungs.

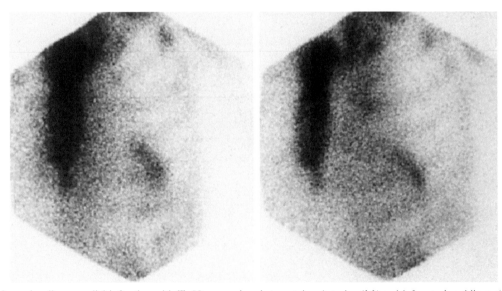

FIGURE 16-45. Lateral wall myocardial infarction with Tc-99m pyrophosphate uptake. Anterior *(left)* and left anterior oblique *(right)* images. The amount of myocardial uptake is greater than rib uptake but less than sternal uptake.

bound. Highest uptake is at the periphery of infarction. In large infarctions, with neither direct flow nor diffusion to the central area, no tracer is delivered and a characteristic ring or doughnut pattern is seen as a result of uptake around the margin of the infarction.

Uptake is highest for detecting infarction at 24 to 48 hours after the acute event. Significant uptake is seen at 12 hours. Maximum localization occurs at 48 to 72 hours. Thereafter uptake begins to diminish as the infarcted area heals. The scan usually reverts to normal within 14 days.

▬ INVESTIGATIONAL CARDIAC RADIOPHARMACEUTICALS

Iodine-123 Meta-iodo-benzyl-guanidine

Iodine-123 meta-iodo-benzyl-guanidine (MIBG), a nor-epinephrine analog, has been used to study the adrenergic status of the heart. The heart is richly innervated, and MIBG has been used to provide prognostic insights. Uptake of MIBG is blocked in patients taking drugs (e.g., guanethidine, cocaine) that compete for uptake into the presynaptic storage vesicles of the adrenergic system. Decreased uptake is seen after myocardial infarction and in some patients with cardiomyopathies.

MIBG can be used in risk stratification in patients who have advanced heart failure. Normal uptake has a high negative predictive value for cardiac events, especially death and arrhythmias. It may have a role in guiding therapy by helping select patients unresponsive to conventional medical therapies who might benefit from device therapies, such as an implantable cardioverter defibrillator, cardiac resynchronization therapy, left ventricular assist devices, or cardiac transplantation. It has potential in assessing patients after cardiac transplantation, with primary arrhythmic conditions, coronary artery disease, diabetes mellitus, and cardiotoxic chemotherapy.

Fatty Acid Radiopharmaceuticals

Fatty acids supply the majority of the heart's metabolic requirements under normal aerobic conditions. With ischemia, energy metabolism shifts to anaerobic metabolism and the main energy substrate changes from free fatty acids to glucose metabolism. Radiolabeled fatty acids can be used to image myocardial aerobic metabolism.

PET imaging with carbon-11 palmitic acid uptake reflects fatty acid metabolism. C-11 acetate allows for good images of the heart. Decreased uptake and delayed clearance indicates ischemia. Because of its rapid metabolism, cardiac turnover is inferred from dynamic analysis of its myocardial clearance pharmacokinetics. Controversy exists regarding the significance of the metabolic information provided. An onsite cyclotron is required.

I-123 beta-methyl-p-iodophenyl-pentadecanoic acid (BMIPP) is a single-photon branching free fatty acid radiopharmaceutical with slow metabolism. Decreased uptake occurs with ischemia. The uniqueness of this radiopharmaceutical is that it demonstrates a persistent disturbance of fatty acid metabolism, even when blood flow has been reestablished, such as with unstable angina and stunned myocardium.

▬ SUGGESTED READING

Allman KC, Shaw LJ, Hachamovitch R, et al. Myocardial viability testing and impact of revascularization on prognosis in patients with coronary artery disease and left ventricular dysfunction: a meta-analysis. *J Am Coll Cardiol.* 2002;39(7):1151-1158.

Bacharach SL, Bax JJ, Case J, et al. PET myocardial glucose metabolism and perfusion imaging. I. Guidelines for patient preparation and data acquisition. *J Nucl Cardiol.* 2003;10(5):543-554.

Bateman T, Heller G, McGhie I, et al. Diagnostic accuracy of rest/stress ECG-gated rubidium-82 myocardial perfusion PET: comparison with ECG-gated Tc-99m sestamibi SPECT. *J Nucl Cardiol.* 2006;13(10):24-33.

Cerqueira MD, Weissman NJ, Disizian V, et al. Standardized myocardial segmentation and nomenclature for tomographic imaging of the heart. *Circulation.* 2002;105(4):539-549.

Di Carli MF, Asgarzadie F, Schelbert HR, et al. Quantitative relation between myocardial viability and improvement in heart failure symptoms after revascularization in patients with ischemic cardiomyopathy. *Circulation.* 1995;92(12):3436-3444.

Di Carli MF, Davidson M, Little R, et al. Value of metabolic imaging with positron emission tomography for evaluating prognosis in patients with coronary artery disease and left ventricular dysfunction. *J Am Coll Cardiol.* 1994;3(8):527-533.

Dilsizian V, Narula J. *Atlas of Nuclear Cardiology.* 3rd ed. Philadelphia: Current Medicine; 2009.

Eitzman D, Al-Aouar Z, Kanter HL, et al. Clinical outcome of patients with advanced coronary artery disease after viability studies with positron emission tomography. *J Am Coll Cardiol.* 1992;20(3):559-565.

Hendel RC, Berman DS, Di Carli MF, et al. Appropriate use criteria for cardiac radionuclide imaging. *Circulation.* 2009;199(22):561-587.

Jaroudi WA, AJ, Iskandrian AE. Regadenoson: a new myocardial stress agent. *J Am Coll Cardiol.* 2009;54(13):1123-1130.

Ji SY, Travin MI. Radionuclide imaging of cardiac autonomic innervations. *J Nucl Cardiol.* 2010;17(4):655-666.

Machac J, Bacharach S, Bateman T, et al. ASNC guidelines: positron emission tomography myocardial perfusion and glucose metabolism imaging. *J Nucl Cardiol.* 2006;13(6):e121-e151.

Nandalur KR, Dwamena BA, Choudhri AF, et al. Diagnostic performance of positron emission tomography in the detection of coronary artery disease: a meta-analysis. *Acad Radiol.* 2008;15(4):444-451.

Sampson UK, Dorbala S, Limaye A, et al. Diagnostic accuracy of rubidium-82 myocardial perfusion imaging with hybrid positron emission tomography/computed tomography in the detection of coronary artery disease. *J Am Coll Cardiol.* 2007;49(10):1052-1058.

Shelbert HR, Beanlands RB, Engel F, et al. PET myocardial perfusion and glucose metabolism imaging. II. Guidelines for interpretation and reporting. *J Nucl Cardiol.* 2000;10(5):557-571.

Underwood SR, Anagnostopoulos C, Cerqueira M, et al. Myocardial perfusion scintigraphy: the evidence. *Eur J Nucl Med and Mol Imaging.* 2004;31(2):261-291.

Yoshinaga K, Chow BJ, Williams K, et al. What is the prognostic value of myocardial perfusion imaging using Rb-82 positron emission tomography? *J Am Coll Cardiol.* 2006;48:1029-1039.

Zaret BL, Beller GA. *Clinical Nuclear Cardiology.* 3rd ed. Philadelphia: Elsevier; 2010.

CHAPTER 17

Pearls, Pitfalls, and Frequently Asked Questions

This chapter reinforces concepts presented in this textbook. Students of medicine gather pearls of wisdom from their mentors that may not fit well into a didactic treatment of a subject but are valuable in day-to-day practice. Likewise, we all learn to avoid pitfalls that arise but have escaped our formal education. Interpretative questions require assembling multiple bits of information for a correct answer, and these questions are not usually asked in quite the same way that subject material was presented didactically. This chapter is neither comprehensive nor weighted toward the relative importance of the topics.

RADIOPHARMACEUTICALS

A PEARL: *Radiopharmaceuticals are radioactive molecules comprised of a radionuclide, which permits external detection, and a biologically active molecule or drug that acts as a carrier, determining localization and biodistribution. Exceptions to this are radioiodine, gallium, thallium, and oxygen-15, in which the radioactive atoms themselves confer the desired localization properties.*

Q: What is the relationship between the half-lives of a parent radionuclide and a daughter radionuclide in a generator system?

A: The parent radionuclide must have a long enough half-life to permit formulation and distribution of the generator. The daughter half-life must be long enough for the clinical application. A longer-lived parent decays to a shorter-lived daughter in all clinical generator systems.

Q: How are parent and daughter radionuclides separated in generator systems?

A: Because the parent and daughter are different elements, they can be chemically separated, (e.g., molybdenum-99 and technetium-99m).

A PEARL: *The most common radionuclide contaminant in the generator eluate is the parent radionuclide, Mo-99. Tc-99, the daughter product of the isomeric transition of Tc-99m, is also present but is not considered an impurity or contaminant, although significant Tc-99 can be a problem from a radiolabeling standpoint.*

Q: What quality-assurance procedure is used to detect radionuclide impurities?

A: Thin-layer chromatography is the procedure used to detect impurities.

A PEARL: *If 5% of Tc-99m activity remains as free pertechnetate in a radiolabeling procedure, the radiochemical purity is reported as 95%.*

Q: What is the legal limit for Mo-99 in Tc-99m–containing radiopharmaceuticals?

A: The Nuclear Regulatory Commission (NRC) limit is 0.15 microcurie of Mo-99 activity per 1 mCi of Tc-99m activity in the administered dose.

Q: How does the ratio of Mo-99 to Tc-99m change with time?

A: In any preparation in which the radionuclidic contaminants have longer half-lives than the desired radionuclide label, the relative activity of the contaminant increases with time.

Q: What is the purpose of stannous ion in Tc-99m labeling procedures?

A: Stannous ion is used to reduce technetium pertechnetate from a +7 valence state to lower valence states necessary for labeling a wide range of agents.

Q: What constitutes a medical event, formerly known as a misadministration of a radiopharmaceutical?

A: In the past, a *misadministration* was defined by the NRC as a radiopharmaceutical given to the wrong patient, receiving the ordered radiopharmaceutical by the wrong route of administration, or the administered dose differing from the prescribed dose by greater than an allowable standard. Although these are all of concern and need discussion of quality assurance within a department and institution, as well as a record of the event, the NRC now requires reporting only *medical events*, defined as a medical event in which the effective dose equivalent to the patient exceeds 5 rem to the whole body or 50 rem to an individual organ.

Q: Describe the general response to the spill of radioactive material.

A: The person who recognizes that a spill has occurred should notify all persons in the vicinity, and the area should be restricted. If possible, the spill should be covered. For *minor spills*, cleanup using appropriate disposable and protective clothing can be accomplished until background or near-background radiation levels are observed. For *major spills*, the source of the radioactivity should be shielded. For both major and minor spills, all personnel potentially exposed in the area should be surveyed, with appropriate removal of contaminated clothing and decontamination of skin. The radiation safety officer should be notified of all spills and has the primary responsibility for supervising cleanup for major spills and determining what reports must be made to regulatory agencies.

NUCLEAR MEDICINE PHYSICS

A PEARL: *Positrons are positive electrons, and thus they are particles. With radioactive decay, an emitted positron travels 2 to 10 mm in tissue (depending on the radionuclide) before losing its kinetic energy, then interacts with an electron. The two particles annihilate each other and emit two 511-keV gamma photons at approximately 180-degree angles from each other. The gamma photons can be detected by positron emission tomography (PET) coincidence detectors. This conversion of mass to energy is predicted by Einstein's well-known formula: $E = mc^2$.*

Q: What is the difference between x-rays and gamma rays?
A: Both x-rays and gamma rays are ionizing radiation. X-rays originate outside the atomic nucleus, and gamma rays originate inside the atomic nucleus. The respective energy spectra for x-rays and gamma rays substantially overlap at the high-energy end of the spectrum for all forms of electromagnetic radiation.

Q: What is the energy equivalent of the rest mass of an electron?
A: The energy equivalent is 511 keV. This is also the energy equivalent of a positron (positive electron).

Q: What is the difference among the rad, roentgen, and rem?
A: These terms are frequently confused with each other but have important distinctions.
The *roentgen* is a unit of radiation exposure, defined as the quantity of x-radiation or gamma radiation that produces one electrostatic unit of charge per cubic centimeter of air at standard temperature and pressure. In the International System of Units (SI) radiation exposure is expressed in terms of coulombs per kilogram (C/kg). One roentgen is equal to 2.58×10^{-4} C/kg air.
A radiation absorbed dose, or *rad*, is equal to the absorption of 100 ergs of energy per gram of absorbing material and is the traditional unit of absorbed dose. The gray (Gy) is the unit of absorbed dose in the SI system. 1 Gy = 100 rads.
A *rem* is an acronym for *r*oentgen *e*quivalent *m*an. The rem is calculated by multiplying the absorbed dose in rads by a factor to correct for the *relative biological effectiveness* (RBE) of the type of radiation in question. In the SI system, one *sievert* (Sv) = 100 rem.

Q: Which is more penetrating in soft tissues—alpha or beta particles of the same kinetic energy?
A: Alpha particles have very low penetration in soft tissue because of their rapid loss of kinetic energy through interaction of their electrical charge with electrons in the tissues. Beta particles of the same respective kinetic energy of alpha particles have higher velocity, lower mass, and a single negative charge. They demonstrate significantly greater penetration in soft tissues, although penetration still is typically measured in millimeters.

Q: Define the two systems for expressing radioactive decay.
A: The traditional unit of radioactive decay is the *curie* (Ci). One curie is equal to 3.7×10^{10} disintegrations per second (dps). This number was derived from the decay rate of 1 g of radium. (Modern measurements indicate that the actual decay rate for 1 g of radium is 3.6×10^{10} dps.) In the SI system, decay is expressed in becquerels (Bcq). One becquerel equals one disintegration per second. 1 mCi = 37 MBq.

Q: How are the half-life and the decay constant related?
A: The physical *half-life* ($T_{1/2}$) of a radionuclide is defined as the time for half the atoms in a sample to decay. The $T_{1/2}$ is expressed in units of time, typically seconds, minutes, hours, days, or years. The *decay constant* indicates the fraction of the sample decaying in a unit of time. The units of the decay constant are "per unit time" (per second, per hour). Mathematically, the $T_{1/2}$ and the decay constant (λ) are related by the following equation:

$$T_{1/2} = \frac{\ln 2}{\lambda}$$

Q: After a photon has undergone Compton scattering, how does the energy of the scattered photon compare to the original photon energy?
A: In Compton scattering, the photon gives up energy to a recoil or Compton electron. The "scattered" photon has correspondingly lower energy. The amount of energy lost increases as the angle of scattering increases.

Q: What factors speed up or slow down radioactive decay?
A: Unlike chemical reactions, radioactive decay is a physical constant that cannot be sped up or slowed down by heating or cooling a specimen or by applying other physical or chemical influences.

Q: What special term is used to designate the electrons in the outermost shell of an atom?
A: They are called *valence* electrons and are responsible for many of the chemical characteristics of the element.

Q: What is the binding energy of an electron?
A: *Binding energy* refers to the amount of energy required to remove that electron from the atom. Electrons in shells close to the nucleus have higher binding energy than electrons farther from the nucleus. This energy is typically expressed in terms of electron volts (eV). The binding energy for each electron shell and subshell is characteristic for the respective element; the higher the atomic number

of the element, the greater is the binding energy for each shell and subshell.

RADIATION DETECTION AND INSTRUMENTATION

Q: What are some examples of the uses of ionization chambers in nuclear medicine?

A: Ionization chambers are used for radiation survey meters and some pocket dosimeters. The radionuclide dose calibrator incorporates an ionization chamber.

Q: What is the purpose of the thallium impurity added to sodium iodide crystals in gamma detectors?

A: The thallium is used to "activate" the sodium iodide crystal. The thallium impurity provides "easier" pathways for the return of electrons from the conduction band of the crystal to the valence bands of atoms.

Q: What is the relationship between photon energy and detection efficiency in a sodium iodide crystal?

A: For a given crystal size, detection efficiency decreases with increasing photon energy.

Q: Why do photopeaks appear as bell-shaped curves in pulse height spectra rather than as discrete spikes corresponding to the energy of the gamma ray?

A: Although gamma rays have discrete energies, the detection process is subject to statistical factors at each step of the process. The bell-shaped curve corresponding to the gamma ray photopeak reflects these statistical variations, which results in different events being measured as having slightly different energies. The better the "energy resolution" of a pulse height analyzer, the narrower the bell-shaped curve.

Q: In using a gamma scintillation camera, what does it mean to "set" the energy window?

A: Gamma cameras are equipped with pulse height analyzers that allow the operator to select a range of observed energies for accepting photons to be used in making the scintigraphic image. The window is usually described by giving the photopeak energy of interest and a percentage range that defines the limits of acceptance above and below the photopeak energy. A typical window for the 140-keV photon of Tc-99m is 20%, or ±14 keV.

Q: What are the causes of inhomogeneous flood field images in gamma camera quality control?

A: Causes include improper photomultiplier tube voltage adjustment, off-peak camera pulse height analyzer setting, crystal imperfections or damage, poor coupling of the crystal and the photomultiplier tubes, and inadequate mixing of radiotracer in the flood phantom.

Q: What effects do Compton-scattered photons have on scintigraphic image quality?

A: Compton-scattered photons are the enemy! Scattered photons that fall within the acceptance limits of the energy window are included in the image. They represent false data because they are recorded in a different spatial location than the origin of the primary photon. Thus

Compton scattering reduces image contrast and spatial resolution. Compton-scattered photons falling outside the energy window still must be processed by the gamma-camera pulse-height analyzer circuitry. These rejected events contribute to dead time and reduce the count rate capability of gamma cameras.

Q: What photons are desired in the scintigraphic image?

A: Primary (unscattered) photons that arise in the organ of interest in the body and travel parallel to the axis of the gamma-camera collimator field of view are the photons desired in the image. Intuitively, one may think of these as "good" photons. All other photons are "bad" photons. These good photons include (unscattered) photons that arise in the object or organ of interest but travel "off axis," primary photons that arise in front of or behind the organ of interest (background photons), and all scattered photons.

Q: What is the purpose of the collimator?

A: The collimator defines the geometric field of view of the gamma-camera crystal. Off-axis photons, whether they are primary photons or scattered photons, are absorbed in the septa of the collimator and do not get to the crystal.

A PEARL: *Pinhole collimators allow resolution of objects below the spatial resolution of the gamma camera through geometric magnification.*

Q: What is the construction difference between a low-energy, all-purpose collimator and a low-energy, high-resolution collimator?

A: A high-resolution collimator has more holes that are smaller and deeper.

Q: How does poor energy resolution degrade spatial resolution?

A: Gamma cameras with poor energy resolution have reduced ability to reject scattered photons on the basis of pulse height analysis, as well as reduced ability for accurate determination of x and y coordinates for spatial localization of events.

SINGLE-PHOTON EMISSION COMPUTED TOMOGRAPHY AND POSITRON EMISSION TOMOGRAPHY

A PEARL: *Most nuclear medicine departments use 180-degree single-photon emission control tomography (SPECT) acquisition for cardiac studies and 360 degrees for imaging most other organs, including the brain.*

A PEARL: *For SPECT imaging the highest resolution collimator that provides sufficient count rate should be selected.*

A PITFALL: *Besides equipment factors, patient motion is the most important cause of image degradation in SPECT and PET studies.*

Q: What special importance does the biological half-life of a radiotracer have in SPECT imaging?

A: In SPECT imaging, data are acquired sequentially from sequential sampling angles. If significant biological redistribution of a radiopharmaceutical takes place between the start of data acquisition and completion, the reconstruction of tomographic images can be significantly distorted.

Q: What is a filter?

A: Filters are special mathematical functions applied to SPECT and PET data that enhance desired characteristics in the image, such as background subtraction, edge enhancement, and suppression of statistical noise. The ramp filter is designed to eliminate or reduce the star artifact during reconstruction.

A PEARL: *With SPECT and PET, flexible reformatting of image data can be performed in multiple image planes. For cardiac imaging, short-axis, vertical long-axis, and horizontal long-axis views of the heart are typically obtained.*

A PEARL: *Two quick ways of assessing patient motion during SPECT imaging are to view the projection images as a cinematic closed-loop display or to create slice sinograms. In the cinematic display, patient motion is seen as a flicker from one projection image to another. On sinograms, patient motion is seen as a discontinuity in the stacked projection profiles.*

A PITFALL: *SPECT is subject to various artifacts. Field flood nonuniformity can result in ring artifacts. Center-of-rotation misalignment results in loss of image resolution and, if severe, also ring artifacts.*

A PITFALL: *The higher the overall count rate in PET imaging, the more likely is the recording of "false" events because of the presence of paired random events that appear to the detection circuitry as paired annihilation photons.*

A PEARL: *The spatial resolution of PET is twice or greater than that of SPECT.*

A PITFALL: *Spatial resolution in PET is limited by positron travel distance in soft tissue before annihilation and photon emission.*

A PEARL: *PET imaging with transmission attenuation correction and detector sensitivity calibration allows for absolute quantitative uptake determinations.*

A PEARL: *Positron emitters, such as carbon, nitrogen, oxygen, and fluorine (as replacement for hydrogen) make possible the potential radiolabeling of any biological compound. The chemistry for developing and radiolabeling single-photon radiopharmaceuticals is often considerably more complex.*

ENDOCRINE

Q: What is the origin of lingual and sublingual thyroid tissue?

A: The main thyroid anlage begins as a downgrowth from the foramen cecum. Thyroid tissue may be seen anywhere along the tract of the thyroglossal duct from the foramen cecum to the usual location of the gland. However, with lingual thyroid tissue, usually a failure of normal development occurs, with no tissue in the normal location of the thyroid.

Q: What is the difference in mechanism of thyroid uptake between Tc-99m pertechnetate and radioiodine?

A: Radioiodine is taken up or extracted (trapped) by the thyroid follicular cell and organified, binding to tyrosine residues on thyroglobulin, and stored in colloid of the follicle. Tc-99m pertechnetate is trapped but not organified.

Q: What has happened to the range for normal percent thyroid uptake of radioiodine in the United States over the last 50 years?

A: The normal range has dropped significantly as a result of iodination of salt and the use of iodine in foods. The normal 24-hour range was 20% to 45% in the 1960s, but is now 10% to 30%.

A PEARL: *Radioiodine is administered orally. Tc-99m pertechnetate is administered intravenously.*

A PITFALL: *A potentially serious pitfall is to confuse microcuries with millicuries.*

A Pearl: *The following are the approximate adult doses of iodine-123 and iodine-131 used for uptakes, scans, and therapy. Serious consequences can result from confusing these doses, particularly if a therapeutic dose is administered instead of a diagnostic dose.*
I-123 scan (400 microcuries [μCi]), I-131 scan substernal goiter (50 μCi)
I-131 uptake (10 μCi), I-123 uptake (100 μCi)
I-131 therapy for Graves disease (7-15 mCi),
I-131 therapy for thyroid cancer (50-200 mCi)

Q: What is the normal distribution of radioiodine and Tc-99m pertechnetate?
A: Radioiodine is taken up by the thyroid, salivary glands, and stomach and excreted by the kidneys. Tc-99m pertechnetate has identical uptake and clearance, except that because it is not organified, it remains in the thyroid and salivary glands for a much shorter time.

A Pearl: *After injection of the radiopharmaceutical, routine I-123 thyroid scans are acquired at 4 hours and Tc-99m pertechnetate scans are acquired at 15 to 20 minutes. The delayed imaging for I-123 is to allow background clearance; Tc-99m is not organified like I-123 and thus is imaged earlier because of the rapid washout.*

Q: What are common causes of falsely low thyroid uptakes?
A: Patients taking thyroid hormones, iodine-containing drugs, organification blockers such as propylthiouracil, or recent administration of intravenous iodine containing radiographic contrast.

A Pearl: *Levothyroid (Synthyroid) should be discontinued for 4 weeks before a thyroid uptake or scan and liothyronine (Cytomel) for 2 weeks before. Computed tomography (CT) intravenous iodine contrast should not have been received within 6 to 8 weeks.*

Q: Which drug is used clinically to block unwanted thyroid uptake of radioiodine—for example, from administered diagnostic I-123 metaiodobenzylguanidine (MIBG), I-123 DaTscan, or therapeutic I-131 tositumomab (Bexxar)?
A: Iodine as supersaturate potassium iodide (SSKI) is used to block unwanted thyroid uptake.

Q: How does the methodology differ for a thyroid scan and thyroid uptake?
A: A thyroid uptake is a nonimaging study using a gamma-detector probe, whereas a thyroid scan results from gamma-camera imaging.

A Pearl: *Swallowed activity from salivary secretions on radio-pertechnetate scans occasionally remains in the esoph-*

agus and can confuse interpretation. The nature of the activity can be determined by having the patient drink water, followed by reimaging of the thyroid gland.

Q: How can a thyroid uptake test differentiate the two most common causes of thyrotoxicosis—Graves disease and subacute thyroiditis? Why?
A: In the initial phase of subacute thyroiditis, thyroid hormones are released from the inflamed gland, causing thyrotoxicosis. Both radioiodine and Tc-99m uptake require thyroid-stimulating hormone (TSH) stimulation for uptake. As a result of pituitary feedback, TSH is suppressed. Thus the uptake of radioiodine or Tc-99m pertechnetate is suppressed. With Graves disease, although TSH is suppressed, the gland is autonomous, and the uptake is high.

Q: What is the mechanism of action of antithyroid drugs propylthiouracil (PTU) and methimazole (Tapazole)?
A: Both PTU and methimazole are thiourea antithyroid drugs that block the organification of iodine.

Q: What medical conditions are associated with an increased incidence of paragangliomas (pheochromocytomas)?
A: Both forms of multiple endocrine neoplasia type II are associated with pheochromocytoma, as are von Hippel-Lindau disease and neurofibromatosis.

A Pitfall: *Autonomous nodules are not synonymous with toxic nodules. Patients with small autonomous nodules (<2.5 cm in diameter) are often euthyroid.*

A Pearl: *The incidence of thyroid cancer in a patient with a single cold nodule is 15% to 20%, a multinodular goiter, 5%, and a hot nodule, less than 1%.*

Q: Which radiopharmaceutical is used most commonly to localize a clinically diagnosed parathyroid adenoma? Describe its characteristic and diagnostic pharmacokinetics.
A: Tc-99m sestamibi is taken up by both thyroid and hyperfunctioning parathyroid tissue; however, it is typically cleared faster by the thyroid, thus the rationale for early (15 minutes) and delayed (2 hour) imaging. At early imaging, uptake in the thyroid is dominant. A hyperfunctioning parathyroid may not be apparent or may be seen as focal hot uptake, particularly if adjacent to the thyroid. On delayed imaging, the parathyroid uptake is dominant and the thyroid has mostly washed out.

A Pearl: *The most common false positive for parathyroid scanning is a thyroid adenoma. Benign and malignant tumors are other potential causes for false positive scintigraphy.*

▬ BONE

Q: What are the potential impurities in technetium-labeled diphosphonate compounds, based on their biodistribution?

A: Activity in the oropharynx, thyroid gland, and stomach suggests free unlabeled Tc-99m pertechnetate. Activity in the liver suggests a colloidal impurity. Rarely, activity is seen in the gut, the result of excretion of activity through the biliary system. The mechanism is not understood. Other increased soft tissue or renal activity is usually caused by a disease process rather than tracer impurity.

Q: What percentage of Tc-99m–labeled compounds is retained in the skeleton at the usual time of imaging?

A: In normal adult subjects, 40% to 60% of the injected dose is in the skeleton 2 to 3 hours after tracer administration.

A PITFALL: *The greatest pitfall in interpreting a bone scan is failure to appreciate its nonspecificity. The bone scan is very sensitive; however, its specificity is considerably lower. The most common pitfalls are diagnosing areas of arthritis or prior trauma as metastases. Correlative anatomical imaging is advisable.*

Q: Which factors favor osteoarthritis versus metastatic disease as the cause of increased activity?

A: Osteoarthritis has characteristic locations in the extremities. Because metastatic lesions are relatively rare below the proximal femurs or beyond the proximal humeri, osteoarthritis should be considered first in the elbows, wrists, hands, knees, and feet of older patients. Involvement of both sides of a joint is common in arthritis but unusual in metastatic disease. The lower lumbar spine is the most problematic area because both arthritis and metastases are common there. Degenerative disease is often more posterior and lateral, compared to metastases. Anatomical imaging is advised to differentiate.

Q: What is the distribution of metastatic deposits from epithelial primary malignancies in the skeleton?

A: A rule of thumb is that 80% of metastases are found in the axial skeleton (spine, pelvis, ribs, and sternum). The remaining metastases are distributed equally between the skull (10%) and the long bones (10%).

A PEARL: *The majority of epithelial tumor metastases localize first in the red marrow. The skeletal tracers do not localize in the tumor tissue but rather in the reactive bone around the metastatic deposits.*

A PITFALL: *A small amount of activity is frequently seen at the injection site; this should not be confused with a metastatic lesion. Extravasation at the injection site can result in proximal nodal uptake. Variable degrees of urinary contamination on the skin may be superimposed on skeletal structures and confused with activity caused by metastatic disease.*

A PEARL: *In many diseases, the bone scan has a very high sensitivity for detection of bone metastases. Sensitivity is lower in tumors with a lytic rather than blastic response, such as multiple myeloma, thyroid cancer, renal cell carcinoma. The bone scan is also less sensitive for tumors that preferentially go to bone marrow, such as lymphoma.*

Q: How can the radiation dose to the bladder, ovaries, and testes be reduced?

A: The radiation dose to these structures is largely caused by radioactivity in the bladder. Frequent voiding reduces the radiation dose.

A PEARL: *Faint or absent visualization of the kidneys should alert the observer to the possibility of a superscan. This may be misinterpreted as indicating lack of excretion of tracer through the kidneys. In cases of superscan resulting from metastatic disease, visualization of the kidneys is faint (1) because the skeleton accumulates more tracer than usual, leaving less available for renal excretion, and (2) because of the increased skeletal tracer uptake, the renal activity may actually fall below the gray scale threshold. The presence of renal activity is readily established by adjusting the intensity setting window.*

Q: What factors distinguish a superscan resulting from metastatic disease from a superscan resulting from metabolic disease?

A: In the usual superscan caused by metastatic disease, the increased uptake is usually restricted to the axial skeleton and the proximal parts of the femurs and humeri, the red marrow–bearing areas. In metabolic bone disease, the entire skeleton is typically affected, with increased uptake seen in the extremities and axial skeleton.

Q: What is the mechanism of the "flare" phenomenon?

A: In some patients treated with chemotherapy for metastatic disease, regression of the tumor burden is associated with increased osteoblastic activity, presumably caused by skeletal healing in response to chemotherapy. This can appear on skeletal scintigrams as a paradoxical increase or apparent worsening of the abnormal tracer. This may last for up to 6 months after therapy.

Q: What is the postmastectomy appearance of the thorax?

A: With radical mastectomy, the majority of the soft tissue is removed from the corresponding anterior thorax. The ribs appear "hotter" than on the contralateral side. This is caused by less attenuation of rib activity by soft tissue. Note, however, that if the patient is imaged with a breast prosthesis in place, the rib activity may be attenuated.

Q: What factors contribute to prolonged fracture positivity on scintigrams?

A: Displaced and comminuted fractures and fractures involving joints tend to have prolonged positivity scintigraphically. Elderly patients have delayed healing.

Q: What factors favor shin splints versus stress fracture scintigraphically in the tibia?

A: *Stress fractures* are classically focal or fusiform. The uptake can involve the entire width of the bone but more commonly extend partially across the shaft of the bone. *Shin splints* are classically located along the posterior medial tibial cortex and involve a third or more of the length of the bone. In pure shin splints, a focal component should not be present and superficial linear activity runs parallel to the long axis of the bone.

Q: The three-phase bone scan is used to diagnose osteomyelitis. What are other causes for a positive three-phase scan?

A: Recent fracture, tumor, Charcot's joint, and soft-tissue infection overlying chronic noninfectious bone disease.

A PITFALL: *False negative scintigrams may be seen in neonates with osteomyelitis. Sometimes the lesions appear photopenic.*

▬ HEPATOBILIARY

Q: What are the two U.S. Food and Drug Administration (FDA)-approved Tc-99m iminodiacetic acid (IDA) analog radiopharmaceuticals in clinical use and how are they different?

A: Tc-99m DISIDA (disofenin) and Tc-99m mebrofenin (Choletec) are the approved agents. Mebrofenin has better hepatic extraction, 98% versus 88%, and less renal excretion, 1% versus 9%. The higher extraction of mebrofenin is preferable in patients with hepatic insufficiency.

A PEARL: *Tc-99m IDA is extracted by the same cellular mechanism as bilirubin, but it is not conjugated. The radiopharmaceutical then follows the path of bile through the biliary system into the bowel.*

A PEARL: *The alternative route of excretion for Tc-99m IDA radiopharmaceuticals is via the kidneys. The amount of excretion is usually small but increases with hepatic dysfunction.*

Q: What is the most important question to ask a patient before starting cholescintigraphy for suspected acute cholecystitis and why?

A: When did the patient last eat? If the patient has eaten in the last 4 hours, the gallbladder may be contracted secondary to endogenous stimulation of cholecystokinin, and

therefore radiotracer cannot gain entry into the gallbladder. If the patient has not eaten for more than 24 hours, the gallbladder may not have had the stimulus to contract and will contain thick, concentrated bile, which may prevent tracer entry. Sincalide is indicated to empty the gallbladder.

A PEARL: *If the patient receives sincalide before the study to empty the gallbladder, the hepatobiliary iminodiacetic acid (HIDA) radiopharmaceutical should not be administered until at least 30 minutes later to allow time for the gallbladder to relax.*

Q: What are other common indications for sincalide infusion than mentioned here?

A: Other common indications are as follows. (1) To differentiate common duct obstruction from functional causes, as an alternative to delayed imaging. (2) To exclude acute acalculous cholecystitis if the gallbladder fills in a patient strongly suspected of having the disease. A diseased gallbladder will not contract from either acute or chronic disease. (3) To confirm or exclude chronic acalculous gallbladder disease (gallbladder dyskinesia).

Q: Cholescintigraphy is a very sensitive and specific test for acute cholecystitis. In what clinical settings can an increased number of false positive study findings for acute cholecystitis be seen?

A: An increased number of false positive results can be seen in patients who have fasted less than 4 hours or more than 24 hours, those receiving hyperalimentation, and patients who have chronic cholecystitis, hepatic dysfunction, or concurrent serious illness.

Q: What is the *rim sign* seen during cholescintigraphy and what is its significance?

A: The rim sign is increased activity in the liver adjacent to the gallbladder fossa. This finding has been associated with severe acute cholecystitis, and there is an increased incidence of the complications, such as perforation and gangrene.

Q: At what time after Tc-99m IDA injection is nonfilling of the gallbladder diagnostic of acute cholecystitis?

A: One hour is defined as abnormal. However, the diagnosis of acute cholecystitis cannot be made unless the gallbladder does not fill by 3 to 4 hours after radiopharmaceutical injection or 30 minutes after morphine administration.

A PEARL: *The cause of delayed gallbladder visualization is most commonly chronic cholecystitis. It also may occur with severe hepatic dysfunction because of altered pharmacokinetics—that is, delayed uptake and clearance.*

Q: What is the mechanism of morphine-augmented cholescintigraphy?

A: Morphine increases tone at the sphincter of Oddi, producing increased intraductal pressure. This results in bile flow preferentially through the cystic duct, if patent.

Q: What is acute acalculous cholecystitis?
A: Acute acalculous cholecystitis occurs in sick hospitalized patients who have sustained trauma, burns, or sepsis or have other serious illness. It is associated with a high morbidity and mortality. The cystic duct may be obstructed by debris or inflammatory changes. In some cases, the acute cholecystitis is caused by direct inflammation of the gallbladder wall as a result of infection, ischemia, or toxemia, without cystic duct obstruction.

A PEARL: *The sensitivity of cholescintigraphy for acute acalculous cholecystitis is approximately 75% to 85% compared with 95% to 98% for acute calculous cholecystitis.*

A PEARL: *If the clinical suspicion for acute acalculous cholecystitis is high but the gallbladder can be visualized (e.g., if the cystic duct is not obstructed), sincalide can be helpful diagnostically. Cholecystitis can be excluded if the gallbladder contracts. If it does not contract, the cause could be acute or chronic acalculous cholecystitis. A radiolabeled leukocyte study can confirm acute disease.*

Q: The diagnosis of common duct obstruction is often made by sonographic detection of a dilated common duct. In what clinical situations would cholescintigraphy be diagnostically helpful?
A: Cholescintigraphy would be helpful in early acute obstruction before the duct has had time to dilate (24-72 hours) and in patients with previous obstruction who have baseline dilated ducts.

Q: What are the cholescintigraphic findings of high-grade common duct obstruction?
A: Prompt hepatic uptake but a persistent hepatogram without clearance into biliary ducts, caused by high backpressure are seen on cholescintigraphy.
Q: What are the cholescintigraphic findings of partial common duct obstruction?
A: Retention of activity in the biliary ducts, delayed biliary-to-bowel clearance, and poor ductal clearance on delayed imaging or after sincalide are seen.

A PEARL: *Delayed biliary-to-bowel transit is an insensitive and nonspecific finding for common duct obstruction. Delayed biliary-to-bowel transit is seen in only 50% of patients with partial biliary obstruction. On the other hand, delayed biliary-to-bowel transit may be seen in up to 20% of healthy patients. It often occurs in patients pretreated with sincalide.*

A PEARL: *Administration of sincalide will cause sphincter of Oddi relaxation, prompt biliary duct clearance, and biliary-to-bowel transit in patients with functional causes of delayed transit, but will remain abnormal in patients with partial common duct obstruction.*

A PITFALL: *The methodology used for administering sincalide is important. A bolus infusion may cause spasm of the neck of the gallbladder and ineffective emptying. Similarly, 1- to 3-minute infusions may result in poor contraction of the gallbladder in approximately one third of normal subjects. A multicenter investigation comparing 15-, 30-, and 60-minute sincalide infusion methods showed that 0.02 µg/kg infused over 60 minutes is the optimal methodology (abnormal is <38%).*

Q: What ancillary maneuver increases the sensitivity of cholescintigraphy for detection of biliary atresia?
A: The administration of phenobarbital for 5 days before the HIDA study activates liver enzymes and increases biliary excretion.

Q: How is the diagnosis of biliary atresia made with cholescintigraphy?
A: No clearance of Tc-99m IDA tracer is seen by 24 hours. The various causes of neonatal hepatitis usually have clearance by that time.

Q: What is the postcholecystectomy syndrome and what are common causes for it?
A: This is a recurrent biliary, coliclike pain in patients who have had a cholecystectomy. Causes include a retained or recurrent stone, inflammatory stricture, sphincter of Oddi dysfunction, or cystic duct remnant.

A PEARL: *Sphincter of Oddi dysfunction is a partial biliary obstruction at the level of the sphincter without stone or stricture. Cholescintigraphy shows a pattern of partial biliary obstruction. The diagnosis is ultimately made by excluding stones or stricture with endoscopic retrograde cholangiopancreatography (ERCP).*

Q: What is the sensitivity and specificity of Tc-99m–labeled red blood cells for diagnosis of cavernous hemangioma?
A: Specificity is very high, greater than 98%. The sensitivity is lower, particularly for small hemangiomas, those adjacent to major vessels, and those that are deep to the surface of the liver. SPECT or SPECT/CT should be routine.

Q: What are the characteristic scintigraphic findings in liver hemangioma?
A: Blood flow is normal. Immediate images show a cold defect, whereas delayed images acquired 1 to 2 hours after

tracer administration show increased uptake within the lesion compared with that in the normal liver, often equal to uptake in the spleen and heart.

GENITOURINARY

Q: What percentage of renal plasma flow is filtered through the glomerulus, and what percentage is secreted by the tubules?

A: Twenty percent of renal plasma flow is cleared by glomerular filtration and 80% by tubular secretion.

Q: What are the mechanisms of renal uptake for Tc-99m diethylenetriaminepentaacetic acid (DTPA), Tc-99m mercaptylacetyltriglycine (MAG3), and Tc-99m dimercaptosuccinic acid (DMSA)?

A: The mechanisms are Tc-99m DTPA, glomerular filtration; Tc-99m MAG3, tubular secretion; Tc-99m DMSA, cortical proximal tubular binding.

Q: What is the percent cortical binding of Tc-99m DMSA?

A: The percent cortical binding is 40% to 50%.

A Pearl: *Dehydration will delay uptake and clearance. All patients undergoing renal scintigraphy should be hydrated.*

Q: What time interval is used to calculate differential renal function for dynamic renal scintigraphy?

A: Because cortical uptake of the renal radiopharmaceutical is of interest, the optimal interval is after the initial flow but before the collecting system activity appears, usually 1 to 3 minutes. With good function, activity may be seen before 3 minutes, especially in children. Thus the 1- to 2-minute interval may be optimal overall.

Q: What are the general methods for calculating absolute glomerular filtration rate (GFR)?

A: Blood sampling, blood sampling and urine collection, and camera-based methods are used to calculate the absolute GFR.

Q: What is the proper renal region of interest selection for diuresis renography?

A: The region of interest should include the dilated collecting system and exclude the cortex.

Q: Which of these factors affects the accuracy of diuresis renography: state of hydration, renal function, diuretic dose, choice of radiopharmaceutical, bladder capacity?

A: All of these affect the accuracy. Adequate hydration is required for good urine flow and adequate response to the diuretic. A full bladder may cause a functional obstruction. Intravenous hydration and urinary catheterization are strongly suggested in patients who cannot void and in children. Because of its high extraction efficiency and good image resolution, Tc-99m MAG3 is the radiopharmaceutical of choice. Tc-99m DTPA works well only in patients with good renal function. Renal insufficiency

is a limitation to diuresis renography. The kidney must be able to respond to the diuretic challenge. Therefore the dose of diuretic must be increased in renal insufficiency, but the exact dose required is only an educated estimate.

Q: What is the most sensitive technique for diagnosing scarring secondary to reflux?

A: Tc-99m DMSA cortical imaging is the most sensitive. CT may be similar, but with considerably higher radiation dose. Ultrasonography has lower sensitivity.

Q: How can radionuclide imaging differentiate upper from lower urinary tract infection and why is this differentiation important?

A: With upper tract infection or pyelonephritis, Tc-99m DMSA shows tubular dysfunction, manifested by decreased uptake. This is a reversible process. With appropriate therapy, tubular function will return in 3 to 6 months. Upper tract infection has prognostic implications because it may lead to subsequent renal scarring, hypertension, and renal failure.

Q: What is the advantage of radionuclide versus contrast cystography?

A: The radionuclide test is more sensitive for detection of reflux than contrast-enhanced voiding cystourethrography and results in much less radiation exposure, by a factor of 50- to 200-fold. The exception is in the first evaluation of a male patient, when the better resolution of the contrast study can permit the diagnosis of an anatomical abnormality such as posterior urethral valves.

A Pearl: *Scintigraphy allows for calculation of bladder volumes and residuals. The residual activity in the bladder is calculated by one of two methods using a region of interest around the bladder:*

$$\text{Residual volume (mL)} = \frac{[\text{Voided urine volume (mL)} \times \text{Postvoid bladder counts}]}{[\text{Initial bladder counts} - \text{Postvoid bladder counts}]}$$

or

$$\text{Residual bladder volume (mL)} = \frac{[\text{Postvoid bladder counts} \times \text{Volume infused (mL)}]}{\text{Initial bladder counts}}$$

ONCOLOGY: POSITRON RADIOPHARMACEUTICALS

Q: What is the difference in uptake mechanism between glucose and F-18 FDG?

A: After initial cellular uptake via glucose tranporters, both are phosphorylated by hexokinase. Unlike glucose-6-phosphate, F-18 FDG-6-phosphate does not undergo further metabolism. Thus it is trapped within cells. F-18 FDG is cleared via the kidneys.

Q: The sensitivity of FDG PET is high for detection of many malignancies. For which tumors is the sensitivity of FDG PET often not as high?

A: FDG PET has poor sensitivity for primary hepatocellular carcinoma, renal carcinoma, and prostate cancer. This is less true of metastatic disease than primary tumors.

A PEARL: *For thyroid cancer imaging, I-131 is more sensitive than F-18 FDG for well-differentiated papillary or follicular thyroid carcinoma. In patients who have been treated with I-131 and have a negative I-131 whole-body scan on follow-up evaluation but have an elevated serum thyroglobulin value, F-18 FDG PET has good sensitivity for detection of malignancy. The reason is that the tumor has dedifferentiated into a higher grade malignancy.*

A PEARL: *With PET/CT, misregistration caused by patient motion, respiratory motion, or organ movement (bowel) can introduce potential false positive interpretations. PET is acquired at normal tidal volume breathing. The CT with PET is acquired with breath-hold or shallow breathing. Artifacts result from errors in anatomical registration and attenuation correction occur.*

Q: What are some limitations of FDG PET in tumor staging?

A: PET imaging does not detect microscopic metastases, tumor involvement in local lymph nodes may be obscured by activity in an adjacent tumor, concurrent infection/inflammatory processes may cause false positive results, and sensitivity for intracranial metastases is low.

Q: What are limitations of tumor restaging by FDG PET?

A: Posttherapy effects of surgery, chemotherapy, and especially radiation therapy may cause increased F-18 FDG uptake, which can be confused with tumor uptake. Even patients scheduled for imaging after an appropriate delay after therapy may require follow-up imaging. If activity is diminishing, this helps confirm a benign process.

A PEARL: *The usual recommended FDG PET imaging time to evaluate response to chemotherapy is 3 weeks, but longer for radiation therapy, at least 2 to 3 months. It is not always possible from a clinical standpoint to follow these guidelines, but an awareness of the potential problem is critical for interpretation.*

A PEARL: *FDG PET can help direct biopsy to the most metabolically active area of a mass to help avoid sampling areas of necrosis.*

Q: Which is the most accurate method for the detection of osseous metastases?

A: This depends. Magnetic resonance imaging (MRI) is highly sensitive and often detects lesions not seen on bone

scan because it can visualize changes in the marrow and does not depend on secondary reactive cortical bone changes to develop. Bone scan, on the other hand, can image the whole body in a cost-effective manner. It is particularly helpful for sclerotic metastases. FDG PET scanning is more sensitive than bone scan for detection of lytic tumors. At times, the modalities complement each other by detecting different lesions in the same patient. F-18 sodium fluoride PET is a very sensitive bone scan agent, and some feel that it may replace Tc-99m methylene diphosphonate (MDP) imaging. Each of these methods is more sensitive than CT or radiographs.

Q: What are some differences between non–attenuation-corrected and attenuation-corrected FDG PET images?

A: The noncorrected image has an appearance very different from that of the corrected image. Structures near the surface appear more intense because fewer photons are attenuated before hitting the detector. This explains why the skin looks like it is outlined with a charcoal pencil. The air-filled lungs are also intense. Because fewer counts are seen in central areas, lesions may be missed. For accurate quantification (standard uptake value [SUV]), attenuation corrected images must be used.

Q: What is the most significant type of scatter experienced in PET?

A: Compton scatter is most common in the energy range of PET (511 keV). It is particularly a problem with three-dimensional (3-D) mode (no septa) acquisition. 3-D is highly sensitive and faster than 2-D but also accepts more scatter counts, which reduce image quality.

ONCOLOGY: SINGLE-PHOTON RADIOPHARMACEUTICALS

Q: Which of the following are true statements regarding indium-111 OctreoScan?
a. It is a somatostatin receptor imaging agent.
b. The sensitivity for all neuroendocrine tumors is very high.
c. Highest uptake is seen in the spleen and kidneys.
d. Only neuroendocrine tumors have somatostatin receptors.

A: *a, c.* Although its sensitivity for detection of most neuroendocrine tumors is high, it has a poorer sensitivity for insulinomas and medullary carcinoma of the thyroid. Somatostatin receptors are found on a variety of nonneuroendocrine tumors, including astrocytomas, meningiomas, malignant lymphoma, and breast and lung cancer.

Q: Which radiopharmaceutical is used for melanoma lymphoscintigraphy? What is the injection methodology?

A: Filtered Tc-99m sulfur colloid is the usual agent, because unfiltered Tc-99m sulfur colloid does not migrate well from the site of injection. It is injected intracutaneously at four sites around the primary lesion site.

Q: In which patients with melanoma is sentinel node lymphoscintigraphy indicated and why?

A: Patients with a primary lesion less than 1 mm in thickness are at low risk for recurrence and have a good prognosis. Patients with a primary lesion thickness greater than 4 mm are at high risk for metastatic regional and distant metastases. Lymphoscintigraphy is indicated for patients with primary lesions greater than 1 mm and less than 4 mm thickness.

Q: What information does sentinel node lymphoscintigraphy provide in patients with intermediate-thickness malignant melanoma?

A: Sentinel node lymphoscintigraphy can pinpoint lymphatic flow and the sentinel node for the surgeon that can be localized easily at surgery with a gamma probe. After immunohistochemical staining of tissue from this lymph node, the presence of metastases can be determined. The results will determine which patients require further nodal bed dissection and adjuvant chemotherapy.

Q: In what other malignant disease is sentinel node lymphoscintigraphy commonly performed and how is it injected?

A: Breast cancer. The method of Tc-99m sulfur colloid injection varies. At some hospitals, it is injected intratumorally. Others inject it subdermally, whereas some inject in the periareolar region. The rationale for the latter is that all lymphatics drain to the areolar region before drainage to the axillary region. Lymphatic drainage to the internal mammary or supraclavicular nodes is occasionally detected.

A PEARL: *Many experts recommend using two methods to ensure optimal breast lymphatic transit. Massaging the site of injection vigorously after injection promotes migration of the dose.*

A PEARL: *The membrane-specific antigen that In-111 ProstaScint localizes to is not prostate-specific antigen (PSA) but rather prostate specific membrane antigen (PSMA), a glycoprotein expressed by prostate epithelium, which is not expressed on any other adenocarcinomas.*

A PEARL: *In patients with acquired immunodeficiency syndrome (AIDS) and an intracerebral mass, thallium-201 can differentiate malignancy, usually lymphoma, from inflammatory causes, commonly toxoplasmosis. Tl-201 is rarely taken up in inflammation, but is taken up by malignant tumors. Predictive value is greater than 85%.*

A PEARL: *The dose of yttrium-90 ibritumomab (Zevalin) is adjusted based on the patient's platelet count: 0.4 mCi/kg for patients with platelet count greater than 150,000 and 0.3 mCi/kg for platelets between 149,000 to 100,000. If the platelet count is below 100,000, patients should not be treated.*

GASTROINTESTINAL

Q: Which of the following statements in regard to reflux and aspiration studies are true or false:
a. The milk study is a sensitive method for diagnosing gastroesophageal reflux.
b. The milk study is a sensitive method for diagnosing aspiration.
c. Frequent image acquisition improves the sensitivity of the milk study.
d. The "salivagram" is a more sensitive method for diagnosing aspiration.

A: True: *a, c, d.* False: *b.* Aspiration is seen infrequently on the milk study. A "salivagram," or esophageal transit study, is more sensitive for aspiration.

Q: What is the functional role of the proximal and distal stomach?

A: The proximal stomach, or fundus, is responsible for liquid emptying and receptive relaxation and accommodation of a large meal. The distal stomach, or antrum, is responsible for the grinding and sieving of solid food and solid emptying.

Q: Describe the difference in emptying patterns between solids and liquids.

A: Liquids empty exponentially. Solid emptying is biphasic, with an initial lag phase before linear emptying begins. The lag phase is due to the time required for food to be broken down into small enough pieces to allow passage through the pylorus.

Q: Which of these factors will affect the rate of gastric emptying: meal content, time of day, position (standing, sitting, lying), stress, exercise?

A: All. The gastric emptying study should be standardized for the meal, time of day, patient position, methodology of acquisition, and processing. A standardized meal is recommended.

Q: Which of the following statements are true regarding the need for variable attenuation correction of gastric emptying studies?
a. Gastric emptying may be underestimated when an anterior acquisition alone is obtained.
b. The characteristic pattern of attenuation effect on a solid gastric emptying time-activity curve is a rise in activity after meal ingestion before emptying begins.
c. The geometric mean method is considered the standard method for attenuation correction.

A: All. Both anterior and posterior acquisitions are required to best correct using the geometric mean calculation (square root of the product of the anterior and posterior views).

Q: List in increasing order the labeling efficiency of methods to label Tc-99m red blood cells: in vivo, in vitro, and in vivtro labeling methods.

A: Labeling efficiency is 75% for in vivo, 85% for modified in vivo, and 97% for the in vitro method. An in vitro commercial kit method (Ultra-Tag) for labeling Tc-99m erythrocytes is the method of choice, particularly for gastrointestinal bleeding studies.

Q: What are the essential criteria needed to confidently diagnose the site of active bleeding on a radionuclide study?
A: A radiotracer "hot spot" appears where there was none and transits in a pattern conforming to bowel anatomy; the activity increases over time; and it moves antegrade or retrograde.

A PITFALL: *A poor label for a GI bleeding study can result in activity that might be construed as gastrointestinal bleeding.*

A PEARL: *Look for thyroid and salivary gland uptake when in doubt about the presence of free Tc-99m pertechnetate.*

A PEARL: *A lateral view of the pelvis should be routine at the end of the acquisition to differentiate bladder, rectal bleeding, and penile activity.*

A PITFALL: *Focal activity in a GI bleeding study that does not move may be anatomical—for example, kidney, accessory spleen, hemangioma, varices, aneurysm.*

A PEARL: *The red blood cell gastrointestinal bleeding study can detect bleeding rates of about 0.1 mL/min versus contrast angiography, which can detect bleeding rates of about 1 mL/min.*

A PEARL: *The mucin cells in the stomach are primarily responsible for gastric uptake of Tc-99m pertechnetate, not the parietal cells.*

Q: What is the origin of Meckel diverticulum?
A: This most common congenital anomaly of the gastrointestinal tract results from failure of closure of the omphalomesenteric duct of the embryo, which connects the yolk sac to the primitive foregut via the umbilical cord.

A PEARL: *This true diverticulum (Meckel) arises on the antimesenteric side of the bowel, usually 80 to 90 cm proximal to the ileocecal valve, although it can occur elsewhere.*

A PEARL: *Gastric mucosa is present in 10% to 30% of all Meckel diverticula, in 60% of symptomatic patients, and in 98% of those with bleeding.*

A PITFALL: *False positive study results have been reported (mostly case reports) over the years for Meckel scans, including urinary tract origin (e.g., horseshoe kidney, ectopic kidney), those resulting from inflammation (e.g., inflammatory bowel disease, neoplasms), bowel obstruction (seen most often with intussusception and volvulus), and other areas of ectopic gastric mucosa.*

INFECTION AND INFLAMMATION

Q: Which photopeaks are used for In-111 leukocyte imaging and what is their abundance?
A: The photopeaks are 173 keV (89%) and 247 keV (94%).

Q: Which collimator should be used for In-111 and gallium-67?
A: A medium-energy collimator should be used. A high-energy collimator can be used, although its sensitivity is less, image acquisition time is longer, and image quality is inferior.

Q: Ga-67 is taken up by the lungs because of drug toxicity. With which other drugs is uptake seen?
A: Bleomycin is the most common; uptake is also seen with cytoxan, nitrofurantoin, and amiodarone toxicity.

A PEARL: *Characteristic scintigraphic patterns of uptake of sarcoidosis with Ga-67 are (1) the "panda" sign, caused by uptake in the salivary glands, parotids, and nasopharyngeal region, and (2) the "lambda" sign, which results from paratracheal and hilar lymph node uptake. This is also seen with FDG PET.*

Q: Which subtypes of leukocytes are labeled with In-111 oxine and Tc-99m hexamethylpropyleneamine oxime (HMPAO)?
A: In-111 binds to neutrophils, lymphocytes, monocytes, erythrocytes, and platelets. Tc-99m HMPAO binds to neutrophils.

Q: Which of the following statements is true regarding In-111 oxine leukocytes?
a. It is diagnostically useful for evaluating inflammatory lung disease.
b. It has a high sensitivity for detecting osteomyelitis of the spine.
c. It should not be used when the peripheral leukocyte count is less than 3000/mm³.
d. It is the radiopharmaceutical of choice for intraabdominal infection.
A: *c* and *d*

a. Response *a* is false. Ga-67 is the agent of choice.
b. The sensitivity for vertebral osteomyelitis is poor, with a 40% to 50% false negative rate.
c. Fewer than 3000/mm³ leukocytes are inadequate for radiolabeled leukocyte studies.
d. The lack of intraabdominal hepatobiliary and genitourinary clearance makes In-111 leukocytes ideal for detecting intraabdominal infection and superior to Tc-99m HMPAO.

A PEARL: *Tc-99m HMPAO is the preferred agent for localizing infection in children because of In-111 leukocyte's high radiation dose to the spleen of 30 to 50 rads (15-20 rads in adults).*

Q: What is the optimal imaging time for In-111–labeled and Tc-99m HMPAO–labeled leukocytes?
A: In-111–labeled leukocytes are imaged at 24 hours. Imaging at 4 to 6 hours is less sensitive for detection of infection. Tc-99m HMPAO–labeled leukocytes should be imaged by 2 hours for intraabdominal infection before biliary and renal clearance occurs. Extraabdominal infection can be imaged later, usually at 4 hours, allowing time for background clearance.

A PEARL: *The one exception to 24-hour imaging for In-111–labeled leukocytes is for inflammatory bowel disease, in which imaging should be done at 4 hours, because intraluminal shedding of inflamed cells may result in inaccurate localization at 24 hours.*

A PITFALL: *Leukocytes may accumulate at the site of inflammation without infection, such as intravenous catheters; nasogastric, endogastric, and drainage tubes; tracheostomies; and colostomies. Leukocytes may accumulate at postoperative surgical sites for 2 to 3 weeks, and low-grade uptake may be seen at healing fracture sites. Accessory spleens may be misinterpreted as infection, and renal transplants accumulate leukocytes.*

A PITFALL: *Intraluminal intestinal radioactivity can be the result of swallowed or shedding cells from pharyngitis, sinusitis, pneumonia, herpes esophagitis, or gastrointestinal bleeding.*

A PITFALL: *A radiolabeled leukocyte study for suspected osteomyelitis may have a false positive result because of displaced bone marrow. The addition of a bone marrow study (Tc-99m sulfur colloid) can be diagnostic. Uptake resulting from displaced marrow will have matched studies. Osteomyelitis will have increased uptake on the leukocyte study and normal or decreased uptake on the bone marrow study.*

CENTRAL NERVOUS SYSTEM

Q: How is the diagnosis of brain death made?
A: This is mainly a clinical diagnosis, typically made in a patient in deep coma with total absence of brainstem reflexes and spontaneous respiration. Reversible causes must be excluded (e.g., drugs, hypothermia), the cause of the dysfunction must be diagnosed (e.g., trauma, stroke), and the clinical findings of brain death must be present for a defined period of observation (6-24 hours). Confirmatory tests such as electroencephalography (EEG) and radionuclide brain flow imaging may be used to increase diagnostic certainty.

Q: Which radiopharmaceuticals are used to evaluate brain death and what are the advantages of each?
A: Tc-99m DTPA is inexpensive but more technically demanding to use and interpret. Tc-99m HMPAO or Tc-99m ethyl cysteinate dimer (ECD) are often preferred because no flow study is required, only delayed planar images to visualize radiotracer fixed in cerebral cortex.

A PEARL: *A "hot nose" may be seen on the flow-phase images and delayed images as a result of shunting of blood from the internal to the external carotid system supplying the face and nose.*

Q: What is the mechanism of uptake for the Tc-99m cerebral perfusion agents?
A: Tc-99m HMPAO and Tc-99m ECD are lipid-soluble cerebral perfusion agents taken up in proportion to regional cerebral blood flow. They fix intracellularly.

A PEARL: *In most clinical situations, cerebral blood flow follows metabolism. An exception is the decoupling of metabolism and blood flow seen during the acute phase of a stroke. Blood flow may be normal or increased for the initial 1 to 10 days (luxury perfusion), but metabolism is decreased.*

Q: How can SPECT brain perfusion or FDG PET imaging be useful in the differential diagnosis of dementia?
A: By noting the distribution pattern. Multiinfarct dementia is characterized by multiple areas of past infarcts, recognized as areas of decreased uptake that correspond to vascular distribution, and changes in the deep structures, such as the basal ganglia and thalamus. Alzheimer disease exhibits a characteristic pattern of bitemporal and parietal hypoperfusion and hypometabolism. Pick disease has decreased frontal lobe uptake.

A PEARL: *Although Alzheimer disease has a characteristic bitemporal-parietal pattern on perfusion imaging, it is often not symmetric and decreased frontal lobe uptake also may be seen in late-stage disease.*

Q: What is the purpose of cerebral perfusion imaging in patients with seizures? What is the expected PET or SPECT pattern?

A: Interictal studies are performed in patients unresponsive to medical therapy, requiring surgery for seizure control. Interictally, a seizure focus will show decreased metabolism on FDG PET and decreased perfusion on SPECT; increased activity is seen during a seizure (ictal). In some surgical seizure centers, depth electrodes are not required preoperatively if the clinical picture, EEG, and SPECT or PET study are all consistent as to the location of the seizure focus.

Q: Name the radiopharmaceutical used for cisternography and the most common clinical indication for this study.
A: In-111 DTPA is the most commonly used. The most common use of this radiopharmaceutical in modern practice is to localize shunt patency or cerebrospinal fluid leaks. Shunt patency studies can use In-111 DTPA or Tc-99m DTPA because of the short duration of the study.

CARDIAC

A PEARL: *Myocardial perfusion scintigraphy, whether performed with SPECT or PET, is a "map" of relative blood flow to viable myocardium. That is, for activity to be recorded in the image, it must be delivered (blood flow) and taken up by a myocardial cell (viable myocardium).*

Q: What percentage of Tl-201, Tc-99m sestamibi, and Tc-99m tetrofosmin localizes in the heart?
A: Tl-201, 3%-4%; Tc-99, sestamibi, 1.5%, and tetrofosmin, 1.2% localize in the heart.

A PITFALL: *Patient motion can cause image degradation, create a defect, or obscure a defect.*

Q: What quality control should be routinely performed to detect patient motion?
A: Review raw data in cinematic display. Review of the sonogram can confirm the extent of the problem.

A PEARL: *The best method for correcting the problem of motion is to repeat the study. If this is not possible, software motion correction programs can be used. However, this software usually corrects for motion only in one axis. Motion typically occurs in all three axes.*

A PITFALL: *Attenuation of photons by soft tissue can result in decreased activity seen in the myocardium that could suggest myocardial infarction if seen on both rest and stress or as ischemia if only apparent on the stress study. With females, breast attenuation results in decreased activity of the anterior, septal, or lateral wall, depending on their size and shape. Males characteristically have attenuation of the inferior wall, so-called diaphragmatic attenuation.*

Q: In what ways can the image interpreter determine if fixed decreased activity is indeed pathological (i.e., infarction) or merely caused by attenuation?
A: Review the raw data in the cinematic display to look for soft attenuation. Review of the gated SPECT can help determine whether ventricular wall motion and thickening are present, which would indicate that it is not an infarction, but probably the result of attenuation. Attenuation correction programs are quite helpful in differentiating attenuation from infarction.

A PEARL: *To correct for attenuation, a transmission map must be acquired. This can be done by acquiring transmission counts from a gamma source—for example, gadolinium-153. With SPECT/CT systems, the acquired CT is used for attenuation correction.*

Q: What is the significance of exercise-induced dilation on SPECT perfusion studies?
A: The normal heart dilates during exercise stress but gated SPECT images are acquired after stress, when normal hearts have returned to baseline size. Poststress dilation suggests cardiac decompensation and three-vessel disease.

A PEARL: *Patients with left bundle branch block may have reversible exercise stress-induced hypoperfusion of the septum. Patients with ischemia do not typically have isolated septal involvement, but also have associated apical and anterior wall ischemia. This potential diagnostic problem can be avoided by performing pharmacological.*

A PEARL: *The primary cause of false negative exercise study results in the diagnosis of coronary artery disease is failure to achieve an adequate exercise level.*

A PEARL: *After exercise stress, significant uptake in the liver usually indicates a poor exercise level was achieved. At peak exercise, blood flow is diverted from the splanchnic circulation.*

A PITFALL: *Quantitative analysis of stress myocardial perfusion that relies on databases of "normals" may not reflect the patient population in a different nuclear medicine department. Care must be taken to not rely too heavily on these databases.*

Q: What is the mechanism of action of dipyridamole?
A: Dipyridamole inhibits the action of adenosine deaminase. By augmenting the effects of endogenous adenosine, dipyridamole is a powerful vasodilator.

Q: What effect can a cup of coffee have on a dipyridamole or adenosine stress test?

A: Caffeine in coffee, tea, soft drinks, or foods such as chocolate are chemically related to dipyridamole and adenosine and can block the effect of pharmacological stress testing.

Q: What percentage of stenosis at rest is necessary in the coronary arteries for resting blood flow to be affected?

A: Coronary artery stenosis greater than 85% to 90% is required before flow is diminished at rest. Not all stenoses are created equal. Long irregular stenotic segments have more effect than discrete short-segment stenoses.

Q: Why is imaging delayed for 30 to 90 minutes after administration of Tc-99m sestamibi or Tc-99m tetrofosmin?

A: Although myocardial uptake is rapid with both Tc-99m sestamibi and Tc-99m tetrofosmin, lung and liver uptake are also prominent. The lung and liver clear with time and the target-to-background ratio improves. The liver clears somewhat more rapidly with Tc-99m tetrofosmin.

Q: What is the name of the pharmaceutical that allows Tc-99m to bind to the red blood cell for blood pool imaging?

A: Stannous (tin) pyrophosphate is the usual agent. Stannous chloride has been used.

Q: To what part of the red blood cell does the Tc-99m label bind?

A: Tc-99m binds to the beta chain of hemoglobin when pretreated with stannous ion.

Q: What are the considerations for selecting the number of frames in a gated blood pool study?

A: Selecting the number of frames to divide the cardiac cycle is a balance between having enough frames to capture the peaks and valleys of the ventricular time-activity curve versus the need to acquire a statistically valid number of counts in each frame. Too many frames increases the imaging time required for a given number of counts per frame. For gated ventriculography (multiple gated acquisition [MUGA]), using 16 frames achieves this compromise. For gated SPECT myocardial perfusion imaging, 8 frames is the usual compromise because of lesser counts. Too few frames will "average out" the peaks and valleys.

A PITFALL: *In calculation of the left ventricular ejection fraction, too high an estimate of the background counts per pixel will result in a falsely high ejection fraction. This can happen if the background area includes activity from the spleen.*

A PEARL: *Variations in the length of the cardiac cycle can be recognized on gated perfusion or blood pool studies if the time-activity curve (ventricular volume curve) trails off or fails to approximate the height of the initial part of the curve.*

Q: What do amplitude and phase images portray?

A: Amplitude and phase images are parametric or derived images. The amplitude image portrays the maximum count difference at each pixel location during the cardiac cycle. High ejection fraction areas have high amplitude, and background areas have low amplitude. The phase image portrays the timing of cyclical activity with respect to a reference standard, usually the R wave.

Q: What is the hallmark of a ventricular apical aneurysm by phase analysis?

A: Aneurysms demonstrate paradoxical motion. Activity in the area of the aneurysm is typically 180 degrees out of phase with the rest of the ventricle.

▬ PULMONARY

Q: What are the two most commonly used radiopharmaceuticals for ventilation imaging? What are their advantages and disadvantages?

A: Xenon-133 and Tc-99m DTPA aerosol are the most commonly used. Xe-133 demonstrates more clearly the physiology of respiration and is very sensitive to detection of obstructive airway disease, manifested by slow washout. The disadvantage is the rapid washout, limiting the views obtainable, and its suboptimal image quality is due to the low photopeak (81 keV) and poor count rate image. Tc-99m DTPA aerosol results in high-count images in all projections; however, the images are comparable to those with Xe-133 only in the inspiratory phase. With obstructive airway disease, particles become impacted in the proximal bronchi, potentially causing interpretation difficulties.

A PITFALL: *Xe-133 will be taken up and cleared slowly from livers with fatty metamorphosis. This should not be confused with pulmonary delayed washout.*

Q: What is the minimum number of particles recommended for pulmonary perfusion imaging?

A: Pulmonary perfusion scanning assumes a statistically even distribution of particles throughout the lung. This requires at least 100,000 particles in normal adults; 300,000 to 400,000 particles are generally administered.

Q: How should the dose of technetium-99m macroaggregated albumin (MAA) be adjusted in pediatric patients?

A: Radiopharmaceutical doses are adjusted with respect to patient size or age in the pediatric population. With Tc-99m MAA it is also necessary to reduce the number of particles.

Q: What is the size range of MAA particles?

A: In commercial preparations, the majority of particles are 20 to 40 μm (range of 10 to 90 μm).

A PITFALL: *Withdrawing blood into a syringe with Tc-99m MAA particles may create a small radioactive embolus that shows up as a "hot spot" on subsequent images.*

A PITFALL: *Failure to resuspend the Tc-99m MAA particles before administration may result in clumping of particles together and the presence of "hot spots" on subsequent imaging.*

Q: What is the biological fate of MAA particles?
A: Tc-99m MAA particles are physically broken down in the lung. Delayed imaging performed several hours after pharmaceutical administration demonstrates activity in the reticuloendothelial system because of phagocytosis of the breakdown particles.

A PEARL: *One way to determine whether radioactivity outside of the lungs is caused by free Tc-99m or right-to-left shunting of Tc-99m MAA is to image the brain. Free pertechnetate should not localize in the brain cortex, but rather in the thyroid, salivary glands, stomach, and soft tissue, whereas Tc-99m MAA particles that gain access to the systemic circulation will lodge in the first capillary bed that they encounter, including the capillary bed in the brain. If no brain uptake is seen, no significant right-to-left shunt exists.*

Q: What is the preferred patient position during administration of Tc-99m MAA?
A: Administering Tc-99m MAA with the patient supine results in a more homogeneous distribution of particles in the lung than when the patient is sitting or standing. Gravitational effects result in more basilar distribution than when injection is accomplished with the patient upright.

A PITFALL: *In lateral views of the lung obtained for a fixed number of counts, "shine-through" from the contralateral lung can give the false impression of activity arising from the side being imaged. This is most dramatically demonstrated in patients who after pneumonectomy show no activity on anterior or posterior views but a near-normal appearance can be seen because of the shine-through phenomenon.*

A PITFALL: *In analysis of perfusion scintigrams, failure to recognize the significance of decreased versus absent activity is a potential pitfall. Not every clot is 100% occlusive of the circulation. Significantly diminished activity needs to be recognized as one of the patterns caused by pulmonary emboli.*

A PITFALL: *The pulmonary hili on lung scans are photon-deficient structures caused by the displacement of lung parenchyma by large vascular and bronchial structures. Failure to remember this can result in false positive interpretations, especially for defects seen on posterior oblique images.*

A PITFALL: *If the patient is placed supine for ventilation-perfusion imaging but the chest radiograph was obtained with the patient upright, it can be difficult to correlate findings on the examinations. For example, free fluid may collect in a subpulmonic location or obscure the lung base in the upright position. With the patient supine, the fluid may layer out posteriorly or collect in the fissures. Also, the apparent height of the lungs may be different, as may the heart size. Ideally, imaging studies should be performed with the patient in the same position for all examinations. On the other hand, if significant pleural fluid is present, it may be desirable to image the patient in more than one position to prove that a defect is caused by mobile fluid.*

Q: What is the "stripe" sign?
A: The stripe sign refers to a stripe or zone of activity seen between a perfusion defect and the closest pleural surface. Because pulmonary emboli are typically pleura based, the stripe sign suggests another diagnosis, often emphysema. Rarely, in the resolution of pulmonary emboli, a stripe sign develops as circulation is restored.

Q: What is the physiological basis for perfusion defects in areas of poor ventilation?
A: The classic response to hypoxia at the alveolar level is vasoconstriction. Shunting of blood away from the hypoxic lung zone maintains oxygen saturation.

Q: What is the classic appearance of multiple pulmonary emboli on lung perfusion scintigraphy?
A: Multiple pleura-based, wedge-shaped areas of significantly diminished or absent perfusion. The size of the defects may vary from subsegmental to segmental or may involve an entire lobe or lung.

Q: What is the sensitivity of the high-probability scan category for detecting pulmonary embolism?
A: In the PIOPED study, 41% of patients with pulmonary embolism had a high-probability scintigraphic pattern. Thus the majority of patients with pulmonary emboli have intermediate or low-probability scans. However, the category of high-probability is a specific finding for pulmonary embolus.

Index

Note: Page numbers followed by *f* refer to figures, by *t* to tables, and by *b* to boxes.